W. B. SAUNDERS COMPANY
Harcourt Brace Jovanovich, Inc.

The Curtis Center
Independence Square West
Philadelphia, PA 19106

Library of Congress Cataloging-in-Publication Data

Aesthetic surgery of the breast / edited by Nicholas G.
Georgiade, Gregory S. Georgiade, Ronald Riefkohl.

    p.   cm.

ISBN 0–7216–3207–6

1. Mammaplasty.   I. Georgiade, Nicholas G., 1918–   .
   II. Georgiade, Gregory S.   III. Riefkohl, Ronald. [DNLM:
   1. Breast—surgery.   2. Surgery, Plastic.   WP 910 A254]
RD539.8.A37   1990
618.1′9059–dc20
DNLM/DLC
                                 90–8408

Editor: Jennifer Mitchell
Designer: W. B. Saunders Staff
Production Manager: Peter Faber
Manuscript Editor: Jessie Raymond
Illustration Coordinator: Walt Verbitski
Indexer: Kathy Garcia

AESTHETIC SURGERY OF THE BREAST   ISBN 0–7216–3207–6

Printed in the United States of America.

Last digit is the print number: 9   8   7   6   5   4   3   2   1

AESTHETIC SURGERY OF THE BREAST

EDITED BY

Nicholas G. Georgiade, M.D., F.A.C.S.

Professor and Former Chairman,
Department of Surgery,
Division of Plastic, Maxillofacial and
Reconstructive Surgery,
Duke University Medical Center,
Durham, North Carolina

Gregory S. Georgiade, M.D., F.A.C.S.

Associate Professor,
Department of Surgery, and
Associate Professor,
Division of Plastic, Maxillofacial and
Reconstructive Surgery,
Duke University Medical Center,
Durham, North Carolina

Ronald Riefkohl, M.D., F.A.C.S.

Associate Professor,
Department of Surgery,
Division of Plastic, Maxillofacial and
Reconstructive Surgery,
Duke University Medical Center,
Durham, North Carolina

1990

W.B. SAUNDERS COMPANY
Harcourt Brace Jovanovich, Inc.

Philadelphia   London   Toronto   Montreal   Sydney   Tokyo

To all our national and international colleagues whose contributions have made this book possible.

To Ruth Georgiade for her penchant for detail and accuracy in editing, which made this fine text what it is.

CONTRIBUTORS

Mehdi N. Adham, M.D.
Clinical Instructor, Georgetown University Hospital, Washington, D.C.

Edgar D. Altchek, M.D., F.A.C.S.
Associate Clinical Professor of Plastic Surgery, Mount Sinai School of Medicine, New York, New York

Louis C. Argenta, M.D., F.A.C.S.
Section Head, Plastic and Reconstructive Surgery, Bowman Gray School of Medicine, Winston Salem, North Carolina

Stephen Ariyan, M.D., F.A.C.S.
Professor of Surgery, Chief, Plastic and Reconstructive Surgery, Yale University, New Haven, Connecticut

Dale P. Armstrong, M.D., F.A.C.S.
Ventura, California

Namik K. Baran, M.D.
Professor and Chief, Plastic and Reconstructive Surgery, Department Dean, Faculty of Medicine, Gazi University, Ankara, Turkey

Ricardo Baroudi, M.D.
Campinas, Sao Paulo, Brazil

Louis Benelli, M.D.
Paris, France

Thomas M. Biggs, M.D., F.A.C.S.
Chairman, Department of Surgery, Saint Joseph's Hospital, Houston, Texas

Bernard Bodin, M.D.
Ancien Interne des Hôpitaux de Paris, Ancien Chef de Clinique à la Faculté Chirurgien à l'Hôpital Saint-Louis, Paris, France

Heinz H. Bohmert, M.D.
Professor of Surgery, Division of Plastic Surgery, Ludwig-Maximilians-Universität München, Klinikum Grosshadern, Munich, Federal Republic of Germany

Jean-Paul Bossé, M.D., F.R.C.S. (C)
Professor of Surgery, University of Montreal, Montreal, Quebec, Canada

T. Ray Broadbent, M.D., F.A.C.S.
Clinical Professor of Plastic and Reconstructive Surgery, University of Utah, Salt Lake City, Utah

Garry S. Brody, M.D., F.A.C.S.
Clinical Professor of Surgery (Plastic), University of Southern California, Chief of Plastic Surgery Research, Rancho Los Amigos Medical Center, Downey, California

Primarius Dr. Hans G. Bruck
F. A. Plastische Chirurgie, Vorstand Abt Plast. Chirurgie, Wilhelminenspital, Vienna, Austria

Boyd R. Burkhardt, M.D., F.A.C.S.
Clinical Associate, University Medical Center, Staff Surgeon, Tucson Medical Center, Tucson, Arizona

Sarah A. Carpenter, M.D.
Department of Pathology, Duke University Medical Center, Durham, North Carolina

Cemalettin Celebi, M.D.
Associate Professor, Plastic and Reconstructive Surgery Department, Faculty of Medicine, Gazi University, Ankara, Turkey

Eugene H. Courtiss, M.D., F.A.C.S.
Assistant Clinical Professor of Surgery, Harvard Medical School, Consultant in Plastic Surgery, Massachusetts General Hospital, Boston, Massachusetts

Melvin I. Dinner, M.B., B.Ch., F.R.C.S., F.A.C.S.
Center for Plastic Surgery, Cleveland, Ohio

G. Stephenson Drew, M.D.
Assistant Professor, Division of Plastic Surgery, Medical College of Georgia, Augusta, Georgia

Ray A. Elliott, Jr., M.D., F.A.C.S.
Clinical Professor of Surgery (Plastic), Associate Clinical Professor of Orthopaedics (Hand), Albany Medical College, Albany, New York

Nabil I. Elsahy, M.D., F.R.C.S.(C)
Riverdale, Georgia

Jorge Fonseca Ely, M.D., F.I.C.S.
Professor and Head of Plastic Surgery, Fundacao Faculdade Federal de Ciencias Medicas, Porto Alegre, Brazil, Professor of Plastic Surgery, Universidade Federal do Rio Grande do Sul, Faculdade de Medicina, Porto Alegre, Brazil, Chief of Plastic Surgery, Santa Casa Hospital, Porto Alegre, Brazil

E. Ronald Finger, M.D., F.A.C.S.
Savannah, Georgia

Robert A. Fischl, M.D., F.A.C.S., F.R.C.S.
Attending Plastic Surgery, The Danbury Hospital, Danbury, Connecticut

Gary D. Friedman, M.D.
Chief of Plastic Surgery, Mount Zion Medical Center, San Francisco, California

David W. Furnas, M.D., F.A.C.S.
Clinical Professor and Chief, Division of Plastic Surgery, University of California—Irvine, Irvine, California

Mario S. L. Galvao, M.D.
Head of Reconstructive Microsurgery Unit, National Cancer Institute, Rio de Janeiro, Brazil

Gregory S. Georgiade, M.D., F.A.C.S.
Associate Professor, Department of Surgery, Associate Professor, Division of Plastic, Maxillofacial and Reconstructive Surgery, Duke University Medical Center, Durham, North Carolina

Nicholas G. Georgiade, M.D., F.A.C.S.
Professor of Plastic and Reconstructive Surgery, Division of Plastic and Reconstructive Surgery, Duke University Medical Center, Durham, North Carolina

Kenna S. Given, M.D., F.A.C.S.
Professor and Chief, Division of Plastic Surgery, Medical College of Georgia, Augusta, Georgia

Marcia K. Goin, M.D., Ph.D.
Los Angeles, California

Robert M. Goldwyn, M.D., F.A.C.S.
Clinical Professor of Surgery, Harvard Medical School, Head, Division of Plastic Surgery, Beth Israel Hospital, Boston, Massachusetts

Ronald P. Gruber, M.D., F.A.C.S.
Clinical Instructor in Surgery, Stanford University Medical Center, Oakland, California

Yaron Har-Shai, M.D.
Resident, Department of Plastic Surgery, Rambam Medical Center, Haifa, Israel

John H. Hartley, Jr., M.D., F.A.C.S.
Assistant Clinical Professor of Plastic Surgery, Emory University School of Medicine, Atlanta, Georgia

Ulrich T. Hinderer, M.D.
Former Professor of Plastic Surgery, Universitas Complutensis Madrid, Director, Clinica Mirasierra de Cirugia Plástic-Éstetica, Madrid, Spain

Bernard Hirshowitz, M.D., F.R.C.S.
Professor and Head, Department of Plastic Surgery, Rambam Medical Center and Faculty of Medicine, Technion-Israel Institute of Technology, Haifa, Israel

Saul Hoffman, M.D.
Clinical Professor of Surgery (Plastic), Mount Sinai School of Medicine, New York, New York

Hans Holström, M.D.
Professor of Plastic Surgery, Göteborg Universitet, Plastikkirurgiska Kliniken, Göteburg, Sweden

Linda C. Huang, M.D.
The Plastic Surgery Center, Denver, Colorado

Norman E. Hugo, M.D., F.A.C.S.
Professor and Chairman, Division of Plastic and Reconstructive Surgery, College of Physicians and Surgeons, Columbia University, New York, New York

Michael E. Jabaley, M.D., F.A.C.S.
Clinical Professor of Plastic Surgery and Orthopaedic Surgery, University of Mississippi School of Medicine, Jackson, Mississippi

Ulrich K. Kesselring, M.D.
Centre de Chirurgie Plastique, Lausanne, Switzerland

Jean-Pierre Lalardrie, M.D.
Neuilly, Paris, France

Claude Lassus, M.D.
Attaché des Hôpitaux de Nice et Cannes, Nice, France

Gordon Letterman, M.D., F.A.C.S.
Clinical Professor of Surgery (Plastic Surgery), The George Washington University School of Medicine, Washington, D.C.

Carson M. Lewis, M.D., F.A.C.S.
Senior Staff, Scripps Memorial Hospital, Associate Professor, University of California, San Diego, California

Sarah S. Linden, M.D.
Assistant Professor of Radiology, Department of Radiology, University Medical Center, Jacksonville, Florida

William R. N. Lindsay, M.D.
Plastic, Reconstructive and Hand Surgery, Toronto, Canada

Clas Lossing, M.D.
Göteborg Universitet, Plastikkirurgiska Kliniken, Göteborg, Sweden

Gaston F. Maillard, M.D.
Privat-Docent à la Faculté de Médecine, Lausanne, Switzerland

Daniel Marchac, M.D.
Ancien Chef de Clinique à la Faculté et Assistant de l'Hôpital Saint-Louis, Chirurgien att. Consultant des Hôpitaux de Paris, Paris, France

Malcolm W. Marks, M.D., F.A.C.S.
Associate Professor of Plastic and Reconstructive Surgery, Bowman Gray School of Medicine, Wake Forest University, Winston Salem, North Carolina

G. Patrick Maxwell, M.D., F.A.C.S.
Assistant Clinical Professor, Department of Plastic Surgery, Vanderbilt University School of Medicine, Nashville, Tennessee

Kenneth S. McCarty, Jr., M.D., Ph.D.
Associate Professor, Department of Pathology and Medicine, Duke University Medical Center, Durham, North Carolina

Rodolphe Meyer, M.D.
Former Associate Professor, University Lausanne, Centre de Chirurgie Plastique, Lausanne, Switzerland

D. Ralph Millard, M.D., F.A.C.S., Hon. F.R.C.S. Ed.
Light-Millard Professor of Plastic Surgery, Chief, Division of Plastic Surgery, University of Miami School of Medicine, Miami, Florida

Richard A. Mladick, M.D., F.A.C.S.
Plastic Surgery Center, Inc., Virginia Beach, Virginia

A. R. Moscona, M.D.
Deputy Head, Department of Plastic Surgery, Rambam Medical Center, Haifa, Israel

Richard Moufarrège, M.D., F.R.C.S.
Hôtel-Dieu de Montréal, University of Montréal, Montreal, Canada

Roger Mouly, M.D.
Professeur Associé au College de Médecine, Hôpitaux de Paris, Paris, France

Walter R. Mullin, M.D., F.A.C.S.
Associate Professor of Plastic Surgery, University of Miami School of Medicine, Miami, Florida

Henry W. Neale, M.D., F.A.C.S.
Professor of Surgery (Plastic), Director, Division of Plastic and Reconstructive Surgery, University of Cincinnati Medical Center, Cincinnati, Ohio

Frederick Nicolle, M.Chir., F.R.C.S.
Consultant Plastic Surgeon, London, England

Naoyuki Ohtake, M.D.
Department of Plastic and Reconstructive Surgery, School of Medicine, Kitasato University, Kitasato, Japan

John Q. Owsley, M.D., F.A.C.S.
Clinical Professor of Surgery (Plastic Surgery), University of California—San Francisco, San Francisco, California

Jean-Marie Parenteau, M.D., F.A.C.S., F.R.C.S.(C)
Montreal, Canada

Gerardo Peixoto, M.D.
Department of Plastic Surgery, Catholic University of Salvador, Bahia, Brazil

Ivo Pitanguy, M.D., F.B.C.S., F.A.C.S., F.I.C.S.
Professor of Plastic Surgery, Catholic University of Rio de Janeiro, Chief, Plastic Surgery Department, Santa Casa de Misericordia General Hospital, Rio de Janeiro, Brazil

Jaime Planas, M.D.
Director, Clinica de Cirugia Plástica y Éstetica Dr. Planas, Associate Professor of Plastic Surgery, Universidad Automnoma de Barcelona, Barcelona, Spain

Ronaldo Pontes, M.D.
Rio de Janeiro, Brazil

Charles L. Puckett, M.D., F.A.C.S.
Professor and Chairman, Division of Plastic Surgery, University of Missouri Medical Center, Columbia, Missouri

Paule Regnault, M.D., F.R.C.S.
Chirurgie Plastique, La Tour de la Cité, Montreal, Canada

Liacyr Ribeiro, M.D.
Attending Surgeon and Director, Clinica Fluminense de Cirurgia Plástica, Niteroi, Rio de Janeiro, Brazil

Ronald Riefkohl, M.D., F.A.C.S.
Associate Professor of Plastic Surgery, Division of Plastic and Reconstructive Surgery, Duke University Medical Center, Durham, North Carolina

O. Gordon Robinson, Jr., M.D., F.A.C.S.
Birmingham, Alabama

Leonard R. Rubin, M.D., F.A.C.S.
Professor, Clinical Plastic Surgery, Stony Brook School of Medicine, Director, Plastic and Maxillofacial Surgery, Nassau County Medical Center, New York

Richard C. Schultz, M.D., F.A.C.S.
Clinical Professor of Surgery (Plastic), University of Illinois, College of Medicine, Chicago, Illinois

Maxine Schurter, M.D., F.A.C.S.
Clinical Professor of Surgery (Plastic Surgery), The George Washington University School of Medicine, Washington, D.C.

Alan E. Seyfer, M.D., F.A.C.S.
Professor and Chairman, Division of Plastic and Reconstructive Surgery, Oregon Health Science University, Portland, Oregon

Nobuyuki Shioya, M.D., F.A.C.S.
Department of Plastic and Reconstructive Surgery, School of Medicine, Kitasato University, Kitasato, Japan

Gilbert B. Snyder, M.D., P.A., F.A.C.S.
Clinical Assistant Professor of Plastic Surgery, University of Miami School of Medicine, South Miami, Florida

Michael C. Stalnecker, M.D., F.A.C.S.
Assistant Professor of Surgery (Plastic), College of Physicians and Surgeons, Columbia University, New York, New York

Jan Olof Strömbeck, M.D.
Assisting Professor (Docent) of Plastic Surgery, Chief, Department of Plastic Surgery, Sabbatsbergs Sjukhus, Stockholm, Sweden

Daniel C. Sullivan, M.D.
Associate Professor, Department of Radiology, Duke University Medical Center, Durham, North Carolina

Bahman Teimourian, M.D., F.A.C.S.
Associate Clinical Professor, Georgetown University School of Medicine, Washington, D.C., Faculty Member, George Washington University School of Medicine, Washington, D.C., Chairman, Department of Surgery, Surburban Hospital, Bethesda, Maryland

Edward O. Terino, M.D., F.A.C.S.
Director, Plastic Surgery Institute of Southern California, Agora Hills, California

I. Richard Toranto, M.D.
Plano, Texas

Trudy Vogt, M.D.
Plastische und Wiederherstellungschirurgie FMH, Bellevue Klinik, Zurich, Switzerland

R. C. A. Weatherley-White, M.D., F.A.C.S.
Associate Clinical Professor of Surgery, University of Colorado, The Plastic Surgery Center, Denver, Colorado

FOREWORD

According to the most up-to-date statistics in 1990, aesthetic breast surgery is still the most frequently performed surgical procedure in the armamentarium of plastic, reconstructive, and aesthetic surgeons.

This same statement and generalization could have been made similarly in 1983 when Nick Georgiade first published the volume *Aesthetic Breast Surgery,* which then included 58 contributors from North America, South America, and Europe. At that time there was so much good and concise information contained in its seemingly slim 402 pages and 30 chapters that I recommended it to the entire resident and attending staff at New York University's Institute of Reconstructive Plastic Surgery as the most valuable up-to-date volume at that time dealing with all aspects of aesthetic breast surgery with which they might be confronted and the problems that they might be asked to solve in both their clinical teaching patients and their private patients. I might add that our resident staff was particularly pleased to have this volume in their hands to use in studying for their Boards and other examinations.

Now Nick Georgiade, and his co-editors, Gregory Georgiade and Ronald Riefkohl, present us in 1990 with a larger, expanded, and even more complete text, *Aesthetic Surgery of the Breast,* with 93 contributors from 13 countries, representing North America, South America, Europe, the Middle East, and Asia, presenting their material in 49 chapters, including, thus, an additional 18 chapters and encompassing almost eight hundred pages. These additional chapters are certainly a reflection of the greater variation of procedures employed by plastic surgeons today. They also represent the increasing number of noteworthy papers that have appeared in the literature in the past 6 years dealing with an even larger variety of problems that face the plastic surgeon at the end of this ninth decade of the twentieth century.

The recent rapid expansion of interest in aesthetic surgery itself has created a considerable stimulus in the improvement of this surgical art. And it might also be said that these internationally recognized editors have now published chapters in this encyclopedic text that encompass almost the entire gamut of aesthetic breast surgery, thereby bringing to the readers what could be called the "state of the art."

It goes without saying, therefore, that these 49 chapters markedly enhance the intrinsic value and the depth of our knowledge in this area of aesthetic breast surgery. In this single volume, readers of plastic, reconstructive, and aesthetic plastic surgery advances now have available a wealth of information covering almost every conceivable aspect of aesthetic breast surgery. Most of the chapters are accompanied by extremely good, high-quality illustrations, as well as very satisfactory preoperative and postoperative photographs, and valuable up-to-date bibliographies with accurate reference material.

As a medical historian and editor, it would seem to be appropriate for me to draw the attention of the reader, at the very beginning of this book, to the fact that he can look forward to entirely new chapters not included in the 1983 book, covering such important subjects as the history of the treatment of augmentation mammaplasty, the history of reduction mammaplasty, and the history of the treatment of sagging breasts (mastopexy). Other chapters include the preoperative evaluation of the patient for breast surgery; the use of biomaterials in augmentation mammaplasty; of mammography for augmentation mammaplasty patients; congenital and acquired breast abnormalities; the triple areolar approach to augmentation mammaplasty; reduction mammaplasty utilizing the sliding nipple technique; use of the medial pedicle flap for reduction mammaplasty; reduction mammaplasty utilizing the inferior glandular "pyramid" pedicle; the total dermoglandular pedicle technique; use of the vertical dermal pedicle in breast reduction; the bipedicle vertical dermal flap in reduction mammaplasty; Z-plasty with minimal scarring; a physiological reduction mammaplasty; reduction mammaplasty utilizing a single vertical scar for breast reduction; a reduction mammaplasty technique using the inferior areola longitudinal incision; reduction mammaplasty utilizing the short inframammary scar technique; modified technique for reduction mammaplasty; preservation of sensation in the nipple areola complex; comparison of various reduction mammaplasty techniques; aesthetic breast surgery in Japan; the management of ptosis; general considerations; the management of various degrees of ptosis; and anomalies of the nipple and areola. An entirely new concept utilizing the "round block" technique for the correction of ptosis and breast hypertrophy, which limits the scar to only the circumareolar area, is also described.

When one stops to consider the magnitude of editing these many chapters contributed by international authorities and the thoroughness, exactness, and refinement this volume presents to the reader, it is not surprising for anyone who knows these three editors that there has probably been behind the scenes the always steady collaborative effort of Ruth Georgiade. Representing the plastic surgery community at large, I would like to take the opportunity in this Foreword to thank them all for their admirably successful efforts.

It is probably not too much of an understatement to believe that this textbook can now be considered the hallmark for all future texts in this field. It has not been difficult for me in any manner whatsoever, therefore, to overpraise this all-encompassing text, because I think it represents the most up-to-date unabridged source of contemporary thought and practice in this select and fascinating field of aesthetic breast surgery as we know it today.

Blair O. Rogers, M.D., F.A.C.S.
Professor of Clinical Surgery (Plastic Surgery)
New York University Medical Center
Editor, Aesthetic Plastic Surgery

ACKNOWLEDGMENTS

We wish to thank the excellent Duke University Medical Art Department for their skills in producing much of the art for this textbook; the Medical Center Library Staff for their assistance in producing the multilingual references we checked for accuracy in the many chapters; the publishers, W. B. Saunders Company, for their expertise in putting together this finished textbook; our hard-working secretarial staff for carefully producing the final accurate manuscripts, regardless of country of origin; the many international authors who contributed their valuable time and expertise; once again, Ruth Georgiade for her untiring efforts in striving for excellence in this publication; and Ms. Jessie Raymond, of the Saunders editorial staff, for her penchant for accuracy and perfection and remarkable equanimity in dealing with many problems.

CONTENTS

GENERAL CONSIDERATIONS

Kenneth S. McCarty, Jr.
Sarah A. Carpenter
Gregory S. Georgiade

1

The Breast: Embryology, Anatomy, and Physiology

A knowledge of the basic embryology, anatomy, and physiology of the human breast is a prerequisite for one interested in diseases of the breast. This chapter reviews these areas of breast biology and integrates them with concepts concerning the physician in the diagnosis and treatment of diseases of the breast.

EMBRYOLOGY

Mammary development begins in the fifth week of embryonic life with the formation of the milk line. This thickened epithelial band is derived from ectoderm and extends from each axilla to the groin. During the sixth week, the line widens to form the mammary ridge. The milk hill arises from the midthoracic portion of the ridge; simultaneously, the remainder of the ridge involutes. Incomplete involution of the mammary ridge results in accessory mammary tissues (gland, nipples, or both). Such accessory breast tissue is noted in 2% to 6% of women and 1% to 3% of men (Haagensen, 1986; Vorherr, 1974). More rarely, accessory tissue is found outside the embryonal mammary lines (Haagensen, 1986). Most supernumerary nipples or accessory breasts have no physiologic function and are not subject to disease, but some may become enlarged and secrete milk during pregnancy and lactation or become involved by conditions that affect the ectopic breasts.

In the 7-week embryo, the ectodermal milk hill starts to invaginate the underlying mesenchymal tissue. It continues to descend; and by the tenth to fourteenth week, the breast anlage has formed a sunken cone with an overlying nipple groove. Stimulated by the inward epithelial growth, the surrounding mesenchymal cells differentiate into primitive blood vessels and the smooth muscle fibers of the nipple and areola. At 12 weeks, three vascular zones around the mammary anlage are defined (Dabelow, 1957). The inner zone contains the smallest vessels and is in close contact with the basal layer of the anlage. An intermediate vascular zone lies in the connective tissue surrounding the breast anlage and supplies the deeper layer of the skin. The outer zone contains the largest vessels, which supply peripheral mammary structures and fat.

By 15 weeks, epithelial buds develop at the tip of the invading parenchymal tissue and subsequently branch into 15 to 25 epithelial stalks. Simultaneously, hair, sweat, and sebaceous gland development appears in the surrounding subcutaneous tissues. While the hair and sweat glands regress, the sebaceous glands fully develop. Additionally, special apocrine glands, the Montgomery glands, develop around the mammary anlage (Vorherr, 1974).

The early stages of mammary development are independent of sex steroid hormones, but at 15 weeks the breast tissue is sensitive to testosterone. This sensitivity is transitory, with loss of androgen responsiveness occurring shortly after its acquisition. The target of testosterone appears to be the mesenchyme (Topper and Freeman, 1980). In the presence of testosterone, the mesenchyme condenses around the epithelial stalk, which leads to its rupture. This results in isolation of the mammary bud subdermally, where further development does not occur. Epithelial sprouts not exposed to testosterone during this window of sensitivity begin to canalize, which leads to formation of milk ducts between 20 and 32 weeks (Vorherr, 1974). From week 32 to week 40, the milk glands branch into lobuloalveolar structures (Vorherr, 1974). It has been suggested that this morphologic change is largely a consequence of mesenchymal influences and may be independent of specific hormonal effects (Topper, 1980). Near term, however, maternal and placental sex steroids stimulate the fetal mammary gland, and the monolayered alveoli become secretory. At birth, with withdrawal of sex steroids, fetal prolactin stimulates colostrum secretion until 3 to 4 weeks of age (in both male and female infants). Upon further withdrawal of maternal steroids and an eventual decline in fetal prolactin, the glandular tissues revert to ductular organization (Vorherr, 1974). These regressional epithelial changes are minor, compared with postlactational involution of the adult breast. The 15 to 25 milk ducts merge in the indented center of the areola, the location of the nipple, which will be formed at puberty. The mammary tissues remain quiescent throughout childhood until puberty and adolescence.

3

CONGENITAL BREAST ANOMALIES

True anomalies of the breast, other than accessory breasts or nipples, include those in which a breast is absent, rudimentary, or structurally abnormal. Defective embryonic mammary development may result in a complete lack of breast tissue (amastia) and is one of the more unusual breast anomalies. Rudimentary breasts are very small, often unilateral, and are less rare. Mammary aplasia is a condition in which breast tissue is absent but the areola and nipple develop. The rarest of breast anomalies appears to be absence of the nipple. Conversely, polythelia indicates the existence of more than one nipple per breast. Differences in the size of normal breasts or extension of breast tissue into the axilla or midline are frequent enough that they should not be considered anomalies, although individual patients may be disturbed by the cosmetic consequence.

ADOLESCENCE

Alterations in gonadotropin (follicle-stimulating hormone and luteinizing hormone) secretion at the onset of puberty stimulate ovarian primordial follicles to mature into graafian follicles. The growing follicles secrete estrogens, which, in the presence of growth hormone or prolactin, restimulate breast ductal growth. Neither sex steroid nor peptide hormone is effective alone, and more specifically, the ductal growth is independent of progesterone (Topper and Freeman, 1980). Elongation of mammary ducts, thickening of ductal epithelium, formation of lobular buds from terminal ductular parts, and increases in periductal connective tissue all follow under the influence of estrogens. This growth continues until a characteristic ductal spacing, apparently governed by local factors, is reached (Topper and Freeman, 1980). Differentiation into lobuloalveolar structures requires progesterone in addition (Topper and Freeman, 1980). The dark brown pigmentation of the areolae and nipples is also only observed when both female sex steroids are present (Dabelow, 1957), although pituitary peptide hormones may also play a direct role. Multiple hormones influence different components of mammary ductal and alveolar formation (Table 1–1). Under the stimulation of cyclic ovarian hormones, mammary lobuloacinar development and connective tissue growth continue up to the third decade of life, contributing to the appearance of the mature female breast.

DEVELOPMENTAL ABNORMALITIES

Abnormalities of breast development are found in conjunction with various disease states. Breasts fail to develop in Turner's syndrome (ovarian agenesis), congenital adrenal hyperplasia, and delayed menarche (Haagensen, 1986). In these patients estrogen therapy usually makes the breasts develop. Precocious development of the female breasts occurs in constitutional precocious puberty, a state of elevated sex steroids in which no causative lesion is found (Haagensen, 1986). More rarely, aberrations in sex steroid secretion due to childhood ovarian tumors, lutein cysts, or lesions of the third ventricle cause precocious hypertrophy of the female breast. Biopsy and surgery are not indicated, because the tissue is normal and the procedures can be damaging to a developing breast (Haagensen, 1986). The most frequent type of female breast hypertrophy occurs during adolescence in girls with apparently normal hormonal function (Haagensen, 1986). Sometimes affecting one breast more than the other, the excessive

TABLE 1–1
Major Hormonal Influences on the Human Breast

HORMONE	EFFECTS
Estrogen	Required for ductal growth during adolescence Required for lobuloalveolar growth during pregnancy Stimulates pituitary secretion of thyroid stimulating hormone + prolactin Stimulates protein, lactose synthesis with prolactin + thyroid hormone Not necessary for maintenance of lactation
Progesterone	Required for lobuloalveolar differentiation and growth Not necessary for ductal formation
Testosterone	Causes mesenchymal destruction of mammary epithelium during critical period of testosterone sensitivity
Glucocorticoid	Required for maximal ductal growth Nonessential but enhances lobuloalveolar growth during pregnancy Stimulates rough endoplasmic reticulum formation in lactogenesis
Insulin	Stimulates replication of mammary epithelium Nonessential but enhances ductal and alveolar growth Required for secretory activity with glucocorticoid + prolactin Stimulates rough endoplasmic reticulum formation in lactogenesis
Prolactin	Required for lactogenesis and maintenance of lactation Stimulates epithelial growth after parturition
Human placental lactogen	Able to substitute for prolactin in epithelial growth and differentiation Stimulates alveolar growth and lactogenesis in second half of pregnancy
Growth hormone	Required for ductal growth in adolescence May contribute to lobuloalveolar growth during pregnancy
Thyroid hormone	Increases epithelial secretory response to prolactin Nonessential for ductal growth; may enhance alveolar growth
Oxytocin	Causes contraction of myoepithelial cells

growth is of the connective tissue and fat, not of the epithelial elements. If bothersome to the patient, the excessive tissue can be excised.

ANATOMY OF THE MATURE BREAST

The mature female breast has a unique dome-shaped form. Its size may vary from under 30 gm to over 500 gm. Obesity is an important factor influencing size (Haagensen, 1986). The majority of the breast parenchyma extends over the third to seventh intercostal spaces from the edge of the sternum to the anterior axillary line. The mammary tissue also extends variably into the axilla as the glandular tail of Spence.

Approximately 75% of the breast rests on the pectoralis major muscle (superior and medial portions). The lateral portion of the breast extends over the third and fourth digitation of the serratus anterior muscle. The inferior portion of the breast is partly over the serratus anterior muscle, external oblique muscle, and most medially over the superior rectus muscle fascia.

The breast parenchyma is made up of 15 to 25 lobes, each emptying into a separate milk duct terminating in the nipple (Haagensen, 1986). These lobes are surrounded by connective tissue and are divided into many lobules. The lobule is subdivided into 10 to 100 alveoli, which are enveloped by a sheath, forming the basement membrane. The sheath extends to invest the collecting duct. The lobule is the basic structural unit of the breast and as a whole is enclosed by a somewhat thicker connective tissue envelope.

The ectodermally derived nipple is located in the fourth to fifth intercostal space. The skin of the nipple contains numerous sebaceous and apocrine sweat glands but relatively little hair. The 15 to 25 parenchymal milk ducts enter the base of the nipple, where they dilate to form the milk sinuses. Slightly below the nipple's surface, the sinuses terminate in cone-shaped ampullae. In the resting breast, these ampullae are filled with epithelial debris. During lactation they function as temporary milk repositories. Collagenous and elastic connective tissue intermeshes with the nipple's milk ducts, but the bulk of the nipple is comprised of circular and longitudinal smooth muscle fibers. Muscular contraction results in local venous stasis, nipple erection, and emptying of the milk sinuses.

The circular pigmented areola surrounds the nipple and varies between 15 and 60 mm in diameter. The skin of the areola contains lanugo hair, sweat glands, small sebaceous glands, and Montgomery's glands. Montgomery's glands are large sebaceous glands with miniature milk ducts that open into Morgani's tubercles in the epidermis of the areola. They enlarge and secrete with pregnancy and, unlike sebaceous glands, undergo involution postmenopausally (Vorherr, 1974). The areola, too, contains smooth muscle fibers arranged circularly and radially. They function to contract the areola and compress the base of the nipple.

The skin overlying the breast is thin and creates a flexible and elastic cover adherent to the subcutaneous tissues. It contains hair follicles, sebaceous glands, and eccrine sweat glands (Osborne, 1987). Beneath the dermis, the mammary tissues are enveloped by the superficial and deep layers of the superficial fascia, continuous above with the cervical fascia and below with Cooper's superficial abdominal fascia. The breast is fixed by Cooper's ligaments, fibrous and elastic bands that link the deep layers of epidermis to the superficial fascia and give suspensory support. Fibrosis or displacement by mass may cause traction on these fibrous bands, resulting in skin dimpling or nipple retraction. The superficial layer of the superficial fascia is very delicate but defines an avascular plane just below the dermis. The deep layer of the superficial fascia is better developed, lying partly on the pectoral fascia that covers the underlying pectoralis major muscle. Between these two fasciae, there is a retromammary space filled with loose tissue that allows the breast to move freely over the chest wall. Projections of the deep layer of the superficial fascia cross this retromammary space, fuse with the pectoralis fascia, and form the posterior suspensory ligaments of the breast (Fig. 1–1). Breast parenchyma may accompany these fibrous processes into the pectoralis major muscle itself (Stiles, 1936). Therefore, com-

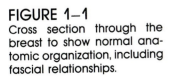

FIGURE 1–1
Cross section through the breast to show normal anatomic organization, including fascial relationships.

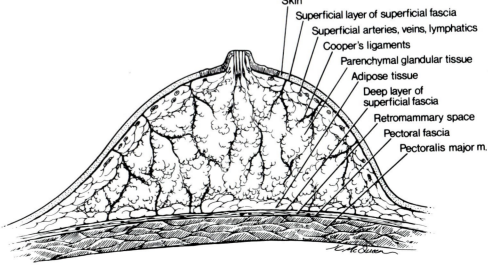

Skin
Superficial layer of superficial fascia
Superficial arteries, veins, lymphatics
Cooper's ligaments
Parenchymal glandular tissue
Adipose tissue
Deep layer of superficial fascia
Retromammary space
Pectoral fascia
Pectoralis major m.

plete removal of breast parenchyma necessitates excision of a portion of the muscle as well.

The pectoralis fascia encases the pectoralis major, extends medially to the contralateral pectoral fascia, and continues cephalad with the deltoid and clavicular fasciae. Although it is common to consider the entire breast as lying upon the pectoral fascia, only approximately half overlies this fascia, and the remainder lies upon other muscles of the chest wall (Haagensen, 1986). These include the serratus anterior, the external oblique, and the rectus abdominis, all covered by the same deep fascia that blends them together. An axillary fascia encloses and separates the two pectoral muscles and forms a bridge from the deltoid and clavicle to the muscles of the chest wall. Its superficial layer invests the pectoralis major muscle. The costocoracoid fascia is the deeper and thicker portion that invests the pectoralis minor muscle. The importance of this layer, however, is that it guards the nerves, vessels, and lymphatics of the axilla. In so doing, it provides the supporting structure that permits the surgeon to remove the axilla *en bloc*.

BLOOD SUPPLY

The arterial supply to the breast is provided by three main routes: the internal mammary artery, the lateral

thoracic artery, and the intercostal arteries (Maliniac, 1943, 1950) (Fig. 1–2). Approximately 60% of the breast receives blood from the anterior and posterior perforating branches of the internal mammary artery. This artery arises from the subclavian artery and descends behind the clavicle and first rib. It usually sends two branches at each interspace via the anterior perforating arteries. The anterior perforating branches exit their respective intercostal spaces approximately 2 cm lateral to the sternum and run within the subcutaneous tissue of the breast (Fig. 1–3). These branches supply the medial breast and course laterally to anastomose with branches of the lateral thoracic artery at the nipple. Anastomoses with the intercostal arteries occur less frequently (Vorherr, 1974). The posterior perforating branches exit more laterally from the intercostal spaces and supply the posterior aspect of the breast (Serafin, 1979).

The lateral thoracic artery arises from the axillary artery, or rarely from the thoracoacromial or subscapular artery, or is absent (Haagensen, 1986; Maliniac, 1943, 1950). The lateral thoracic artery approaches the breast lateral to the superior portion of the pectoralis minor muscle and sends perforating branches through and around the lateral aspect of the pectoralis major muscle into the base of the breast tissue. It courses inferomedially within the subcutaneous tissue and supplies up to 30% of breast blood flow to the lateral and

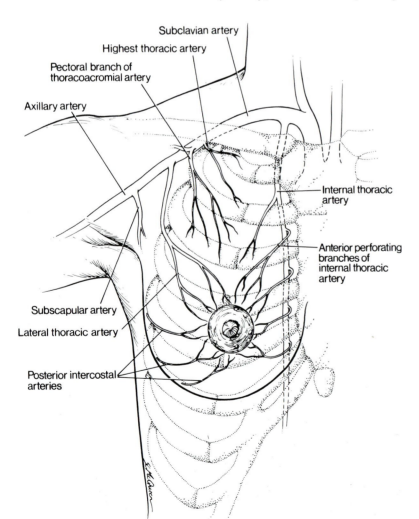

Subclavian artery
Highest thoracic artery
Pectoral branch of thoracoacromial artery
Axillary artery

Internal thoracic artery

Anterior perforating branches of internal thoracic artery

Subscapular artery
Lateral thoracic artery

Posterior intercostal arteries

FIGURE 1–2
Arterial supply to the breast.

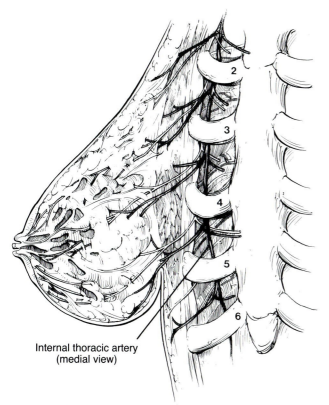

FIGURE 1–3
Arterial supply to the breast with perforation of breast parenchyma via internal thoracic artery.

upper outer portions of the breast. There is also quite often a direct branch of the axillary artery to the superior portion of the breast, which perforates the superior aspect of the pectoralis major muscle.

The anterior and lateral branches of the third to fifth posterior intercostal arteries are the least important of the arteries supplying the breast. Originating from the aorta, they course in the intercostal spaces and chiefly supply the lower outer quadrant. Additional minor sources of arterial supply to the breast include the highest thoracic artery, the pectoral branch of the thoracoacromial artery, the subscapular artery, and its continuation, the thoracodorsal artery.

The blood supply to the nipple has been extensively studied, and much controversy exists regarding the design of operations that preserve the best circulation to the nipple, yet result in aesthetic contours and minimal scars. The blood supply to the nipple and periareolar area appears to be mainly from the lateral thoracic branches, with anastomosis from the internal mammary vessels forming a plexus around the areola. In summary, ensuring viability of both the nipple and glandular tissue, the nipple-areola complex cannot be separated from its dermal blood supply, and the glandular tissue must remain in continuity with the cutaneous blood supply (Serafin, 1979).

For the most part, mammary venous drainage follows the arterial distribution pattern and is divided into superficial and deep systems (Fig. 1–4). Lying just below the superficial layer of the superficial fascia, the superficial system has been classified into two main types:

transverse and longitudinal (Massopust, 1950). The transverse veins (91%) run medially in the subcutaneous tissues, then deeply, to join perforating vessels that empty into the internal thoracic veins. Longitudinal vessels (9%) ascend to the suprasternal notch and empty into the superficial veins of the lower neck. Anastomoses of these superficial venous systems across the chest midline are frequent (Haagensen, 1986). The superficial veins may become clinically obvious in certain diseases of the breast, including some highly malignant and rapidly growing tumors. Thrombophlebitis of a superficial vein may resemble breast cancer by causing skin edema and retraction over a firm mass.

There are three groups of veins to consider in the deep drainage system of the breast. The perforating branches of the internal thoracic vein are the largest vessels of the deep system and empty into the corresponding innominate veins. The axillary vein has many irregular tributaries that drain the chest wall, pectoral muscles, and deep breast tissue. The third deep drainage system is posteriorly directed through the intercostal veins. These veins communicate with the vertebral veins and the azygos vein, which leads to the superior vena cava. All three of these venous pathways lead to the pulmonary capillary network and provide a route for metastatic carcinoma emboli to the lungs (Haagensen, 1986). The vertebral system of veins connected to the intercostal drainage at each vertebral segment provides an entirely different metastatic route. These veins form vertebral venous plexuses and provide a direct venous pathway for metastases to bones of the spine, pelvis, femur, shoulder girdle, humerus, and skull (Haagensen, 1986).

INNERVATION

Innervation of the breast is supplied by somatic sensory and sympathetic autonomic nerves (Vorherr, 1974). The skin of the upper breast receives sensory innervation from the supraclavicular nerves, branches C3 and C4 of the cervical plexus. The intercostal nerves supply the skin of the lower breast, including the nipple-areola complex (Serafin, 1979) (Figs. 1–5 and 1–6). These nerves give off lateral cutaneous branches and then continue anteriorly to terminate as anterior cutaneous branches. Lateral cutaneous branches from the fourth to sixth intercostal nerves further divide into anterior and posterior branches. The anterior branches send forth the lateral rami mammarii, which innervate the lateral portion of the breast and the nipple-areola complex. The fourth intercostal nerve appears to be the dominant innervation to the nipple (Cooper, 1840; Goldwyn, 1976). The medial and inferior aspect of the breast is innervated by the medial rami mammarii from the anterior cutaneous branches of the second to sixth intercostal nerves (Fig. 1–7).

The lateral cutaneous branch of the second intercostal nerve (intercostobrachial nerve) does not divide into anterior and posterior divisions. Rather, it crosses the axilla laterally and forms a plexus with the medial brachial cutaneous nerve and the posterior division of the third lateral cutaneous nerve (Haagensen, 1986).

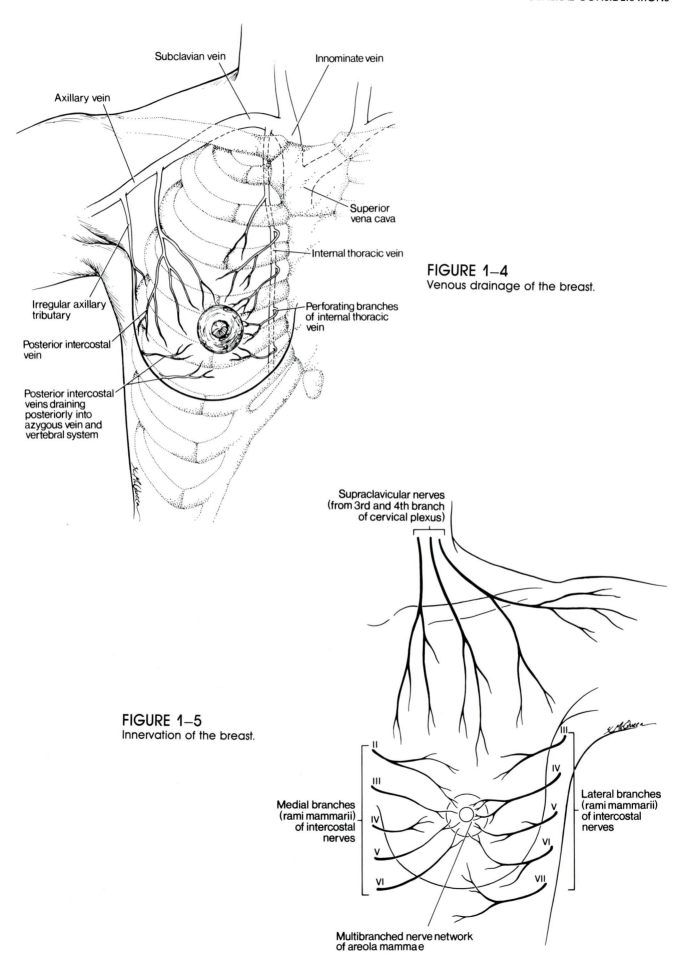

Subclavian vein

Innominate vein

Axillary vein

Superior vena cava

Internal thoracic vein

Irregular axillary tributary

Perforating branches of internal thoracic vein

Posterior intercostal vein

Posterior intercostal veins draining posteriorly into azygous vein and vertebral system

FIGURE 1–4
Venous drainage of the breast.

FIGURE 1–5
Innervation of the breast.

Supraclavicular nerves
(from 3rd and 4th branch
of cervical plexus)

II

III

III

IV

Medial branches
(rami mammarii)
of intercostal
nerves

IV

V

V

VI

VI

Lateral branches
(rami mammarii)
of intercostal
nerves

VII

Multibranched nerve network
of areola mammae

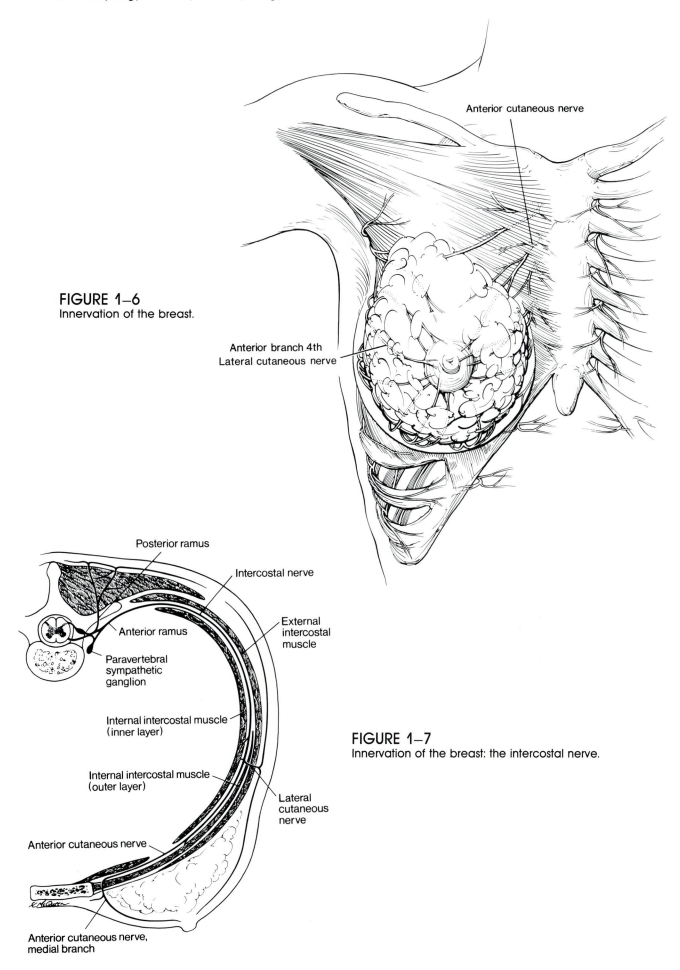

FIGURE 1–6
Innervation of the breast.

Anterior cutaneous nerve

Anterior branch 4th
Lateral cutaneous nerve

Posterior ramus

Intercostal nerve

External
intercostal
muscle

Anterior ramus

Paravertebral
sympathetic
ganglion

Internal intercostal muscle
(inner layer)

Internal intercostal muscle
(outer layer)

Lateral
cutaneous
nerve

Anterior cutaneous nerve

FIGURE 1–7
Innervation of the breast: the intercostal nerve.

Anterior cutaneous nerve,
medial branch

The nerve and the plexus it forms innervate the medial aspect of the upper arm. The thoracodorsal nerve crosses the axilla to enter the latissimus dorsi muscle, which it supplies (Grant, 1958). Because the nerve traverses the central and scapular groups of axillary lymph nodes, attempts to save it in an axillary dissection can be hazardous. The long thoracic nerve emerges from beneath the axillary vein and lies in the areolar tissue upon the serratus anterior muscle (Grant, 1958). This nerve, in contrast to the above two, should not be sacrificed, because lymph nodes are not ordinarily seen along it (Haagensen, 1986).

The epidermis of the areola, nipple, and bordering dermal parts is poorly innervated, which is evidenced by a limited sensory discrimination including light touch, stereognosis, and two-point discrimination (Courtiss and Goldwyn, 1976; Vorherr, 1974). Alternatively, the deeper portions of the dermis and skin appendages are well innervated (Cathcart et al., 1948). The relatively large number of dermal nerve endings provide a high mammary responsiveness toward stimuli (Vorherr, 1974). Specifically, Krause- and Ruffini-like endings located in the dermis of the nipple-areola complex are extremely sensitive to mechanical stimulation that can initiate the suckling reflex. This induces release of pituitary prolactin and oxytocin. Oxytocin causes contraction of myoepithelial cells and, in the lactating gland, milk ejection.

Autonomic nerves are the second type of innervation in the breast. Postganglionic sympathetic fibers (gray rami) traveling through the second to sixth intercostal nerves and the supraclavicular nerves innervate the smooth musculature of the areola, nipple, and mammary blood vessels; parasympathetic fibers are absent in the breast (Grant, 1958). Stimulation of the various end organs in the nipple-areola complex can initiate neural transmission through the afferent limb of the reflex arc and cause smooth muscle contraction of the nipple and areola (nipple erection) as well as of the mammary blood vessels (decreased blood flow) through the efferent α-adrenergic sympathetic limb. Simultaneously, β-adrenergic sympathetic excitation releases norepinephrine, causing relaxation of myoepithelial cells. Because parasympathetic fibers are lacking, no vasodilation or myoepithelial contraction due to postganglionic acetylcholine release is observed. A minor inhibitory effect on the mammary myoepithelium by norepinephrine may exist that is overcome by oxytocin release during suckling, causing myoepithelial contraction (Vorherr, 1974). It has been suggested that no parasympathetic activity in the breast is necessary (Vorherr, 1974).

LYMPHATICS

Knowledge of the lymphatic drainage of the breast is of particular clinical importance. Four principal lymphatic pathways drain the breast: cutaneous, axillary, internal thoracic, and posterior intercostal (Edwards, 1976; Haagensen, 1986). Lymphatics in general accompany blood vessels and, therefore, extend in all directions from the breast (Fig. 1–8). Furthermore, autoradiographs of surgical specimens found "no striking

tendency for any particular quadrant to drain in one direction" (Turner-Warwick, 1959). Lymphatic vessels empty into lymph nodes; the mammary gland is associated with an average of 35 nodes. If a lymph node is blocked, as by cancer, retrograde lymph flow can occur, leading to widespread dispersal of cancer through lymphatic channels (Edwards, 1976).

The cutaneous lymphatics consist of a superficial plexus without valves that sends branches around the dermal papillae and a perilobular deeper network with valves that follows the mammary ducts in the subareolar area of the breast (Haagensen, 1986). Some superficial lymphatics from the medial breast may cross the midline and continue with contralateral lymphatics (Vorherr, 1974). Most of the cutaneous lymphatics of the superior, medial, and inferior breast, including the subareolar plexus, drain laterally to the axilla. From the lower border of the breast, cutaneous lymph vessels may drain to the epigastric plexus in the rectus abdominis sheath (Gerota's pathway) and empty into the subdiaphragmatic and subperitoneal lymph plexuses. Flow can then continue to the lymphatics of the liver and intra-abdominal nodes, providing a route by which metastases from breast carcinoma can reach the liver.

The axilla receives the majority of the lymphatic flow from the breast, ranging from 75% (shown by autoradiographs of surgical specimens) (Turner-Warwick, 1959) to 97% (demonstrated by postradical mastectomy with radioactive colloidal gold uptake studies (Hultborn et al., 1955). There are six groups of axillary nodes, and they all lie beneath the costocoracoid fascia, which encloses them with the blood vessels and nerves of the axilla (Haagensen, 1986). The external mammary nodes lie beneath the lateral edge of the pectoralis major muscle adjacent to the lateral thoracic artery from the sixth to second rib. The scapular nodes are closely applied to the subscapular vessels and their thoracodorsal branches. The intercostobrachial and thoracodorsal nerves are also intimately associated with these nodes, necessitating their sacrifice in an axillary dissection. The nodes most easily palpated, the central nodes, lie embedded in the center of the axilla. They receive the greatest proportion of the axillary lymph flow and represent the group of nodes in which metastases are most often found. The interpectoral (Rotter's) nodes lie between the pectoralis major and minor muscles. If these nodes must be excised, removal of the pectoralis major is necessary (McCarty et al., 1983). The axillary vein nodes lie on the lateral, caudad, and ventral aspects of the axillary vein, separated from it by a delicate layer of fascia. The subclavicular nodes are the most medial group, situated along the ventral and caudad aspects of the axillary vein. They extend from the origin of the thoracoacromial vein to the apex of the axilla and represent the highest point to which the surgeon can carry an axillary dissection. The lymphatic drainage from all the other groups of axillary nodes empties into these subclavicular nodes. One or more large lymphatic trunks arise from the plexus of lymphatic vessels and conduct the subclavicular lymph upward and medially to the junction of the jugular and subclavian veins. The subclavicular nodes are beyond "regional" nodes, and involvement by tumor is a grave sign (Haagensen, 1986).

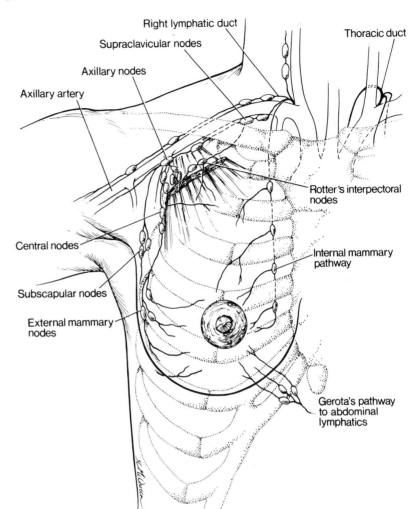

FIGURE 1–8
Lymphatic pathways of the breast.

The internal thoracic lymphatic route carries from 3% to 25% of breast lymph flow (Hultborn et al., 1955; Turner-Warwick, 1959). The lymphatics of the internal thoracic route emerge from the deep aspect and the medial edge of the breast. Lying upon the pectoral fascia, they run medially to reach the medial ends of the intercostal spaces. The lymphatic vessels then turn inward and penetrate the pectoralis major and intercostal muscles to reach the internal mammary nodes. These nodes are interspersed along the course of the internal thoracic trunk lymphatics and number three to four per side of the sternal edge. The internal thoracic trunks eventually empty into the great veins in one of several ways: (1) via the thoracic duct on the left and right lymphatic duct; (2) via lower cervical nodes, or (3) directly into the jugular-subclavian confluence.

The posterior intercostal lymphatics empty into the posterior intercostal lymph nodes, which lie within the thorax in front of the junction of ribs and vertebrae. The posterior intercostal nodes receive lymph sparsely and irregularly from the breast via perforating intercostal lymphatics as well as lymphatics from the external intercostal muscles, the parietal pleura, the vertebrae, and the spinal muscles. Efferent lymphatic vessels from the posterior intercostal nodes vary in their destination, depending on the interspace in which they are located (Haagensen, 1986). These nodes become significant when the other pathways are obstructed (Serafin, 1979).

MICROSCOPIC ANATOMY OF THE BREAST PARENCHYMA

Microscopically, the breast parenchyma consists of the ductulolobuloalveolar structures surrounded by basement membrane, stroma with connective tissue and vessels, and fat. During childhood, the mammary ductular and alveolar lining consists of a 2-cell-layered basal cuboidal and low cylindrical surface epithelium (Vorherr, 1974). The cells of the duct epithelium, as opposed to mammary alveolar cells, contain few mitochondria and sparse endoplasmic reticulum. Under hormonal influence, especially estrogens, the alveolar epithelium proliferates and specializes into A, B, and myoepithelial cells. Columnar, basophilic, luminal A cells are rich in ribosomes and are actively involved in the process of milk synthesis and secretion during lactation. B cells, thought to be the precursors of A and myoepithelial cells, are basal cells with clear cytoplasm and round nuclei. Myoepithelial cells are apposed to the inner aspects of the basement membrane of alveoli and the small ducts. They have starlike branching and contain myofibrils and oval, dense nuclei. As contractile ectodermal smooth muscle cells, myoepithelial cells are 10 to 20 times more sensitive to oxytocin than mesodermal myometrial cells (Vorherr, 1974). No innervation of myoepithelial cells can be observed. Surrounding the epithelial elements is a specialized structure, the epithelial stromal junction. It is composed of the plasma membranes of the epithelial and myoepithelial cells, a lamina lucida, a basal lamina, and delimiting fibroblasts (McCarty et al., 1983) (Fig. 1–9).

PHYSIOLOGY AND ENDOCRINOLOGY

Changes occur in mature breasts throughout an individual's lifetime and include those associated with the menstrual cycle, pregnancy and lactation, and menopause. As an integral part of the reproductive system, the breast and its changes are largely under tightly regulated hormonal control. An understanding of the normal changes in the breast is necessary to distinguish physiologic versus pathologic states encountered by the physician.

The Menstrual Cycle

Clinically, breast size, density, and nodularity are closely correlated with the menstrual cycle (Haagensen, 1986). The nodularity can be so marked during the premenstrual (postovulatory) phase of the cycle that it can be mistaken for clinically significant tumors of the breast. Biopsy should be withheld, however, until the breasts are re-examined near the midpoint of the next menstrual cycle, when physiologic nodularity is minimized.

Attempts to correlate these cyclic physical changes with histologic changes in the breast have produced conflicting results. Although some authors maintain that the nongravid breast is essentially a resting gland (Haagensen, 1986), morphologic changes in the mammary epithelial and stromal components have been identified as they relate to specific pituitary-ovarian events in the menstrual cycle (Longacre and Bartow, 1986; Vogel et al., 1981). Vogel and associates (1981) described five phases of cyclic morphologic alterations in the breast associated with the menstrual cycle (Table 1–2). From day 3 to 7 of the menstrual cycle, the epithelium is oriented in acini lined by 2- to 3-cell layers with relatively poorly defined lumina. The acinar epithelial cells are of one type, small and polygonal, with pale eosinophilic cytoplasm and a dark, centrally located nucleus. As a whole, the lobules and their acini are relatively compact. The stroma is a dense cellular mantle with plump fibroblasts (Fig. 1–10A). Maximal mitotic activity occurs in a later phase of the cycle, according to the studies of Ferguson and Anderson (1981), although some activity is seen in this phase and throughout the cycle (Longacre and Bartow, 1986; Vogel et al., 1981).

During the follicular phase, days 8 through 14, three morphologically distinct cells become apparent. The most basal cells, myoepithelial cells, have clear cytoplasm and small, dense nuclei. The intermediate pale cells of the proliferative phase, B cells, persist. The third type of cells, A cells, begin to border well-defined lumina and have basophilic cytoplasm and a dense basal nucleus. The basophilia of this cell correlates with increasing ribonucleic acid and ribosome content, observed by electron microscopy (Fanger and Ree, 1974). The stroma remains dense but is less cellular and more collagenous than in the proliferative phase.

With ovulation and increasing progesterone, days 15 through 20, the breast enters the luteal phase of differentiation. The hallmark of this phase is vacuolization and ballooning of the basal cell layer due to an increase

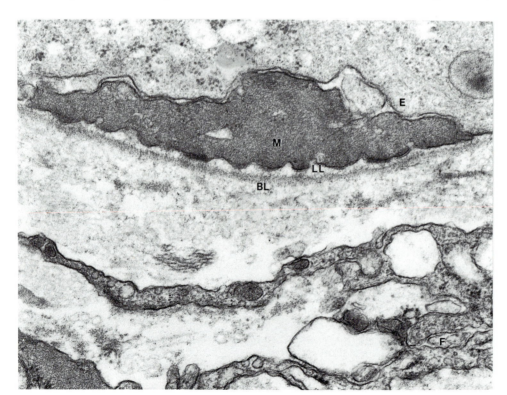

FIGURE 1–9

Epithelial stromal junction of the breast acinus. Electron micrographs of the epithelial stromal junctions demonstrating the epithelial plasma membrane (E), myoepithelial cell (M), lamina lucida (LL), basal lamina (BL), and delimiting fibroblast.

Table 1–2
Morphologic Criteria for Menstrual Phase Assignment

PHASE	STROMA	LUMEN	EPITHELIUM		
			Cell Types	Orientation	Secretion
Early follicular	Dense, cellular	Tight	Single predominant pale eosinophilic cell	No stratification apparent	None
Late follicular	Dense, cellular-collagenous	Defined	1) Luminal columnar basophilic cell 2) Intermediate pale cell 3) Basal clear cell with hyperchromatic nucleus (myoepithelial)	Radial around lumen	None
Early luteal	Loose, broken	Open, slight secretion	1) Luminal basophilic cell 2) Intermediate pale cell 3) Prominent vacuolization of basal clear cell (myoepithelial)	Radial around lumen	Minimal
Late luteal	Loose, edematous	Open with secretion	1) Luminal basophilic cell 2) Intermediate pale cell 3) Prominent vacuolization of basal clear cell (myoepithelial)	Radial around lumen	Active apocrine secretion from luminal cell
Menstrual	Dense, cellular	Distended with secretion	1) Luminal basophilic cell with scant cytoplasm 2) Extensive vacuolization of basal cells	Radial around lumen	Resorbing

in glycogen content of the myoepithelial cells. The lumina are enlarged over previous phases and contain some secretory product with minimal evidence of active secretion. There is an overall increase in size of lobules and number of terminal duct structures (Longacre and Bartow, 1986). The stroma loosens, and the basal lamina becomes less prominent.

The secretory phase, days 21 through 27, is characterized by apocrine secretion from the luminal epithelial cells into dilated lumina. The apical budding also ap-

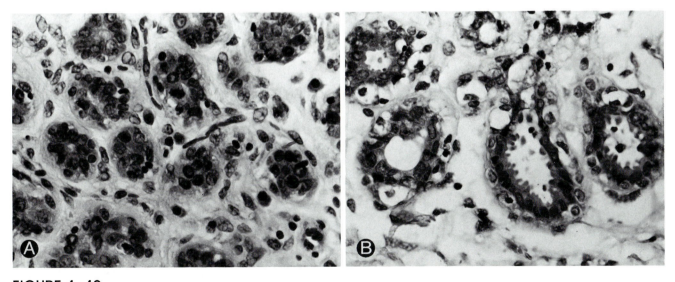

FIGURE 1–10
Menstrual cycle–associated changes in breast morphology. *A,* Menstrual cycle phase I, during the proliferative phase (days 3 to 7). The stroma is dense and cellular, with numerous plasma cells. The alveolar epithelial cells are of one dominant type, have poorly defined cell borders, and are irregularly arranged about the tight lumen. Mitoses are present. *B,* Menstrual cycle phase IV, during the secretory phase (days 21 to 27). The stroma is loose and edematous. Three epithelial cell types surround open, secretion-filled lumina in a radial arrangement. Apocrine secretion by the luminal basophilic cell is seen as well as the intermediate pale cell and the prominent vacuolization of the basal myoepithelial cell.

pears to be a progestational effect. Ultrastructurally, there is a marked increase in polysomes, rough endoplasmic reticulum, enlarging Golgi, and secretory vacuoles, supporting this phase as one of active protein synthesis and secretion (Fanger and Ree, 1974). The maximum size of lobules and number of acini are expressed during this time (Longacre and Bartow, 1986). Another prominent feature of this phase is the onset of stromal edema with fluid-filled spaces that disrupt lobular borders. The edematous change has been attributed to sex steroid–induced histamine effect on mammary circulation (Vogel et al., 1981). Large, congested venous spaces are present in the mantle tissue as well (see Fig. 10B). As mentioned above, peak mitotic activity is seen during this phase of the menstrual cycle (Ferguson and Anderson, 1981; Longacre and Bartow, 1986). Such activity occurs shortly after the progesterone peak and second estradiol peak at cycle days 22 through 24 and is highly suggestive of a progestational effect or a combined estrogenic and progestational effect (Longacre and Bartow, 1986).

The menstrual phase, days 28 through 32, is associated with estrogen and progesterone withdrawal. Apocrine budding abates, but the acinar lumina remain distended with eosinophilic granular secretions. The luminal cells have scant basophilic cytoplasm, whereas the basal cells remain extensively ballooned with glycogen. The lobules are decreased in size and the acini slightly less numerous than in the previous phases (Longacre and Bartow, 1986). The stroma is again compact and cellular. As the tissue reenters the proliferative phase, the luminal cells become less basophilic, the vacuolization diminishes in the basal cells, acinar lumina become tighter, and the cycle is reinitiated. The breast volume is at a minimum 5 to 7 days after menstruation but never returns to that of the previous cycle; each cycle furthers mammary development. That these morphologic changes are related to various hormones present in cycling women is evident from comparison with mammary tissue from postmenopausal women, where no changing epithelial and stromal features are observed (Longacre and Bartow, 1986).

In an attempt to understand the morphologic changes in the breast accompanying the menstrual cycle, many investigators have studied the receptors for estrogen and progesterone. An abundance of evidence for the presence of estrogen and progesterone receptors in breast carcinoma tissue exists, but there is controversy concerning sex steroid receptors in nonneoplastic breast tissues. Several studies have found low levels of estrogen receptor in breast tissue, whereas others have been unable to demonstrate measurable levels of estrogen receptor. The study of progesterone receptor is even more limited. A few studies have evaluated whether receptor expression varies with the menstrual cycle. Silva and associates (1983) measured estrogen and progesterone receptor with biochemical assays in epithelial enriched preparations obtained from normal premenopausal women. Maximum estrogen receptor values occur on days 5 to 8, with a small second peak on days 25 and 26; and two peak values of progesterone receptor are noted on days 13 and 14 and 21 to 23. Thus estrogen receptor values are highest during the proliferative

phase, and progesterone receptor levels are highest during the follicular phase of differentiation. The menstrual cycle variation may account for some of the discrepancies among levels of estrogen and progesterone receptors reported in normal breast tissue. It may also have significance in evaluating premenopausal women with breast cancer.

The development of highly specific monoclonal antibodies to estrogen and progesterone receptor allows study of menstrual cycle variation of receptor expression in intact tissue (Greene and Press, 1987). Studies have found receptor concentration greatest for estrogen receptor in the follicular phase, with a less distinct maximal period for progesterone receptor (Carpenter et al., 1988). Both estrogen and progesterone receptors localize to the nuclei of the epithelium, and no staining is seen in surrounding stroma or myoepithelium (Carpenter et al., 1988; Fabris et al., 1987; Petersen et al., 1987). Furthermore, estrogen and progesterone receptor localization is often heterogeneous between lobules but tends to be uniform within a lobule of a given specimen. This observation correlates with the variation in lobular architecture within any single breast reported in morphologic studies (Longacre and Bartow, 1986; Vogel et al., 1981).

The functional significance of the cyclic alterations observed in stromal connective tissue is not well understood. Important interactions of collagen and mucopolysaccharides with glandular epithelium in embryonal morphogenesis are well recognized, and they may not be restricted to the embryonic period (Longacre and Bartow, 1986). Specifically, cyclic stromal alterations might play an important local role in cyclic epithelial changes and estrogen and progesterone receptor expression.

Pregnancy and Lactation

In pregnancy, mammary epithelial cell replication resumes and differentiation begins, leading to remarkable increases in lobuloalveolar structures at the expense of fibrofatty stroma. Stromal changes associated with epithelial growth include increased vascularization and fat cell depletion. The intensified lobuloalveolar growth requires estrogen, progesterone, prolactin, and growth hormone and is enhanced by adrenal corticosteroids and insulin (Topper and Freeman, 1980). Within the first 3 to 4 weeks of gestation, ductular sprouting, branching, and lobule formation exceed the respective premenstrual glandular changes (Vorherr, 1974). A definite enlargement of the breast with dilation of the superficial veins occurs from week 5 to week 8. At the same time, nipple and areolar pigment intensifies, and fibroblasts and inflammatory cells become prominent in the stroma. By the end of the third month, colostrum has begun to collect in the alveoli.

At the beginning of the second trimester, the mammary alveoli become monolayered, whereas the ducts maintain their 2-cell layer. While the rate of mammary epithelium proliferation begins to decline around midpregnancy, the alveolar epithelium differentiates to assume a presecretory function requiring the presence of prolactin, human placental lactogen or growth hormone, insulin, and glucocorticoid (Topper and Freeman, 1980). Secretory machinery, stimulated by insulin and glucocorticoid, appears within the epithelial cells, rough endoplasmic reticulum appears basally, and the Golgi apparatus becomes apical. Golgi vacuoles, cytoplasmic fat droplets, mitochondria, and microvilli all increase. From midpregnancy on, alveolar mammary cells are actively synthesizing milk fat and proteins, but only small amounts are released into the acinar lumina. The continued increase in breast size during pregnancy is attributable to progressive dilation of mammary alveoli by continued secretion of colostrum and enhanced mammary vascularization. Fat and connective tissue are relatively decreased (Vorherr, 1974). By term, each breast gains approximately 12 oz in weight and becomes full, firm, and ready for lactation.

Prolactin secretion increases throughout pregnancy, but it appears that luteal and placental sex steroids (especially progesterone) antagonize the full secretory prolactin effect on mammary epithelium (Topper and Freeman, 1980). The prolactin effect on mammary secretory cells is supported by glucocorticoids, growth hormone, insulin, and thyroid hormone. After postpartum withdrawal of sex steroids and placental lactogen, prolactin-induced lactation sets in. Presecretory mammary glandular cells are converted into actively milk-synthesizing and milk-releasing cells. Complex protein, milk fat, and lactose synthetic pathways are activated. Large fat vacuoles and Golgi vesicles containing lactose, protein, and water ascend to the secretory cell's apex. The epithelial cells release fat, lactose, and protein by apocrine secretion and lactose and protein by merocrine secretion. With synthesis and secretion, the cells alternate between columnar and cuboidal. Ions (primarily potassium, calcium, and chloride and, to a lesser extent, sodium, magnesium, and iron) enter the milk at the apical secretory cell membrane by diffusion and active transport (Linzell and Peaker, 1971). Drug excretion into milk depends on the drug's solubility in fat and water, the degree of ionization, and the extent of active transport mechanisms. Its concentration in milk usually does not exceed 1% of the ingested dose (Vorherr, 1974). The final product of secretion and subsequent dilution from interstitial fluid is milk: fat and protein suspended in lactose solution. The concentration of fat, protein, and electrolytes may vary, but the lactose concentration remains constant. As the major osmole of the aqueous phase of milk, lactose may be the controlling factor for the volume of milk secreted (Vorherr, 1974). Approximately 1 to 2 ml of milk per gram of breast tissue per day is produced.

Continued synthesis of milk is maintained during nursing, because suckling releases both prolactin and adrenocorticotropic hormone. The stimulus of suckling or breast stimulation also releases oxytocin. This posterior pituitary hormone induces myoepithelial contraction and thus ejection of contents from alveoli and smaller ducts into lactiferous sinuses. The initial secretion, colostrum, contains nutritional elements as well as immunoglobulins, transferring passive immunity to the newborn. After the period of colostrum secretion, transitional milk (with a lower concentration of immunoglobulins and total protein) and then mature milk are elaborated.

Lactation is usually stopped around 4 to 6 months post partum when secretory activities diminish. Cessation of lactation causes mammary involution, a process that encompasses nearly 3 months. Milk accumulates and distends alveoli, causing epithelial compression and eventual rupture of alveolar walls. Distended alveoli also lead to mammary capillary compression and resultant diminished nutrient, oxygen, prolactin, and oxytocin delivery. Milk secretion is greatly decreased. Epithelial cells degenerate, desquamate, and are phagocytized, reducing the number and size of glandular elements (Vorherr, 1974). The remaining alveolar lining returns to a nonsecretory 2-cell-layered epithelium. As the lobuloalveolar structures become smaller and fewer, the breast returns to a more ductular system. New connective tissue and fat are formed between the involuted mammary alveolar structures. The postlactational involution encompasses all breast tissues and leads to less dense, less nodular, and less protuberant breasts than in the prepregnant state. Breast-feeding does not seem to influence the degree of involution and thus the final breast form and consistency (Haagensen, 1986).

Menopause

Unlike postlactational mammary involution, in which there is principally a reduction of mammary alveoli, postmenopausal breast involution is characterized by regression of the parenchymal lobuloalveolar structures. At menopause ovarian secretion of estrogen and progesterone declines, whereas ovarian secretion of androgens such as androstenedione, testosterone, and dihydroepiandrosterone becomes predominant. Specifically, the plasma levels of estrone, estradiol, estriol, and progesterone in postmenopausal women are 53%, 16%, 8%, and 30%, respectively, of those found at the midfollicular phase of cycling women and 27%, 5%, 6%, and 10% of those found in women at midcycle (Vorherr, 1980). Plasma levels of testosterone, in contrast, are similar in premenopausal and postmenopausal women. The declining levels of estrogen and progesterone are associated with menopausal breast involution. In the climacteric phase, between 35 and 45 years of age, a moderate decrease in glandular epithelium with round-cell infiltration occurs. The postmenopausal phase, after approximately age 45, has a marked reduction of glandular tissue with an increase in fat deposition and relative predominance of connective tissue. Parenchymal vascularity and round-cell infiltration diminish. At the end stage of menopausal mammary involution, only small islands of an epithelial ductular system embedded in dense, hyalinized fibrous tissue remain. While this glandular involution is striking, remarkably little is known about the factors contributing to this process other than the observation that estrogen and progesterone appear to be necessary for maintenance of the mammary gland.

THE MALE BREAST

Until puberty, the mammary glands of both sexes are alike in structure. The lack of a sustained pubertal surge of estrogen in males results in the breast's remaining rudimentary. The mammary tissue in the adult male is about 2 cm in diameter and 4 mm in thickness. The parenchyma consists of short ducts only, with no true acini, and is surrounded by connective tissue and fat. Blood supply, innervation, and lymphatics are similar to those of the female breast (Vorherr, 1974).

Gynecomastia is the transient or permanent enlargement of the male breast, usually exceeding 2 cm in diameter. In a significant proportion of normal boys, increased mammary growth around puberty occurs. Growth of ducts is seen, but the bulk of the lesion is formed by an increase in fibrous stroma (Haagensen, 1986). Pubertal gynecomastia is attributed to an abnormally high ratio of estradiol to testosterone or increased levels of testosterone binding globulin, leading to a decline in free testosterone (Vorherr, 1974). The condition tends to subside spontaneously within 3 years (usually in the first 4 to 6 months) in over 90% of cases and rarely requires surgical intervention (Haagensen, 1986). In senescent gynecomastia, ages 50 to 70, a similar enlargement of breast tissues occasionally occurs. It is associated with declining serum testosterone levels and an unchanged estrogen level (Osborne, 1987). Although the condition often regresses within 6 months to a year, a biopsy may be indicated because of the cancer incidence in this age group.

Other causes of estradiol/testosterone imbalance can cause gynecomastia. These include hypogonadotropic states like Klinefelter's syndrome and other special syndromes and diseases and conditions affecting the testes, such as mumps orchitis, trauma, tuberculosis, and radiation (Osborne, 1987). Neoplasms of the testis or adrenal gland may result in gynecomastia as a result of hormone secretion by the tumor. Gynecomastia may occur in systemic diseases, including chronic liver, renal, or pulmonary disease, colon or prostate cancer, and hyperthyroidism, and in malnutrition and starvation (Osborne, 1987). Additionally, numerous drugs have been implicated in gynecomastia. In these several causes of gynecomastia, the mammary proliferation consists of stroma and ducts; developed acini are rarely seen. The stimulus for breast growth is therefore not complete (Haagensen, 1986).

Gynecomastia *per se* does not require specific therapy, but in a number of cases there is an underlying reversible cause. Initial treatment consists of removing known causes, such as drugs or hyperthyroidism. Suspected estrogen/testosterone imbalances may be treated with antiestrogens or androgens. If removal of causes or correction of causes does not result in regression of gynecomastia and the patient is symptomatic, surgical treatment may be indicated. Most surgical treatments are requested for psychologic reasons and are appropriate to help restore a healthy concept of body image.

SUMMARY

The embryology, anatomy, and physiology of the human breast have been reviewed and correlated with common clinical entities encountered by the physician.

An understanding of these areas of breast biology should enhance the physician's ability in managing diseases of the breast.

References

Carpenter, S. A., Greene, G., Konrath, J., et al.: Menstrual cycle variation of sex steroid receptors in human breast by immunocytochemistry. Abstract, Canadian and United States Academy of Pathology, Washington, D.C., March, 1988.

Cathcart, E. P., Gairns, F. W., and Garven, H. S. D.: The innervation of the human quiescent nipple, with notes on pigmentation, erection and hyperneury. Trans. R. Soc. Edinb. Trans. 61:699, 1948.

Cooper, A. P.: *On the Anatomy of the Breast.* Vol. 2. London, Longmans, 1840.

Courtiss, E. H., Goldwyn, R. M.: Breast sensation before and after plastic surgery. Plast Reconstr Surg 58:1, 1976.

Dabelow, A.: Die Milchdruse. In Bargmann, W. (ed.): *Handbuch der Mikroskopischen Anatomie des Menschen (Haut und Sinnesorgane).* Vol. 3, Part 3. Berlin, Springer-Verlag, 1957, p. 277.

Edwards, E. A.: Surgical anatomy of the breast. In: Goldwyn, R. M. (ed.): *Plastic and Reconstructive Surgery of the Breast.* Boston, Little, Brown, 1976, p. 37.

Fabris, G., Marchetti, E., Marzola, A., et al.: Pathophysiology of estrogen receptors in mammary tissue by monoclonal antibodies. J. Steroid Biochem. 27:171, 1987.

Fanger, H., Ree, H. J.: Cyclic changes of human mammary gland epithelium in relation to the menstrual cycle: An ultrastructural study. Cancer 34:574, 1974.

Ferguson, D. J. P., Anderson, T. J.: Morphological evaluation of cell turnover in relation to the menstrual cycle in the "resting" human breast. Br. J. Cancer. 44:177, 1981.

Goldwyn, R. M.: *Plastic and Reconstructive Surgery of the Breast.* Boston, Little, Brown, 1976, p. 52.

Grant, J. C.: *A Method of Anatomy.* Baltimore, Williams & Wilkins, 1958.

Greene, G. L., Press, M. F.: Immunochemical evaluation of estrogen receptor and progesterone receptor in breast cancer. In: Ceriano, R. (ed.): *Immunological Approaches to the Diagnosis and Therapy of Breast Cancer.* New York, Plenum Press, 1987.

Haagensen, C. D.: *Diseases of the Breast.* 3rd ed. Philadelphia, W. B. Saunders, 1986.

Hultborn, K. A., Larsson, L. G., Ragnhult, I.: The lymph drainage from the breast to the axillary and parasternal lymph nodes, studied with the aid of colloidal Au[198]. Acta Radiol. 43:52, 1955.

Linzell, J. L., Peaker, M.: Mechanism of milk secretion. Physiol. Rev. 51:564, 1971.

Longacre, T. A., Bartow, S. A.: A correlative morphologic study of human breast and endometrium in the menstrual cycle. Am. J. Surg. Pathol. 10:382, 1986.

McCarty, K. S., Jr., Glaubitz, L. C., Thienemann, M., et al.: The breast: Anatomy and physiology. In: Georgiade, N. G. (ed.): *Aesthetic Plastic Surgery.* Philadelphia, W. B. Saunders, 1983, p. 1.

Maliniac, J. W.: Arterial blood supply of the breast. Arch. Surg. 47:329, 1943.

Maliniac, J. W.: *Breast Deformities and Their Repair.* New York, Grune & Stratton, 1950.

Massopust, L. C., Gardner, W. D.: Infrared photographic studies of the superficial thoracic veins in the female. Surg. Gynecol. Obstet. 91:717, 1950.

Osborne, M. P.: Breast development and anatomy. In: Harris, J. R., et al. (eds.): *Breast Diseases.* Philadelphia, J. B. Lippincott, 1987.

Petersen, O. W., Hoyer, P. E., van Deurs, B.: Frequency and distribution of estrogen receptor-positive cells in normal, nonlactating human breast tissue. Cancer Res. 47:5748, 1987.

Serafin, D.: Surgical anatomy of the breast. In: Georgiade, N. G. (ed.): *Breast Reconstruction Following Mastectomy.* St. Louis, C. V. Mosby, 1979.

Silva, J. S., Georgiade, G. S., Dilley, W. G., et al.: Menstrual cycle-dependent variations of breast cyst fluid proteins and sex steroid receptors in the normal human breast. Cancer 51:1297, 1983.

Stiles, H. J.: Uber Eine Neue Methode der Mammaplastic. Wien Med. Wochenschr. 86:100, 1936.

Topper, Y. J., Freeman, C. S.: Multiple hormone interactions in the developmental biology of the mammary gland. Physiol. Rev. 60:1049, 1980.

Turner-Warwick, R. T.: The lymphatics of the breast. Br. J. Surg. 46:574, 1959.

Vogel, P. M., Georgiade, N. G., Fetter, B. F., et al.: The correlation of histologic changes in the human breast with the menstrual cycle. Am. J. Pathol. 104:23, 1981.

Vorherr, H.: *The Breast: Morphology, Physiology, and Lactation.* New York, Academic Press, 1974.

Vorherr, H.: *Breast Cancer, Epidemiology, Endocrinology, Biochemistry, and Pathobiology.* Baltimore, Urban & Schwarzenberg, 1980.

2

Marcia Kraft Goin

Psychologic Aspects of Aesthetic Surgery of the Breast

The woman who has an aesthetic breast operation is an enigma to most people. Her motivations seem an inexplicable riddle. It is generally assumed that her wish is to enhance her sexual allure. To subject oneself to a surgical operation for such a frivolous reason is perceived as evidence of a shallow character. Few women (and fewer men) are familiar with the conscious and unconscious feelings, fantasies, and symbolic meanings that women attach to their breasts. Nonetheless, it is a complex mixture of these that plays the major part in a woman's decision to have any operation that changes the appearance of her breasts. These feelings, fantasies, and symbolic meanings have a long history. All of the events of her life—her childhood experiences, the reactions of her family, friends, and of society in general—play a part in their formation.

Much of what we have learned about these complex psychologic meanings of the breast comes from the reactions of women who have had breast operations. Formal studies of women who undergo augmentation or reduction mammaplasty have contributed valuable data, as have reports from women who have had to undergo mastectomies for cancer. After a mastectomy, some patients express surprise at the intensity of their emotional reaction to the loss. Examples of such reactions reported in an ongoing study of breast reconstruction patients (Goin and Goin, 1981) are as follows: "I never thought of myself as a 'breast conscious person,' and yet I feel devastated by the loss," and "It's like the loss of a loved one . . . you don't go around thinking about how much he or she means or in what particular way they are important while they're alive. It's only when they're gone that you realize the depth and pervasiveness of the attachment." The reactions of both breast cancer patients and of others who elect to have a desired change made have taught us that women's breasts are linked with feelings about femininity, sexuality, womanliness, and the ability to nurture and to be nurtured.

In discussing the psychologic aspects of aesthetic surgery, the question is often asked, Are we a breast-oriented society? Are we controlled by television, newspapers, magazines, films, and advertisements? Are women's views of themselves and their bodies dominated by men's attraction to large-breasted women? What does it mean that pictures of buxom women are used in advertisements to attract the attention of potential buyers of used cars, decaffeinated coffee, dental floss, and suppositories? Such questions are sometimes asked angrily, sometimes quizzically, by those who are trying to understand why a woman would have an operation to change the size or shape of her breasts. I do not think we have complete answers to these questions. I do know that while these media-influenced factors may play a part in a woman's decision and desire for breast surgery, they are only a part of a larger picture.

A woman who desires an aesthetic operation on her breasts usually feels emotionally traumatized by her breast size. Whether she is small- or large-breasted, her self-perceived physical deficiency or overendowment troubles her. Her reaction is primarily an intrapersonal one, not uninfluenced by society but likewise not dominated by it.

ADOLESCENCE

The psychologic impact of too much or too little breast development begins in adolescence. At this time, young girls must also cope with hormonal changes, growth spurts, and all of the complexities of pubertal separation and individuation. The strengthening of emotional ties to peers facilitates the consolidation of an identity separate from but ultimately equal to that of the parents. However, the resultant peer pressure and the need to conform produces an additional stress of intense competition with both peers and parents. Thus, we see the complex importance of breast development as it relates to a young girl's sense of self-worth and her struggle to find newer and more mature ways to interact with her mother, father, other girls, and boys. The struggle over adequacy and competition is reflected in one of the findings in the study by Beale et al. (1980) of women requesting augmentation mammaplasty. Seventy-nine percent of the small-breasted women reported being afraid to appear naked in front of their husbands, but 100% were afraid to appear naked in front of other women.

Not every small-breasted girl emerges from adolescence self-conscious and unhappy about her breast size, but those who do may appear in the plastic surgeon's office requesting an augmentation mammaplasty. Neither does every woman with large breasts feel self-conscious, but those who do are socially and psychologically uncomfortable.

Women with large breasts have problems very different from those of small-breasted women. As Rosenbaum (1980) reported in her study of adolescent girls (which seems not to have included any with large breasts), all of the girls wanted their features to be less obtrusive with the exception of breasts, "where bigger was seen as better." This desire on the part of the adolescent girl causes those girls with larger breasts to feel isolated from their peers. Other girls, unaware of the physical and psychologic discomfort, envy them. Boys are fascinated and leer self-consciously, often making lewd comments and assuming that sexual promiscuity is linked with this developmental precocity. Self-consciousness is not always a part of being large-breasted. Sometimes sisters in the same family who are equally overendowed may have very different reactions to their breasts. As one woman reported, "My sister, who is even larger than I am, doesn't seem to mind at all. I tell how bad I feel and she just doesn't have any of those feelings. I don't know whether she doesn't feel bad because she is happily married or whether she's happily married because she doesn't feel bad." This is an excellent example of Which comes first?—so prevalent in the search for an understanding of the feelings of people who request aesthetic plastic surgery. However, the attitude of the sister who does not feel bad is more the exception than the rule. More often, other siblings with a similar problem will also request a reduction after a surgically successful breast reduction performed for one family member with large breasts.

PSYCHOLOGIC STUDIES

Although the literature is not flooded with reports of psychologic studies of women requesting augmentation mammaplasty, there are a respectable number of publications (Baker et al., 1974; Druss, 1973; Edgerton et al., 1958; Edgerton et al., 1961; Goin and Goin, 1981; Hetter, 1979; Shipley et al., 1978). However, at the time of writing, there has been only one report of those who have had reduction mammaplasties (Goin et al., 1977). Perhaps this is due to the fact that breast reduction falls somewhere in between elective and required surgery. Plastic surgeons aware of the physical incapacities that large breasts cause have felt under less pressure to understand the psychologic meaning of the operation. Psychologic questions arise more often with decisions about procedures done for purely aesthetic reasons.

Most of the psychologic studies of women undergoing augmentation mammaplasty have indicated that these women have more problems with their sense of self-esteem and self-confidence than women with normal-sized breasts. In the study by Beale et al. (1980) comparing 64 women who underwent augmentation mammaplasty with a matched control group, the psychologic test scores of the small-breasted women revealed a personality pattern of outward confidence masking an inner sense of inferiority. Although Beale's findings are generally consistent with those of Baker et al. (1974)

and Edgerton and associates (1958, 1961), another study by Shipley et al. (1978) did not uncover a measurable decrease in self-esteem in women requesting augmentation mammaplasty. Because different testing methods were used in these studies, it is unclear whether the differing findings were real or merely a product of the research method. In Hetter's (1979) study of 165 women who underwent augmentation mammaplasty, 91% reported an improved self-image. Baker et al. (1974) reported that 84% had strong feelings of increased adequacy and 93% reported increased self-confidence. A large number of these latter patients also described a decrease in sexual inhibition with more enjoyment, and some became orgasmic for the first time.

Considering these findings, it is noteworthy that the woman who usually requests augmentation mammaplasty is not an unattached, dating woman in her early twenties. In fact, in the 1974 report by Baker et al. of 132 women who underwent augmentation mammaplasty, the mean age was 32, 66% were married, and 84% stated that they had made the decision to have surgery on the basis of their "personal needs." These findings are commensurate with those of Edgerton et al. published in 1961. The change in feelings about sexuality appears to be due to a decrease in self-consciousness about physical appearance. Feeling more attractive diminishes inhibitions and allows a woman to behave more freely in the presence of others.

Druss (1973), in his intensive psychoanalytic study of a small number of augmentation mammaplasty patients, described an interesting phenomenon. The women he talked with often found that after the operation they enjoyed touching their newly enlarged breasts. The gratification derived from this was not erotic but instead was described as having a self-nurturing quality. These women all had childhoods lacking in maternal support. Psychologically, they experienced their newly enlarged breasts as providing the feeling of nurturing that they did not receive as children. In this same vein of psychologic experience, one woman in another case study (Seitlman and Goin, 1983) reported the loss of a sense of being nurtured after bilateral mastectomy for cancer. This loss of the sense of being nurtured was the most psychologically traumatic part of her postmastectomy experience. Such reports demonstrate the symbolic significance of a woman's breasts as they are linked to nurturing. Sometimes breast augmentation reinforces the feelings of nurturing that she had as an infant; at other times it is a substitute for the deprivations that resulted from having a mother who was incapable of mothering or was physically absent.

POSTOPERATIVE DILEMMAS AND DISTURBANCES

Both enlargement and reduction of breast size can give rise to body image disturbance. The body image is a person's mental and psychologic picture of himself. The individual may like or dislike this mind's eye picture. Although it never totally matches the realities of the person's physical appearance, it is usually a fairly close representation. However, at times, the correspondence between the real body and its representation in the body image can be extremely distorted. Distortions of the body image occur with regularity following an actual change in the person's body. There is a lag period during which the mental image attempts to catch up with reality. This is particularly true if the physical change is virtually instantaneous, as is the case with mammaplasty. The lag time varies in length, depending upon many factors: the abruptness of the change, the desirability of the change, psychologic comfort with the change, and a whole group of reasons that fall under the heading "individual variations." Some women who undergo augmentation mammaplasty leave the operating table experiencing their newly enlarged breasts as their own; others take weeks, months, or years to assimilate the breasts into their body image as "theirs." Occasionally the assimilation fails to occur altogether.

Following breast reduction, some women have described the fear that their nipples will fall off. Seeing them perched in an unfamiliar place at the tip of their breasts, whereas previously they had been hidden from sight beneath large, pendulous breasts, has even evoked anxious fantasies that in the shower the nipples would come off and go down the drain (Gifford, 1976).

One woman with feelings of guilt and anxiety about her sexuality described a strange postoperative experience. For the first 6 months after her reduction mammaplasty, her body image was that of a woman with no breasts at all—this despite the conscious intellectual awareness that she did in fact have moderately large breasts. As her sexual conflict resolved and she was able to accept herself psychologically, so, too, did her body image change and take on the realistic picture of a woman with B-cup–sized breasts. Another woman had hated her breasts since their early development when she was 11 years old. However, she did not realize until she had them reduced that she had also felt them to be a buffer and protection from the world around her. This is similar to the reactions of some overweight people who may also experience their bodies as buffers against psychologic intrusions. People who lose weight can feel anxious and vulnerable when this adipose defense against the world is lost. The patient had similar feelings after her reduction mammaplasty. She was keenly aware of this vulnerability, especially when her mother, whom she feared and hated, came to visit. Until she adjusted to her new smaller self, she would have her husband sit between her mother and herself, providing the physical barrier previously supplied by her large breasts.

Body image disturbances are not fatal. But their unexpected and unexplained appearance can cause a great deal of anxiety. Patients may interpret these sensations as a sign of mental illness. The primary treatment is to let the patient know that they are not unexpected nor unexplainable. The surgeon's reassurance that sometimes it takes a while to get used to being a new size and shape provides valuable information that relieves patients' anxiety and allows them to relax while their body image catches up with the reality of their body size.

It would follow from what has been written about the many psychologic meanings attached to breasts that a woman who has a breast reduction might suffer a sense of loss even though she is losing a part of her body that has been cumbersome, inhibiting, uncomfortable, and sometimes hated. Because breasts are linked with feelings of being nurtured, there is the potential for transient feelings of loss and depression. This reaction was found to exist in a few of the patients studied (Goin et al., 1977). One woman found herself looking with longing and envy at others who had large breasts similar in size to those she had had preoperatively. This surprised her because she had wanted the operation very much, was delighted with the result of the operation, and was feeling a sense of physical freedom and absence of embarrassment that she had not enjoyed since childhood. The explanation that reactions of this sort are neither unexpected nor unexplainable is usually sufficient to reassure and relieve these patients, who admit that such reactions are confusing and make them wonder if they are "going crazy."

Social adjustment may also prove to be a problem after breast operations. Considering the fact that a woman who undergoes augmentation mammaplasty probably has been shy and sexually inhibited because of self-consciousness about her breasts and that after the operation she is likely to feel self-confident and less sexually inhibited, we can see there is potential for interpersonal problems. The patient may have had a paucity of social experience because of her previous inhibition, which interfered with but also protected her from experiencing the adolescent trials, tribulations, and excitement of new relationships, including the ups and downs of dating. Problems with promiscuity and reports that patients suddenly find themselves "in over their heads" following rhinoplasties have been noted by Linn and Goldman (1949). New-found self-confidence and a subsequent quest for new experiences stimulated by such elective procedures can cause some patients great anxiety. It is useful to alert patients to the fact that the good feelings they have after surgery may cause them to act impulsively. Patients should be advised to take their total situation into account before they act on what may be new desires and impulses. The physician should explain that such feelings are not unexpected but may not be appropriate at the patient's age. The experiences the patient desires are typically those that the patient missed out on because of her intense inhibitions, lack of self-confidence, and shyness during adolescence. This type of common-sense approach can help a woman pause and give thought to what she really wants, rather than launching off thoughtlessly into some impulsive behavior that might later be regretted.

Psychologic reactions to aesthetic surgery of the breast can be very positive. The plastic surgeon who is also aware of the possible disturbances can offer understanding, counseling, and reassurance that will help potentiate these results.

References

Baker, J. L., Jr., Kolin, I. S., Bartlett, E. S.: Dynamics of patients undergoing mammary augmentation. Plast. Reconstr. Surg. 53:652, 1974.

Beale, S., Lisper, H., Palm, B.: A psychological study of patients seeking augmentation mammaplasty. Br. J. Psychiatry 136:133, 1980.

Druss, R. G.: Changes in body image following augmentation breast surgery. J. Psychoanal. Psychother. 2:248, 1973.

Edgerton, M. T., McClary, A. R.: Augmentation mammaplasty: Psychiatric implications and surgical indications. Plast. Reconstr. Surg. 21:279, 1958.

Edgerton, M. T., Meyer, E., Jacobson, W. E.: Augmentation mammaplasty: II. Further surgical and psychiatric evaluation. Plast. Reconstr. Surg. 27:279, 1961.

Gifford, S.: Emotional attitudes toward cosmetic breast surgery: Loss and restitution of the "ideal self." In: Goldwyn, R. M.: *Plastic and Reconstructive Surgery of the Breast.* Boston, Little, Brown, 1976, p. 103.

Goin, J., Goin, M. K.: Augmentation mammaplasty. In: *Changing the Body: Psychological Effects of Plastic Surgery.* Baltimore, Williams & Wilkins, 1981.

Goin, M. D., Goin, J. M.: Psychological reactions of breast reconstruction patients. Unpublished.

Goin, M. K., Goin, J. M., Gianini, M. H.: The psychic consequences of a reduction mammaplasty. Plast. Reconstr. Surg. 59:530, 1977.

Hetter, G. P.: Satisfaction and dissatisfactions of patients with augmentation mammaplasty. Plast. Reconstr. Surg. 64:151, 1979.

Linn, L., Goldman, I. B.: Psychiatric observations concerning rhinoplasty. Psychosom. Med. 11:307, 1949.

Rosenbaum, M.: Girls seem to underestimate their looks. Clinical Psychiatric News, December 1980, p. 38.

Seitlman, J., Goin, M. K.: One woman's breast-mother equation revealed following mastectomy. Unpublished, 1983.

Shipley, R. H., O'Donnell, J. M., Bader, K. F.: Psychosocial effects of cosmetic augmentation mammaplasty. Aesthetic Plast. Surg. 2:429, 1978.

3

Ricardo Baroudi

Preoperative Evaluation for Breast Surgery

During a woman's lifetime her breasts are subjected to continuous modification in shape, volume, and structure. The more important factors causing these changes include genetics, age, extensive body weight variation, lactation, pregnancy, and hormones and, combined or separate, determine the flaccidity and ptosis of the breasts, compromising them aesthetically and functionally.

Human history is rich with information on behavior relative to the breasts. The interrelationship of sex, the breasts, and the psyche is very important. Therefore, unaesthetically pleasing breasts can often cause insecurity, depression, and inhibition.

The modern woman has shown a propensity to expose her body, mostly in the tropical regions. To show what is beautiful has become natural. Thus, distortions in the shape or volume of the breasts prevent the use of minimal bathing suits and dresses that expose an unappealing body contour in public.

A lack of dietary control produces a disproportion between weight and height, which becomes more evident in gynecoid and android types of body shape. It is often quite difficult for some women to attain sufficient weight loss to obtain localized benefits. Gynecoid women have excess volume in the lower segment of the trunk and thighs, and small breasts. In an attempt to reduce the volume of these regions by weight loss, the breasts and the face also are reduced. Android women have the problem in reverse.

All these involvements have brought great concern to specialists over the past century. The literature registers an extensive number of techniques for reducing, rebuilding, and performing augmentation of the breasts. The great number of different procedures is conclusive in showing that mammaplasty is a difficult technique, with unpredictable results, as determined by medium- and long-term follow-up studies.

The modern techniques and their specific refinements are based on older techniques. The ideal technique, suitable for all types of cases, is still unknown.

This chapter covers the scope of indications for breast surgery, taking into account all the aspects presented in this introduction.

THE IDEAL BREAST SHAPE

The breast has basically a conical shape with the nipple-areola complex located in the vertex (Fig. 3–1A). It is divided in two upper and two lower quadrants, with medial and lateral aspects. These aspects can be observed in a young woman in the standing position and with her arm elevated. The base contour is more evident in the lower lateral and medial quadrants through the inframammary sulcus (Fig. 3–1B). The pectoralis muscle edge limits the upper lateral quadrant. Medially the contour becomes evident when the upper and lower lateral breast quadrants are pressed with the hand (Fig. 3–1C). The thickness of the breast tissue versus the thin skin texture of the surrounding area makes this contour even more evident. In the standing position and with the arm abducted, the breast is displaced inferiorly over the pectoralis muscle aponeurosis, limited by the respective skin elasticity. A slight breast ptosis can be seen. The upper hemisphere remains less evident, and the lower bulges. In the profile view a lazy concave line from the superior pole to the nipple projection and a convex one from this point to the inframammary sulcus can be observed (Fig. 3–2). The areola has a circular shape, with an average diameter of 4 to 5 cm. The nipple shows a cylindrical projection around 5 to 15 mm in length. The ideal volume of the breasts is difficult to estimate. Within the normal aesthetic limits they should be proportional to the lower segment of the trunk. In general, the circumference of the chest should be the same as that of the hips.

TYPES OF BREASTS

Breasts have different volumes, from amastia to gigantomastia, through all the intermediate steps from hypomastia to marked hypertrophy. Within this considerable variation, shape and symmetry also may be distorted. The breasts may have only slight asymmetry, unnoticed even by the woman herself; or there may be a considerable difference, difficult to correct. Finally, the continuous change in size and volume during life

23

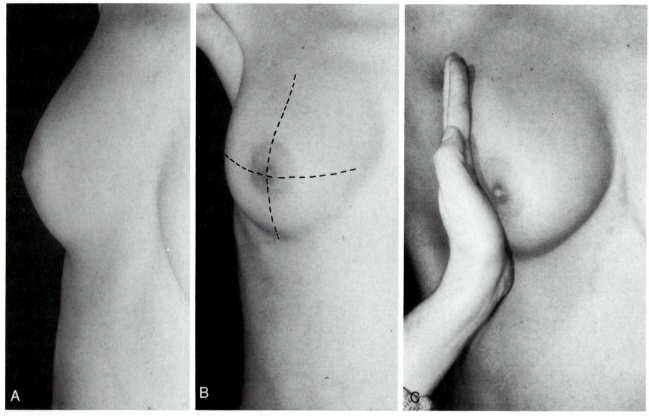

FIGURE 3–1

A, Typical conical breast with the nipple-areola complex located in the vertex in a 23-year-old woman. *B,* The breast is divided in two upper and two lower quadrants. The base of the breast is more evident in the inframammary sulcus. *C,* Medially the contour is more evident when the breast is pressed with the hand.

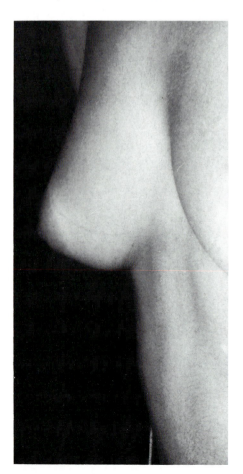

FIGURE 3–2

In a young woman, in standing position, the normal breast shows a discrete concave line in the upper hemisphere and a mild convex line in the lower hemisphere. The nipple-areola complex and the breast remain above the inframammary sulcus.

explains the importance of mammaplasty for women in different decades of life (Fig. 3–3).

Paintings and sculptures from different civilizations substantiate the ethnic, religious, and aesthetic concepts of human behavior relative to women's breasts. Over the centuries, the breasts have been both exposed and hidden by clothes from the eyes of the observer. In the last few decades the following tendencies have evolved: (1) Breast exposure has gone from mild to almost completely uninhibited. (2) This exposure is more evident in tropical countries or in cities near the ocean. (3) The criteria for beauty of the breast are governed by ethnic and regional sensibilities. In other words, breasts of small or medium volume are considered beautiful in some countries. In others with a different cultural bias, hypertrophic breasts are considered more beautiful than small breasts. (4) The breast continues to be a determinant of female beauty and a symbol of sexual importance. (5) Distortion still can be corrected only by surgery.

CLASSIFICATION OF BREASTS

There are several academic classifications relative to the shape and volume of the breasts. These classifications will not be adopted in this chapter. We will consider the following main classifications.

Classification of Breast Volume

Based on the volume, the breast can be divided into four groups:

Amastia. Amastia is a complete absence of breast projection over the chest wall, with the lack of even a minimal amount of parenchymal tissue. The areolae are small and less than 4 cm in diameter. The nipple is the only projection. In some cases it is disproportionately long. Amastia may be unilateral or bilateral. In Poland's syndrome the problem is even more complex aesthetically because of atrophy of the pectoralis muscle and the nipple-areola complex (see Fig. 3–3C). Amastia is more frequently seen in Asian women and in the gynecoid type of body shape, in which the upper segment of the trunk is smaller than the lower (Fig. 3–4).

Hypomastia. In hypomastia, the volume of the breasts falls between that in amastia and that in normomastia. For practical evaluation, women with this type of breast wear brassieres that are two to four sizes smaller than the size of the hips (Fig. 3–5). In exceptional situations there are women with hypomastia in whom the brassiere size is the same as the size of the hips, but the breasts are small and do not fill the cups.

Normomastia. This type of breast has ideal volume relative to the proportion of the upper and lower trunk segments (Fig. 3–6). Women with this breast volume have a better body shape and can easily wear all types of dresses. Often they take pride in their bodies and are self-confident. The use of tight clothes and exiguous

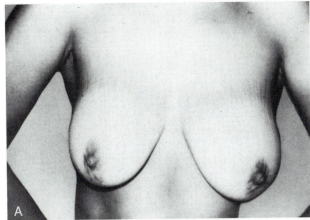
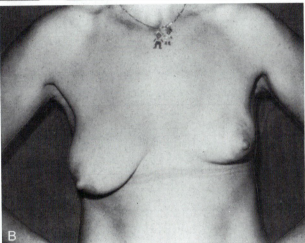
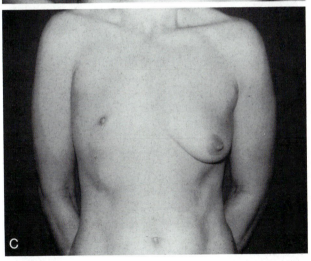

FIGURE 3–3
The breasts present great diversification in shape and volume. Asymmetry may range from unnoted *(A)* to evident *(B)*. In Poland's syndrome *(C)* complete atrophy of one of the breasts makes the asymmetry of the chest unacceptable aesthetically.

bathing suits to expose themselves is also common. To show what is beautiful is natural. During the course of life, this type of breast may undergo various distortions in shape and volume, from atrophy to hypertrophy, and varying degrees of ptosis may also occur.

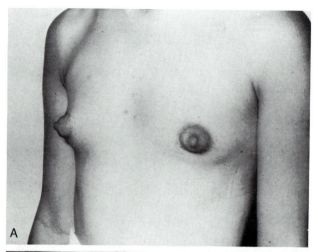

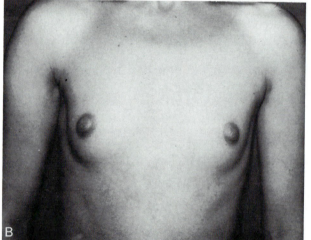

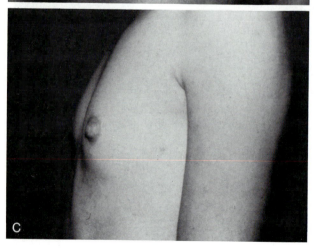

FIGURE 3–4
A, Typical case of amastia. No glandular tissue is evident. Only the nipple-areola projection is seen. *B* and *C,* Another illustrative case with minimal projection of breast contour can be seen.

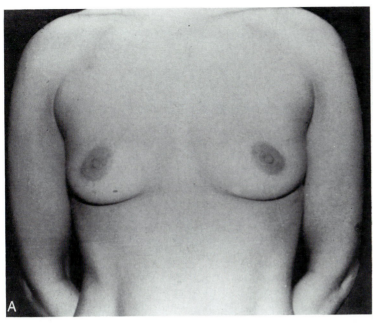

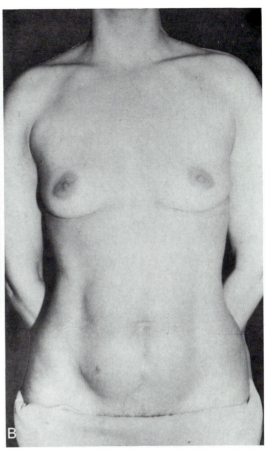

FIGURE 3–5
A, Common aspect of hypomastia in an adult woman after pregnancies. *B*, The breasts are proportionally smaller relative to chest and trunk size and do not fill brassiere cups entirely.

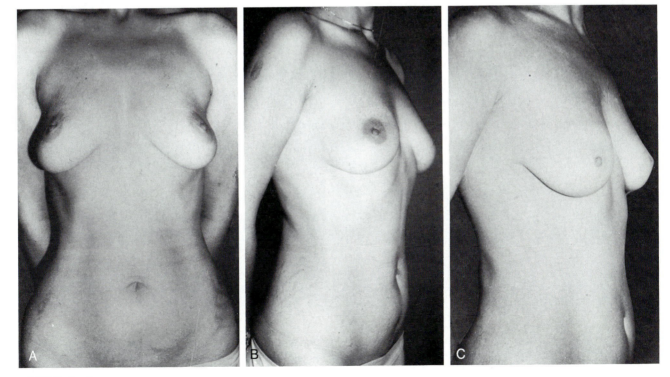

FIGURE 3–6
A and *B*, Front and lateral views of a 32-year-old Caucasian woman with normomastia. The volume of the breast is in proportion to the chest circumference and the lower trunk segment. Breast ptosis may or may not exist. *C*, Lateral view of a 30-year-old woman with normomastia relative to chest and trunk size.

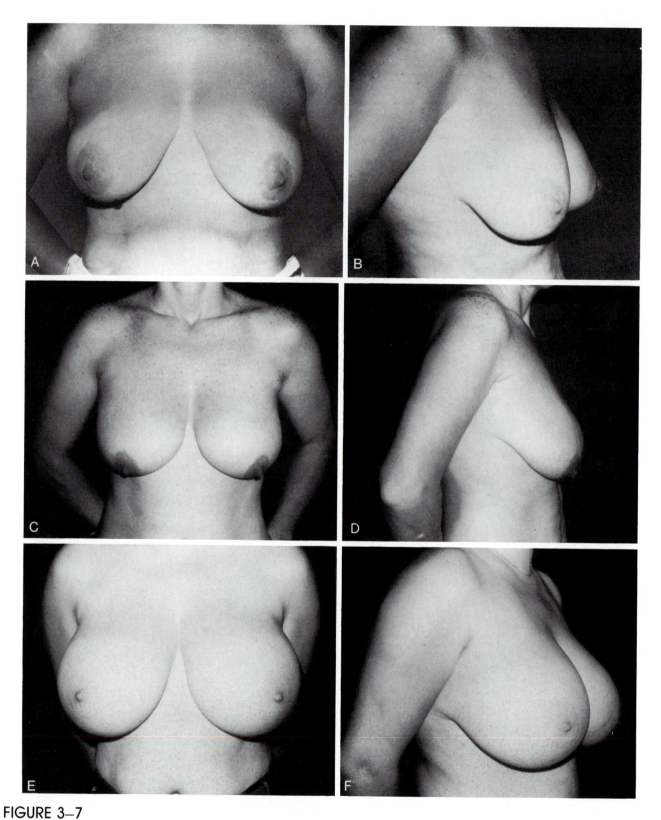

FIGURE 3–7
Hypertrophic breast volume is always more than the volume in normomastia. The chest, in both circumference and breast volume, is larger than the pelvic segment of the trunk. All types of hypertrophic breasts may exist. Three main sizes can be considered: small (A and B), medium (C and D), and large (E and F). The different size of brassiere and the amount in grams of breast tissue resected during a breast reduction are the reference points to be taken into account in this type of clinical classification.

Hypertrophy. Women with this type of breast have disproportionate upper and lower trunk segments. In general, they have an android body shape. The shoulders, the chest, and the breasts are larger than the hips and thighs. From normomastia to marked hypertrophy, there are several types of intermediate situations, almost impossible to classify. Whatever the volume variation, each author may have his or her own criteria for classifying breast hypertrophy. My colleagues and I usually classify such cases simply as *small, medium,* or *marked* hypertrophy.

The amount of breast resection from each breast during a mammaplasty for small hypertrophy ranges up to 300 gm; for medium hypertrophy, from 300 to 700 gm; and for marked hypertrophy, from 700 to 1200 gm (Fig. 3–7). Above 1200 gm can be considered gigantomastia (Fig. 3–8).

Another criterion is based on brassiere size. There are three main patterns. The first one, mostly used in North America, Central America, and some countries of South America, is based on the size of the circumference of the chest wall measured in inches. The sizes of the brassieres are 32, 34, 36, 38, 40. Numbers 34, 36, and 38 also have three sizes for the cup, A, B, and C. Cup A is small, B is medium, and C is large.

A second type of classification used in some countries in South America and Europe uses three brassiere sizes: small, medium, and large. Finally, in the third classification, the brassiere numbers are 38, 40, 42, 44, 46, 48, and 50.

Comparing these different measures with the breast sizes and the upper trunk segment, one can summarize as follows: Women with amastia, hypomastia, and normomastia may use the small brassiere size, the number 38 or 40 or the North American size 32 A, B, and C. Women with normomastia and small hypertrophy use the size medium, the number 42 or 44, or the size 34 A, B, and C. Women with medium and large hypertrophy may use the size large, the numbers 46 or 48, and

the size 36 A, B, and C. Women with gigantomastia use the number 50 or larger or size 38 or 40 in the North American classification.

Classification of Breast Ptosis

Based on the inframammary sulcus, breast ptosis can be divided in two groups: (I) the nipple-areola complex is below the sulcus; (II) the complex remains above the sulcus, but the lower quadrants are below it.

Group I. In this group, in which the nipple-areola complex and the upper and lower quadrants are below the sulcus, the ptosis is evident. Whatever the extent of the problem, there is dissatisfaction. Women who have normal and aesthetically pleasing breasts can be affected by factors like age, pregnancies, lactation, body weight variation, and so forth, which determine natural ptosis, with or without breast hypertrophy. These changes may occur from the beginning of puberty to the later decades, when ptosis becomes more common (Fig. 3–9).

Group II. Ptosis in this group is located in the lower quadrants. The nipple-areola complex remains above or at the level of the inframammary sulcus. There is a downward dislocation of the upper pole of breast tissue over the pectoralis muscle, filling the lower quadrants. The breast shows a teardrop shape. The ribs become more evident and the chest wall empty (Fig. 3–10).

AESTHETIC BREAST SURGERY—WHEN TO SAY YES AND WHEN TO SAY NO

The previous clinical study of breast distortions can now be used for the selection of candidates for mammaplasty.

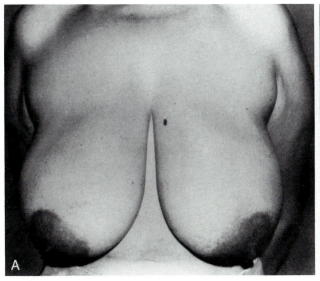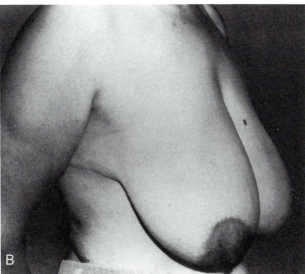

FIGURE 3–8

A and *B,* Front and lateral views of typical gigantomastia in a 42-year-old Caucasian woman. In general, these types of breasts are pendulous, adipose, and heavy and cause discomfort.

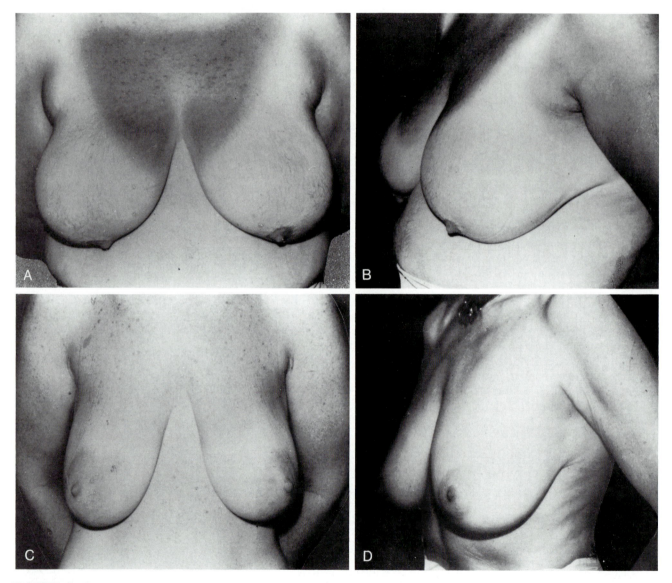

FIGURE 3–9

Group I: Universal breast ptosis, where the upper and the lower quadrants and the nipple-areola complex remain below the inframammary sulcus. This type of aesthetic problem may occur in teenage girls as a genetic aspect of breast development *(A and B)*, adult women after multiple pregnancies and lactation *(C)*, and older women *(D)*.

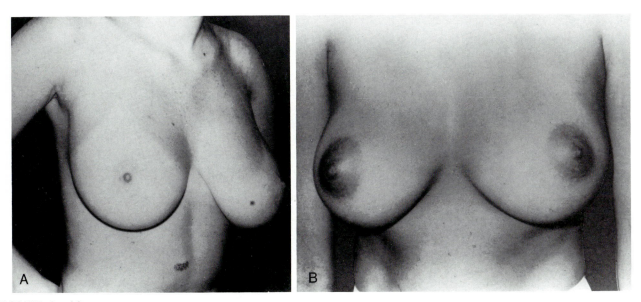

FIGURE 3–10
Group II: Ptosis of only the lower breast quadrants. The nipple-areola complex remains above the inframammary sulcus. It is more commonly seen in young women. A and B, Two teenage girls with similar breasts.

Amastia and Hypomastia

The anatomic and the aesthetic aspects already described may lead one to conclude that the silicone implant prosthesis is the practical solution to the problem of amastia and hypomastia. Surgery is indicated for these two mammary problems on the basis of the patient's emotional behavior. There are women who cannot accept the absence of, or minimal, breast volume (Fig. 3–11). Over decades additional different types of ptosis may occur in hypoplastic breasts, in which case mastopexy combined with a silicone implant in the same surgical stage is recommended. Patients with amastia will never have ptosis. Skin flabbiness, however, may exist after pregnancies with or without lactation, becoming more evident after the fourth decade. These patients still remain as candidates for breast augmentation with silicone implants. Surgical indication in cases of hypomastia, with or without ptosis, is always difficult to determine: mastopexy, implants, or both. The best

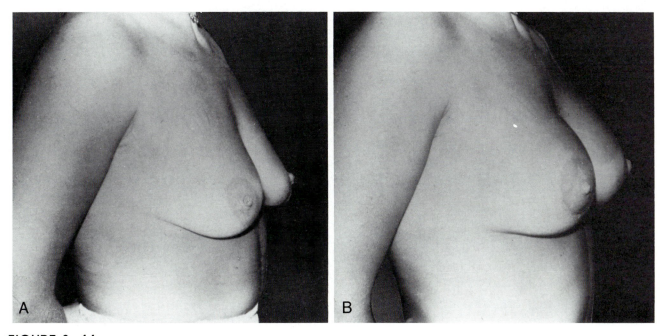

FIGURE 3–11
A and B, Routine preoperative and postoperative lateral views of a 35-year-old patient after silicone breast implantation. The hypomastia and the breast ptosis limits are within implantation indications, and no extra surgical procedure is necessary.

surgical program depends on the patient's wishes and the doctor's aesthetic sensibilities. The resultant scars, the risks of capsular contracture, and the anxiety related to the wish to have the breasts augmented will determine what to do. The doctor should provide the best information possible, but the decision is the patient's (Fig. 3–12).

Normomastia

Mastopexy is an elective procedure. Almost all patients with normomastia accept their breast size, but they want to eliminate the ptosis commonly observed (Fig. 3–13).

Patients often believe that there is always a definitive solution for breast ptosis. The realities should be clearly explained before surgery so that there is no misunderstanding. It is better to reject surgery when the quad-

rants or the nipple-areola complex does not reach the level of ptosis for which surgery is recommended. Minimal or mild ptosis may not justify the procedure.

Hypermastia (Hypertrophy)

The previous discussion of breast hypertrophy reveals two main indications for breast reduction: hypertrophy with ptosis and hypertrophy without ptosis. It is easy to decide in favor of routine surgical reduction with typical hypertrophy *with* ptosis. Deciding in the case of hypertrophy *without* ptosis becomes quite difficult.

The patient's age, emotions, profession, and so forth, should be taken into consideration by the doctor before the surgery. The physician should advise the patient of disadvantages relative to scarring and the long-term follow-up relative to breast modification and even decline to perform the surgery if he or she is not convinced

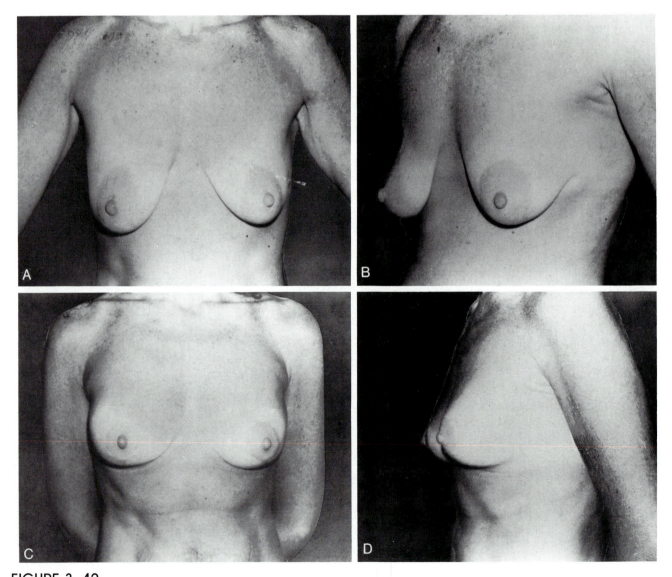

FIGURE 3–12

A and *B*, Preoperative views of a 44-year-old patient with universal breast ptosis combined with hypomastia. Shape and volume asymmetry can also be observed. *C* and *D*, Postoperative front and lateral views. Mastopexy and silicone breast implantation were performed in the same surgical stage.

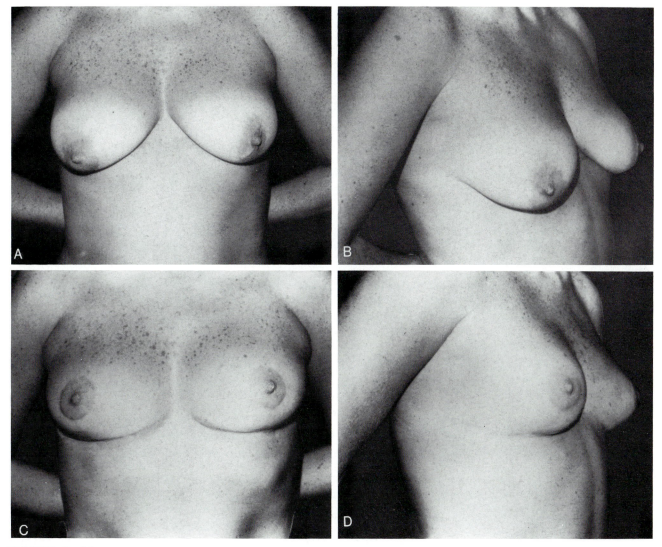

FIGURE 3–13
A and *B*, Routine case of normomastia and ptosis in a 42-year-old patient. Moderate shape and volume asymmetry can be seen. Preoperative front and lateral views of the patient. *C* and *D*, Postoperative front and lateral views illustrating a mastopexy procedure using the inverted-T surgical technique.

that the final result will improve on the preoperative appearance of the breasts.

Based on these concepts, two situations can now be described.

Hypertrophy without Ptosis

Patients with this type of breast wear a brassiere size a minimum of two sizes larger than the size of the lower trunk segment. The breasts are aesthetically pleasing, and the nipple-areola complex is in the correct position. With the lack of proportion between the upper and the lower trunk segment, the breasts are too big for the body contour. The patient's main complaint is related to the problem of dressing, mostly with regard to bathing suits. Her other problems are relative to the psychologic aspect of exposing herself and the excess volume of the breasts and the upper trunk segment (Fig. 3–14).

There is no plastic surgeon who does not have some discomfort in recommending surgery for this type of breast. Surgical selection becomes even more difficult when the patient's age, profession, psychologic behavior, and so forth, are taken into account.

My personal and specific surgical procedure for hypertrophy without ptosis is based on Cloutier's technique (1979).

Because the shape of the breast is perfect, and volume is the problem, the main emphasis of surgery is on reduction; the shape should be kept, with a minimum of scarring. The literature indicates that Cloutier was the first to publish this method. Basically, the breast tissue is undermined from the pectoralis major fascia, through a 6-cm incision in the inframammary sulcus. According to the breast volume, a glandular resection is performed like a cone segment from the base of the breast tissue. The amount and the thickness, with or without axillary breast tissue resection, differ from case to case. The important aspect is how to manage the volume of gland to be resected to obtain a good final breast volume following the shrinkage of the skin envelope after a minimum of 8 weeks (Fig. 3–15).

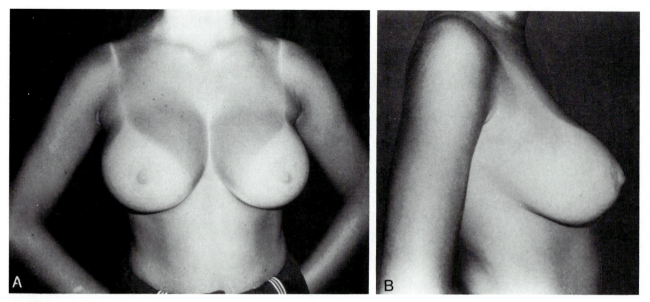

FIGURE 3–14

A and *B*, Front and lateral views of hypertrophic nonptotic breasts in a teenage patient. The breasts are aesthetically pleasing. The patient's major complaints were the lack of proportion between the upper and lower trunk segments and the problems involved in wearing tight clothes and bathing suits.

The final result should maintain the same preoperative shape with an average reduction of 25% to 30% of the prior volume. No ptosis and no flabby breast skin should be observed. In any attempt to reduce more than 30% of the breast volume, secondary problems may start to be seen. In some cases, to avoid future small skin redundancies in the lower breast quadrants, a small additional horizontal fusiform skin resection with 2 cm of excess vertical skin resection is also performed (Fig. 3–16).

Any other technique for the reduction of this type of breast that manipulates the nipple-areola complex should be avoided. The scars that are left are not justified in light of the prior appearance of the breasts. There are cases between hypertrophy with no ptosis and hypertrophy with minimal ptosis in which such a technique might be indicated, however. After the normal period of skin retraction, if evidence of breast flaccidity, loss of the normal primitive cone shape, a more ptotic aspect, or any type of combination occurs, a second surgical stage after a minimum of 6 months should be part of the treatment program. Patients should be warned previously about this possibility. This inframammary scar is preferable to a good vertical or periareolar scar.

Hypertrophy with Ptosis

The different types of hypertrophy, with all degrees of ptosis, have been described. The two main groups of ptosis were also discussed (see Figs. 3–11 and 3–12).

The techniques used for the reduction mammaplasty are based on the resection of skin, gland, and fat from the different quadrants, preserving as much as possible the physiology of the breast and the vitality of the nipple-areola complex. The extension of the upward

areola migration depends on the prior degree of ptosis and the aesthetic result to be obtained. The most common type of final scar has an inverted-T or L shape, beside the circular scar that surrounds the areola. The length of the horizontal scar may be different from one breast to its opposite, and from case to case. The surface of the breast base, the axillary breast extension, the amount of skin and breast reduction, and finally the surgeon's expertise are some of the factors that may determine it.

Gigantomastia

Reduction mammaplasty is highly recommended in the cases of gigantomastia. Multiple complaints from these patients are frequent. These complaints include the hygienic aspect, weight on the shoulders, pain in the back, discomfort in sleeping, and problems related to buying and wearing clothes.

Skin flaccidity, ptosis, and excessive glandular volume make the operation a difficult process. Special care should be taken with nipple-areola complex manipulation. The extent of the upward dislocation may involve different degrees of subsequent necrosis. In general, the scars are long, and very often they join at the midsternal line.

COMMENTS
Adipose versus Glandular Breast Tissue

From pure gland to a preponderance of adipose tissue, the palpation method can detect the consistency and the

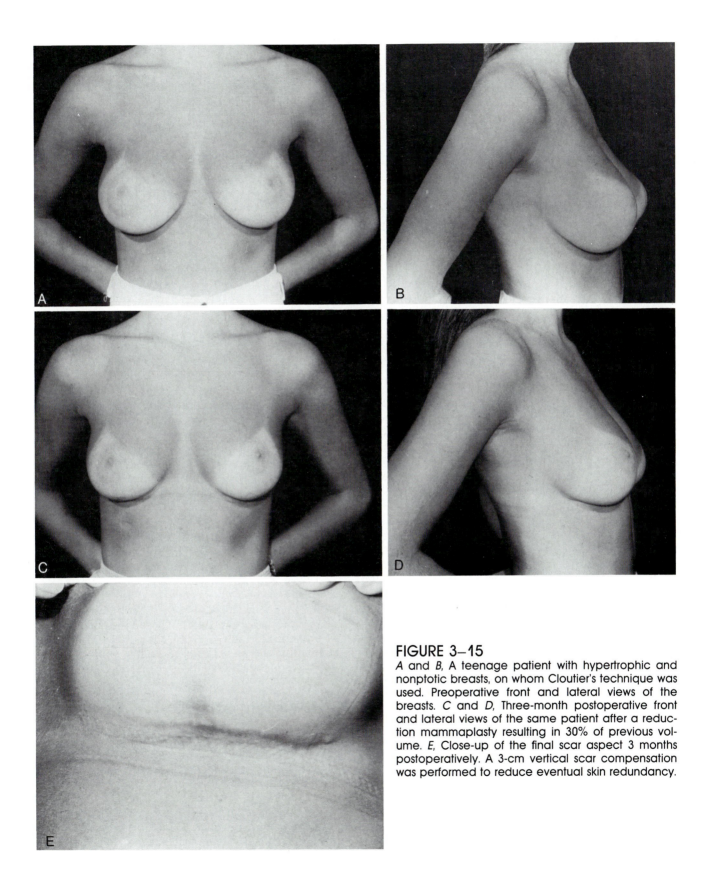

FIGURE 3–15

A and *B*, A teenage patient with hypertrophic and nonptotic breasts, on whom Cloutier's technique was used. Preoperative front and lateral views of the breasts. *C* and *D*, Three-month postoperative front and lateral views of the same patient after a reduction mammaplasty resulting in 30% of previous volume. *E*, Close-up of the final scar aspect 3 months postoperatively. A 3-cm vertical scar compensation was performed to reduce eventual skin redundancy.

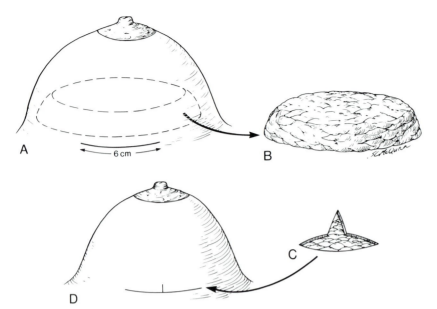

FIGURE 3–16
Schematic aspects *(A to D)* of Cloutier's technique for breast reduction, based on the shrinking skin involvements after the resection of a conical breast tissue segment near the breast base. Access is through a 6-cm skin incision in the inframammary sulcus. To avoid skin ptosis above the sulcus, a 3-cm vertical resection of the skin can be performed. A final small inverted-T scar will remain.

structure of the breast. The proportion of these tissues can also be observed by means of other types of technology. The amount of glandular tissue or fat may indicate precociousness and flabbiness of the breasts over the years.

In the clinical setting, teenagers are sometimes seen with breast ptosis, as are women past their 40s with nonptotic breasts. There are also women with small breasts with a long lactation period and women with voluminous breasts who do not produce milk more than a week *post partum*. The conclusion is obvious. Fat tissue does not produce milk, and the breasts lack consistency. Precocious breasts become ptotic. The reverse is observed with glandular breasts.

In addition, glandular atrophy and its gradual substitution by fat tissue can explain the occurrence of variation in breast volume and shape. Already known endogenous factors also contribute to this dysmorphosis.

The same technique used for breast reduction in patients at the same age, with similar breast volume and ptosis, but with different breast structure with regard to gland and fat will yield different results in these patients. Distortions and ptosis will occur more precociously in adipose breasts.

In conclusion, glandular tissue or adipose tissue, or both, can be easily observed by palpation and by other types of tests (mammography, xerography, ultrasound, etc.). On the basis of the results of such studies, the physician should be able to predict and advise the patient of the quality of the result in medium- and long-term follow-up, so as to avoid any misunderstanding in the relationship with the patient.

When to Say Yes and When to Say No to Aesthetic Breast Surgery

Human imagination and fantasy have no limits. A woman's aesthetic sense regarding her breasts is also

unpredictable. The results of the mammaplasty may go from the unaesthetic problems of asymmetry, shape, and volume to a psychologic involvement in which the breasts are a type of "organ of emotional shock." In other words, the breasts may be within the limits of normality, but the patient does not accept them aesthetically. In her imagination, her breasts should be even smaller or bigger, or with the nipple 1 or 2 cm above its position. Another aspect is related to the use of bathing suits, tight blouses, or the disproportion of the upper and the lower segments of the trunk. The degree of ptosis, the type of dysmorphosis, the psychologic involvement, body weight variation, age, profession, and so forth, should all be evaluated by the physician.

It is important to say No before than to say Sorry after! Based on all these criteria, the final aesthetic result in medium and long-term follow-up should justify the surgery and the resultant scars.

Patients who do not accept even mild ptosis, small breast volume, or any other type of moderate distortion usually are highly emotional. These cases are difficult, and prudence dictates the denial of performing surgery. Patients like these usually have a high complaint level, even for a minimal detail.

Body Weight Loss

Surgery is better indicated when the patient is of normal body weight. Patients who are 4 to 5 kg overweight should lose weight before surgery. The breasts support up to 5 kg of weight loss after mammaplasty without significant shape change or ptosis. This support is better observed in glandular than in adipose breast. In weight loss greater than 5 kg, signs of ptosis, flabbiness, and volume reduction become more evident. There are patients who are unable to lose body weight. Several factors contribute to this. Many diets fail. Psychologically, some patients do not have the ability to continue on a long-term diet. Breast surgery may be recommended for such patients whatever the excess weight. After surgery, many of them become stimulated to lose weight. The new breast volume and shape psychologically motivate the patient, in a behavior pattern relative to her new image, to start a diet program. Therefore, the patient should be warned in advance about the possible risks of compromising the results of the breast reduction procedure. Revision of the initial surgery may be a part of the program of weight loss when necessary.

Breast Surgery Before and After Marriage, Pregnancy, and Lactation

It is impossible to avoid the involvement of the breasts in pregnancy and lactation. Candidates for a mastopexy or a breast reduction should avoid surgery until the end of their childbearing plans.

Teenagers with breast distortion may undergo specific breast surgery prior to marriage. It is not logical to live with breast discomfort for years, waiting for a possible marriage and future babies and lactation. Candidates for breast augmentation may have the surgery even a few months before their marriage. The distortions of an eventual pregnancy will not ruin the results.

Candidates for surgery and those who have already undergone surgery should finish their childbearing program, lactation period, and the return of the body weight to the normal condition before breast surgery or breast surgical revision. A minimum of 4 to 6 months is recommended after the end of lactation.

Surgical Scars

The great number of factors that interfere in the structure of the breast makes the quality of the scars and the results quite unpredictable, whatever the technique used and whatever the surgeon's expertise. Age, body weight variation, skin quality, breast tissue structure, hormones, and so forth, are some of the factors that interfere with the results of breast surgery in long-term follow-up.

Patients should be aware of these possibilities. They should estimate the risks before making the decision to accept surgery. Scars continue to be a great problem in breast surgery. There have been attempts to shorten the incisions, but there are limitations in the quality of the results. These are more regularly seen in ptotic breasts with or without hypertrophy, especially when the nipple-areola complex must be moved more than 5 cm. Hypertrophic or keloid scars should receive surgical revision after a 1-year postoperative period.

CONCLUSIONS

Everything taken into consideration, the physician should agree to perform mammaplasty if he or she anticipates that the results after long-term follow-up will be better than the preoperative condition. Unpredictable and unacceptable results in the long-term postoperative course should not be considered a malpractice problem. Patients should be warned about these possibilities so that misunderstandings can be avoided. Also, the patient contemplating surgical revision of breast surgery performed elsewhere must have a realistic attitude, as should the physician, who should know his or her limitations.

Aesthetic breast surgery is complicated. Creating a satisfactory breast is difficult; creating a balanced symmetric mound on the opposite breast is even more so.

References

Arié, G.: Una nueva técnica de mastoplastia. Rev. Latinoam. Cir. Plast. 3:23, 1957.
Baroudi, R.: The present and future aspects of the sculpturing surgery. In: *Transactions of the VII International Congress of Plastic Surgeons.* Montreal, R. B. T. Printing, 1983.
Biggs, T. M., Cukier, J., Worthing, L. F.: Augmentation mammaplasty. Plast. Reconstr. Surg. 69:445, 1982.
Cloutier, A. M.: Volume reduction mammaplasty. Ann. Plast. Surg. 2:475, 1979.
Franco, T., Rebello, C.: *Cirurgia Estetica.* Rio de Janeiro, Livraria Atheneu., 1977.
Grazer, F., Klingbeil, J. M.: *Body Image.* St. Louis, C. V. Mosby, 1980.
Lewis, J. R., Jr.: *Atlas of Aesthetic Plastic Surgery.* Boston, Little, Brown, 1973.
Peixoto, G.: Reduction mammaplasty: A personal technique. Plast. Reconstr. Surg. 65:217, 1980.
Pitanguy, I.: *Aesthetic Plastic Surgery of the Head and Body.* Berlin, Springer-Verlag, 1981.
Pontes, R.: A technique of reduction mammaplasty. Br. J. Plast. Surg. 26:365, 1973.
Regnault, P., Daniel, R. K.: *Aesthetic Plastic Surgery.* Boston, Little, Brown, 1984.

BREAST AUGMENTATION

Gordon Letterman
Maxine Schurter

4

A History of Augmentation Mammaplasty

The demand for breast augmentation has increased tremendously throughout the twentieth century. Concomitantly, surgical management of the small breast has been plagued with numerous complications. Despite the odds, the search for the perfect prosthesis continues along with the demand. The methods of augmentation that have been used to date may be divided into three categories: (1) injectables, (2) autogenous tissue transplantation, and (3) prostheses.

INJECTABLES

Paraffin

Gersuny (1900) appears to have been the first to propose paraffin injection to fill out soft tissue deformities, but he did not extend the indications to the breast. Lagarde (1903) summarized the reports of paraffin injections to that date and found no breast augmentation among them. He is credited with suggesting, however, that paraffin could be used for breast reconstruction.

The injection of paraffin for the augmentation of body contour was done not only by physicians but also by a variety of lay persons. Case reports concerned with the complications of paraffin injections into the breast began to appear in the early literature of this century. Höllander (1912) described a woman who had undergone paraffin injection 8 years previously and who was seen for treatment of hard lumps and draining fistulas. Kolle (1911) devoted a large section of his textbook on cosmetic surgery to this subject. Complications included blindness, pulmonary embolism, inflammation, and necrosis. Schmorl (1922) described the late appearance of granulomas (paraffinomas). He also described a patient in whom scirrhous carcinoma developed in a paraffinoma.

Despite these complications, paraffin injections were continued for a time. Tucked away in a paper on aesthetic surgery of the breast is mention of such injections by Dartiques (1928). As late as the 1950s and 1960s patients were seen with late complications. Memorable are two of our patients, one an elderly Chinese woman (Fig. 4–1) and one a young nurse, who had melted paraffin and injected it into their own breasts. Each had hard masses, and surgical treatment was impossible unless some form of mastectomy was performed.

Silicone

In the 1950s and 1960s some turned to the injection of liquid silicone. All of the complications that had been seen with paraffin injections were again seen with silicone injections. Some of the results were even worse, because persons who were not physicians often performed the injections and medical-grade silicone was not always used. Therefore, both impurities and additives were injected with the silicone. In addition to granulomas, extensive calcification was seen, which often necessitated adenomammectomy (Figs. 4–2 and 4–3). Ellenbogen et al. (1975) reported these complications.

Autogenous Fat Injections

As liposuction became popular, the idea was conceived of injecting that fat back into the patient where there were tissue defects. Bircoll (1987) has described his use of collected fat from liposuction in improving contour in both a reconstructed breast and the unaffected breast. While the use of autogenous fat would

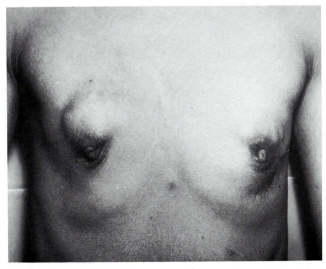

FIGURE 4–1
Patient who performed self-injection of paraffin many years previously, showing multiple paraffinomas.

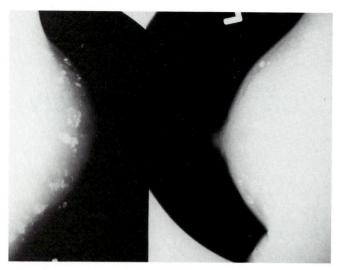

FIGURE 4–2
Mammogram of a patient who had silicone injections performed in a beauty salon.

seem to be a good answer to augmentation of the breast, the procedure has been condemned because of the late deposition of calcium, which would lead to confusing mammographic findings.

AUTOGENOUS TISSUE TRANSPLANTATION

Free Grafts

Czerny (1895) was probably the first to use free fat as a breast implant. After performing a subcutaneous sub-

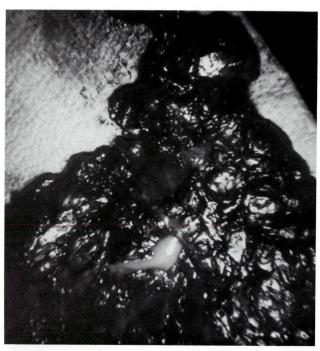

FIGURE 4–3
Specimen from subcutaneous mastectomy of the patient shown in Figure 4–2, showing nodules and greasy material throughout the gland.

total mastectomy to remove a fibroadenoma and hypertrophic breast tissue (underlying interstitial mastitis), Czerny transplanted a lipoma the size of his fist from the lumbar area to augment the breast. Lexer (1914) described free transplantation of skin, mucous membrane, muscle, fat, nerve, vessels, tendon, fascia, periosteum, peritoneum, cartilage, joint, limbs, and organs. His only reference to breast augmentation was the work of Czerny. Bartlett (1917) transplanted fat from the anterior abdomen, the outer aspect of the thigh, and the buttocks to reform breasts in six patients who underwent adenomammectomy for fibrocystic mastitis.

Bames (1953) used free dermofat fascia grafts for the specific purpose of building up an undeveloped breast. He harvested the grafts from the buttocks. The graft was placed in the submammary space with the fascial side of the graft resting on the pectoral fascia. His estimated survival of the grafts was about 90% (Fig. 4–4).

Serafin et al. (1982) have presented beautiful results in reconstruction after mastectomy. They used groin flaps, latissimus dorsi musculocutaneous flaps, tensor fasciae latae musculocutaneous flaps, and gluteus maximus musculocutaneous flaps vascularized by microsurgical anastomosis. It would probably never be practical to apply this extensive a procedure to augmentation of the small breast.

Flaps

Longacre (1954) designed adjacent flaps for the specific purpose of correction of the hypoplastic breast. A dermofat pedicle flap was prepared from inframammary tissue, split, and inserted into a pocket beneath the gland. Longacre (1956) also used these dermofat flaps with a wide attachment to the inferior aspect of the breast. The flaps were inserted into a pocket beneath the gland, then anchored to the periosteum over the third rib (Fig. 4–5).

Zavaleta and Marino (1963) described the use of omental flaps for breast augmentation.

PROSTHESES

Sponges

Autogenous tissue transplantation was not adopted by many for augmentation of the small breast; and as the era of paraffin and silicone injections came to an end, the insertion of sponge prostheses was introduced. Edgerton and McClary (1958) described a group of patients who had had Ivalon prostheses used for breast augmentation. Many plastic surgeons followed suit and did the same. It was found that the prostheses became very hard, a result that at the time was thought to be due to invasion of fibrous tissue (Figs. 4–6 and 4–7). Pangman and Wallace (1955) advocated the use of their compound prosthesis, which incorporated a polyethylene sac around the Ivalon. The incidence of infection was high, and the use of Ivalon was discontinued. Other sponges were tried, among them Etheron (Fig. 4–8),

FIGURE 4–4

Donor site is outlined and closed with tension sutures *(A)*. The free graft of fascia, fat, and dermis *(B)* is inserted with fascia to fascia and dermis to gland *(C)*.

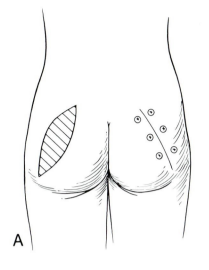

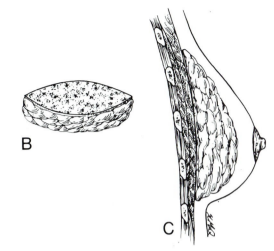

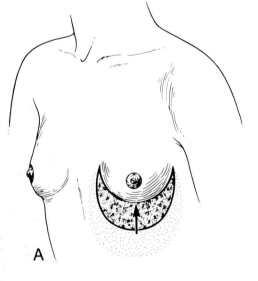

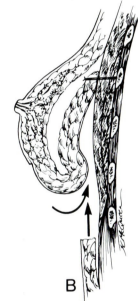

FIGURE 4–5

Dermofat flaps based on abdomen *(A)* and breast *(B)*.

FIGURE 4–6

Extrusion of Ivalon prosthesis following a long period of drainage.

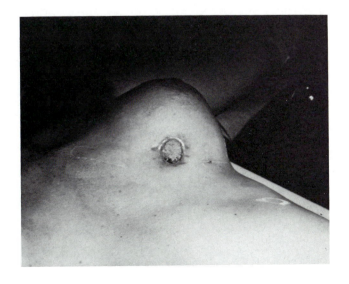

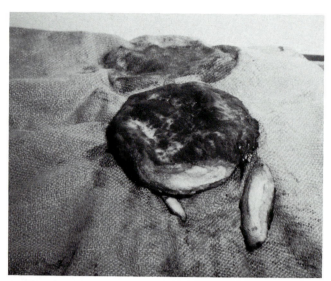

FIGURE 4–7
Ivalon prosthesis after removal from the patient shown in Figure 4–6.

polystan, polyurethane, and Teflon. Because of the high rate of infection and extrusion, sponges were discontinued.

Silicone Prostheses

New impetus was given to prosthetic implantation for breast enlargement when Cronin and Gerow (1963) reported on their use of a silicone gel prosthesis.

The interesting story behind this gel prosthesis was told by Biggs (1988) at the PSEF/ASAPS* symposium on plastic surgery of the breast in Santa Fe. Frank Gerow was a resident in Houston on the service of Dr. Thomas Cronin in 1959. While working late in the operating room one night, he looked up and saw a

*Plastic Surgery Educational Foundation/American Society of Aesthetic Plastic Surgery.

plastic bag filled with blood to be used as a transfusion. It occurred to him that it resembled a breast. It was known that Silas Braley was knowledgeable about silicone chemistry, and he was contacted to make such a sac out of silicone. He made some that Gerow implanted into dogs. Dr. Cronin then designed an implant made of clay, which was sent to Dow Corning at Midland, Michigan. In March 1962 the first implant, filled with saline, was given a clinical trial. It broke. One week later a silicone sac filled with silicone gel was given a clinical trial, and it was successful. The paper was ultimately presented at the Third International Congress of Plastic Surgery in Washington, D.C., in 1963.

Scales (1953) had outlined the properties of an ideal soft tissue implant as follows:
1. Not physically modified by soft tissue
2. Chemically inert
3. Produces no inflammation or foreign body reaction
4. Noncarcinogenic
5. Produces no stage of allergy or hypersensitivity
6. Capable of resisting mechanical strains
7. Capable of fabrication in the form desired
8. Capable of sterilization

Blocksma and Braley (1965) summarized a large volume of research work on silicones and felt that silicone fulfilled these requirements. Today we know that in the strictest sense that this is not entirely true. Vistnes (1978) points out that nothing is truly inert and that fibrous encapsulation around a prosthesis is to be expected.

Patients soon rushed to the plastic surgeons' offices for breast augmentation with silicone prostheses, and plastic surgeons likewise were enthusiastic about their use (Fig. 4–9). When the patient was healed and happy, there seemed to be little need to follow the case closely. Therefore, it was not until much later that it was realized that many of these prostheses had become hard. From that day until the present time there has been a tremendous amount of both laboratory and clinical research aimed at the etiology and prevention of the condition. It was found that the gel had not hardened, but that the capsule had contracted and forced the prosthesis into a smaller space, with resulting deformities.

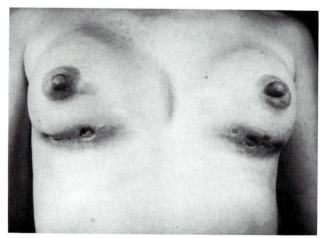

FIGURE 4–8
Draining fistulas from Etheron prostheses.

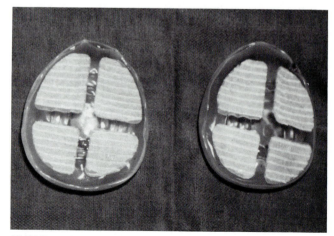

FIGURE 4–9
An early Cronin prosthesis made by Dow Corning.

ETIOLOGY OF CONTRACTED CAPSULES

Various aspects of this very provocative subject have been studied simultaneously, and therefore the following evolution of concepts is not necessarily chronologic.

The Prosthesis

Williams (1972) and others felt that the Dacron patches on the backs of the prostheses, which were designed for fixation, were probably the cause of a reaction in the capsule that led to hardness. The patches were decreased in size and ultimately discontinued, but the problem of hardness remained.

In his historical review, Braley (1973) indicated that it became evident that the device should be softer and have less palpable edges. The seams were inverted and then discarded altogether. A thinner sac was manufactured, making for a much softer prosthesis. The softer the covering and gel, the harder the prosthesis became.

Teardrop designs were added to the original oval prostheses. Some surgeons, including Watson (1976), believed that the teardrop designs caused more capsular contraction, and discoid prostheses then came into favor. On the other hand, some felt that round prostheses were more prone to spherical contracture of the capsule.

Ashley (1970) introduced the polyurethane covering for gel prostheses in an effort to reduce the contracture rate. While there are those who continue to use polyurethane covers, most believe that is an unsuitable prosthesis because of degeneration with marked foreign-body reaction, as shown by Smahel (1978).

Shortly after the introduction of silicone gel prostheses, Arion (1965) presented the inflatable prosthesis, using polyvinylpyrrolidone (dextran) as the liquid filler. Jenny (1971) was also an early advocate of a saline inflatable prosthesis. He did not publish his early work, but he did present a paper at the Fifth International Congress of Plastic and Reconstructive Surgery in Paris entitled "Areolar Incision for Augmentation Mammaplasty." The paper was listed in the Appendix and was unfortunately not published in the *Transactions*.

Regnault et al. (1972) evaluated the saline prostheses that had been used over a 2-year period. There was a lower incidence of capsular contracture than with gel implants, and this was also shown by Jenny and Smahel (1981). Many surgeons turned to the inflatable prosthesis because they were discouraged by the inadequacies of closed capsular fracture. In time, however, the inflatable prosthesis was also discarded by most because of the high incidence of deflation. This was documented by Worton et al. (1980).

Leakage was not usually due to valve failure, but to the shearing force exerted by the body's motion on the inside of an underfilled sac. The resulting fold flaw eventually tore and leaked saline. To prevent this fold flaw, Colon (1982) created a double-lumen implant with saline on the inside and a layer of silicone gel on the outside. While this might correct leakage, the fibrous contracture problem was still there.

By this time several investigators, among them Baker et al. (1982), showed that silicone was present in capsules surrounding gel prostheses. The term "silicone bleed" came into existence, and an effort was made by the manufacturers to create a shell that would prevent the leakage of silicone molecules into the body's capsule; unfortunately, capsular contracture continued. Price and Barker (1983) thought that Dow Corning Silastic II was helpful but that McGhan Intrashiel was not. Some believe that a double-lumen implant with saline in the outer compartment remains a double-sac barrier. This double-lumen implant was designed for a different reason by Hartley (1976). He thought that when a contracture developed, the saline could be removed percutaneously, making the implant smaller and disguising the capsular contracture.

There has been interest in the surface of the prosthesis and the interface between the surface and the body tissues. Wilflingseder et al. (1976) suggested that a grazing effect of the rough surface might initiate contracture of the capsule. The current trend of the implant manufacturers is to fabricate a textured surface designed to diminish fibrous capsule formation. Picha (1988) discussed random discontinuous, milled, and pillared surfaces at the PSEF/ASAPS plastic surgery of the breast symposium in Santa Fe. The first is McGhan's Biocell. The second has a highly irregular surface contour with 10- to 50-μm spikes. The capsule is less dense and more vascular, and the fibers are aligned. The third is experimental. The Misti prosthesis seems to have the most suitable configuration in the microtexturing of the outer shell in order to minimize the occurrence of scar contracture. It has pillars 500 μm high and shows very little fibrous capsular formation.

Surgical Technique

From time to time various faults associated with the operation itself have been implicated as etiologic in the formation of contracted capsules. They are all in violation of good surgical practice and should be avoided in any type of operation. If the following steps are adhered to, these causes can be eliminated: prevent deposition of particulate material into the pocket; use meticulous sterile technique; be sure surgery is atraumatic; use accurate hemostasis; and make the pocket of adequate size. There have been many articles written on this subject. Some of the most comprehensive papers have been by Wilflingseder et al. (1974), Biggs et al. (1982), and Burkhardt (1983, 1984, 1985). The latter bibliography has been compiled by Dr. Burkhardt but has not been published.

It should be noted that various incisions have been employed for approaching the cavity for reception of the prosthesis. Their importance to the problem of capsular contracture is not always clear. Incisions have been inframammary, as described by Lewis (1965); axillary, as described by Hoehler (1973), transareolar, as described by Pitanguy (1978); periareolar, as described by McKinney et al. (1974); and suprapubic when augmentation of the breast is combined with abdominoplasty, as described by Barrett and Kelly (1980) (Fig. 4–10).

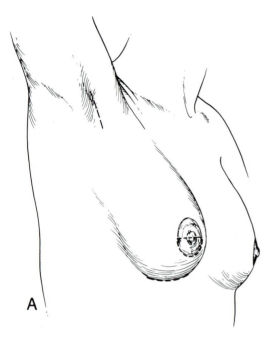

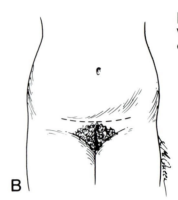

FIGURE 4–10
Various incisions used for breast augmentation.

Treatment of an Established Capsular Contracture

At first no one knew what to do with the hard augmented breast. Surgical exploration revealed that the prosthesis itself was not hard, but that the space in which it was contained had become much smaller. The capsule was incised, excised, or injected with cortisone. These possibilities were enumerated by Baker et al. (1976). Prostheses were removed or exchanged for newer models. They were placed behind the posterior wall of the old capsule, as described by Silver (1972), or in front of the old capsule, as described by Mladick (1977). Today surgical correction often leads to the finding of a ruptured prosthesis, many times with calci-

fication, particularly if the prosthesis has been in place for a long time (Figs. 4–11 and 4–12). At present the prosthesis is replaced and usually put behind the pectoralis major muscle, as described by Reddick (1984).

It was quite by chance that the so-called closed capsular fracture was discovered. Baker et al. (1976) had a patient who was embraced by a big football player, whereupon there was a loud pop. When she went to the ladies' room, she found that the breast that had been squeezed was soft. This suggested the concept and led to the procedure of intentional closed capsulotomy. It provided a solution to the problem of the hard breast and eliminated the hospitalization, confinement, and cost necessary for open capsulotomy. Unfortunately, there was a high recurrence rate. In addition, surgeons tired of repetitive painful episodes for the patient and,

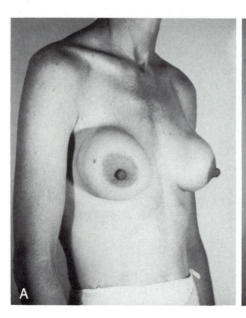

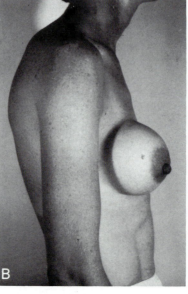

FIGURE 4–11
Front (A) and side (B) views of patient who had free silicone gel placed on top of the pectoralis major muscle, showing marked capsular contracture.

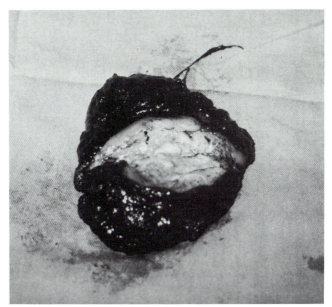

FIGURE 4–12
Specimen from the patient shown in Figure 4–11, showing encapsulation and severe calcification.

incidentally, trauma and pain to their own thumb joints; and if the fracture of the capsule was not complete, the shape of the breast was distorted.

Soon reports began to appear about the complications of closed capsulotomy. Ruptured prostheses with migration of silicone gel into the axilla were reported by Hueston et al. (1979). Zide (1981) showed silicone drainage from the nipple after closed capsulotomy, and Edmond (1980) found silicone granuloma over the biceps muscle after closed capsulotomy. Bleeding was reported by Laughlin et al. (1977). As the capsule tore, breast vessels also tore. Sometimes the bruise extended all the way down the flank and into the groin. Complications other than capsular contracture have been listed by Letterman and Schurter (1985).

This was one of the darkest moments in the history of prosthetic breast augmentation. Both open and closed treatments of capsular contracture were largely unsuccessful. Vistnes et al. (1978) made a wise comment: "The purposeful manual rupture of the capsule around a breast implant, a capsule which represents the final establishment of an equilibrium between the organism and the foreign body implant, creates a deliberate upset of this equilibrium."

Many modalities have been tried for preventing capsular contracture. They all had loyal proponents, but many have been discarded. One of the longest lived has been the local use of steroids around the prosthesis, as described by Peterson and Burt (1974), or in the saline compartment of a double-lumen prosthesis, as described by Hartley (1976). There appears to be a decrease in percentage of contracted capsules, but they do still sometimes occur. Steroid-related complications such as streaking, thinning, and extrusion prevented most surgeons from continuing their use. Cohen and Carrico (1980) described some of the untoward results of steroid therapy.

Perhaps the use of local antibiotics has had more followers. Burkhardt (Burkhardt et al., 1981) was an early proponent of local antibiotic use and continues to be one. The compression exercises of Foerster (1978) and the use of vitamin E by Baker (1981) and Diapulse by Silver (1982) are among other forms of prevention.

One of the most significant factors in decreasing capsular contracture has been the positioning of the prosthesis behind the pectoralis major muscle, rather than anterior to it. Why this is successful is debatable. It could be that the continuous motion of the rib cage prevents the contracture. Or it could be that the muscle separates the prosthesis from the breast, which is basically a bacterium-contaminated organ. Details of the procedure have been discussed by many, some of whom are Dempsey and Latham (1968), Regnault (1977), and Truppman and Ellenby (1978).

For those who wish to study the subject further, information may be found in the following references: Grossman (1976), Letterman and Schurter (1978), and Georgiade (1983).

References

Arion, H.: Présentation d'une prothèse retromammaire. Soc. Fr. Gynecol. 35:427, 1965.

Ashley, F. L.: A new type of breast prosthesis: Preliminary report. Plast. Reconstr. Surg. 45:421, 1970.

Baker, J.: The effectiveness of alpha-tocopherol (vitamin E) in reducing the incidence of spherical contracture around breast implants. Plast. Reconstr. Surg. 68:696, 1981.

Baker, J. L., Jr., Bartels, J., Douglas, W. M.: Closed compression technique for rupturing a contracted capsule around a breast implant. Plast. Reconstr. Surg. 58:137, 1976.

Baker, J. L., Jr., LeVier, R. R., Spielvogel, D. E.: Positive identification of silicone in human mammary capsular tissue. Plast. Reconstr. Surg. 69:56, 1982.

Bames, H.: Augmentation mammaplasty by lipotransplant. Plast. Reconstr. Surg. 11:404, 1953.

Barrett, B. M., Jr., Kelly, M. V., II: Combined abdominoplasty and augmentation mammaplasty through a transverse suprapubic incision. Ann. Plast. Surg. 4:286, 1980.

Bartlett, W.: An anatomic substitute for the female breast. Ann. Surg. 66:208, 1917.

Biggs, T. M.: The gel implant: Day one to the present. Presented at the PSEF/ASAPS Third Annual Plastic Surgery of the Breast Symposium, Santa Fe, New Mexico, September 1988.

Biggs, T. M., Cukier, J., Worthing, L. F.: Augmentation mammaplasty: A review of 18 years. Plast. Reconstr. Surg. 69:445, 1982.

Bircoll, M., Novack, B. H.: Autologous fat transplantation employing liposuction techniques. Ann. Plast. Surg. 18:327, 1987.

Blocksma, R., Braley, S.: The silicones in plastic surgery. Plast. Reconstr. Surg. 35:366, 1965.

Braley, S. A.: The use of silicones in plastic surgery. Plast. Reconstr. Surg. 51:280, 1973.

Burkhardt, B., Fried, M., Schnur, P., Tofield, J.: Capsules, infection, and intramural antibiotics. Plast. Reconstr. Surg. 68:43, 1981.

Burkhardt, B. R.: Augmentation mammaplasty and capsular contracture 1963–1983. 1984 Supplement. 1985 Supplement. Tucson, Arizona.

Cohen, I. K., Carrico, T. J.: Capsular contracture and steroid-related complications in augmentation mammaplasty. Aesth. Plast. Surg. 4:267, 1980.

Colon, G.: The reverse double-lumen prostheses: A preliminary report. Ann. Plast. Surg. 9:293, 1982.

Cronin, T., Gerow, F.: Augmentation mammaplasty: A new "natural feel" prosthesis. In: Broadbent, T. R. (ed.): *Transactions of the Third International Congress of Plastic Surgery.* Amsterdam, Excerpta Medica Foundation, 1963, p. 41.

Czerny, V.: Drei plastischen Operationen. Arch. Klin. Chir. 50:544, 1895.

Dartigues, L.: État actuel de la chirurgie esthétique mammaire: Les différentes procédés de mastoplastie en général et de la greffe aréolo-mammelonnaire en particulier. Monde Méd. 38:75, 1928.

Dempsey, W., Latham, W.: Subpectoral implants in augmentation mammaplasty. Plast. Reconstr. Surg. 42:515, 1968.

Edgerton, M., McClary, A.: Augmentation mammaplasty. Plast. Reconstr. Surg. 21:279, 1958.

Edmond, J. A., Versaci, A. D.: Late complication of closed capsulotomy of the breast (Letter). Plast. Reconstr. Surg. 66:478, 1980.

Ellenbogen, R., Ellenbogen, R., Rubin, L.: Injectable fluid silicone therapy. JAMA 234:308, 1975.

Foerster, D.: "False bursa" concept in augmentation mammaplasty. Aesth. Plast. Surg. 2:419, 1978.

Georgiade, N. G.: Aesthetic Breast Surgery. Baltimore, Williams & Wilkins, 1983.

Gersuny, R.: Ueber eine subcutane Prosthese. Z. Heilk. 21:199, 1900.

Gersuny, R.: Harte und Weiche Paraffinprothesen. Zentralbl. Chir. 30:1, 1903.

Grossman, A. R.: Augmentation Mammoplasty. Springfield, Ill., Charles C Thomas, 1976.

Hartley, J. H., Jr.: Specific applications of the double lumen prosthesis. Clin. Plast. Surg. 3:247, 1976.

Hoehler, H.: Breast augmentation: The axillary approach. Br. J. Plast. Surg. 26:373, 1973.

Höllander, E.: Abstract from Berliner Gesellschaft für Chirurgie. Münch. Med. Wochenschr. 59:2842, 1912.

Hueston, J., Hare, W.: Rupture of subpectoral prostheses during closed compression capsulotomy. Aust. J. Surg. 49:564, 1979.

Jenny, H.: Areolar incision for augmentation mammaplasty. Presented at the Fifth International Congress of Plastic and Reconstructive Surgery, Melbourne, February 1971.

Jenny, H., Smahel, J.: Clinicopathologic correlations in pseudocapsule formation after breast augmentation. Aesthetic Plast. Surg. 5:63, 1981.

Kolle, F. S.: Plastic and Cosmetic Surgery. New York, Appleton, 1911.

Lagarde, M.: Les Injections de Paraffine. Paris, Jules Rousset, 1903.

Laughlin, R., Raynor, A., Habal, M.: Complications of closed capsulotomies after augmentation mammaplasty. Plast. Reconstr. Surg. 60:362, 1977.

Letterman, G., Schurter, M.: History of augmentation mammaplasty. In: Owsley, J. Q., Peterson, R. A. (eds.): Symposium on Aesthetic Surgery of the Breast. St. Louis, C. V. Mosby, 1978, p. 243.

Letterman, G., and Schurter, M.: Suggested nomenclature for aesthetic and reconstructive surgery of the breast: Part II. Augmentation mammoplasty and mastopexy. Aesthetic Plast. Surg. 9:293, 1985.

Lewis, J. R., Jr.: The augmentation mammaplasty. Plast. Reconstr. Surg. 35:51, 1965.

Lexer, E.: Free transplantation. Ann. Surg. 60:166, 1914.

Longacre, J.: Correction of the hypoplastic breast with special reference to reconstruction of the "nipple type breast" with local dermo-fat pedicle flaps. Plast. Reconstr. Surg. 14:431, 1954.

Longacre, J.: Surgical reconstruction of the flat discoid breast. Plast. Reconstr. Surg. 17:358, 1956.

McKinney, P., Shedbalker, A.: Augmentation mammaplasty using a non-inflatable prosthesis through a circum-areolar incision. Br. J. Plast. Surg. 27:35, 1974.

Mladick, R.: Treatment of the firm augmented breast by capsular stripping and inflatable implant exchange. Plast. Reconstr. Surg. 60:720, 1977.

Pangman, J., Wallace, R.: The use of plastic prosthesis in breast plastic and other soft tissue surgery. West. J. Surg. Obstet. Gynecol. 63:503, 1955.

Peterson, H. D., Burt, G. B.: The role of steroids in prevention of circumferential capsular scarring in augmentation mammaplasty. Plast. Reconstr. Surg. 54:28, 1974.

Picha, G. J.: The biology of silicones, polyurethanes and texturing. Presented at the PSEF/ASAPS Third Annual Plastic Surgery of the Breast Symposium, Santa Fe, New Mexico, September 1988.

Pitanguy, I.: Transareolar incision for augmentation mammaplasty. Aesthetic Plast. Surg. 2:363, 1978.

Price, J. E., Jr., Barker, D. E.: Initial clinical experience with "low bleed" breast implants. Aesthetic Plast. Surg. 7:255, 1983.

Reddick, L. P.: Combatting capsular contracture. Plast. Reconstr. Surg. 74:731, 1984.

Regnault, P.: Partially submuscular breast augmentation. Plast. Reconstr. Surg. 59:72, 1977.

Regnault, P., Baker, T. J., Gleason, M. C., et al.: Clinical trial and evaluation of a proposed new inflatable mammary prosthesis. Plast. Reconstr. Surg. 50:220, 1972.

Scales, J. T.: Discussion on metals and synthetic materials in relation to soft tissues: Tissue reaction to synthetic materials. Proc. R. Soc. Med. 46:647, 1953.

Schmorl: Paraffingranulome. Münch. Med. Wochenschr. 69:215, 1922.

Serafin, D., Voci, V., Georgiade, N. G.: Microsurgical composite tissue transplantation: Indications and technical considerations in breast reconstruction following mastectomy. Plast. Reconstr. Surg. 70:24, 1982.

Silver, H.: Treating the complications of augmentation mammaplasty. Plast. Reconstr. Surg. 49:637, 1972.

Silver, H.: Reduction of capsular contracture with two-stage augmentation mammaplasty and pulsed electromagnetic energy (Diapulse therapy). Plast. Reconstr. Surg. 69:802, 1982.

Smahel, J.: Tissue reactions to breast implants coated with polyurethane. Plast. Reconstr. Surg. 61:80, 1978.

Truppman, E., Ellenby, J.: A 13-year evaluation of subpectoral augmentation mammaplasty. In: Owsley, J. Q., Peterson, R. A. (eds.): Symposium on Aesthetic Surgery of the Breast. St. Louis, C. V. Mosby, 1978, p. 344.

Vistnes, L. M., Ksander, G. A., Kosek, J.: Study of encapsulation of silicone rubber implants in animals. Plast. Reconstr. Surg. 62:580, 1978.

Worton, E. W., Seifert, L., Sherwood, R.: Late leakage of inflatable silicone breast prostheses. Plast. Reconstr. Surg. 65:302, 1980.

Watson, J.: Some observations on breast augmentation procedures over the past two decades. Aesthetic Plast. Surg. 1:89, 1976.

Wilflingseder, P., Propst, A., Mikuz, G.: Constrictive fibrosis following silicone implants in mammary augmentation. Chir. Plast. 2:215, 1974.

Wilflingseder, P., Propst, A., Mikuz, G., Hoinkes, G.: Constrictive fibrosis post augmentation mammoplasty. In: Marchac, D. (ed.): Transactions of the Sixth International Congress of Plastic and Reconstructive Surgery. Paris, Masson, 1976, p. 535.

Williams, J. E.: Experiences with a large series of Silastic breast implants. Plast. Reconstr. Surg. 49:253, 1972.

Zavaleta, D., Marino, E.: Hipoplasia mamaria unilateral: Relleno mamario con epiplón mayor transplantado. Prensa. Méd. Argent. 50:639, 1963.

Zide, B.: Complications of closed capsulotomy after augmentation. Plast. Reconstr. Surg. 67:697, 1981.

5

Garry S. Brody

Silicone Technology for the Plastic Surgeon*

The purpose of this chapter is to bring to the attention of the readers of this comprehensive textbook dealing with aesthetic breast surgery a better understanding and clarification of some of the important synthetic materials used in aesthetic breast surgery. Today's state of the art in this area is directly related to the use of silicons.

In order to understand the properties of silicone, one needs an explanation of terms.

Silicon (Si) is the basic metallic element.

Silica (SiO_2) is common sand. Sand and glass are crystalline forms of SiO_2, in contrast to fumed (amorphous or noncrystalline) silica, used as a filler for the solid forms of silicone elastomer.

Silicates are a group of minerals including clay, feldspar, talc, and bauxite, among others.

Silica gel is a mineral with powerful hygroscopic properties, commonly seen packed with such devices as new cameras in order to absorb excess humidity.

Silicone is the generic name for a host of silicon-based polymers. For medical uses the predominant monomeric building block is dimethyl siloxane.

$$\left[\begin{array}{c} CH_3 \\ | \\ Si-O- \\ | \\ CH_3 \end{array} \right] +$$

Silicone oil is formed when the molecules are arranged in linear chains of silicone monomer with trimethyl end blocks. The viscosity depends upon the chain length.

Silicone gel is formed when the polymer branches and becomes semiliquid. As the branching increases, such gels progressively thicken into gums, resins, and waxes.

Silicone elastomer is formed when long chain polymer oils are joined by side bonding and become solid—a process known as vulcanization. ("Elastomer" is a generic name for all rubberlike polymers. Properly "rubber" should be reserved for the familiar organic carbon-based material. However, in common usage, silicone elastomers are frequently referred to as rubber.) Silicone elastomers are much purer compounds than organic rubbers.

Silastic is a trade name for the Dow Corning brand of silicone.

Silicones are polymers based on the element silicon, an elemental metal adjacent to carbon on the periodic table. Silicon is one of the most abundant elements on the earth's surface. The silicone polymers are structured very much like their carbon-based relatives and use much the same terminology. Linear, short-chain, lighter weight molecules form oils. The viscosity increases with increasing molecular weight and, with additives, becomes greaselike. With catalysts and/or heat, the chains can be branched and form gels, gums, and waxes. With side bonding of the linear chains, the oils are vulcanized into various elastomers. As with carbon-based compounds, the silicones can be formulated into an almost unlimited number of compounds such as adhesives, lubricants, caulks, sealants, water repellents, and rubbers. In contrast to their carbon-based counterparts, the silicone rubbers are extremely temperature-resistant. They stay flexible when very cold and resist degradation at relatively high temperatures. Most silicone rubbers are quite weak and are easily torn or abraded, as compared with the carbon-based materials (Jakubczak, 1987).

The major value of silicone for medical usage is its extreme biologic inertness. This is in part due to its hydrophobic properties. If water is repelled, chemicals, enzymes, and so forth cannot gain sufficient contact to affect the material. In fact, the United States Pharmacopeia (Pharmacopeia, 1975) uses medical grade silicone as its standard for biocompatibility against which all other compounds are compared. Medical grade silicones are highly purified and free of toxic catalysts and contaminants. When a broken implant is removed from a pocket, the shell may seem to have disappeared and may be reported as having disintegrated. A broken shell that is crumpled and immersed in the gel becomes invisible, which leads to the misconception that it has somehow degraded. A careful search through the silicone will always locate the envelope. This is not unlike looking for a contact lens in a glass of water. Although the physical properties of silicone may change, such as occurs with lipid absorption and calcification, biochemical disintegration does not appear to occur. Even the hydrophobic silicones are not, however, resistant to ingestion by macrophages.

OILS

The silicone oils can be formulated for use as a coating for needles and syringes or as a lubricant for surgical instruments. As a surfactant, silicone oil is available in

*Modified from Brody, G. S.: Silicone Technology for the Plastic Surgeon. Clin. Plast. Surg. 15(4):517, 1988.

many medications to control gastrointestinal gas. Injectable silicone is made of highly purified oil. Because it is not practical to produce a fluid wherein all of the molecules are of the same chain length, all oils available for use are blends of multiple-length chains with the viscosity determined by the particular mix of the product in hand.

GELS

In plastic surgery, gels are used exclusively in breast implants and as fill for one type of chin implant. Like the oils, the gels are also made of a blend of various chain lengths. The earliest implants were quite viscous; but in response to the request of the plastic surgical community for what was considered to be more natural-feeling implants, the "responsive" gels containing shorter-chained diluent became available in the mid 1970s. The earlier gels were quite cohesive and were relatively easy to remove from an implant pocket if ruptured. The price paid for the more responsive gels was a decrease in cohesiveness, making removal of a ruptured implant more challenging.

RUBBERS

As a rubber, silicones are available in a wide variety of medically useful products ranging from catheters and drains to hydrocephalic shunts, coatings for pacemakers, and the shells of breast implants. Medical grade silicone elastomer is vulcanized by one of two basic processes. With a catalyst such as stannous octuate the reaction occurs at room temperature (RTV).* With a platinum-containing or peroxide compound catalyst, high temperatures are required for vulcanization (HTV). Silicone in sponge form was not available for many years because the manufacturing process was hazardous as a result of the use of hydrogen gas as a foaming agent. After an explosion in one of the manufacturer's plants, the foam was considered too dangerous to make and was withdrawn from the market by all producers. Advances in technology have resulted in the safe manufacture of foams, and they are again available. The rubber is often formulated with fumed silica as a filler to give it strength and body. Fumed silica must not be confused with sand, although both are basically silicon dioxide (SiO_2). Sand is the crystalline form of the molecule, whereas the fumed silica is amorphous. (It should be noted that it is the physical crystalline structure that is primarily responsible for stimulating the intense fibrosis seen in silicosis, as opposed to the chemistry of the SiO_2.) The fumed silica is tightly bound to the silicone molecule and, contrary to speculation, is not independently available for direct biologic activity.

The basic silicone breast implant is manufactured by dissolving the silicone in a dispersant and repeatedly

dipping a mandril of the desired shape into the liquid. The mandril can also be coated by spraying. The elastomer is then cured and peeled from the mandril as a rubber. This produces as smooth a surface and as uniform a shell thickness as is practical. The envelope is then filled with gel, sealed with a glued patch, tested, and packaged. Inflatables tend to have thicker walls for strength, and the valve is appropriately attached. Sterilization is usually accomplished with ethylene oxide gas. All of the manufacturers have their own particular technology, the details of which are trade secrets, but the basic technology is similar.

ADHESIVES

A self-curing adhesive (Medical Adhesive AR) is commercially available for gluing and sealing silicone assemblages. When exposed to air, this one-component elastomer slowly absorbs water and releases acetic acid, curing to a densely cross-linked rubber. The acetic acid is tissue-reactive but disperses in air in a few hours. Therefore, the adhesive should not be implanted until the acid is gone, usually within 4 to 24 hours, depending on the quantity and thickness of the adhesive segment.

PHYSICAL PROPERTIES OF SILICONE RUBBER

While silicone approaches the ideal as a compatible material because of its chemical inertness in the biologic environment, its physical shortcomings must be accepted in compromise.

Strength

Compared with their carbon-based counterparts, ordinary silicone elastomers formulated with the classic dimethyl siloxane are not very strong. When these materials are scratched or damaged, any stress will tend to concentrate at the site of injury, causing the flaw to propagate until the device fails. If the silicone is formulated with regional cross-linking (such as in Dow Corning's Silastic HPR), flaw propagation is greatly diminished and tear strength improved. The solid rubbers also resist abrasion and flexing motions poorly, shedding tiny shards of silicone from prosthetic parts and tubing. Patients with silicone wrist bone prostheses have been shown to develop synovitis with silicone particles found within the synovium, bone, and axillary nodes (Christie et al., 1977; Peimer et al., 1986; Smith et al., 1985). Autopsies of renal dialysis patients have shown a high percentage of silicone particles in the liver if silicone dialysis tubing was used (Bommer et al., 1981; Leong et al., 1981, 1982; Parfrey et al., 1981). (Silicone tubing has largely been replaced by other materials for use in cardiac pump tubing and dialysis membranes.) Breast prosthesis shells are fortunately not subject to

---

*Stannous octuate has recently been discontinued as a catalyst because of some theoretic uncertainty over the safety of some of the residuals. No human health problem has ever been documented as due to this catalyst (Jakubczak, 1987).

the same stresses as joint implants or tubing, and there is only one report of sharding noted in the literature.

Another problem, however, besets the inflatable device. If underinflated, creases will form in the shell and the rubber will abrade itself. A phenomenon known as cold flow occurs, leading to rupture at the site of the fold flaw. This does not occur in gel or double-lumen implants because the gel lubricates the shell surfaces, which minimizes abrasion. Internal lubrication of the molecules of rubber within the wall by gel also results in greater elasticity.

Elasticity

Silicone prostheses are relatively elastic. This elasticity permits their insertion through small incisions and allows significant overinflation of tissue expanders. Understanding the mechanism of damage during closed capsular rupture requires an appreciation of the physics involved and the difference between stress and strain: *stress* is force per unit area; *strain* is the percentage of elongation.

If one thinks of the implant in its scar capsule as similar to an inner tube in a tire, it can be appreciated how the prosthesis can withstand tremendous pressure as long as it is constrained. If the capsule ruptures and the tear propagates widely, the forces are spread relatively evenly over the surface of the shell and there is no significant stretching at any given point. Additionally, such wide capsular tears result in the desired softness, and no further force is applied. If, however, as too often happens, a small tear is made, and the surrounding tissue is less resistant than the remaining scar capsule, a knuckle of implant will bulge through, with severe stretching of a small area of implant. This excessive stretching, coupled with a concentration of stress at the ring, can cause the implant to fail at that point. It is therefore recommended that if such limited tears develop, one should either cease to attempt further rupture or try to prevent that area from enlarging by protecting it with the hand and directing the tear forces elsewhere. These small pockets can result in unsightly bulges in the breast contour. Thus, it is not the force of capsular compression that can rupture the implant, but the stretching of follow-through.

Silicone elastomers, like connective tissue, are viscoelastic materials (Ferry, 1980). As such, their elastic properties are rate-dependent. A large force applied rapidly and briefly will produce little deformity, whereas small forces over a period of time can significantly distort the material. Although there are no studies available concerning the effect of high-impact trauma on an implant, conventional intuition suggests that a powerful blow to a broken implant will drive the silicone into the tissues and even into remote locations. An understanding of viscoelastic flow, however, suggests that the gel is quite cohesive under high impact and flows better when chronically deformed by low forces. Thus, although we tend to relate migration of gel to an acute traumatic episode, it is more probably caused by the minor repetitive, steady deformations of everyday life.

Permeability

Silicone rubbers are selectively permeable to various materials. They behave like typical semipermeable membrane to electrolytes. They are very permeable to gases. The yellow color of explanted prostheses is due to lipids, which diffuse easily through the shell.* Amino acids and proteins such as albumin, fibrinogen, and gamma globulin are known to be absorbed onto the surface. The elastomers are very permeable to the lower-molecular-weight fractions of oils and gels, resulting in so-called gel bleed (Brody, 1977). The greater the cross-linking of the rubber, the less porous it becomes. Fluorinated or phenyl-containing silicones are relatively nonporous and are used in Low Bleed devices (Dow Corning).

Silicones are variously permeable to many drugs and are being used increasingly in implantable or skin-surface drug delivery systems. The silicone container must be individually formulated for the drug and the delivery rate selected. Breast implants are *not* designed as drug delivery devices and should not be used as such. It is foolhardy and hazardous to place any medication in the implant lumen, because its diffusibility and rate are totally unknown. Some drugs have a limited shelf life after they have been reconstituted, and the degradation products that develop when stored in an implant for prolonged periods at body temperature are unknown and possibly hazardous (Brody and Latts, 1981).

SUMMARY

There are considerable misconceptions about the properties of silicone gels and envelopes among plastic surgeons, partly because of the characteristics of this unique material. It should be appreciated that the material is relatively weak as rubbers go, its deformation characteristics are time-related, and its permeability varies with the substance involved. Closed capsular rupture should be handled with caution, and current prostheses are not designed to be—and never should be—used as drug delivery systems.

References

Bommer, J., Ritz, E., Waldherr, R., Gastner, M.: Silicone cell inclusions causing multi-organ foreign body reaction in dialysis patients. Lancet 1:1314, 1981.

Brody, G. S.: Fact and fiction about breast implant "bleed." Plast. Reconstr. Surg. 60:615, 1977.

Brody, G. S., Latts, J. R.: Capsules, infection and intraluminal antibiotics. Plast. Reconstr. Surg. 68:48, 1981.

Christie, A. J., Weinberger, K. A., Dietrich, M.: Silicone lymphadenopathy and synovitis: Complications of silicone elastomer finger joint prostheses. JAMA 237:1463, 1977.

Dow Corning: Breast implant product brochure for mammary implant H.P. #1834967-0885. Midland, Michigan.

---

*Heart valve leaflets are no longer made of silicone, because the absorbed lipids tended to calcify, causing the leaflets to crack and fail.

Ferry, J. D.: *Viscoelastic Properties of Polymers.* 3rd ed. New York, John Wiley & Sons, 1980.

Frisch, E. E.: Technology of silicone in biomedical applications. In: Rubin, L. R. (ed.): *Biomaterials in Reconstructive Surgery.* St. Louis, C. V. Mosby, 1983, p. 73.

Jakubczak, G.: Personal communication, 1987.

Leong, As.-Y., Disney, A. P. S., Gove, D. W.: Refractile particles in liver of hemodialysis patients. Lancet 1:889, 1981.

Leong As.-Y., Disney, A. P. S., Gove, D. W.: Spallation and migration of silicone from blood-pump tubing in patients on hemodialysis. N. Engl. J. Med. 306:135, 1982.

Parfrey, P. S., O'Driscoll, J. B., Paradimas, F. J.: Refractile material in the liver of hemodialysis patients. Lancet 1:1101, 1981.

Peimer, C. A., Medige, J., Eckert, B. S., et al.: Reactive synovitis after silicone arthroplasty. J. Hand Surg. [Am.] 11:624, 1986.

Pharmacopeia of the United States of America (The United States Pharmacopeia). 19th revision. Rockville, Md., United States Pharmacopeial Convention, Inc., 1975.

Smahel, J.: Histology of the capsules causing constrictive fibrosis around breast implants. Br. J. Plast. Surg. 30:324, 1977.

Smith, R. J., Atkinson, R. E., Jupiter, J. B.: Silicone synovitis of the wrist. J. Hand Surg. [Am.] 10:47, 1985.

6

Daniel C. Sullivan
Sarah S. Linden

Imaging of Augmentation Mammaplasty Patients

Radiographic imaging of the breast has been a valuable diagnostic tool for decades. However, techniques for breast imaging in women with implants are still evolving and have not yet been studied in large numbers. The presence of prostheses does present certain technical and diagnostic challenges to the radiologist. Nevertheless, we believe that carefully done mammography is important both preoperatively and postoperatively in the breast augmentation patient.

TECHNIQUES

There are two accepted imaging techniques for mammography: xeromammography and film-screen mammography. In the former, a photosensitive selenium-coated plate, rather than x-ray film, is exposed by x-rays passing through the breast. The resulting image is transferred to paper by a process analogous to that used in photocopying machines. The advantages of xeromammography include (1) more uniform imaging of the entire breast from the thicker posterior region to the thinner anterior region and (2) edge enhancement of mass lesions and fine calcifications. Disadvantages include low soft tissue contrast and higher radiation dose to the breast tissue.

Modern film-screen technology has overcome many of its earlier limitations and now provides excellent soft tissue contrast with a very low radiation dose to the breast. With vigorous compression, image exposure is uniform from anterior to posterior in the breast. For high-quality film-screen mammography it is considered essential to use a dedicated x-ray unit with rigid compression plates that have a 90-degree angle against the chest wall. High-speed, high-resolution screens and film developed especially for breast imaging should be used. With the equipment described above, the dose to the breast is in the range of 0.1 rad per film, or 0.2 rad per breast for the standard two-view examination.

The key to successful detection and characterization of lesions in the breast is adequate compression of the breast parenchyma. The presence of prostheses can interfere with tissue compression. Only the tissue that is peripheral to the prosthesis can be seen on the mammogram; the remainder is superimposed on and obscured by the prosthesis. Furthermore, the prosthesis bulges anteriorly, crowding the parenchymal structures in the subareolar region (Fig. 6–1A). In addition, when the compression plates are positioned against the chest wall, the prosthesis prevents full compression of the breast tissue anterior to it, compounding the problem.

These problems can be minimized by pulling the breast forward as compression is applied and excluding the prosthesis from compression. The prosthesis is flattened posteriorly against the chest wall, and most of the breast parenchyma is imaged between the compression plates (Fig. 6–1B). We have used this approach successfully for the past few years, and similar results have been reported by Eklund et al. (1988). The technique can be used for both saline- and silicone-filled prostheses and for both subglandular and submuscular placements. Patients with submuscular implants may experience more discomfort because of pressure on the pectoral muscle. In women with a firm, fibrous capsule around the prosthesis, this technique of displacing the implant posteriorly is more difficult to accomplish. Nevertheless, the results are better than those obtained by including the entire prosthesis within the compression plates. Although patients and clinicians may worry about rupture of the implant from mammographic compression, Eklund's and our own experience suggests that these fears are unwarranted.

In normal women with implants, mammograms performed as described above show most of the parenchymal tissue peripheral and anterior to the prosthesis (Figs. 6–2 to 6–4). The posterior portion of the prosthesis is rarely imaged, and some of the tissue peripherally may not be projected free of the prosthesis on the standard views, even when the prosthesis is pushed back as illustrated here. However, if a palpable mass or other clinical evidence suggests a lesion in an area that might be obscured on standard views, supplemental films can usually be obtained for evaluation of the tissue in question.

Some of the literature over the past 20 years regarding breast imaging for patients with implants is no longer applicable to current mammographic techniques. For example, one study of 20 patients concluded that implants do not interfere with mammographic interpretation and may in fact aid it, by pushing breast tissue forward off the chest wall (Rintala and Svinhufvud, 1974). However, the technique used in those patients involved no compression of breast tissue at all, so that visualization of parenchymal detail was poor. Such a

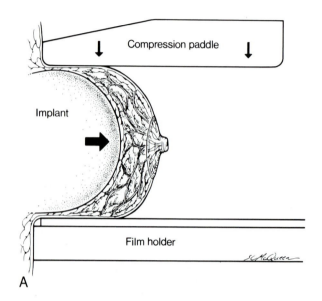

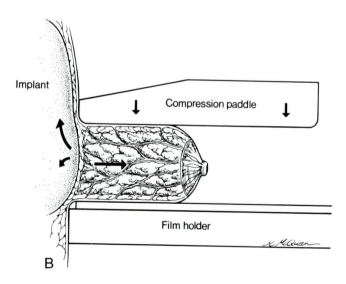

FIGURE 6-1

A, Diagram showing that conventional positioning results in compression primarily of the prosthesis. The implant prevents compression from being applied to the breast tissue anterior to the prosthesis. Tissue structures remain superimposed on each other or on the implant. Also, the implant bulges forward, which further crowds the parenchymal structures together in the retroareolar area. This combination of crowding and lack of compression leads to poor radiographic detail for most of the breast tissue. *B,* Diagram showing the advantages of applying compression selectively to the breast parenchyma and excluding the implant posteriorly. Tissue structures are spread out and brought into close contact with the radiographic film. With this technique, lesions are much less likely to be obscured by superimposition of the prosthesis or parenchymal densities.

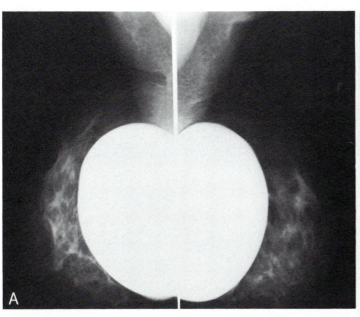

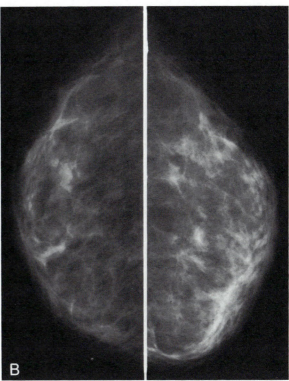

FIGURE 6–2

A, Lateral views of each breast in a 40-year-old woman with silicone prostheses. The entire breast and prosthesis have been included between the compression plates. *B,* Same positioning as in *A,* except that the prosthesis has been pushed back, and full compression is applied to the glandular tissue. Note that islands of dense parenchymal tissue are now spread out and easier to evaluate.

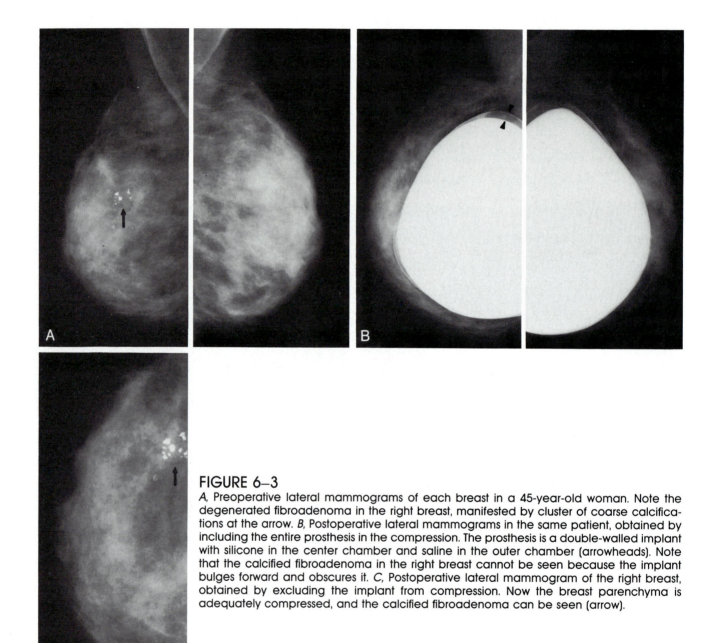

FIGURE 6–3

A, Preoperative lateral mammograms of each breast in a 45-year-old woman. Note the degenerated fibroadenoma in the right breast, manifested by cluster of coarse calcifications at the arrow. B, Postoperative lateral mammograms in the same patient, obtained by including the entire prosthesis in the compression. The prosthesis is a double-walled implant with silicone in the center chamber and saline in the outer chamber (arrowheads). Note that the calcified fibroadenoma in the right breast cannot be seen because the implant bulges forward and obscures it. C, Postoperative lateral mammogram of the right breast, obtained by excluding the implant from compression. Now the breast parenchyma is adequately compressed, and the calcified fibroadenoma can be seen (arrow).

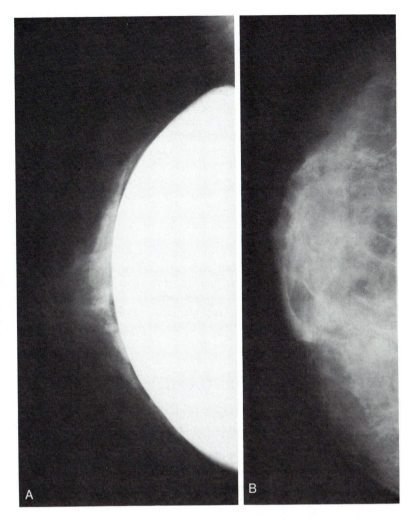

FIGURE 6–4

A, Lateral mammogram in a 38-year-old woman, obtained by including the prosthesis within the compression paddles. Note that there is a small amount of parenchymal tissue anterior to the implant, with little apparent crowding. This might give one a false impression that the parenchyma was well evaluated. *B,* Same view, obtained by excluding the prosthesis from compression. Note the dramatic improvement in spreading out the parenchyma. There is considerably more parenchymal tissue to evaluate than one might think from inspecting the mammogram in *A.*

technique is outdated today, because it has been recognized that vigorous compression is essential for optimal evaluation of the breast. These authors also discussed thermography, which today is considered of little or no value for cancer detection. Other authors reported that implants interfered to some extent with mammographic interpretation, by obscuring portions of the breast parenchyma and by causing crowding and superimposition of other tissue structures (Hoopes et al., 1967; Cohen et al., 1977; Wolfe, 1978; Rosenbaum, 1981; Jensen and Mackey, 1985). With the improved positioning being done today, many of the conclusions in these earlier papers will need re-evaluation.

Some mammographers have advocated xeromammography as superior to film-screen mammography in augmented patients because certain lesions can be seen through saline prostheses with xeromammography (Cohen et al., 1977; Wolfe, 1978; De Waal et al., 1987), whereas in film-screen mammography both saline and silicone prostheses cast an opaque shadow. Other mammographers, however, believe that modern film-screen techniques with improved compression as described in this chapter lead to comparable or better results. No large-scale controlled trials have yet been done to establish whether one technique is superior to the other for augmented patients. We routinely use the film-screen technique for patients with implants, as do the majority of mammographers at present.

There has also been discussion about the relative merits of saline versus silicone gel prostheses from an imaging standpoint. The consensus is that while any implant decreases visibility of parenchymal detail, gel implants do so to a greater extent than saline implants (Eklund et al., 1988; Cohen et al., 1977; Wolfe, 1978). While this has been our own experience, we do not believe the difference to be of much practical importance. Likewise, there are no data to indicate whether submuscular or subglandular placement of the implant leads to better visualization of breast parenchyma by mammography.

Imaging studies other than mammography play adjunctive roles in certain situations. Ultrasound is the most commonly used supplementary study (Hilton et al., 1986). The primary value of ultrasound is in determining whether a mass is cystic or solid. Both palpable and nonpalpable masses can be evaluated by ultrasound, but for reliable differentiation the nodule must be approximately 1 cm in diameter or larger. Ultrasound is not reliable for distinguishing solid benign lesions from malignant lesions.

Computed tomography (CT) is occasionally helpful, especially for evaluating the relationship between the breast and other chest wall structures. In women with prostheses, CT is useful in visualizing the posterior portion of the implant and occasionally for imaging parenchyma that cannot be projected free of the implant with mammographic compression (Hahn and Hoeffken, 1985).

Magnetic resonance imaging (MRI) has not yet been widely applied to breast imaging. In selected cases MRI would offer advantages similar to those described above for CT (Heywang et al., 1985). In the future it is conceivable that MRI may provide histopathologic information in addition to anatomic data.

Cyst aspiration, fine-needle aspiration of solid lesions, and needle localization of nonpalpable lesions can be carried out on patients with prostheses by means of radiographic or ultrasonic guidance. Puncture of the prosthesis can be avoided by carefully choosing the needle entry site and direction of needle travel.

Women who in previous years had silicone injections for augmentation present no special problems in terms of mammographic positioning or compression. However, the density of the silicone and surrounding tissue reaction makes a higher kilovoltage technique necessary. Furthermore, multiple dense silicone deposits can obscure small lesions and make interpretation extremely difficult (Koides and Katayama, 1979; Morgenstern et al., 1985).

DETECTION OF BREAST CANCER

Multiple studies have established the value of mammography in the early detection of breast cancer (Baker, 1982; Seidman et al., 1987; Tabar et al., 1985). Until recently, however, mammography was limited to symptomatic women because of concern over the possible carcinogenic risk of radiation to breast tissue. Technical advancements over the past 20 years have reduced the absorbed radiation dose to the point that routine screening mammography is now recommended at various intervals for all asymptomatic women over age 40. Guidelines concerning the frequency of screening mammograms have been established by several different organizations. There are minor differences in some of these sets of guidelines, and these differences have led to confusion in the minds of some clinicians. The most widely accepted guidelines at present are those promoted jointly by the American Cancer Society and the American College of Radiology, who recommend annual or biannual mammography for women 40 to 49 years of age, depending on risk factors, and annual mammography for women over 50.

Many women requesting augmentation mammaplasty have never had a mammogram. Preoperative mammograms probably have little value as baseline examinations for comparison with postoperative studies, but they have been advocated to exclude unsuspected cancer (Rintala and Svinhufvud, 1974; Perras and Papillon, 1973). Although there have been no large studies for determining the value of preoperative mammography in excluding occult cancer in candidates for aesthetic breast surgery, the incidence of cancer in these patients at the time of surgery has been estimated as 0.3% and 1.5%, respectively, in two studies (Snyderman and Lizardo, 1960; Pitanguy and Torres, 1964). Källen et al. (1986) reported that preoperative mammograms detected two cancers in 159 patients undergoing reduction mamma-

plasty. We believe that it would be prudent for surgeons to obtain a preoperative mammogram in all prospective augmentation patients over 30 years of age. This may be particularly important in light of the question that has been raised about foreign materials in the breast changing the usual growth patterns and/or natural history of breast cancer (Hoopes et al., 1967; Morgenstern et al., 1985).

In patients with augmentation there is still controversy about the value of mammography in the early detection of breast cancer because the implant may interfere with compression of the breast and may obscure some of the parenchyma. Silverstein et al. (1988) reviewed 20 patients in whom cancer had developed 6 months to 15 years after having augmentation mammaplasty. All of these patients had a palpable mass; none had an occult lesion detected by routine mammography. Fifteen patients had prebiopsy mammograms, but only 10 of these examinations showed the cancer. All 20 cancers were invasive, and 13 of the 20 patients had axillary node involvement. On the basis of the advanced state of these cancers, the authors concluded that early detection of breast cancer in augmented patients is impaired and that mammography is less sensitive in these patients than in others. They suggest that, as part of informed consent, patients be advised that the presence of a prosthesis may delay diagnosis of breast cancer by mammographic means. They further suggest that high-risk patients be advised against having augmentation mammaplasty. Despite the disappointing results of mammography in their study, they continue to advocate preoperative mammograms in women over 30 and annual mammography after augmentation.

On the basis of their data and our own experience, we agree with the conclusions and suggestions of Silverstein et al. However, we believe that the number of occult cancers detected by mammography will improve as radiologists devote more attention to technique in augmented patients and use modified forms of compression as described in this chapter (Fig. 6–5). Early detection of cancer in women who had injections of silicone or other foreign material will probably continue to be extremely difficult (Fig. 6–6).

OTHER CONDITIONS

In addition to routine screening for breast cancer, mammography and other imaging techniques are useful in patients with implants in further evaluating palpable abnormalities or symptomatic areas. Imaging studies frequently resolve diagnostic problems resulting from complications of implantation, such as hematoma, seroma, infection, herniation, rupture, displacement, and fibrous capsule formation (Jensen and Mackey, 1985; Hahn and Hoeffken, 1985; Heywang et al., 1985; Grant et al., 1978; Cole-Beuglet et al., 1983; Smith, 1985; Ho, 1987; Theophelis and Stevenson, 1986).

If a mass is found by physical examination or mammography, it can be further characterized by ultrasound, which distinguishes solid from cystic lesions (Fig. 6–7). Cysts need no further evaluation, unless symptomatic, in which case they can be drained by needle aspiration.

FIGURE 6–5

A, Lateral view of the breast, obtained in the standard manner by applying compression to the prosthesis. This causes the prosthesis to bulge forward, crowding the parenchyma anteriorly. Suspicious calcifications (arrow) are difficult to see and could be overlooked. *B,* Same view as in *A,* obtained by excluding the prosthesis posteriorly and applying compression directly to the parenchyma anterior to the implant. Suspicious calcifications (arrow) are much easier to see. The white dot is a metal marker on the skin to indicate the needle entry site for localization. About 40% of calcifications such as these are malignant. Biopsy in this case was benign.

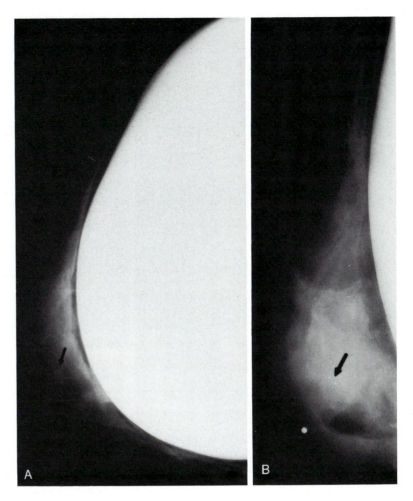

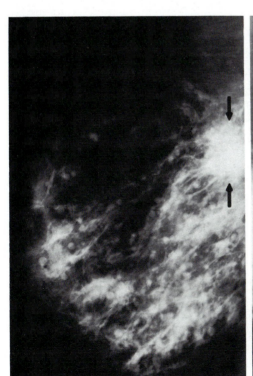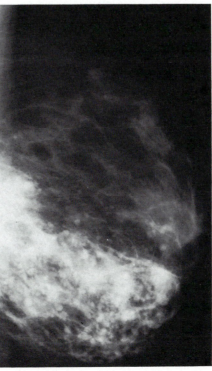

FIGURE 6–6

Lateral views of both breasts in a 46-year-old patient who had had silicone injections more than 10 years previously. The small, round, dense nodules are siliconomas and are more numerous in the lower portion of each breast because of gravity. There is a dense, speculated mass (arrows) in the upper right breast that is of concern. Although it may simply represent a large siliconoma with surrounding chronic inflammatory changes, it could also represent cancer. Biopsy is the only way to distinguish between the two possibilities.

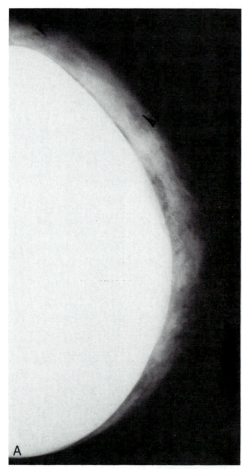

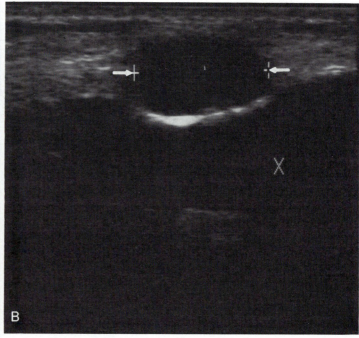

FIGURE 6–7

A, Craniocaudal mammogram of the left breast in a woman with a palpable mass laterally. The mass (arrowheads) is poorly seen on this view because compression was applied to the implant, rather than the tissue in question. The mass is immediately adjacent to the prosthesis. *B*, Ultrasound image confirms the presence of a mass (arrows) and indicates that it is a cyst. Area marked by X is the prosthesis posterior to the cyst.

FIGURE 6–8

Lateral xeromammograms of a patient who presented with a palpable mass in the superior aspect of the left breast. Mammograms reveal a herniated portion of the left implant superiorly (arrowheads). No soft tissue mass was demonstrated on the films. (R, right breast; L, left breast).

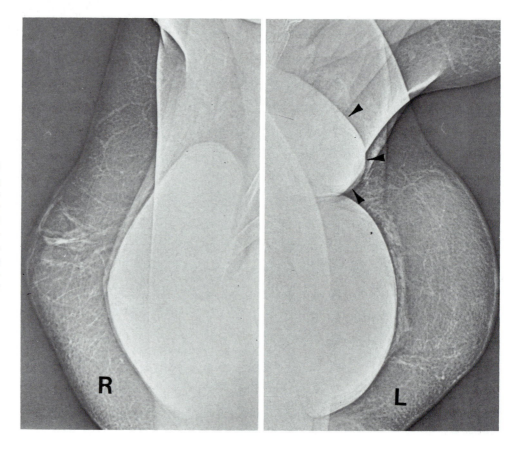

It may be advantageous to perform needle drainage under ultrasonic or radiographic guidance if there is concern about puncturing the prosthesis.

Solid masses remain a diagnostic problem because neither mammography nor ultrasound can differentiate benign and malignant tissue with complete certainty. Many mammographers suggest that well-defined nodules smaller than 1 cm in diameter can be followed by periodic physical examinations and mammograms and that masses larger than 1.5 cm should undergo biopsy. Cases in which the lesion is between 1 and 1.5 cm in diameter may be followed, or a biopsy may be performed, depending on the radiographic or clinical findings and the level of concern.

Occasionally, the appearance of a palpable mass in an augmented patient is due to either displacement or herniation of the prosthesis (Fig. 6–8). Mammography can be helpful in these cases (Grant et al., 1978). Although there have been reported cases in which herniation was mistaken for rupture, we believe that as radiologists gain experience with mammography of augmented patients, this mistake will be uncommon (Smith, 1985).

Rupture of a saline-filled prosthesis leaves an empty, collapsed bag, because the saline is completely resorbed (Fig. 6–9). Silicone implant rupture or leakage presents a different problem because of the irritative effect of free silicone on tissue. On mammography, small, dense nodules of silicone ("siliconomas") are seen in the breast parenchyma (Ho, 1987). These may initially be accompanied by signs of acute inflammation, such as skin thickening and increased parenchymal density, repre-senting edema. Later, signs of chronic inflammation may be seen, such as scarring (Fig. 6–10). In some cases the silicone may be contained by fibrous adhesions or a capsule and give an appearance similar to that of herniation (Theophelis and Stevenson, 1986).

Infection around a prosthesis producing inflammation of the breast makes mammography very unsatisfactory because the patient cannot tolerate much compression. Ultrasound, CT, and MRI are all more feasible in such patients, and any of these examinations will give diagnostically useful information about the prosthesis, the surrounding structures, and possible abscess formation (Fig. 6–11).

Fibrous capsules form around most implants (Speirs and Blocksma, 1963; Lilla and Vistnes, 1976). Occasionally the fibrous capsule has nodular components that may suggest a developing mass. If imaging studies indicate that the nodule is indeed in the capsule, conservative management may be chosen with an increased level of confidence (Fig. 6–12). Calcification in the capsule is commonly seen on mammography. This is a benign finding and, in the absence of any abnormality on clinical examination, requires no further investigation (Fig. 6–13).

SUMMARY

Improvements in mammography equipment and technique over the past two decades have made it a safe and valuable method for detailed evaluation of the breast. Although patients with implants do present spe-

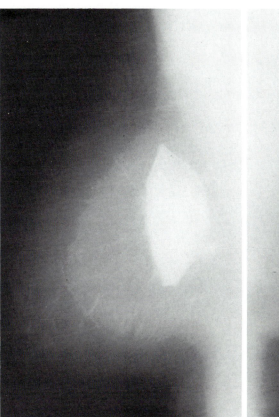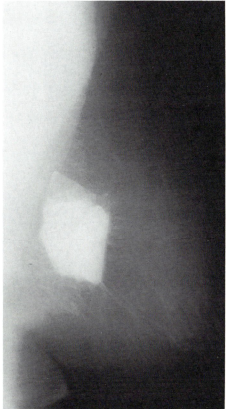

FIGURE 6–9
Lateral mammograms of each breast, demonstrating deflated saline implants. The patient was a 42-year-old male transsexual who had had saline implants and estrogen therapy to create a feminine appearance. When he decided to return to a male role, the implants were deflated percutaneously and estrogen therapy was discontinued. Note the infolded implants and the large amount of fat in the breast, due to the patient's large body habitus and also probably to estrogen. Mammograms were obtained because of the patient's concern that estrogen therapy could have caused cancer.

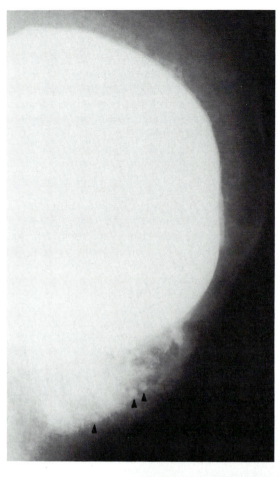

FIGURE 6–10

Lateral mammogram from a 75-year-old woman who noted a firm palpable mass, measuring about 2 cm in diameter, in the lower medial quadrant of her right breast. Prostheses had been inserted 10 years earlier. In the palpable area there are multiple, small, dense nodules representing siliconomas (arrowheads). Note also the localized skin thickening and the generalized, poorly defined increased density due to edema. Biopsy revealed inflammation and fibrosis due to leakage of silicone. No cancer was present.

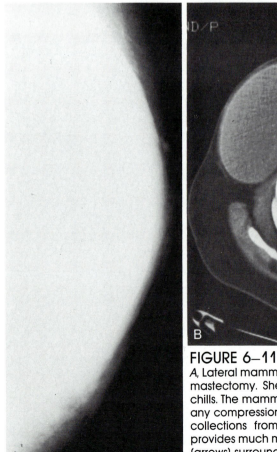

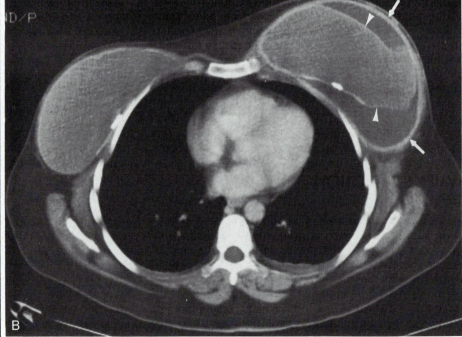

FIGURE 6–11

A, Lateral mammogram in a 36-year-old woman with implants following subcutaneous mastectomy. She presented with diffuse inflammation of the left breast, fever, and chills. The mammogram is of poor quality because of the patient's inability to tolerate any compression. It is not possible to evaluate the parenchyma or to distinguish fluid collections from the implant. B, Computed tomographic scan in same patient provides much more information. A collection of fluid is seen within the fibrous capsule (arrows) surrounding and compressing the prosthesis (arrowheads). Infection was due to a typical mycobacterium.

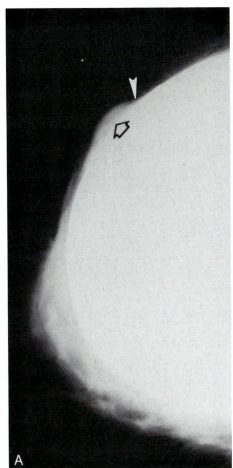

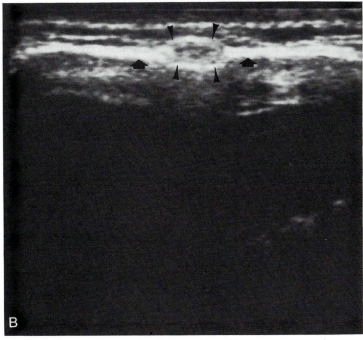

FIGURE 6-12

A, A 48-year-old woman presented with a small palpable nodule firmly adjacent to the implant. An oblique mammogram revealed a smooth-walled nodule (open arrow) adjacent to the prosthesis. The fibrous capsule (white arrowhead) is seen to envelop the nodule. *B*, Ultrasound scan of the nodule (arrowheads) shows that it is solid and that it is located within the fibrous capsule (arrows). This capsular nodule has been followed conservatively with no biopsy obtained.

FIGURE 6-13

Lateral view of the right breast, demonstrating calcification in a fibrous capsule. The patient was 40 years old and had had bilateral silicone implants placed 11 years prior to this study. Because of capsular contracture, the implants were removed 4 months before this study. Note that the fibrous capsule persists and is demarcated by numerous curvilinear calcifications (arrowheads). It is filled with fluid, creating a "natural" augmentation. The left breast had an identical appearance. A follow-up mammogram 1 year after this study showed no change in the fibrous capsules or the seromas they contained. (Courtesy of Edward A. Sickles, M.D., University of California, San Francisco.)

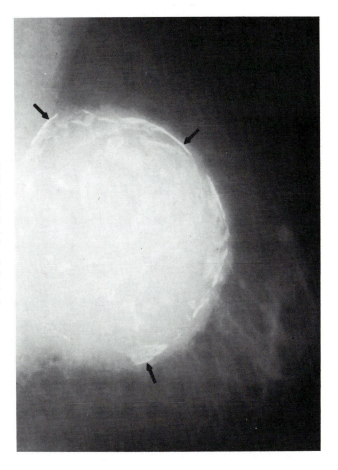

cial challenges to the radiologist, they can be successfully imaged, especially if a modified procedure, in which the prosthesis is excluded from compression, is used. We believe mammography is important in aesthetic breast surgery patients preoperatively for excluding occult malignancy, in asymptomatic women postoperatively for routine screening for occult cancer as recommended by the American Cancer Society, and for symptomatic women as an aid in clinical management. Other imaging techniques, specifically ultrasound, CT, and MRI, may be useful in this latter group.

References

Baker, L. H.: Breast cancer detection demonstration project: Five year summary report. CA 32:194, 1982.

Cohen, I. K., Goodman, H., Theogaraj, S. D.: Xeromammography: A reason for using saline-filled breast prostheses. Plast. Reconstr. Surg. 60:886, 1977.

Cole-Beuglet, C., Schwartz, G., Kurtz, A. B., Patchefsky, A. S., Goldberg, B. B.: Ultrasound mammography for the augmented breast. Radiology 146:737, 1983.

De Waal, J. C., Vaillant, W., Baltzer, J., Zander, J: A carcinoma of the breast behind a breast prosthesis (Letter). Comput. Radiol. 11:207, 1987.

Eklund, G. W., Busby, R. C., Miller, S. H., Job, J. S.: Improved imaging of the augmented breast. A.J.R. 151:469, 1988.

Grant, E. G., Cigtay, O. S., Mascatello, V. J.: Irregularity of Silastic breast implants mimicking a soft tissue mass. A.J.R. 130:461, 1978.

Hahn, H., Hoeffken, W.: Computerized tomography of breast cancer and regional lymph nodes. Diagn. Imag. Clin. Med. 54:165, 1985.

Heywang, S. H., Eiermann, W., Bassermann, R., Fenzl, G.: Carcinoma of the breast behind a prosthesis: Comparison of ultrasound, mammography and MRI (case report). Comput. Radiol. 9:283, 1985.

Hilton, S. W., Leopold, G. R., Olson, L. K., Wilson, S. A.: Real-time breast sonography: Application in 300 consecutive patients. A.J.R. 147:479, 1986.

Ho, W. C.: Radiographic evidence of breast implant rupture. Plast. Reconstr. Surg. 79:1009, 1987.

Hoopes, J. E., Edgerton, M. T., Shelley, W.: Organic synthetics for augmentation mammaplasty: Their relation to breast cancer. Plast. Reconstr. Surg. 39:263, 1967.

Jensen, S. R., Mackey, J. K.: Xeromammography after augmentation mammoplasty. A.J.R. 144:629, 1985.

Källen, R., Broomé, A., Mühlow, A., Forsby, N.: Reduction mammoplasty: Results of preoperative mammography and patient inquiry. Scand. J. Plast. Reconstr. Surg. 20:303, 1986.

Koides, T., Katayama, H.: Calcification in augmentation mammoplasty. Radiology 130:337, 1979.

Lilla, J. A., Vistnes, L. M.: Long-term study of reactions to various silicone breast implants in rabbits. Plast. Reconstr. Surg. 57:637, 1976.

Morgenstern, L., Gleischman, S. H., Michel, S. L., Rosenberg, J. E., Knight, I., Goodman, D.: Relation of free silicone to human breast carcinoma. Arch. Surg. 120:573, 1985.

Perras, C., Papillon, J.: The value of mammography in cosmetic surgery of the breasts. Plast. Reconstr. Surg. 52:132, 1973.

Pitanguy, I., Torres, E. T.: Histopathological aspects of mammary gland tissue in cases of plastic surgery of the breast. Br. J. Plast. Surg. 17:297, 1964.

Rintala, A. E., Svinhufvud, U. M.: Effect of augmentation mammaplasty on mammography and thermography. Plast. Reconstr. Surg. 54:390, 1974.

Rosenbaum, J. L., Bernadino, M. E., Thomas, J. L., Wigley, K. D.: Ultrasonic findings in silicone augmented breasts. South. Med. J. 74:455, 1981.

Seidman, H., Gelb, S. K., Silverberg, E., LaVerda, N., Lubera, J. A.: Survival experience in the breast cancer detection demonstration project. CA 37:258, 1987.

Silverstein, M. J., Handel, N., Gamagami, P., Waisman, J. R., Gierson, E. D., Rosser, R. J., Steyskal, R., Colburn, W.: Breast cancer in women after augmentation mammoplasty. Arch. Surg. 123:681, 1988.

Smith, D. S.: False-positive radiographic diagnosis of breast implant rupture: Report of two cases. Ann. Plast. Surg. 14:166, 1985.

Snyderman, R. K., Lizardo, J. G.: Statistical study of malignancies found before, during or after routine breast plastic operations. Plast. Reconstr. Surg. 25:253, 1960.

Speirs, A. C., Blocksma, R.: New implantable silicone rubbers: An experimental evaluation of tissue response. Plast. Reconstr. Surg. 31:166, 1963.

Tabar, L., Gad, A., Holmberg, L. H., Ljungquist, U., Fagerberg, C. J. G., Baldetorp, L., Grontoft, O., Lundstrom, B., Manson, J. C., Eklund, G., Pettersson, F., Day, N. E.: Reduction in mortality from breast cancer after mass screening with mammography. Lancet 1:829, 1985.

Theophelis, L. G., Stevenson, T. R.: Radiographic evidence of breast implant rupture. Plast. Reconstr. Surg. 78:673, 1986.

Wolfe, J. N.: On mammography in the presence of breast implants. (Letter). 62:286, 1978.

7

Thomas M. Biggs

Augmentation Mammaplasty: Inframammary Approach

The female breasts, long recognized as a badge of femininity, have for many centuries received notable attention and likewise efforts toward their enhancement. Corset makers, brassiere manufacturers, swimsuit designers, and all other creators of women's apparel have focused attention on the breasts and their role in the overall feminine mystique. Because of the emphasis our current society places on the breasts in cinema, television, periodicals, advertising, popular music, and the trend toward youth and vigor, any woman who sees herself with breasts smaller than those she perceives society expects may feel some degree of inadequacy. If this feeling of inadequacy is sufficient, she may seek surgical means to correct it.

Surgical correction for small breasts is not new. Early efforts toward breast enhancement included, among other things, implantation of foreign materials such as ivory, stainless steel, paraffin, rubber, and various plastic sponges (Gonzales-Ulloa, 1960). Either these efforts failed to create an aesthetically satisfactory result or the foreign body was rejected, or both. Dermal fat grafts were attempted but failed because of fat absorption (Conway and Smith, 1958). It was not until 1963, with the introduction of the Silastic gel prosthesis, that augmentation mammaplasty became an operation that could be performed with an expectation of minimal morbidity and some hope of a pleasing enhancement of the appearance of the breast (Cronin and Gerow, 1964). Since its introduction, the Silastic implant has been refined many times over, and the technique for its placement has evolved so that now the plastic surgeon and the patient can proceed with an augmentation mammaplasty with an even greater expectation of minimal morbidity and a much more reasonable expectation of a longer-lasting good appearance.

PREOPERATIVE CONSULTATION

The role of a physician is to extend the length of life or enhance the quality of life, or both. The woman who comes to a plastic surgeon for augmentation mammaplasty is actually coming with the hope that surgery will improve her quality of life. If it does not, she will be unhappy with her surgery and her surgeon. For this reason, accomplishment of the satisfactory result everyone seeks begins with the initial consultation. During this time, the surgeon can ascertain the patient's motivations and her expectations and can explain the operation and its potential shortfalls. If the patient's motivation is solely to please someone else, great caution should be entertained, because it is the author's experience that situations such as this often lead to disappointment when the third party then finds something else to be "wrong." When the patient's expectations exceed what the surgeon can produce, disappointment can occur; and when previously unmentioned complications occur, a very negative attitude can result. If, on the other hand, her motivation and her expectations are reasonable, and she has been suitably apprised of the various potential problems and is, therefore, prepared to deal with them if they should occur, the operation can be a very positive experience for both the patient and the surgeon.

After the nurse has taken an extensive medical history, which the surgeon reviews, the preoperative consultation begins with a few questions such as "Do you know much about this surgery?" or "Why do you want this operation?" Such questions prompt the patient to talk, and thereby both motivation and expectation can be determined. Upon completion of the history taking, the author leaves the examining room while the nurse drapes the patient; upon his return, an examination of the patient ensues that will determine whether augmentation mammaplasty will be of benefit (many patients would do better with mastopexy and some with augmentation mammaplasty and mastopexy). The author begins a small monologue by saying, "I prefer to do this operation in the operating room at the hospital with you sound asleep." The author explains why he prefers this approach and proceeds with a discussion of the location of the incision, the length of the scar, the location of the space to be dissected, the choice of implants, the type of closure, and the dressing. Explanations should be given regarding the recovery room and subsequent discharge, along with the regimen for postoperative care. Finally comes a discussion of the potential problems of hematoma, infection, hypertrophic scarring, nipple hypoesthesia, malposition, and firmness from contracture and their possible causes, methods employed to avoid them, and steps taken to correct them should they occur. The role of aspirin in bleeding is discussed and why it is mandatory to avoid aspirin for 10 days before surgery.

Before closing the discussion, the author mentions the possibility of malignancy and stresses that this operation does not prevent cancer but has not been implicated clinically as a cause of cancer. He further emphasizes the need for regular examination and routine xeromammography. At this point in the discussion it is explained that some controversy exists regarding the completeness of xeromammographic studies in implanted breasts but that many competent radiologists believe these limitations can be in great part overcome if the patient informs the radiologist of her previous surgery and special views are obtained.

The author believes it important to discuss these matters personally with the patient, because in addition to educating her, such a discussion gives the surgeon an opportunity to express the fact that he cares and that the patient's happiness (i.e., enhancement of her quality of life) is of the utmost importance. After this rather lengthy discussion, the patient is encouraged to ask questions so that when she leaves the examination-consultation room, she has as complete an understanding as possible of the surgery. She is sent to Photography, the Business Office for discussion of the economic aspect of the surgery, and finally to Scheduling, where a date for surgery is selected and instructions are given as to when and where she should go. Upon leaving the office, she is again asked whether she has any questions and told that if she should think of any later, she should call the surgeon's nurse or return for another consultation with the surgeon. If her scheduled date of surgery is more than 4 to 6 weeks away, she is encouraged to return (at no charge) for a repeat mini-consultation 1 to 3 days before the operation.

SELECTION OF THE IMPLANT

The author uses both the smooth gel and the polyurethane-covered implant. The preference at this time is to place a Silastic II gel implant beneath the pectoral muscle; but in cases of mild ptosis, or in cases of more pronounced ptosis requiring the placement of an implant and mastopexy, it is preferred to place the implant in a retroglandular position (Figs. 7–1 to 7–8). Patients who are obese or have a thick chest due to body habitus or muscle hypertrophy from resistance exercises have a better appearance with a retroglandular implant. A very thin soft tissue cover over the muscle would be an indication for retropectoral placement of the implant because of the visibility of a noncontracted capsule around a polyurethane implant. Because of the frequency of capsular contracture around a smooth-walled implant in the retroglandular space, the author prefers to use a polyurethane-covered implant in this area. It has been the experience of others (Hester, 1988) and our own that fibrous capsular contracture around a polyurethane-covered implant is extremely unusual.

Because of the difficulty of insertion of a polyurethane implant in a retroglandular space through the axilla, the axillary approach is reserved for smooth-walled implants behind the muscle.

Because of problems of deflation and the unnatural feeling of a saline-filled implant, the author has avoided

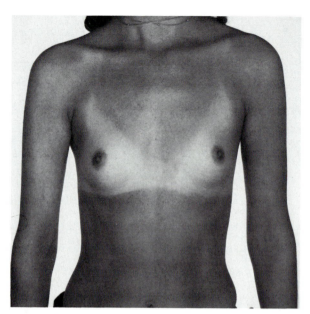

FIGURE 7–1
Preoperative anterior view of a candidate for augmentation mammaplasty using retromuscular placement of a gel implant. A 270-cc low-profile, round, Silastic II gel implant was used.

the use of inflatable implants (Williams, 1972). Because of the associated problems of steroid preparations, the author has avoided the use of these preparations instilled into the implant and avoids their use in the surgically dissected pocket (Carrico and Cohen, 1979).

OPERATIVE TECHNIQUE

The patient is placed in the supine position and a general endotracheal anesthetic is administered. A povi-

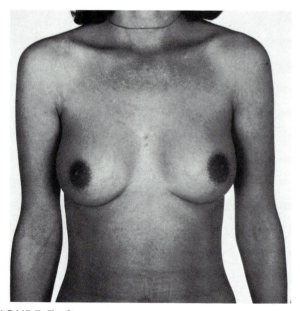

FIGURE 7–2
Anterior view of the patient shown in Figure 7–1, 3 months postoperatively.

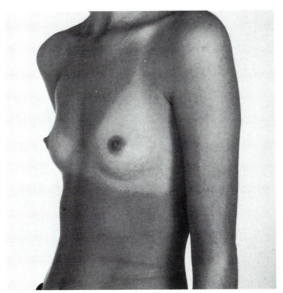

FIGURE 7–3
Preoperative oblique view of the patient shown in Figures 7–1 and 7–2, a candidate for retromuscular augmentation mammaplasty.

done-iodine (Betadine) and alcohol scrub is performed and the patient is draped. The proper location for the incision is determined by finding the true inframammary fold. This is on occasion difficult but can be more accurately found by grasping the breast upward and pushing in a caudal direction simultaneously (Figs. 7–9 to 7–11). If this is not done, the inframammary fold often will be considerably lower than the incision, and the resulting scar will ride up on the breast and will on occasion be hypertrophic. In these cases of high (and also short transversely) inframammary folds, it is imperative that the tissues at and above the fold be incised vertically so as to allow the fold to lengthen. Otherwise,

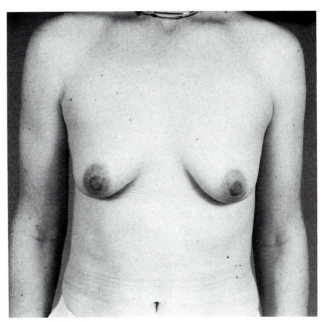

FIGURE 7–5
This patient had a moderate degree of ptosis and was therefore not a candidate for retromuscular augmentation.

a double-bubble effect will be encountered after the implant has been put into proper position. The ideal location for the inframammary fold is 5 to 7 cm below the areola; if this fold is less than this distance, problems can be expected if the preceding precautions are not taken. The angles of the inframammary fold are noted and if found to be obtuse will prompt, on closure, several sutures from the inferior flap to the chest wall to prevent inferior displacement of the implant and subsequent malposition.

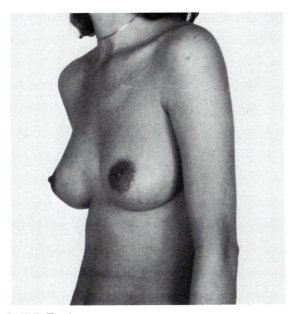

FIGURE 7–4
Oblique view of the patient shown in Figures 7–1 to 7–3, 3 months postoperatively.

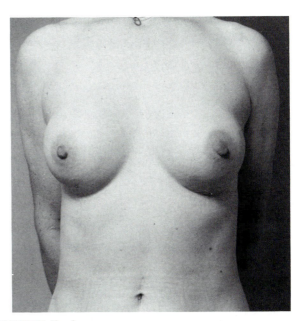

FIGURE 7–6
Patient shown in Figure 7–5, 4 months after augmentation mammaplasty using a 220-gm Même polyurethane-covered implant in the retroglandular position.

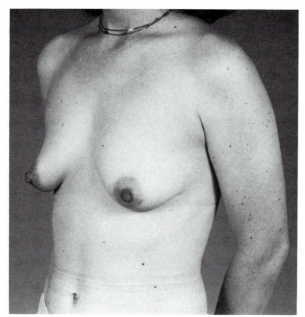

FIGURE 7–7
Preoperative oblique view of the patient shown in Figures 7–5 and 7–6.

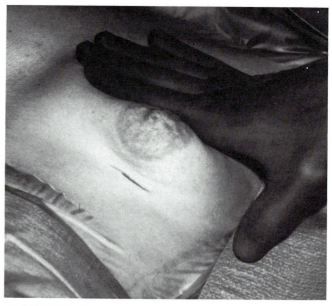

FIGURE 7–9
The apparent inframammary fold is that created by the breast as it falls onto the chest wall by gravity. This is determined by pushing caudally on the breast tissue.

After the sites of incisions are chosen, methylene blue is used to mark their location, and an incision is made on the initial breast 6 cm in length directly below the areola. This incision is made perpendicular to the skin and then in a somewhat cephalad direction to the fascia (again to prevent inferior displacement of the implant). At this point the location of the dissection depends on the type of implant to be used. If a polyurethane-covered implant is chosen (for the reasons mentioned previously), the dissection proceeds along the fascia of the pectoralis major and extends medially to the midline,

stopping short of the emerging vessels from the internal mammary artery, and laterally to the lateral edge of the latissimus dorsi. Careful dissection should be carried out laterally so as to expose and avoid cutting the sensory nerve to the nipple (Fig. 7–12). In a cephalad direction, the dissection extends above the clavicular portion of the pectoralis major but stops short of the clavicle (Fig. 7–13).

All of the dissection is done with either scissors or the cutting current of an electrosurgical unit. The latter

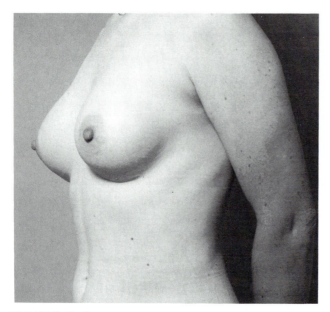

FIGURE 7–8
Oblique view of the patient shown in Figures 7–5 to 7–7, 4 months after retroglandular augmentation mammaplasty using a polyurethane implant.

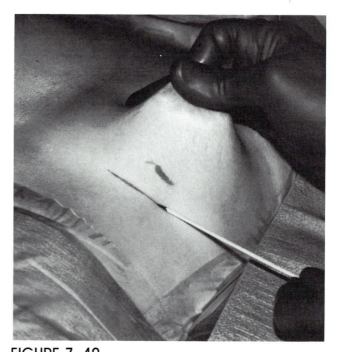

FIGURE 7–10
The true inframammary fold is determined by picking up on the breast tissue and then pushing caudally.

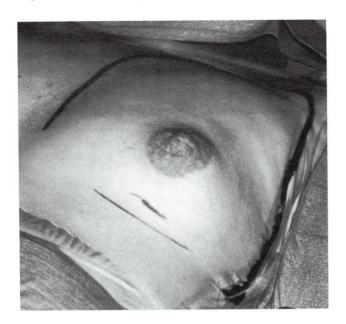

FIGURE 7—11
The relationship of the true to the apparent inframammary folds. If an incision is made in the apparent fold and an implant placed beneath the breast, the true fold will then become obvious and the scar from the incision will lie on the undersurface of the breast and not in the fold. In the author's experience, this contributes more frequently to the formation of hypertrophic scars that are generally more obtrusive.

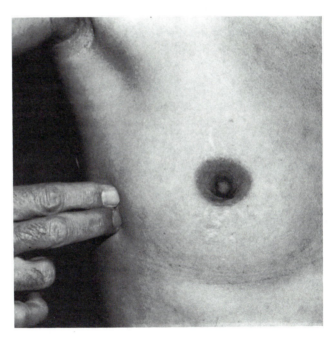

FIGURE 7—12
The anterior edge of the latissimus dorsi muscle and the site of the emergence of the sensory nerve to the nipple. The dissection is carried to this limit but is performed carefully for avoidance of damage to this nerve.

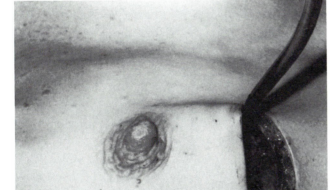

FIGURE 7—13
Dissection is carried to just below the clavicle but over the clavicular head of the pectoralis major muscle. The attachments of this muscle to the overlying tissues are stronger than the muscle itself. Dissection must therefore be sharp, rather than blunt, or the muscle itself will be shredded, leaving a false space and bleeding muscle, which will result in fibrosis and possibly contribute to fibrous capsular contracture and breast firmness.

is particularly efficient, in that hemostasis can be made more complete as one dissects; however, it is especially dangerous because of the ability to be very quickly out of the desired place of dissection, especially as the dissection proceeds near the clavicle. It may also be helpful to have the anesthesiologist administer a short-acting paralytic agent while dissecting in this fashion, for contracture of the muscle with the electric unit can cause a displacement of the edge of the blade and resultant mishap.

If a Silastic gel implant is to be used, the dissection proceeds beneath the pectoralis major muscle. This is accomplished by identifying the lateral edge of this muscle and then elevating it from the underlying ribs in a medial direction (Fig. 7–14). Great care should be taken to identify the serratus anterior muscle and to leave it attached to its origin while raising the pectoralis major. This can be difficult, because these two muscles share a conjoined origin from the ribs. Continued dissection medially and inferiorly separates the muscle from its origin off the fascia of the rectus abdominis inferiorly, and continuation of elevation is carried out in a cephalad direction along its medial border at the sternum. The objective is to raise the muscle from its origin sufficiently so that the inferolateral edge of the muscle will lie above the median of the implant. This prevents the problem of cephalad displacement of the implant with muscle contracture. The extent of cephalad dissection is more limited in the retropectoral pocket than in the retroglandular pocket because upward displacement of the implant under a contracted muscle creates such an unpleasant appearance (Fig. 7–15). Lateral dissection is carried sufficiently to allow ample room to accommodate the implant.

After the initial incision, all sponges are removed from the operating field, and only the suction is used for maintaining a dry space. Particles of sponge material have been found by electron microscopy within the fibrous capsule and may act as a foreign body and thus as a contributing factor in the development of fibrous capsular contracture (Upton and Persoff, 1976).

Direct visualization of the entire dissected space is made possible by the fiberoptic light employed by the surgeon and worn on the head. Lighted retractors offer

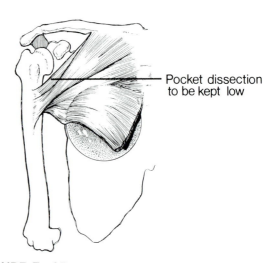

FIGURE 7–15
Extent of cephalad dissection is more limited in the retropectoral pocket than in the retroglandular so that an unpleasant appearance can be avoided upon contraction of the muscle.

advantage over the fixed overhead light, but because of fat and blood occluding the light on the end of the retractor, they are believed to be inferior to those worn by the surgeon and directed wherever he is looking (Fig. 7–16).

After completion of the dissection, hemostasis is made secure by careful visualization of the entire dissected space. This is accompanied by extensive irrigation until the irrigant that is returned is clear. If fresh blood is seen in the irrigant, continued search is carried out until

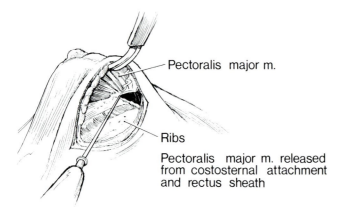

FIGURE 7–14
The pectoralis major muscle released from costosternal attachment and the rectus sheath.

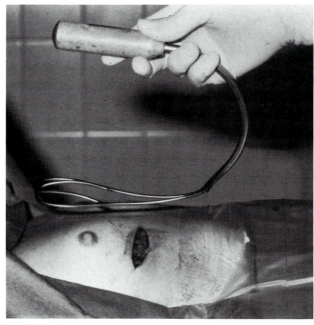

FIGURE 7–16
A good retractor and a fiberoptic light mounted on the surgeon's forehead provide the best visualization possible. The entire operation is performed under adequate direct vision so that hemostasis will be complete and this little trauma will not affect the pectoralis major muscle and sensory nerves to the skin.

all bleeding vessels, regardless of their size, are electro-desiccated. (The electrodesiccation is carried out carefully so that a minimal amount of charred tissue remains in the space, because this also may contribute to subsequent contracture.) Except for the last few drops, the irrigant is allowed to flow out of the wound (not aspirated) so that maximal amount of foreign material, loose fat, or clots will come out with it.

After securing hemostasis and irrigating thoroughly, a trial implant is placed into the cavity and the appropriate size is determined, keeping in mind the patient's wishes and allowing adequate space for the implant to move within the cavity. The trial implant is then removed, the wound irrigated again, and hemostasis determined for the last time. The container holding the selected implant is opened, and the surgeon removes the implant from its package. No one else touches it. The surgeon places it into the space, taking care that it does not touch the paper drapes or the patient's skin (to avoid dust or wood particles from the drapes and bacterial contamination from the skin). The wound is closed in three layers with 3-0 and 4-0 Vicryl and a subcuticular suture of 4-0 Prolene. Steri-Strips are placed over the closure. If a retroglandular dissection has been performed and a polyurethane-covered implant selected, the author prefers a higher-profile prosthesis (Replicon) placed somewhat obliquely with the superior portion of the implant turned somewhat inward so as to achieve minimal step-off deformity where it can be seen most readily, that is, cephalad medially. The slightly teardrop shape of the Replicon seems to give better contour.

Insertion of a polyurethane implant must be done as atraumatically as possible because a tear in the cover can result in a migration of tissue fluid around the inner shell of the implant and fibrous contracture. Gentle insertion is best accomplished with the use of the sleeve provided by the manufacturer (Figs. 7–17 to 7–18).

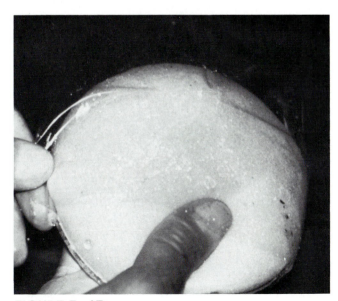

FIGURE 7–17
A polyurethane-covered implant encased in a sleeve provided by the manufacturer.

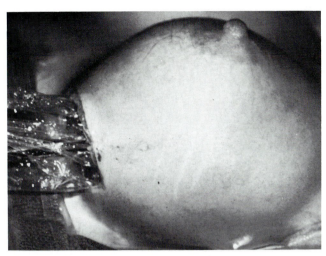

FIGURE 7–18
Insertion of the polyurethane-covered implant shown in Figure 7–17.

In cases of a tight chest in which the dissected space is small and causes limitation of the size of the implant that can be employed, a temporary tissue expander is placed into the space and inflated to approximately 1000 cc. This is left in place on each side for approximately 15 minutes, allowing the tissues to stretch and thereby accept a larger implant. This technique is used both in the retromuscular dissection and in the retroglandular dissection for the polyurethane implant.

POSTOPERATIVE CARE

The patient returns to the office the day after surgery for removal of the bandages. If she has remained in the hospital overnight, they are removed there. The purpose of early bandage removal is twofold. If there is any suggestion of blood in the cavity, the patient is returned to the operating room, where the implant is withdrawn, the blood removed, hemostasis ensured, the wound irrigated, and the implant replaced. The second reason for the bandage removal is to instruct the patient on how to move the implant around the space, a maneuver designed to keep the space open by preventing the superior portion of the dissection from adhering to its underlying surface. This maneuver need only be done once daily. The author feels that "massage" of the breast is possibly counterproductive because bacteria can be displaced from ducts into the breast tissue and mastitis created, which in turn can lead to an increased fibrous capsule thickness and subsequent firmness. If a polyurethane-covered implant is used, no manipulation is recommended.

The patient is advised to refrain from any activity more vigorous than walking for 3 weeks, although many patients return to a sedentary occupation several days after surgery. The running subcuticular Prolene suture is removed 6 to 8 days after surgery. Follow-up visits, at no cost to the patient, are pursued with persistence up to 1 year, although patients who are doing well and are happy with their surgery are reluctant to return for follow-up visits. The need for continued long-term follow-up should be emphasized.

COMPLICATIONS

Although in past years the frequency of problems has dropped and the number of happy and satisfied patients continues to rise, occasionally complications occur. As mentioned earlier, these problems are much more easily managed if they are mentioned beforehand because the patient is more prepared to deal with their resolution in a cooperative way.

Hematoma occurred more frequently when some of our dissection was blind and before the anticoagulant effects of aspirin were understood. It still does occur, however, especially in persons with labile hypertension. The problem is managed aggressively by returning to the operating room for removal of the hematoma; aspiration with a needle or suction in the office is not sufficient. The author has never seen a patient in whom free blood was suspected in the surgical space in whom fibrous capsular contracture was not present within several months. Patients with a suggestion of hypertension are watched closely in the recovery room, and chlorpromazine hydrochloride (Thorazine) may be given at the first suggestion of an increase in pressure or, in select cases, may be given before the patient leaves the operating room.

Infection is a sequela of any surgery and is a particular problem when a foreign material is inserted and left in the body. Improvements in technique and use of antibiotics have reduced the incidence of infection to less than 1%; but when it does occur, removal of the implant usually is necessary for resolution of the infection. In the author's experience, if the implant is not removed, a contracture will occur; and a surgical release will be necessary within several months. The author has, in his experience, seen two cases in which exposure of the polyurethane implant, unlike the Silastic gel implant, was encountered and the wound was allowed to granulate and epithelialize, without infection or fibrous contracture. In the case of exposure of a smooth-walled implant, it has always been necessary to remove the implant and leave the implant out for several months before replacement.

Hypertrophic scarring has resulted at the site of the incision. As in surgery at other sites in the body, hypertrophy of the scar is unpredictable; but in review of those following augmentation mammaplasty, it seemed to occur more often when the implant descended below the level of the inframammary fold and the lower portion of the bra lay below the scar, creating pressure below the scar (and thus impairment of lymphatic drainage). Treatment has been to encourage the patient to massage the scar frequently or to obtain a bra with a broad strap so as to put pressure directly on top of the hypertrophic scar. In more severe cases, excision has been employed, and occasionally steroids have been injected. The author has been reluctant to use therapeutic irradiation because of the concern for the carcinogenic potential of irradiation around the breast tissue.

Hypoesthesia of the nipple has been a more frequent occurrence with more extensive dissection. With careful dissection the nerve that emerges from under the serratus anterior muscle laterally can often be visualized and damage avoided. A return of sensation has been observed in most instances but may be delayed for as long as 6 to 9 months.

Malposition of the implant is usually caused by an inferior descensus. This is caused by dissecting the inferior flap. This dissection may be unplanned, the result of traction. In some patients, the areolar tissue attaching the skin and subcutaneous tissue to the fascia is unduly loose, making this complication more likely. This can be avoided first by dissecting through the subcutaneous tissue in a somewhat cephalad direction, and second by placing several sutures from the subcutaneous tissue of the inferior flap to the fascia at the time of closure. This problem is also more often seen when the angle created by the breast on the chest is obtuse. The problem is, furthermore, more frequent with the use of steroids if administered in high concentration and allowed to pool inferiorly. Once the malposition is noted, some form of pressure may be employed to obliterate this space but must be continued for at least 3 months. If no progress is noted, the patient must be returned to the operating room for an excision of the fibrous sheath lining this space and reclosure. It has been suggested that 5 ml of whole blood injected into this area will obliterate the space naturally, but the author has no experience with this modality (Flowers, 1979). Malposition may also occur from too extensive a dissection cephalad, so that when the woman becomes recumbent the implant rides up onto her shoulder. This problem is not encountered with polyurethane-covered implants. Treatment for a high-riding implant is rarely surgical and often responds to pressure. Lateral drift, like descensus, may need operative correction. Other forms of malposition, if not the result of fibrous capsular contracture, are usually associated with asymmetry that was present preoperatively. It is wise to observe this and to describe it to the patient before the operation. If this has not been done, an examination of the preoperative photograph often will reveal this anomaly (although it must be recognized that nearly all women have some degree of breast asymmetry).

Firmness of the breast from contracture of the fibrous capsule that surrounds the implant has been the most constant and the most disconcerting complication in augmentation mammaplasty. In the author's early experience, this occurred sufficiently to result in at least one breast feeling firmer than one would wish in 64% of the patients after 1 year. Modifications of the implant and refinement in technique have improved the results so that, more recently, grade II to IV contracture developed in only 17% of retroglandular augmentations and only 9% of retromuscular augmentations. It is the author's view that any report on mammaplasty based on patients followed less than 1 year carries doubt as to its validity.

The cause of firmness of the breast following augmentation mammaplasty is the contracture of the fibrous capsule that forms around the implant sufficiently to cause an increased pressure on the implant to change the soft gel feeling to one of a more solid form. The cause of the contracture is the question. If the space into which the implant is placed is of relatively the same size as that of the implant, even the most minimal contracture (and some degree of contracture of any mature fibrous sheet must be considered physiologic) will apply pressure to the prosthesis, resulting in firmness. For this reason, we began making a much more extensive dissection. The clinical observation that all patients with blood in the dissected space developed firmness prompted us to seek and maintain a space void of blood. (Drains have been used at intervals throughout our experience, and each time we have been convinced that they increased problems, rather than decreased them. They are still used, however, in occasional cases of persistent uncontrolled oozing.) Obtaining hemostasis has been far easier since the introduction of the fiberoptic head light. Studies of the fibrous capsule using an electron microscope revealed numerous foreign bodies, which could be avoided by extensive irrigation of the cavity, cleaning of the operator's gloves, and minimal handling of the implants. The cause of contracture most difficult to deal with is infection. If the infection is purulent, the implant must be removed. If the implant stays in with a lower-grade infection responsive to antibiotics, a fibrous capsular contracture usually occurs. An even lower grade infection is probably the most common cause of contracture (Courtiss et al., 1979). Studies revealing the presence of *Staphylococcus epidermidis* in the capsule suggest that this otherwise mild organism may stimulate enough reaction to contract a capsule but not enough to otherwise cause alarm (Burkhardt et al., 1981).

The presence of pain in the breast is the only sign of impending contracture and is often seen several days before the contracture is noted. For this reason, the author promptly initiates antibiotic therapy when a patient complains of pain in an otherwise normal breast. *S. epidermidis*, which is normal flora on the skin, probably infects the tissues around the implant by way of the lactiferous ducts; this is a process that may take months to occur.

Over the course of years, the author has heard patients complain that they had some form of clinical infection such as influenza, gastroenteritis, or cystitis and several days later had a painful breast followed by a fibrous capsular contracture. The author has been unable to culture any organisms from these capsules but believes the contracture is probably related to the same organism that caused the initial problem. Antibiotics are again encouraged and should be considered if the patient contracts some infectious process in other areas. The fact that the implant "bleeds" has been established, and whether this phenomenon is of any significance is yet to be determined (Wickham et al., 1978). In the meantime, principal manufacturers are proceeding with research on and development of a nonbleeding prosthesis.

A complication this author has not seen but which has been mentioned and must be respected is human adjuvant disease following silicone implantation. A review by Sergott et al. (1986) suggests this phenomenon but points out that reports are anecdotal and have little substance. Nevertheless, a conscientious clinician will concern himself with any and all possible problems in his patients; therefore, human adjuvant disease and its variants should be kept in mind.

SUMMARY

Augmentation mammaplasty has undergone an evolution of technique and implant design over the past 25 years. Approximately 2,000,000 women in the United States have undergone the procedure, and 130,000 to 140,000 such procedures are performed annually. Despite complications, which are still present but lessening, satisfaction runs high, in that the procedure accomplishes its purpose, to enhance a woman's sense of well-being by improving the size and shape of her breasts. By enhancing her sense of well-being, the surgeon is successful because he or she thus makes the patient's life better.

References

Biggs, T., Cukier, J., Worthing, L.: Augmentation mammaplasty: A review of eighteen years. Plast. Reconstr. Surg. 69:445, 1982.

Biggs, T., Yarish, R. S.: Augmentation mammaplasty: Retropectoral versus retromammary implantation. Clin. Plast. Surg. 15:549, 1988.

Burkhardt, B., Fried, M., Schnur, P., et al.: Capsules, infection, and intraluminal antibiotics. Plast. Reconstr. Surg. 68:43, 1981.

Carrico, T., Cohen, I.: Capsular contracture and steroid related complications after augmentation mammaplasty. Plast. Reconstr. Surg. 64:377, 1979.

Conway, H., Smith, J., Jr.: Breast plastic surgery: Reduction mammaplasty, mastopexy, augmentation mammaplasty and mammary construction. Plast. Reconstr. Surg. 21:8, 1958.

Courtiss, E., Goldwyn, R., Anastasi, G.: The fate of breast implants with infections around them. Plast. Reconstr. Surg. 63:812, 1979.

Cronin, T., Gerow, F.: Augmentation mammaplasty: A new "natural feel" prosthesis. Transactions of the Third International Congress of Plastic Surgery. Amsterdam, Excerpta Medica Foundation, 1964, p. 41.

Flowers, R.: Personal communication, 1979.

Gonzales-Ulloa, M.: Correction of hypotrophy of the breast by means of exogenous material. Plast. Reconstr. Surg. 25:15, 1960.

Hester, T. R., Jr.: The polyurethane-covered mammary prosthesis: Facts and fiction. Perspectives in Plastic Surgery 2:1, 1988.

Sergott, T., Limoli, J., Baldwin, C., Laub, D.: Human adjuvant disease, possible autoimmune disease after silicone implantation: A review of the literature, case studies, and speculation for the future. Plast. Reconstr. Surg. 78:104, 1986.

Upton, J., Persoff, M.: Personal communication, 1976.

Wickham, M., Rudolph, R., Abraham, J.: Silicone identification in prosthesis-associated fibrous capsules. Science 199:437, 1978.

Williams, J.: Experience with a large series of Silastic breast implants. Plast. Reconstr. Surg. 49:253, 1972.

G. Patrick Maxwell

Transaxillary Subpectoral Augmentation Mammaplasty

Transaxillary subpectoral augmentation mammaplasty is an excellent operative procedure for a select patient population (Peterson, 1984; Tebbetts, 1984, 1988). Its primary advantage is a resultant scarless breast achieved through a straightforward, quickly performed, and reproducible operative approach. Its disadvantage is the difficulty in learning the procedure and its nuances, in placing polyurethane-covered implants through this approach, and in going back through the axilla for a subsequent operation should the need arise. The operation is not difficult to perform, but rather requires a reorientation of thinking for the surgeon who is accustomed to the inframammary approach and has not previously performed the transaxillary technique. At this point I do not attempt to place polyurethane implants through this incision, but it is possible. I advise patients preoperatively that should there arise a need for reoperating upon the breast, an inframammary incision would be made. Textured silicone implants may be inserted via the transaxillary approach.

PATIENT SELECTION

Patients with relatively small breasts and relatively loose inframammary folds are ideal candidates for this operation (see Fig. 8–10). Tight inframammary folds and especially high, tight inframammary folds are potential problems (Maxwell, 1984). With the former, if the operation is performed, it should be done very cautiously; with the latter, this procedure should be strictly avoided. Since dissection is done from a distance, no direct fold scoring is possible, and if dissection is carried below the fold in these cases, an undesirable double-bubble appearance of the lower breast may result. Patients with ptosis and pseudoptosis generally are not candidates for this procedure.

OPERATIVE TECHNIQUE

With the patient in the upright position preoperatively, a line is drawn along the anterior axillary fold at the posterior border of the pectoralis major muscle. A second line is drawn 1.5 cm posterior and parallel to the first line. A dot is then made in the apex of the axilla in the hair-bearing area. The highest transverse natural

skin crease below this point is generally selected for the incision. A line is drawn in this crease beginning at the second line (1.5 cm behind the pectoralis major posterior border) and extending approximately 4.5 cm in length toward the posterior axillary fold (Fig. 8–1).

A mark is then made in each inframammary fold. A second mark is made about 1 to 1.5 cm below the first mark tailored to a point meeting the upper line medially and laterally. This line represents the inferior extent of the pocket dissection (see Fig. 8–1).

The patient is placed on the operating table in the supine position with her arms adducted to a 90-degree angle. The arm boards must be well padded, and the arms are secured to the padded arm boards by straps. General anesthesia is preferable, although local anesthesia is possible. An endotracheal tube is used because the patient will be cranked into an upright position several times during the operation. The patient's position on the operating table must be checked to be certain she will go into the desired straight sitting position. An automatic operating room table is used.

The patient is prepared and then draped, care being taken to secure the drapes in the axilla to avoid contamination. This may be done by stapling or suturing the drapes to the skin or by use of an adherent plastic drape. Lidocaine (0.25% Xylocaine) in 1:400,000 epinephrine in iced solution is injected into the axilla and the inframammary fold area.

The incision is made through the skin, and then subcutaneous undermining is carried out with scissors toward the posterior lateral border of the pectoralis major muscle (Fig. 8–2). This should be done over a relatively wide area and not into the axillary fat pad. Nerves are avoided, and hemostasis is controlled throughout. When the pectoralis major muscle is encountered, the dissection is carried deep to its lateral border for identifying the fascial plane between the pectoralis major and the pectoralis minor muscles. It is crucial to identify this plane accurately, because if the dissection is carried deep to the pectoralis minor, excessive bleeding will occur and correct identification of the desired plane will be even more difficult. Finger dissection is used for the initial and upper dissection (Fig. 8–3). Care is taken to avoid injury superiorly to the thoracoacromial vessels on the underside of the pectoralis major muscle and to the axillary vein and brachial plexus structures in the superiormost extent of the

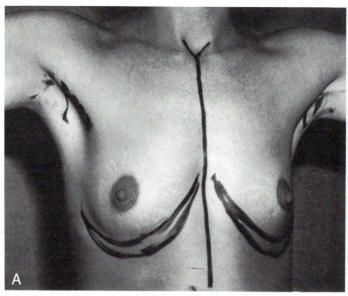
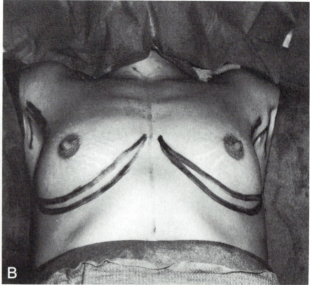

FIGURE 8–1

A, Preoperative markings made in the sitting position: the mark of the anterior axillary fold (pectoralis major muscle border), the mark made posterior to it, the transverse mark in the high axillary crease, the mark in the inframammary fold, and the mark inferior to the inframammary fold. B, These markings are better demonstrated with the patient in the supine position and arms adducted to a 90-degree angle.

pocket. Care should also be taken to avoid injury to the intercostobrachial and pectoral nerves. A Padgett Agris-Dingman axillary dissector (Agris et al., 1976) is used for additional upper pocket dissection and lower pocket dissection. One uses a sweeping motion, working from

medial to lateral and exerting moderately strong forcefulness (Fig. 8–4). This medial-to-lateral movement also protects the intercostal nerves in the low lateral pocket. The pocket should be dissected exactly to the lower of the two inframammary fold marks. Care must be taken to keep the inferior extent of the dissection smooth and accurate. The dissection must not be too low. It will elevate the origin of the pectoralis major muscle such that the implant will be covered by muscle only in its upper portion. Care is taken throughout to avoid excessive retraction or pressure on the anterior incision skin edge in the axilla, because this can be inadvertently lengthened.

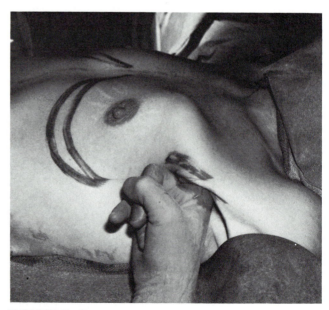

FIGURE 8–2

Following the incision, scissor dissection is carried out in the subcutaneous plane. The surgeon works anteriorly until the posterolateral border of the pectoralis major muscle is identified.

FIGURE 8–3

When the correct plane has been clearly identified, finger dissection initiates the pocket.

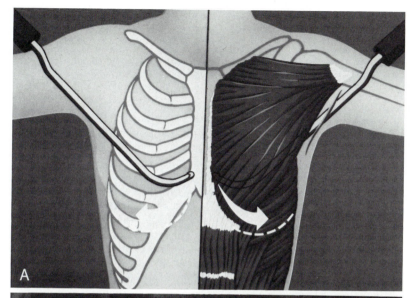

FIGURE 8–4

A, The pocket is dissected inferiorly with the use of the Padgett Agris-Dingman dissector and sweeping medial to lateral strokes. B, Moderate resistance is met medially as the dissection is begun. C, The dissection is extended laterally in the inferior portion, but attachments in the upper lateral pocket (along the anterior axillary fold) are preserved.

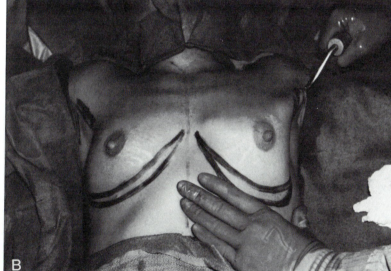

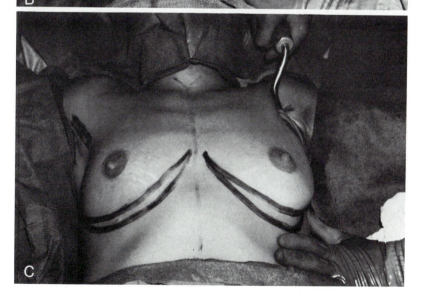

When pocket dissection has been completed, a smooth silicone sizer prosthesis is inserted, and the patient is cranked into an upright sitting position (Fig. 8–5). The implant is pressed inferiorly for demarcation of the inferior pocket dissection. The implant should not cause an upper breast pole convexity. If present, this is alleviated by lowering the pocket dissection inferiorly (if appropriate) or reducing the volume of the prosthesis. A marking pen is used to mark any pocket adjustments that need to be made.

The patient is placed back in the supine position, the sizer prosthesis is removed, and final pocket adjustments are completed. The pocket is then irrigated with saline until clear (to be certain there is no significant bleeding) and then with a 50% povidone-iodine (Betadine) solution (Burkhardt et al., 1986). Drains are rarely used, but may be necessary when there is persistent lower pocket bleeding. A Vacutainer drain would then be used, exited through a small stab wound in the axilla.

A high-profile smooth-wall silicone implant is selected, the volume based on the use of the sizer prosthesis and knowledge of the patient's preoperative wishes (Fig. 8–6). This may be a silicone gel, double-lumen, or saline-filled prosthesis. Textured silicone implants may also be used. Implants are placed in both breasts, and the patient is again elevated to a sitting position and assessed. Final adjustments are made prior to placing the patient again supine and wound closure. Wound closure should be exact. No deep layers are closed. An intradermal running subcuticular suture is utilized (Fig. 8–7), and a longitudinal Steri-Strip is placed over it. The inframammary folds are then taped with Elastoplast for exactness (Fig. 8–8) and a 4-inch Ace bandage is wrapped circumferentially around the upper breasts (superior to the nipples) to keep the implants down in the pockets for the first 24 hours. Cephalosporin is given intravenously intraoperatively and continued orally for 5 days postoperatively.

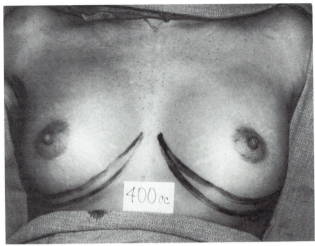

FIGURE 8–6
Final implants (400 cc) used in the patient in Figure 8–5, reevaluated in the upright position.

POSTOPERATIVE CARE

The patient begins implant displacement on the following day (Fig. 8–9). (The Ace bandage is removed for the exercises and rewrapped.) She is seen in the office 2 to 3 days after surgery. Displacement exercises are checked, and the breasts evaluated. Circumferential Ace bandage wrap may be reinstituted if there is any

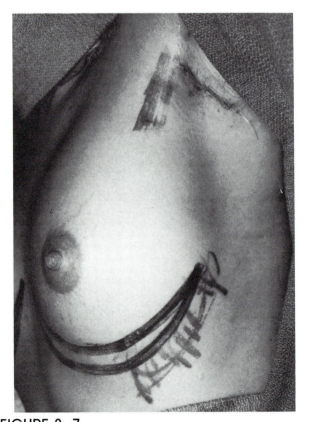

FIGURE 8–7
Wound closure with a single intradermal suture. Note lateral inframammary markings that were made with the patient in the upright position. The need for additional pocket dissection was determined.

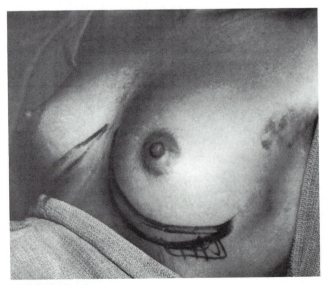

FIGURE 8–5
After sizer prostheses have been inserted, the patient is cranked into an upright sitting position for evaluation of pocket dissection, inframammary fold location and curvature, and implant volume.

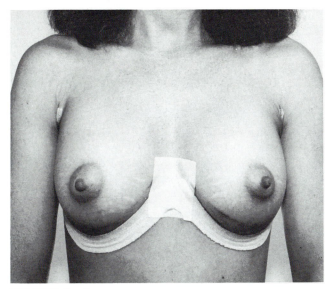

FIGURE 8–8
Appearance in the office on the second postoperative day. Note the original inframammary fold mark and tape-reinforced newly established lower inframammary fold. The dissection has been carried out to (but not below) the lower mark. The tape simply helps ensure its exactness.

upper breast fullness. The patient is seen weekly for 3 weeks, then monthly for 3 months, and finally on a routine 6-month basis (Figs. 8–10 and 8–11).

COMPLICATIONS

The most frequent complications with this operation are resultant inframammary fold irregularities, usually occurring when the operation is performed by a less experienced surgeon and relating primarily to patient selection and secondarily to operative technique. Excessive bleeding and hematoma formation are infrequent

unless the incorrect plane (deep to the pectoralis minor) is entered. Transient sensory loss may be encountered on the undersurface of the arm if sensory nerves are injured. Subcutaneous axillary contracture bands may occur early if the patient does not begin adequate arm and shoulder movement. These disappear with massage. Occasionally, an early scar may be thick (usually in the subcutaneous location), but I have never seen a bad long-term scar from this approach.

ADDITIONAL ISSUES

Intraoperative Expansion
(Maxwell and Fisher, 1988)

Because most patients selected for this operation have relatively small breasts, we have found the use of immediate intraoperative expansion helpful in pocket stretching and the subsequent placement of larger-volume implants. A tissue expander is inserted into the dissected pocket and filled to a volume of 700 to 900 cc and kept in place for around 15 minutes (while the opposite side is dissected) (Fig. 8–12). After its removal, an implant with an average increased volume of 25% can be inserted, as compared with the volume used if the expansion had not been carried out. This is necessary only with breasts having relatively tight skin or when larger-volume resultant breasts are desired.

Selective Pectoral Neurectomy
(Maxwell, 1988)

We have studied clinically the elective intraoperative division of the medial pectoral nerve, which innervates the lower third of the pectoralis major muscle, because the denervated muscle is more flaccid, allowing more anterior pole breast projection and at the same time

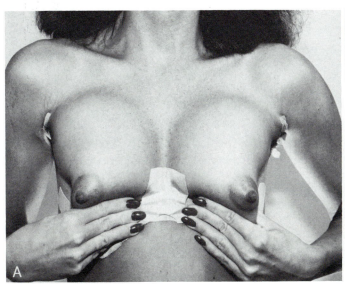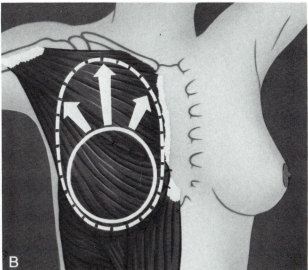

FIGURE 8–9
A, Displacement of the implant is begun on the first postoperative day. This is checked on the first office visit. B, The implant is displaced to the superiormost aspect of the pocket, not simply "massaged."

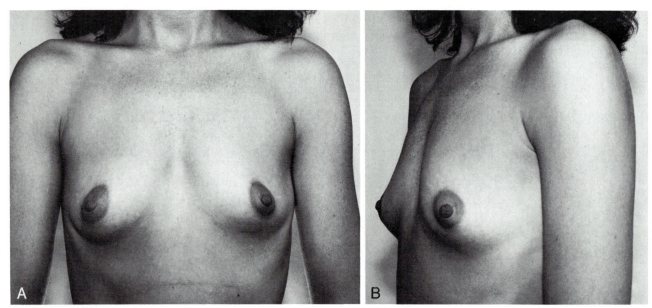

FIGURE 8–10
A and *B*, Preoperative appearance.

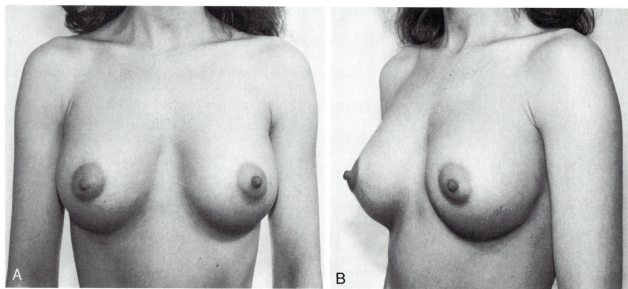

FIGURE 8–11
A and *B*, Postoperative appearance.

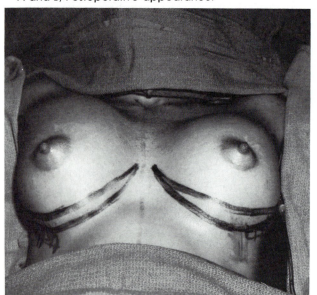

FIGURE 8–12
Immediate intraoperative expansion. For obtaining a larger breast, tissue expanders have been filled to 750 cc in each dissected pocket. (Note intravenous extension tubing going to the left axillary incision.) This tissue manipulation allowed the placement of the 400-cc implants shown in Figure 8–6.

minimizing postoperative flexion-induced breast deformity. Although there may be some validity to this procedure (and we have not encountered any complications), we no longer are performing it in routine transaxillary subpectoral augmentation, because our long-term results do not seem to give conclusive support to the premise.

CONCLUSION

Transaxillary subpectoral augmentation mammaplasty is an excellent operative technique yielding an enlarged breast without a surgical scar. Patient selection is critical, as is attention to operative technical detail.

References

Agris, J., Dingman, R. O., Wilensky, R. J.: A dissector for transaxillary approach in augmentation mammaplasty. Plast. Reconstr. Surg. 57:10, 1976.

Burkhardt, B. R., Dempsey, P. D., Schnur, P. L., Tofield, J. J.: Capsular contracture: A prospective study of the effect of local antibacterial agents. Plast. Reconstr. Surg. 77:919, 1986.

Maxwell, G. P.: Discussion of Tebbetts, J. B.: Transaxillary subpectoral augmentation mammaplasty: Long-term follow-up and refinements. Plast. Reconstr. Surg. 74:648, 1984.

Maxwell, G. P., Fisher, J.: The use of immediate intraoperative expansion in aesthetic and reconstructive breast surgery. Presented at the Annual Meeting of the American Society of Aesthetic Plastic Surgeons, San Francisco, California, March 1988.

Maxwell, G. P., Tornambe, R.: Management of mammary subpectoral implant distortion. Clin. Plast. Surg. 15:601, 1988.

Peterson, R.: Axillary approach. In: Regnault, P., Daniel, R. K. (eds.): *Aesthetic Plastic Surgery*. Boston, Little, Brown, 1984, p. 572.

Tebbetts, J. B.: Transaxillary subpectoral augmentation mammaplasty: Long-term follow-up and refinements. Plast. Reconstr. Surg. 74:636, 1984.

Tebbetts, J. B.: Transaxillary subpectoral augmentation mammaplasty: A 9-year experience. Clin. Plast. Surg. 15:557, 1988.

9

Ronald P. Gruber
Gary D. Friedman

Periareolar Subpectoral Augmentation Mammaplasty

The operation of periareolar subpectoral augmentation mammaplasty grew out of frustration with the high incidence and unpredictability of capsular contracture, breast scars, and inadequate subpectoral visualization. It had been known for some time that postmastectomy breast reconstruction was best accomplished by placing an implant beneath the pectoralis major, if not beneath the serratus anterior as well. The difference in results between suprapectoral and subpectoral implant location was quite dramatic. Submuscular relocation of the implant was also very helpful for those patients who had developed capsular contracture after subcutaneous mastectomy (Fig. 9–1). Many investigators (Biggs, 1983; Mahler and Hauben, 1982) began, therefore, to put the implant under the muscle for routine augmentation mammaplasty following Dempsey and Latham's (1968) lead. Capsular contractures were particularly a problem for the small-breasted patient and one who had thin skin. If capsular contracture occurred in these patients, it gave a very pronounced spherical appearance to the breast that was quite objectionable (McGrath, 1986). The scar that had been used for the inframammary approach to a subpectoral implant placement was reasonable but often not as satisfactory as a periareolar scar (Regnault and Daniel, 1984). Finally, exposure for adequate dissection and hemostasis was lacking in the axillary and inframammary approach. For the above three reasons the authors decided in 1979 to perform subpectoral implantation via the periareolar route. The results of this modification of subpectoral augmentation mammaplasty were first presented by the authors in 1981 (Gruber and Friedman, 1981; Gruber, 1981).

The first patient to undergo this procedure was a woman who was studying to become a court reporter. She had well-shaped breasts that were of medium size. There was a question of whether or not an experimental modification of augmentation mammaplasty should even be done in a sufficiently endowed patient who had some "knowledge of the law." To minimize the chances of capsular contracture, it was clear that the implant should be placed subpectorally. The problem was the potential scar. It was also thought that the axillary approach would not allow insertion of the size implant she requested. The periareolar approach was considered because of its potential for a good scar. However, the concern was the technical difficulty of working through

a small incision, in a deep hole, and relying on a head light for illumination. The final outcome was that the operation was successful, the patient became a court reporter, and periareolar subpectoral augmentation became the authors' operation of choice.

INDICATIONS

The indications for surgery include virtually every patient who is otherwise a candidate for augmentation mammaplasty. One exception would be that patient who has an unusually small areola. However, in some cases with small areola, a decision has been made to make a slight extension lateral to the infra-areolar incision so that a larger opening is possible for the implant insertion. Otherwise, a transaxillary subpectoral approach is used (Peterson, 1983). Extending the areola incision from 2 to 10 o'clock is not employed. An inframammary subpectoral approach is rarely used, simply because there will be a few patients in whom an inframammary scar could not be corrected adequately if correction were indicated. It is generally accepted that inframammary scars (even those that are on the breast side) are usually more visible than periareolar scars.

Where a mild to moderate degree of ptosis occurs, patients are considered for periareolar subpectoral augmentation just as they would be for suprapectoral augmentation mammaplasty. When the ptosis is moderate to severe and the patient refuses mastopexy, if she is willing to ignore the ptosis problem, she is best treated with suprapectoral augmentation, rather than subpectoral periareolar augmentation, because the subpectoral implant can lead to a double-bubble phenomenon, which will be discussed later. Other indications for the use of the periareolar subpectoral procedure include complications following suprapectoral augmentation. The most common example is capsular contracture following a suprapectoral augmentation. In this case, placing the implant beneath the muscle through the periareolar approach (even if the original incision was under the breast) has been an effective use of the periareolar subpectoral approach. Not all will agree with adding an extra scar (periareolar) when there is already an inframammary scar. Justification for doing so is based on the superior quality of the periareolar scar and the need (if

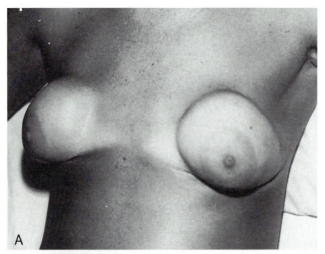

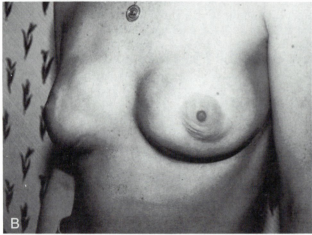

FIGURE 9–1

A, Capsular contracture following prosthetic replacement after subcutaneous mastectomy. B, The capsular contracture was corrected by placing the implant submuscularly.

PREOPERATIVE PREPARATIONS

After the surgeon obtains a brief history, does a physical examination, and makes a general evaluation of the patient's emotional stability, the reasons for augmentation and the surgical options are discussed. The advantages and disadvantages of the procedures are discussed, whether subpectoral or suprapectoral, as are local versus general anesthesia, the type of implant, and the method of insertion (periareolar, inframammary, transaxillary). The authors' preference is subsequently given but not insisted upon. At a second office visit some of this information is repeated, including the potential complications and risks. These include capsular contracture, hematoma, malpositioning, scar formation, and sensory changes. The patient is warned that most patients have temporary sensory changes and that a few may have permanent sensory changes, even though probably minor. The patient is encouraged to try various size implants in her bra to give the surgeon some idea as to her preference, leaving the final decision to the surgeon, based on what appears aesthetically appropriate at surgery. The usual preoperative instructions regarding bathing and avoidance of platelet-inhibiting medication are discussed. Ample literature on the subject of augmentation mammaplasty is also provided.

TECHNIQUE

The patient is placed supine on a table that can be tilted to approximately 40 to 45 degrees (Fig. 9–2). Later in the operation (if necessary) the patient can be tilted to that angle for evaluation of the breasts (i.e., simulate an upright position). Evaluation in the supine position can be misleading. The arms are left at the patient's sides on arm boards (if needed) for evaluation of the true position of the breasts, including the degree of ptosis. More important, with the patient's arms at her sides, the pectoral muscle is looser and is easier to elevate with a retractor during subpectoral dissection; it is also easier to insert a larger implant with the patient in this position.

The type of anesthesia has been almost exclusively general, for the reasons stated. For purposes of hemostasis, a mixture of 50 ml of 0.50% lidocaine (Xylocaine) with epinephrine and 25 ml of 0.25% bupivacaine hydrochloride (Marcaine) with epinephrine is infiltrated into the periareolar area and also inferior and lateral to the edge of the pectoralis major (this is the subcutaneous plane that is common to both the suprapectoral and subpectoral approaches). This greatly facilitates subsequent dissection. Infiltration deep to the muscle is not routinely done because it has a higher risk of causing pneumothorax. However, some Xylocaine and Marcaine with epinephrine is infiltrated along the sternal border. Intraoperative vancomycin, 500 mg intravenously, is given (which covers *Staphylococcus epidermidis* quite well) along with hydrocortisone, 100 mg intravenously. The purpose of the hydrocortisone is threefold: (1) it decreases postoperative edema; (2) it may have a beneficial effect in preventing embolic phenomena; and (3)

such exists) for better exposure. Correction of various deformities or distortions, including minor pectus deformities, have also been good indications for use of the periareolar subpectoral approach.

The size of the desired implant has not been a deterrent to performing the operation. Originally, when the operation was devised, there seemed to be a limitation as to the size of the implant that could be inserted. As experience was acquired, it was found that virtually the same size implant that could be inserted suprapectorally could be inserted subpectorally by simply opening the muscle widely.

General anesthesia is preferred. In the authors' experience, local anesthesia with or without intercostal block has made it more difficult to perform the operation adequately. This, however, has not been the experience of many surgeons, who find it is possible to perform an adequate periareolar subpectoral augmentation with the patient under local anesthesia with or without intercostal blocking (Tebbetts, 1986). Some of these surgeons have found the use of ketamine an invaluable adjunct at the time of muscle release.

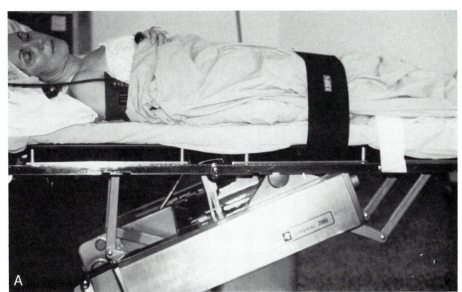

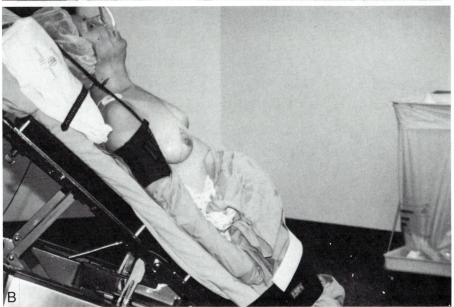

FIGURE 9–2
The operating table (with footboard) *(A)* is adjusted so that during surgery it can be tilted *(B)* to approximately 45 degrees to evaluate the position of the breast. The arms are kept at the sides (on arm boards if needed).

it creates a slight euphoric effect. A one-time dose of this sort certainly has no known effect on potential capsular contracture and does not make the patient more prone to infection.

A periareolar incision is made from the 3 to the 9 o'clock position in the inferior half of the areola (Fig. 9–3). Several other types of areolar incisions have been attempted by the authors over the years, including transareolar, supra-areolar, and medially located incisions, but none has been as effective overall as the infra-areolar incision from the 3 to the 9 o'clock position. The supra-areolar incision and the medial areolar incision were considered because permanent nerve supply was thought to be preserved. As it happens, the cause of the sensory problem is related more to damage to the main nerve (fourth intercostal) or nerves coming out from between the serratus muscle fibers than to transection of the smaller branches at the level of the areola. There is a difference of opinion as to the importance of the location of the periareolar incision (Courtiss and Goldwyn, 1976; Farina et al., 1980).

Furthermore, a medially or superiorly located periareolar scar is more noticeable from the patient's perspective than an infra-areolar (3 to 6 o'clock) scar.

The dissection goes directly vertically toward the pectoral muscle after the parenchyma is adequately released. No attempt is made to circumscribe the parenchymal tissue in an attempt to reach the pectoral muscle. Bleeding is controlled with an electrocoagulator, aided by a head light. When the pectoral muscle is reached, the dissection is extended a short distance over the fascia for good exposure of the pectoral muscle, as for the beginning of a suprapectoral augmentation procedure. An area approximately 7.5 to 10 cm long by 2.5 cm wide in the direction of the muscle fibers is made for a very substantial view of this muscle. This area of exposed muscle is located about 2 to 3 cm medial to the lateral edge of the pectoral muscle. With a tooth forceps and a clamp or Metzenbaum scissors, the muscle is split (Fig. 9–4) until the rib is reached. At this point an Army-Navy type of retractor can be inserted along with a finger in order to split the pectoral muscle for up to

10 cm. Occasionally, there are bleeders within the muscle, and attention has to be paid to hemostasis at this point before going any further. A frequent problem is inadequate splitting of the pectoral muscle (in an attempt to minimize muscle bleeding), resulting in inadequate exposure for the subpectoral dissection and subsequent difficulty in inserting the implant. Therefore, when there is doubt, the muscle-splitting procedure should be longer than necessary. It can always be repaired at the time of closure. After splitting the pectoralis to the length suggested, blunt dissection is done in the superolateral quadrant, where the pectoralis minor is located. The fat pad on the deep side of the pectoralis major is looked for because it distinguishes the pectoralis major from the pectoralis minor. Figure 9–5 demonstrates (on a cadaver) the location of the fat pad on the deep surface of the pectoralis major and the adjacent pectoralis minor. Every attempt should be made not to enter the pectoralis minor, because doing so would cause a great deal of bleeding and prevent adequate dissection of the pocket in the inferolateral quadrant, which is one that requires the most meticulous dissection. The use of cherry sponges—or No. 1 sponges, as they are called—facilitates dissection in the superolateral quadrant, and there are usually no significant blood vessels in this region. After developing the superolateral aspect of the pocket, dissection is continued toward the inferolateral quadrant. A "peanut" dissector (Fig. 9–6) is used to facilitate blunt dissection. One and occasionally two nerve fibers can usually be seen in the inferolateral quadrant and can be preserved by this blunt dissection technique (Fig. 9–7). On occasion, attempts have been made by the authors with the use of long forceps and long Metzenbaum scissors to dissect the nerve laterally and get it out of the way. This has been particularly necessary when the nerve happens to be exiting the serratus muscle more medially, where the implant would be likely to press on the nerve, possibly break it, or cause postoperative hyperesthesia. This requires a great deal of meticulous dissection because the nerves are small and frail. This nerve dissection, therefore, is usually avoided if at all possible. From here the dissection is carried to the inframammary fold area, where the peanut dissector is used to develop a narrow transverse subcutaneous tunnel along and just inferior to the inferiormost aspect of the origin of the pectoralis major muscle. Now that the inferolateral quadrant is complete, the potentially bloody part of the procedure is begun: the muscle fibers of the pectoralis major (originating from the ribs) are transected with the electrocoagulator. Brisk bleeding may be encountered, which requires the use of suctioning and the head light to keep it under control and prevent blood staining of the tissues. The dissection proceeds medially toward the sternum by again transecting muscle fibers that arise from the ribs. Care is taken to avoid entering the rectus muscle by looking for the superiormost edge of the rectus fascia and staying just superficial to it with the peanut dissector or coagulator. When the dissection of the inferior portion of the cavity is complete, one usually sees 1 to 2 cm of the superiormost aspect of the rectus fascia. One may alter the level of this inferior dissection

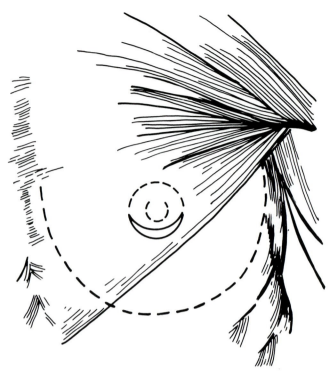

FIGURE 9–3
A periareolar incision is made from the 3 o'clock to the 9 o'clock position.

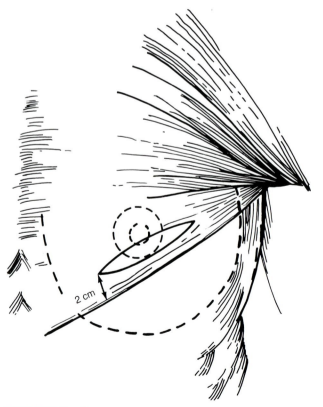

FIGURE 9–4
The muscle is split for a distance of up to 10 cm. The location of the split can be anywhere from 2 to 3 cm from the edge of the pectoralis.

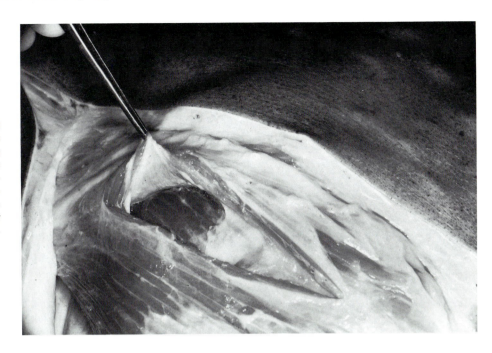

FIGURE 9–5

The pectoralis of this cadaver is split. The fat pad on the deep side of the pectoralis major is noted. It helps one distinguish the pectoralis major from the pectoralis minor. Entering the pectoralis minor at surgery causes unnecessary bleeding and difficulty in completing the remaining dissection.

slightly in order to adjust for a minimal nipple malposition.

Whereas the lateral aspect of the cavity is somewhat limited by the location of the nerves one encounters and by the fact that blunt dissection becomes more difficult laterally, where the tissues fuse, one has more latitude medially. The sternal component of the pectoral muscle can be continuously released toward the midline of the chest. Obviously, it would not be desirable to continue too far, because one could create too much cleavage for the breasts, or the cavities on both sides could inadvertently be merged. Also, one does not want to transect major branches of the internal mammary artery with associated nerve fibers that supply the medial aspect of the breast. Therefore, a compromise is reached by stopping within approximately 1 or 2 cm. from the midline. Oftentimes the peanut dissector is used to sweep the muscle bundles off the ribs and sternum and yet not exert too much pressure, which could break the branches of the internal mammary. Should the surgeon

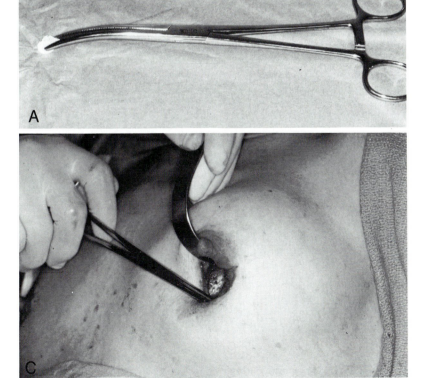

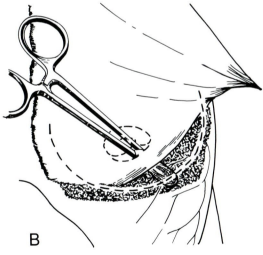

FIGURE 9–6

A, A "peanut" dissector is used to facilitate blunt dissection, especially in the inferolateral quadrant, where nerves are located. *B,* Schematic view. *C,* Intraoperative view.

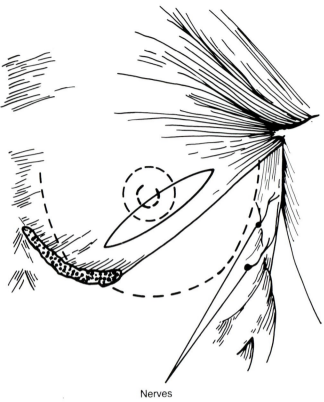

Nerves

FIGURE 9–7
One, if not two, nerve fibers (piercing the serratus) can usually be seen in the inferolateral quadrant and can be preserved by the blunt dissection technique. Subsequently, the pectoralis is extensively released medially to the level of the nipple.

be overzealous in developing either the inferior or the medial components of the cavity, 3-0 nylon sutures can be used to close the compartment to the desired size. Release of the pectoralis and development of the medial cavity proceed superiorly along the sternum, up to approximately the level of the nipple (Fig. 9–7). Very little dissection is required in the superomedial quadrant. At that point the cavity is usually complete. Parenthetically, it is best for a right-handed surgeon to do the left breast first. Dissection is easier, and the peculiarities noted on the first breast are helpful in dissecting the contralateral breast.

All during the procedure absolute hemostasis is obtained with the aid of an electrocoagulator. Cases in which bony abnormalities of the ribs are causing a significant pectus deformity provide an ideal opportunity to use the osteotome and mallet (Fig. 9–8) to make any corrections in the ribs at this time (Spear et al., 1987). Minor concave deformities in the region of the sternum are often correctable as a result of the muscle having been elevated off the sternum, which in turn allows the pectoral muscle to retract medially and fill some of the sternal concavity.

After both cavities are completed, simultaneous bilateral finger palpation indicates the extent of the cavity and indicates the degree of symmetry. Low-profile silicone gel implants of various sizes (125- to 365-cc implants have been used) can be tried for determining

which one gives the best overall appearance to the breast. This usually coincides with the size that the patient selected. High-profile implants have not been used because they tend to produce a firmer breast, the very thing that one tries to avoid. Also, whatever its shape, a soft silicone implant fills the cavity better and forms a teardrop shape (due to gravity) no matter what its preoperative shape is and no matter which way it is placed in the cavity. If difficulty is encountered when one is trying to insert a large implant, it is usually not because of an inadequate opening. It is because the existing cavity has not been enlarged adequately to receive it. Therefore, by applying anterior (upward) traction with two retractors that are placed within the cavity, one usually finds it less difficult to insert a large implant.

One of the frequent problems in performing this operation is in judging the adequacy of inferior pectoral muscle release. One can simply press on the upper half of the breast above the level of the nipple to see whether there is an adequate release of the inferior half of the compartment. By noting whether most of the implant can be compressed into the inferior half of the cavity, one can be fairly certain that the implant will not migrate superiorly in the early postoperative period. It is also advisable to press both breasts toward the midline to evaluate the degree and symmetry of cleavage. Very often not enough cleavage results. A second check of the adequacy of the dissection of the pocket is to simply raise the operating table at this point and see how the breast implants lie. Occasionally it has been found helpful to take a Polaroid picture during the procedure to give the surgeon an additional perspective on the shape and contour of the breast. The Polaroid camera is helpful for both the novice and the experienced surgeon in detecting a subtle asymmetry not appreciated with the naked eye.

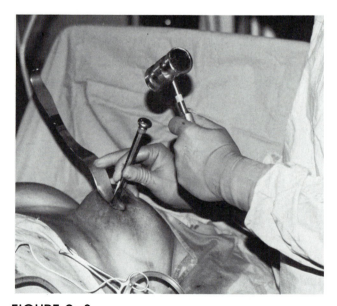

FIGURE 9–8
In cases in which bony abnormalities of the ribs are causing a significant pectus deformity, the periareolar approach provides an ideal opportunity to use the osteotome and mallet to make any corrections.

Before final closure, the wound is irrigated with saline, and an attempt is made to achieve meticulous hemostasis. No intraluminal or intracavity antibiotics, steroids, or antiseptics are used. Whereas drains (Jackson-Pratt) were used for a large number of the patients in the early years of this operation, drains are no longer used. Drains are painful for the patient and have not been shown to lower the incidence of hematoma or capsular contracture. When they were used, they were passed through a separate stab wound incision in the lateral aspect of the inframammary fold. They were left in place for 1 or 2 days.

Closure of the wound consists of absorbable suture such as 3-0 or 4-0 polyglycolic acid for the muscle layer (Fig. 9–9) and for the parenchyma. Usually the muscle is in a satisfactory position to be closed without any difficulty. Seldom will the muscle "bowstring" across the implant to the point of causing a bandlike effect. When a bandlike effect is in fact seen intraoperatively, it is a sign that the muscle has been inadequately released, in which case the surgeon must reexplore the wound and (with his/her finger) pull anteriorly on the pectoral muscle to see what is preventing it from draping adequately around the implant. If the shape of the breast does not look satisfactory at the time of surgery, it is certainly not likely to look better postoperatively.

The subcutaneous tissue is closed with 4-0 polyglycolic acid sutures, followed by interrupted and/or running 5-0 nylon sutures of the skin. The wound is covered with a Xeroform dressing followed by a large roll of cotton and a 6-inch Ace bandage. The operation is approximately 2 hours, longer than most other types of augmentation mammaplasty. This is undoubtedly a discouraging factor for many surgeons. However, extra time spent intraoperatively to prevent postoperative problems is unquestionably worthwhile in the long run.

The patient is usually discharged from the surgery center within hours of the operation, to be seen the next day in the office for evaluation. Postoperative medications include oral antibiotics for 5 days and oxycodone/acetaminophen (Percocet) or hydromorphone hydrochloride (Dilaudid). Discomfort, particularly in the first 24 to 48 hours, is considerably more than that which occurs with a suprapectoral approach (and the patient is warned of this preoperatively). The usual postoperative instructions are given, including observation for severe pain, asymmetry, or swelling. On the first postoperative day, the dressing is changed, and the patient may wear no brassiere or be placed in a stretchable brassiere that does not contain an underwire component. If, as infrequently occurs, the breast implants tend to be somewhat higher than is desired, the patient is asked not to wear a bra and oftentimes asked to wear an Ace bandage to apply a small degree of pressure in the upper half of the breast, above the level of the nipple. This may be necessary for several hours a day for up to 1 to 3 weeks. Fortunately, few patients require this treatment.

RESULTS

The results were critically evaluated during a study in which 178 patients were treated by one of the authors (R.P.G.). In all patients, the breasts were hypoplastic or relatively hypoplastic, without significant ptosis. Low-profile silicone gel implants were used. The patients had follow-up examinations for 2 or more years. In general, an exceptionally soft and natural breast was obtained (Figs. 9–10 and 9–11). The scar was inconspicuous and was not found to be objectionable. Moreover, there was no lateral displacement of the implant resulting from muscle contraction, originally reported with the submuscular approach. The muscle itself, however, could be seen to act as a band across the implant, but only when the patient was asked to squeeze the palms of her hands together or perform some other unusual type of maneuver utilizing the pectoral muscle. Patients seldom found this to be significantly objectionable and considered it a very good trade for a firm breast (Fig. 9–12).

Complications of periareolar subpectoral augmentation in that study are listed in Table 9–1. As can be seen, Baker II capsular contracture (Baker, 1975) occurred in 8.8% of the patients; that is, in 8.8% of the

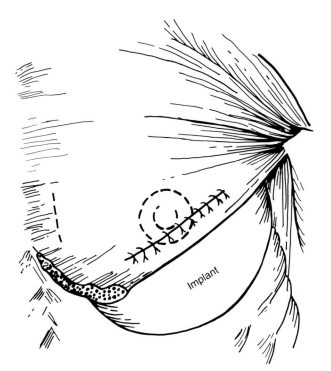

FIGURE 9–9
Closure of the wound consists of absorbable interrupted sutures for the muscular layer.

TABLE 9–1
Complications of Periareolar Subpectoral Augmentation in a Study of 178 Patients

	%
Capsular contracture	
Baker II (firmer than normal to palpation)	8.8
Baker III (firm and visibly contracted)	1.2
Baker IV (firm, visibly contracted, and painful)	0
Scar hypertrophy	1.2
Hematoma	0.6
Infection	0

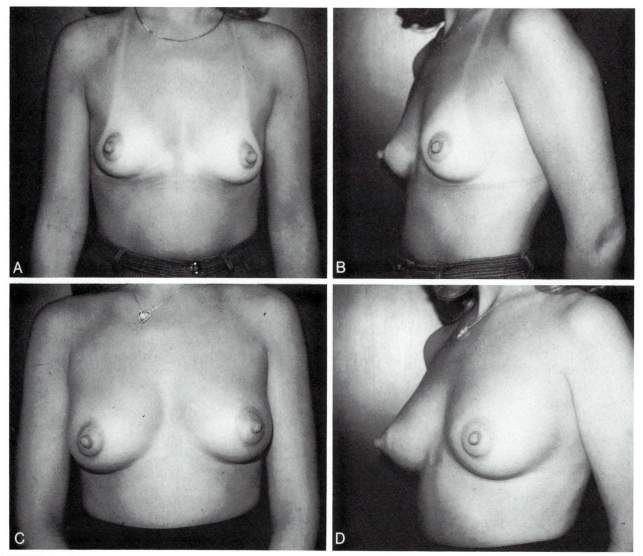

FIGURE 9–10
Typical result after periareolar subpectoral augmentation mammaplasty. *A,* Frontal view (preoperative). *B,* Oblique view (preoperative). *C,* Frontal view (2 years postoperatively). *D,* Oblique view (2 years postoperatively).

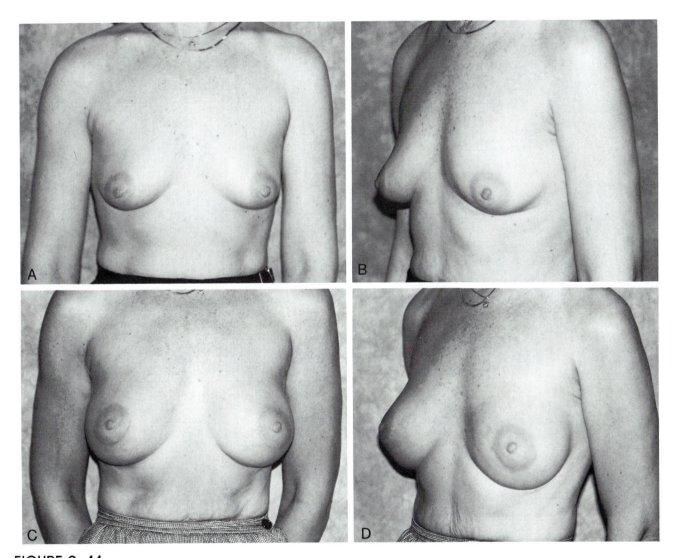

FIGURE 9–11
Typical result after periareolar subpectoral augmentation. *A,* Frontal view (preoperative). *B,* Oblique view (preoperative). *C,* Frontal view (2 years postoperatively). *D,* Oblique view (2 years postoperatively).

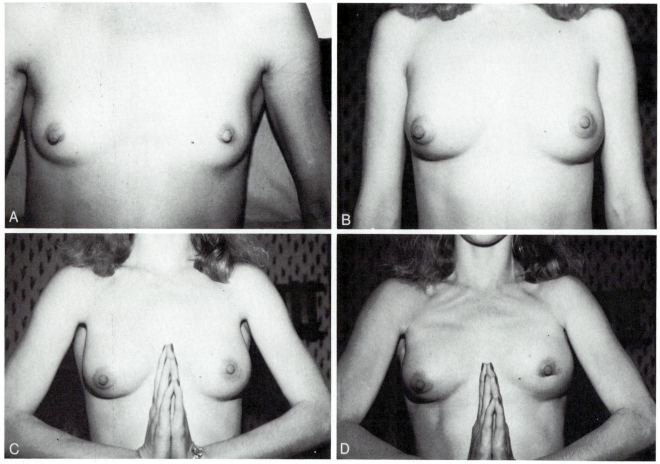

FIGURE 9–12
The muscle itself can be seen to act as a band across the implant (and distort the breasts) only if the patient is asked to squeeze her palms together or perform some other abnormal type of maneuver utilizing the pectoralis. *A,* Preoperative view. *B,* Postoperative view. *C,* Preparing to flex the pectoralis. *D,* Voluntary contraction of the pectoralis, causing a typical degree of distortion.

patients one or both breasts were slightly firm. In evaluating the patient's concern, it appeared that some did not even notice the degree of firmness. Others were aware of it but were unconcerned. A minority were bothered by it to some degree but did not find it so objectionable as to request surgical intervention to correct it. Baker III capsular contracture occurred in 1.2% (two patients). This combination of the spherical appearance of the breast and the abnormal firmness was deemed unsatisfactory. In these patients, open capsulotomy had to be performed, in which the capsule was surgically released at the perimeter and a corticosteroid (triamcinolone acetonide [Kenalog-10, K-10], 10 mg/ml) was injected into the capsule (Fig. 9–13). The K-10 was injected wherever the scar was thickest, usually at the perimeter and dome. As much as 20 to 30 ml of K-10 was injected into the capsule for the purpose of correcting the problem. Hematoma occurred in less than 1% of the patients and required returning to the operating room for evacuation. One patient required surgical correction of a small portion of the periareolar scar. Another patient required K-10 injection into a portion of the periareolar scar that was slightly hypertrophic. No case of implant displacement was noted. No case of infection was noted. Long-term sensory disturbances of

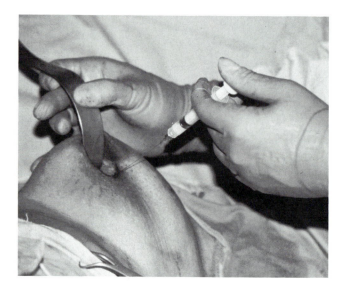

FIGURE 9–13
In patients in whom Baker III capsular contracture develops after periareolar subpectoral augmentation, open capsulotomy is performed and 20 to 30 ml of Kenalog-10 injected into numerous areas of the capsule itself (mostly at the perimeter).

some sort (no matter how minor) were noted in approximately 12% of the patients.

One of the potential problems that can occur with any subpectoral placement of an implant is the double-bubble phenomenon (Fig. 9–14). The breast exhibits two bulges, one from the breast parenchyma itself and another located slightly inferior to that, due to the implant. This phenomenon may result from an attempt to correct ptosis. Obviously, the implant does not fit into the breast parenchyma sac and instead sits behind the bulk of the parenchyma, causing it to sit as a separate mass anterior to the implant. The groove between the two bubbles is of course nothing more than the original inframammary fold that has been anteriorly displaced. In mild cases the groove (and double bubble) becomes less obvious and the ptosis is corrected spontaneously as the inframammary fold stretches over time.

The double-bubble phenomenon can be minor and barely perceptible or can be major, requiring surgical correction (Fig. 9–15). When it is minor, it is considered a much better way of correcting the problem of ptosis than simply putting an implant into the suprapectoral space or adding the scars of a mastopexy. An implant in the suprapectoral space does indeed fill out the tissue but may aggravate the ptosis, in addition causing downward pointing of the nipple. However, the subpectorally placed implant can still lift the entire breast off the chest wall, improving the angle between the breast and the chest. If the double-bubble phenomenon is severe, it means that an attempt to correct ptosis should not have been made by augmentation alone, that an implant of the wrong size was used, or that the implant was placed too low. Correction of the double-bubble phenomenon is done by changing the size of the subpectoral implant, relocating it, or possibly performing a mastopexy (or a combination of the above).

The operation of periareolar subpectoral augmentation has been used for a number of related purposes other than simple augmentation. It has been used to correct problems of capsular contracture by transferring the implant from the suprapectoral pocket to the subpectoral space (Fig. 9–16). Even if the patient has had a previous inframammary incision, it is often deemed advisable to use a new periareolar approach not only to retrieve the implant but to place it in the subpectoral space. A capsulectomy can be considered but of course increases the morbidity of the procedure somewhat and increases the chances of postoperative hematoma.

The pectoralis is split, a submuscular pocket is developed, and the same or a new implant is inserted. Often an implant of a different size (usually larger) will be required to give the proper shape. Soon after surgery some patients require taping (nonallergenic tape and benzoin) of the breasts to prevent the skin and paren-

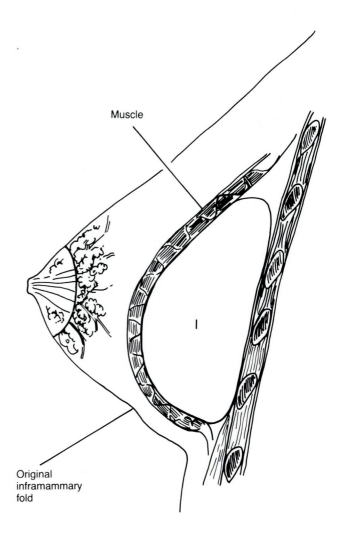

FIGURE 9–14
The double-bubble phenomenon. The bulge of the breast parenchyma is separated from the bulge of the implant by the original inframammary fold. A conspicuous double bubble is avoidable by careful choice of implant size and careful location of the cavity.

Muscle

Original inframammary fold

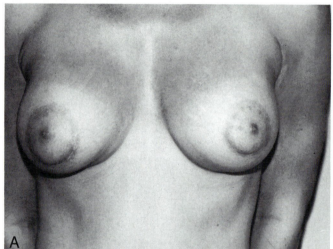

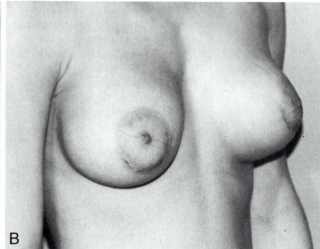

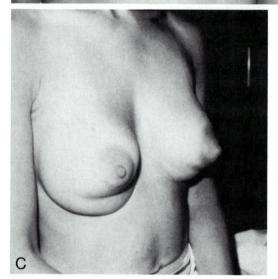

FIGURE 9–15
Front *(A)* and oblique *(B)* views of minor double-bubble phenomena. *C,* Major defect, requiring surgical correction. If severe, it means that the ptosis was not correctable by augmentation, that the wrong size implant was used, or that the implant was placed too low.

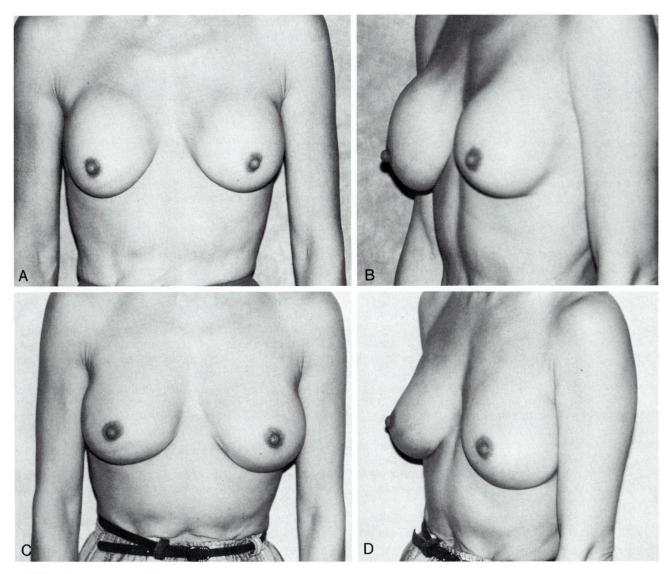

FIGURE 9–16

Correction of Baker III suprapectoral capsular contracture. *A,* Front view. *B,* Oblique view. It is done by placing the implant subpectorally via the periareolar approach. At 1 year postoperatively a Baker class I result was obtained. *C,* Frontal view. *D,* Oblique view.

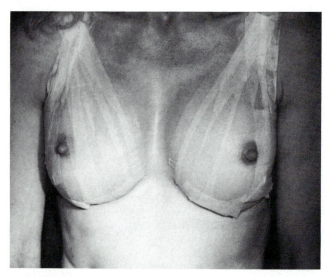

FIGURE 9–17
Patients undergoing correction of suprapectoral capsular contracture by periareolar subpectoral implant placement may need taping of the breast skin for up to 3 weeks postoperatively for preservation of breast shape.

chyma from drooping over the implant (Fig. 9–17). The tape may need to be changed every 4 to 5 days for a total of up to 3 weeks. After that a brassiere will support the parenchyma. A capsulectomy is usually not indicated because the suprapectoral capsule gradually obliterates as the breast parenchyma is "molded" into the desired shape.

One interesting phenomenon was noted in two patients who underwent correction of capsular contracture by periareolar subpectoral replacement. The patients appeared to have capsular contracture early postoperatively (Fig. 9–18). Upon re-exploring the breast, serum under great pressure was found in an otherwise normal suprapectoral cavity. The results of culture were negative. The cavity was drained for several days and remained collapsed after the drain was removed. Because of the resemblance of this tense fluid compartment to capsular contracture, the term "pseudocapsular contracture" may be appropriate.

Periareolar subpectoral augmentation can also be used to improve the difficult problems seen in a thin-skinned patient in whom a suprapectoral augmentation has been performed: (1) when the sternal skin is thin, the implant edges can be seen; and (2) the patient may also complain of "wrinkling of the breast" (Fig. 9–19). This type of skin distortion is correctable by any submuscular approach. However, because of the absolute control of pocket size and hemostasis by the periareolar approach, it has been used by the authors for this particular problem. Most important postoperatively is taping the breast to prevent the thin skin and breast from drooping off the implant mound.

The importance of a periareolar approach and muscle splitting procedure is assumed to be as follows. First, going directly through the nipple and parenchymal tissue provides central exposure of the subpectoral space. This allows better visualization for developing the pocket

than the surgeon has with an inframammary approach. Second, when the pocket is to be closed, the repair is a muscle-to-muscle repair, which is preferable, at least in theory, to a subcutaneous and parenchymal closure, as would occur with an inframammary or axillary approach. One of the hypothetical arguments has been that if capsular contracture is due to *S. epidermidis,* a muscle-to-muscle closure acts as a better barrier to bacteria from the parenchyma and skin. Also, it should be noted that in the event that there is a problem with the superficial portions of the wound, as occurs occasionally from suture reactions, the problem is less likely to have an effect on the cavity if the cavity is well protected by muscle.

With respect to the choice of systemic antibiotics, it should be pointed out that during the study mentioned a cephalosporin was used routinely on all patients (1 gm of cefazolin [Ancef] given intraoperatively followed by cephalexin [Keflex] given orally postoperatively [250 mg q.i.d.]). Since that study, a change was made to vancomycin, 500 mg intraoperatively. The rationale for the use of vancomycin is based on the evidence that if, in fact, *S. epidermidis* is an etiologic factor in capsular contracture, vancomycin is the antibiotic of choice (Aldridge, 1982). *S. epidermidis* is a definite pathogen involving nonsuppurative infections of hip prostheses, cardiac valves, and CNS shunts (Lowy and Hammer, 1983). Vancomycin's effectiveness against *S. epidermidis* has been virtually 100% in comparison with the cephalosporins, which are less effective, and in comparison with erythromycin, which is the least effective of these three antibiotics.

A low-profile silicone gel implant is routinely used. If a patient requests a specific implant such as a double-lumen implant, it is used. The reason for not using saline-filled and double-lumen implants routinely is the potential for leaking. The polyurethane implants also have not been used routinely because (1) there is occasionally a rash associated with them; (2) they are most effective when used suprapectorally; (3) there were initial reports of infection; (4) it is difficult to get them through the periareolar incision; and (5) subsequent implant retrieval, if necessary, is difficult. At this time the polyurethane implant is reserved for the patient who prefers local anesthesia and the suprapectoral approach and who is willing to accept an inframammary scar.

Choosing an implant of the wrong size is a potential problem that has been avoided by the authors in the following manner. The patients are allowed to try on implants of various sizes in the office by inserting them into their brassieres and deciding which implant would be preferred. The patient is instructed to select the larger of the two implants that she believes would give her the appearance she seeks. It has been found that patients generally want only moderate enlargement, to approximately a size B or C cup. Moreover, when asked if they would choose an implant of a different size if the operation were to be done again, they expressed the desire to be only slightly larger if at all. Consequently, suggesting to the patient that she choose the larger of two implants has been found to be the best approach. In the final analysis, however, the surgeon has to modify that decision at surgery if for some reason the size that

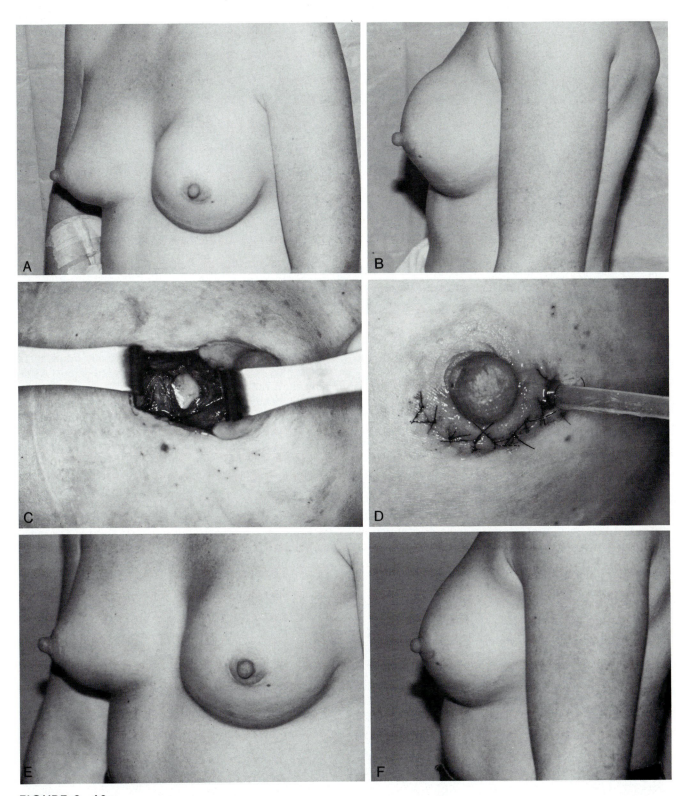

FIGURE 9–18

Pseudocapsular contracture. After suprapectoral capsular contracture is corrected by periareolar subpectoral implant replacement, fluid under tension may form in the remaining capsule and mimic true capsular contracture. *A,* Oblique view. *B,* Profile view. *C,* At surgery the cavity appears normal. Culture results are negative. *D,* Treatment involves simple drainage for several days. *E* and *F,* Oblique and profile views of postdrainage results.

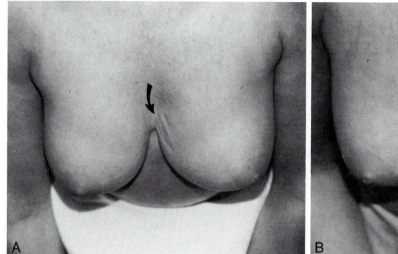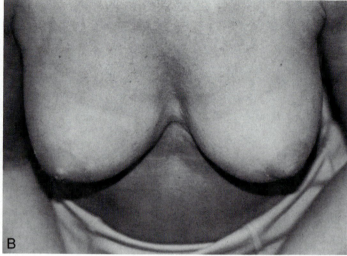

FIGURE 9–19

Wrinkled skin has been reported by some patients after suprapectoral augmentation. It is most noticeable when the patient leans forward. Such patients are candidates for placement of the implant in the subpectoral compartment via the periareolar approach. Note wrinkling of medial breast skin preoperatively *(A)* and improvement postoperatively *(B)*.

the patient picks is inappropriate when viewed intraoperatively. Thus, the Becker type of implant has essentially been restricted to those patients who specifically request it.

A great deal of attention has been given to the problem of muscle banding that occurs in patients who are given subpectoral implants (Fig. 9–20). It is suspected that the greatest single cause of clinically significant muscle banding is inadequate release of the muscle, especially at the inferior and medial portions of the compartment. In the inferior portion, all of the pectoralis fibers originating from the ribs must be released to expose the superior edge of the rectus sheath. Although it is a fact that even after adequate release, contraction of the pectoralis will flatten the breast and distort its shape to some degree, the distortion is seen only under

unusual circumstances. The exceptions to this rule, of course, are in those patients who are body builders, in whom this procedure may be contraindicated. Aside from that, the improvement in the capsular contracture rate has been well worth the price of muscle banding.

Capsular contracture that has resulted from the subpectoral periareolar approach has not been amenable to closed capsulotomy. The tissues are too difficult to rupture by this approach, and there is potential damage due to the amount of pressure that would be required to perform a closed capsulotomy under these circumstances. Therefore, in those circumstances in which correction of capsular contracture is required (Baker III), the only approach that has been used is a surgical one, as previously mentioned.

A comment should be made about the transaxillary

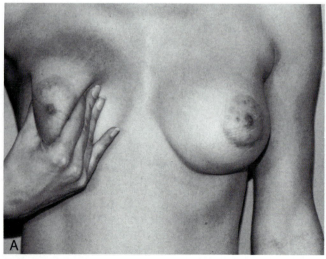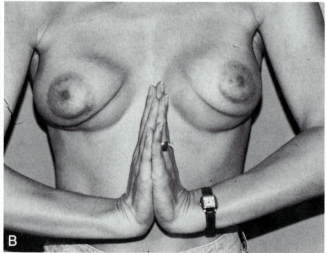

FIGURE 9–20

Severe muscle banding in a patient who received inadequate release during a periareolar subpectoral augmentation. The problem is unnoticeable *(A)* until the patient contracts the pectoralis *(B)*.

approach. In principle, it would seem that the transaxillary approach has everything to offer that the subpectoral approach has, including perhaps a better scar because of its location in the axilla, an area that cannot be seen, and the fact that the operation itself takes less time. However, it should be stressed that whereas the transaxillary approach has a proper place, in the authors' opinion, it has one distinct disadvantage. The transaxillary approach does not lend itself to an extensive and controlled muscle release and therefore does not lend itself to exact placement of the implant nor always allow the use of an implant of the desired size. Theoretically, there is some concern about the fact that the branches of the nerves to the nipple are more likely to be damaged or injured in a blind technique using the transaxillary approach. However, the empirical fact remains that reported cases of sensory changes with the transaxillary approach have not shown that to be the problem once anticipated (Tebbetts, 1986). Furthermore, whereas the hematoma rate with a blind transaxillary approach was once reported to be high, more recent studies show a considerable improvement and an acceptable hematoma range comparable to that of other types of augmentation mammaplasty. The transaxillary approach, therefore, is reserved by the authors for those cases in which the nipple is very small, those in which the patient only requires a small amount of augmentation, and those in which the patient wants no trace of a scar on the breast.

If a subpectoral approach is good, why not use a complete submuscular approach, as advocated by some surgeons (Little and Spear, 1988)? In the authors' experience, elevation of the full-thickness serratus means stripping it off the ribs, with an associated brisk bleeding problem, because there is no well-defined subserratus plane. A partial and superficial serratus elevation would then seem logical if it were not for the problem of the nerves to the nipple, which pierce the serratus and must be preserved. For these reasons the elevation of the pectoralis alone has been considered sufficient.

When the operation of subpectoral augmentation (periareolar or otherwise) was first performed, the reason for the better results was unclear. Some believed that the muscle provided a padding effect (Ksander et al., 1981). Some believed that the results might be due to the constant muscular contracture of the pectoral muscle against the implant, thereby maintaining a soft capsule. It was for this reason that massaging was not recommended as part of the treatment postoperatively. More recently at least one study has suggested the potential harm of massage (Marshall, 1986). Another hypothetical cause of better results was the better hemostasis that is obtainable via the periareolar approach. However, at least one study has shown that hematoma may not play a role in contracture formation (Caffee, 1986). One of the other hypothetical reasons for softer breasts was that the type of tissue in the subpectoral space is qualitatively different from suprapectoral tissue. It is well known that the tissue in this region is more areolar in nature. It was also hypothesized that there might be fewer lymphatics in the subpectoral space, making the subpectoral space a relatively alymphatic plane. Alymphatic spaces are associated with less intense immune responses (specific and nonspecific) to antigen

and foreign bodies. It was fully realized, of course, that part of the pocket created in the so-called subpectoral space is under the muscle and part of it is really just superficial to the serratus muscle (lateral and inferior to the lateral edge of the pectoralis); that is, the "subpectoral pocket" is really only partially submuscular. Nonetheless, it was considered a possibility that the lymphatic drainage may play a quantitative role. If, as has been suggested, capsular contracture is due to a specific or nonspecific immune response to silicone molecules, and if the subpectoral space is alymphatic, one would expect less capsular contracture from the subpectoral location of an implant.

To answer the question of whether the submuscular space is an immunologically privileged site, a small study (Gruber et al., 1984) was undertaken in which a radioisotope technetium-99m antimony chloride, which is picked up by the lymphatics, was inserted into the subpectoral space of one breast and into the suprapectoral space of the other breast. Axillary lymph node scanning (lymphoscintigraphy) was done subsequently to detect the degree of uptake. The results were negative, in that no difference could be appreciated between the lymphatic uptake of the suprapectoral compartment, compared with the subpectoral compartment. Thus, any possibility that the better results seen with subpectoral implant placement were due to the alymphatic ("immunologically privileged") nature of the subpectoral space was rendered unlikely.

The question remains as to why leaving the silicone gel implant in the subpectoral space yields better results. One hypothesis that has yet to be tested at this time is that like skin from different parts of the body, tissues from different anatomic parts of the chest wall vary in their scar response. Perhaps the areolar tissue in the human subpectoral space is less prone to scar formation than is the nonareolar tissue in the suprapectoral space. The area inferior and lateral to the pectoralis is, of course, common to both suprapectoral and subpectoral approaches; and thus scar potential in this vicinity is the same for both procedures. The preceding hypothesis also assumes, of course, that scar thickness does indeed play a role in capsular contracture, which some studies have questioned (Ksander et al., 1981).

SUMMARY

In summary, the periareolar subpectoral augmentation has proved to be a highly effective means of reducing the incidence of capsular contracture. The incidence of significant capsular contracture requiring surgical correction, which has been the overwhelming problem during the last two decades, has been reduced to approximately 1% of patients. Another 9% of the patients will have some degree of firmness of the breasts, but none that is significant enough to require surgical correction. These results are a distinct improvement over those of the suprapectoral approach and are attributed to the surgical technique itself, rather than the type of implant, the choice of antibiotics, or other factors as previously discussed. Moreover, the scar in the periareolar area has been more than satisfactory in most patients. The ability to visualize the nerves to the nipple and avoid them is easiest through the periareolar subpectoral approach, as is the ability to obtain complete hemostasis. The periareolar incision does not usually limit the size of the implant that can be inserted. Muscle banding has not been a significant problem when the muscle is adequately released. Perhaps the one major disadvantage of periareolar subpectoral augmentation, which has stopped a number of surgeons from using this approach more frequently, is the fact that it takes more time than other procedures. The development of the plane requires more tedious dissection, a search for bleeders, and care in avoiding entering the wrong surgical planes. However, failing to develop the adequate plane has probably been a cause of problems about which surgeons have complained: (1) the inability to insert a large implant, (2) muscle banding, and (3) implant displacement. Finally, the subpectoral periareolar approach is ideal for correcting the problems associated with complications following other approaches, including distortion problems, but in particular, capsular contracture due to a suprapectoral approach.

References

Aldridge, K. E.: Topics in clinical microbiology. Infection Control 3:161, 1982.

Baker, J. L., Jr.: Augmentation mammaplasty. In: Owsley, J., Peterson, R. (ed.): *Aesthetic Surgery of the Breast.* St. Louis, C. V. Mosby, 1978, p. 261.

Biggs, T. M.: Augmentation mammaplasty. In: Georgiade, N. G.: *Aesthetic Breast Surgery.* Baltimore, Williams & Wilkins, 1983, p. 50.

Caffee, H. H.: The effect of hematoma on implant capsules. Ann. Plast. Surg. 16:102, 1986.

Courtiss, E. H., Goldwyn, R. M.: Breast sensation before and after plastic surgery. Plast. Reconstr. Surg. 58:1, 1976.

Dempsey, W. C., Latham, W. D.: Subpectoral implants in augmentation mammaplasty: Preliminary report. Plast. Reconstr. Surg. 42:515, 1968.

Farina, M. A., Newby, B. G., Alani, H. M.: Innervation of the nipple-areolar complex. Plast. Reconstr. Surg. 66:497, 1980.

Gruber, R. P.: Periareolar subpectoral augmentation mammoplasty (Video). Presented at the American Society of Aesthetic Plastic Surgery, Houston, Texas, April 1981.

Gruber, R. P., Friedman, G. D.: Periareolar subpectoral augmentation mammoplasty periareolar incision. Plast. Reconstr. Surg. 67:453, 1981.

Gruber, R. P., Perkins, P. J., Chafen, L. T., Shrago, G. G.: Augmentation mammoplasty in the submuscular space: An immunologically privileged site? Unpublished data, 1984.

Ksander, G. A., Vistnes, L. M., Kosek, J.: Effect of implant location on compressibility and capsule formation around mini prostheses in rats and experimental capsule contracture. Ann. Plast. Surg. 6:182, 1981.

Little, J. W., Spear, S.: Totally submuscular augmentation mammaplasty. Presented at the American Society of Plastic and Reconstructive Surgeons Annual Meeting, Toronto, 1988.

Lowy, F. D., Hammer, S. M.: Staphylococcus epidermidis infections. Ann. Intern. Med. 99:834, 1983.

Mahler, D., Hauben, D. J.: Retromammary versus retropectoral augmentation: A comparative study. Ann. Plast. Surg. 8:370, 1982.

Marshall, W. R.: Amelioration of capsular contracture by motion restriction. Ann. Plast. Surg. 16:211, 1986.

McGrath, M. H.: Capsular contracture in the augmented breast. In: Rudolph, R.: *Problems in Aesthetic Surgery.* St. Louis, C. V. Mosby, 1986, p. 405.

Peterson, R.: T-A-S-P-M-A (transaxillary subpectoral mammary augmentation). In: Georgiade, N. G. (ed.): *Aesthetic Breast Surgery.* Baltimore, Williams & Wilkins, 1983, p. 63.

Regnault, P., Daniel, R. K.: Breast augmentation. In: Regnault, P., Daniel, R. K.: *Aesthetic Plastic Surgery.* Boston, Little, Brown, 1984, p. 559.

Spear, S. L., Romm, S., Hakki, A., Little, J. W.: Costal cartilage sculpturing as an adjunct to augmentation mammoplasty. Plast. Reconstr. Surg. 79:921, 1987.

Tebbetts, J. B.: Transaxillary subpectoral augmentation mammaplasty: An integrated surgical-anatomical-clinical instructional course. John B. Tebbetts, M.D., Dallas, Texas, 1986.

A Transareolar Circumthelial Approach to Augmentation Mammaplasty

The ultimate goal in prosthetic breast augmentation is to imitate or recreate normal anatomy. In fact, the ideal in all plastic and reconstructive surgery—head and neck surgery, burn surgery, hand surgery, and aesthetic surgery—occurs when the surgical effort closely reproduces normal anatomy.

The problem with aesthetic breast surgery in the 1970s was that operations were routinely being performed that did not predictably produce breasts that were "real" in either shape or consistency. Moreover, the inframammary or periareolar incisions were frequently obvious. Even more significant was the rapidly developing and persistent problem of constrictive fibrosis, or capsular contracture, which produced an aesthetically unsatisfactory result.

HISTORY

Approaches to the submammary space through the nipple-areola complex are not new. In 1974, Pitanguy et al. (1974), in Brazil, described a transareolar/transnipple incision (Figs. 10–1A and 10–2A). Jenny, in the early 1970s, used a periareolar incision for placement of his saline-inflatable protheses. Other investigators have noted and published experience with similar incisions (see References).

PERSONAL EXPERIENCE

Following tradition, and beginning practice in 1970, I utilized an inframammary incision. I soon found, however, that in Southern California this relatively inconspicuous scar and location was highly unacceptable to the majority of young female patients for this new and captivating cosmetic procedure.

Forced necessarily to satisfy the local populace, I designed a variety of incisions around the nipple and within the areola to obscure a noticeable scar distant from the periareolar margins (see Figs. 10–1 and 10–2). Initially, the transareolar/transnipple incision of Pitanguy (1974) was utilized in approximately 150 patients with perfectly satisfactory results (see Figs. 10–1A and 10–2A). However, hemisection of the nipple appeared to be an unnecessary and unaesthetic manipulation. Moreover, the theoretic concerns were (1) potential

compromise of blood supply, particularly in the protuberant nipple, and (2) duct damage or obstruction with resulting mammary atrophy or mastitis during lactation or nursing. Consequently, several incisions were designed (see Figs. 10–1B to D and 10–2B to E) to avoid damage to the central thelial ducts by circumscribing the nipple and obscuring the remainder of the incision within the confines of the areolar margin (Terino, 1982).

During the period from January 1975 through January 1983, 792 patients underwent prosthetic breast surgery. A transareolar incision of some variety was successfully used in 99.4% and a circumareolar incision in 0.6%.

ADVANTAGES OF AREOLAR INCISIONS

Transareolar approaches to breast augmentation have the following advantages (Table 10–1): First, they are cosmetically superior. The scars may differ according to the individual texture, color, and size of the patient's nipple-areola complex. However, they are universally almost entirely inconspicuous (Figs. 10–3 and 10–4). Unsightly scars (Fig. 10–5), should they occur, can readily be corrected with minor secondary revision. Second, the ease of dissection is facilitated because the nipple-areola complex is central within the breast cone. All limits of the roughly 360-degree submammary space can be reached more readily from this more central approach. Third, sensory disturbances of the breast are minimized. Finally, the transareolar intramammary approach favors early breast manipulations and early patient mobilization for surgeons who advise this postoperative regimen. The thickness of the breast and subcutaneous tissue overlying the implant presents a margin of safety for these exercises. And with the normally erect patient, the weight of the implant does

TABLE 10–1
Advantages of Alveolar Incision

Is cosmetically superior
Facilitates anatomic space dissection
Minimizes sensory disturbances
Favors early manipulation
Favors early patient mobilization

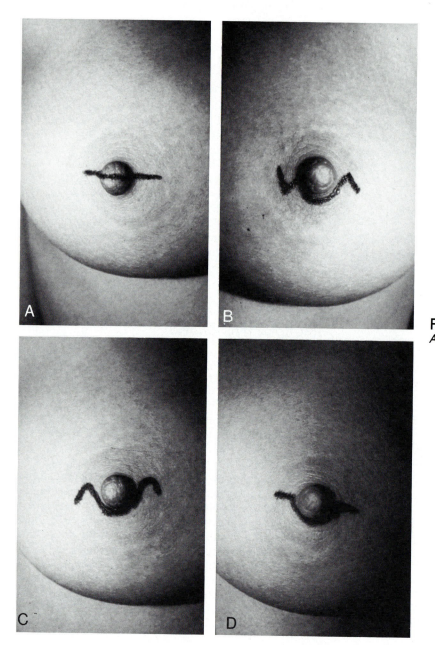

FIGURE 10–1
A to *D*, A variety of transareolar incisions.

FIGURE 10–2
A to *E*, Schematic representation of transareolar incisions.

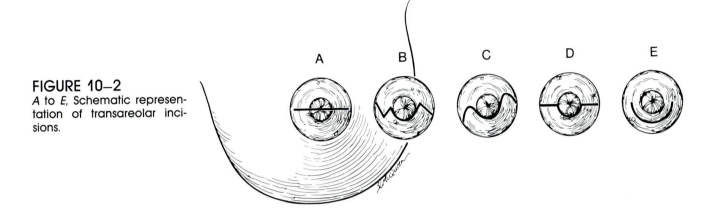

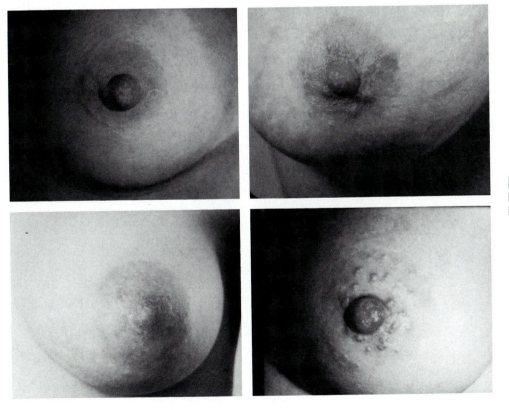

FIGURE 10–3
Postoperative scar results of intra-areolar incisions.

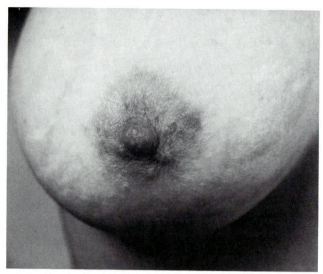

FIGURE 10–4
Postoperative scar results of intra-areolar incisions.

not place gravitational stress on the incision. With the submammary approach there is only a thin covering of skin and subcutaneous tissue between the prosthesis and the external environment. With this approach, unlike the inframammary approach, early movements of the arm and axilla are permissible without undue stress on the incision.

ANATOMIC AND SENSORY FACTORS

There has been a common misconception about incisions in and around the nipple-areola complex. Both patients and physicians have been concerned about disturbance of nipple and areolar sensation from dissection in this anatomic region. Such fears are unfounded.

Anatomically, the nipple-areola complex represents the terminal end of the peripheral nerves that reach this area via thoracodorsal and intercostal end branches, particularly from T4 (Fig. 10–6). As with other peripheral nerves, such as within digits, distal damage facilitates regeneration and rehabilitation of sensation, whereas a more proximal injury limits recuperative capacity.

In augmentation mammaplasty routine dissection of the anatomic submammary space extends from just below the clavicle to just below the inframammary sulcus and from the parasternal border to the midaxillary line. Therefore, it is at the periphery where the possibility is likely of either damaging or transecting the proximal branches of the nerves that ordinarily proceed distally to the center of the breast cone. It is this proximal damage that may severely impair nipple and areolar sensation to the point of complete loss. Incisions within the nipple-areola complex that damage the distal nerve endings do not increase morbidity in this regard and in reality may cause less sensory disturbance than the inframammary dissection. Nonetheless, in all cases, patients are told that (1) there will be a definite, but temporary, change in the sensitivity of the nipple-areola complex and skin over the breasts; (2) there can be no predictability regarding the return of sensitivity—it may return completely to normal or be changed to varying degrees; (3) the sensitivity may ultimately differ from one side to the other. There has been little patient dissatisfaction in this series because of sensory disturbances. Perhaps this is because of the open communication during preoperative consultation.

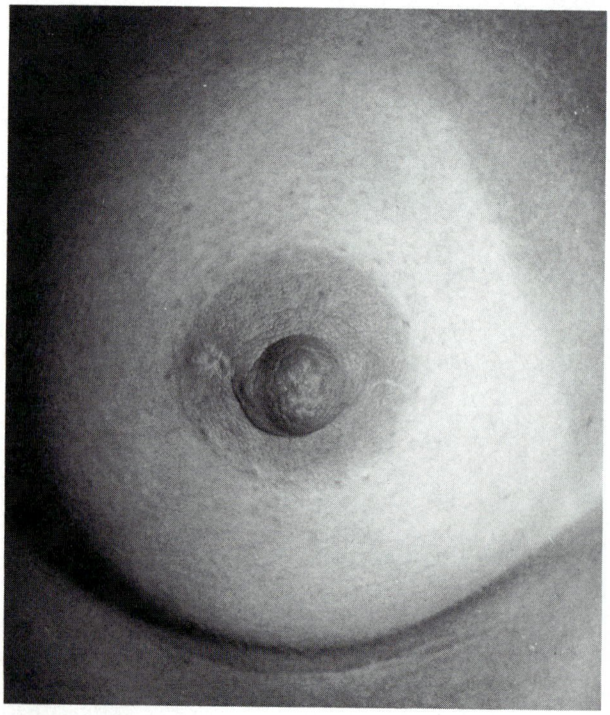

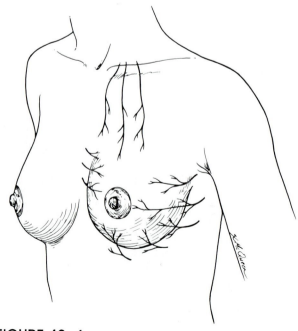

FIGURE 10–5
Example of a postoperative scar.

FIGURE 10–6
Innervation of the nipple-areola complex.

TECHNIQUE

To minimize ductal damage during thelial hemisection, the incision proceeds exactly perpendicular to the nipple base in order to avoid tangential severance of a greater number of ducts over a greater surface area. However, when the incision circumscribes the nipple, the scalpel is slanted inferiorly away from its base at a 45-degree angle to parallel the ducts. This avoids excessive damage to them and to the blood supply of the nipple itself. After this surface incision, deep transection of the breast is accomplished by using two skin hooks and then Army-Navy retractors to separate the breast tissue. Sharp scalpel incision or Bovie's electrodissection then penetrates the breast tissue vertically until the obvious fibroareolar plane between the breast and pectoral fascia is reached.

Entrance into the submammary or subpectoral space via the nipple-areola complex directs the surgeon into the center of the breast cone for ready accessibility to its base circumference. Transaxillary and submammary approaches enter the periphery of the space maximally distant from the opposite limit of the base diameter of the chest wall breast cone, making distal dissection difficult.

The generous elasticity of the areolar skin and muscle permits adequate access to the submammary space. Further access in order to facilitate very large gel prostheses or polyurethane prostheses may be gained by extending the incisions several millimeters laterally or even perpendicularly along the medial and lateral margins of the areola itself.

Very little bleeding is encountered when the tissues are infiltrated adequately with local anesthesia. Three hundred milliliters of a local mixture are used (150 ml for each breast). This consists of one bottle of 1% lidocaine with 1:100,000 epinephrine diluted into 250 ml of sterile normal saline. This greatly attenuated (1:650,000) epinephrine solution produces extremely adequate vasoconstriction. Meanwhile, the very dilute lidocaine (0.2% solution) results in a tissue-level degree of anesthesia that minimizes the other anesthetic drug needs. Injecting this large volume of saline in which the local anesthetic is diluted seems to facilitate demarcation and dissection of the anatomic planes, particularly between the breast and the pectoral fascia. This dramatically lessens the degree of the trauma to the tissues. Based on an 18-year experience (approximately 5000 breasts), it is my belief and observation that excessive damage, particularly to the pectoral fascia or its muscle fibers, definitively precipitates capsule contracture, periprosthetic fibrosis, and myofibroblast activity to a frequently undesirable degree.

Postoperative drainage is routinely used. Despite the meticulous hemostasis that all surgeons strive for, observations over the past 12 years have shown that postoperative Hemovac drainage through a percutaneous axillary site produces generous quantities of blood and serum for up to 5 to 7 days after surgery. Two hundred to three hundred milliliters daily is the rule during the first 48 hours, dropping to 75 ml, then 50 ml daily on days 4 through 7. Significantly less ecchymosis, swelling, and capsular contracture have occurred since 1976, when such drainage was routinely instituted (Terino, 1982).

ANESTHESIA

All surgery is presently performed with the patient under general endotracheal anesthesia. This is in contradistinction to the period from 1970 to 1979, when I personally administered the now rather standard potpourri of intravenous narcotics, tranquilizers, and dissociative agents without inducing a single medical mishap. Since 1980 we have performed nearly 10,000 cosmetic procedures of 2 to 8 hours' duration under general endotracheal anesthesia.

The following observations have been made: (1) Bleeding is significantly more controlled when the systolic blood pressure is maintained between 90 and 110 mm Hg. (2) The constancy and consistency of this parameter are vastly superior when one uses general endotracheal anesthesia. This creates a much greater degree of physiologic safety and control. (3) Such control of blood pressure and bleeding facilitates accuracy of dissection, which greatly minimizes postoperative bruising, swelling, and other more severe complications such as hematoma formation. (4) All of the preceding factors provide a much more suitable environment in which plastic surgeons can perform the meticulous, detailed work necessary for the finest results.

The present regimen used is 10 to 30 µg sufentanil prior to intubation to provide adequate narcosis, followed by constant administration of isoflurane (Forane) (1% to 1.5%) by means of a ventilator. Subsequent small doses of short-acting narcotics such as fentanyl may be given as well as short-acting beta blockers and/or atropine. Nitrous oxide (50%) with oxygen (50%) is optional, depending on the individual philosophy of the anesthesiologist.

As for breast augmentation by any approach, the limits of space dissection are critical, particularly those of the internal level of the inframammary sulcus and the lateral chest corridor. However, the use of fiberoptic retractors clarifies visualization of the limits of the submammary space. This encourages delicate and accurate internal dissection to perfectly define the designated borders inscribed externally by the preoperative skin markings. Again, as with all techniques, it is critical to adjust the final space dissection according to "trial and error" prosthesis spacers or sizers and also by elevating the operating table into an upright position to better define the final anatomic margins of the pocket to suit the individual needs of the patient.

LIMITATIONS AND CONSIDERATIONS

The intra-areolar, perithelial approach has limitations in the case of a breast that requires a very large prosthesis or in a patient with a small nipple-areola complex. In either case, it is possible to extend the incision slightly beyond the margins of the areola to gain necessary access. This should, however, only be done for a distance of approximately 3 to 5 mm. In most instances, the pigmentation of the border presents a diffuse color gradient favoring a totally inconspicuous incision.

Another consideration relates to the issue of ductal transection causing contamination by *Staphylococcus epidermidis*. This potential problem has not been observed in this series. Cultures taken in eight secondary open capsulotomies were negative. Moreover, the spherical contracture rate was not greater than that of the best reported series (Terino, 1982). Instead, it appeared to be statistically less than other published data from this same time period (1975 to 1982).

The transareolar circumthelial approach also facilitates submuscular implantation. With this technique the fibers of the pectoralis are divided in their anatomic direction, obliquely toward the sternum, for dissection beneath the muscle with complete and direct visualization. Depending upon one's philosophy and purpose, either a total submuscular pocket or a partial submuscular space is created. For most augmentations the origins of the pectoralis major must be severed from the third or fourth sternal costal junction inferiorly to include its attachments from the fifth and sixth ribs. Moreover, transection of these origins must be complete until overlying fascia and subcutaneous tissue are clearly visualized.

When this is done adequately, the artificial-looking, high-riding or "axillary breast" is avoided and abnormal unattractive breast twitching caused by residual pectoralis activity is minimized. Our 1984 to 1988 series (437 patients) has a less than 5% incidence of detectable spherical contracture.

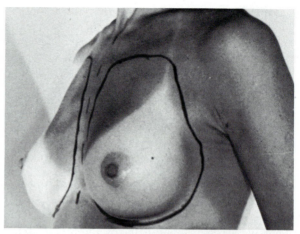

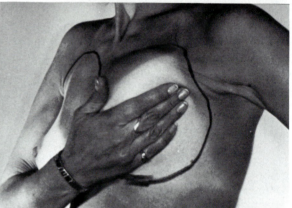

FIGURE 10–7
Example of adequate submammary space.

EVALUATING SPHERICAL CONTRACTURE: A PERSONAL CLASSIFICATION

A workable definition of spherical contracture is anything that diminishes the submammary anatomic space from its original size on the anterior chest wall at the time of dissection. Adequately created, this space should comfortably encompass a mammary prosthesis in order to permit a full two-hand squeeze of the breast, where the thumb and fingers of both hands come together easily with only the thickness of the implant, subcutaneous tissue, and breast tissue intervening.

The prosthesis should naturally lie in an inferior and lateral aspect, yet also have superior space for upward mobility, provided it is not a polyurethane prosthesis. An adequate submammary space will not permit the implants either to uncomfortably intrude upon the patient's prone position or to project above a hand flattened across the sternum and anterior chest (Fig. 10–7). In other words, a natural breast does not recline high on the thorax anterior to the ribs and sternum with the patient supine, but flows more laterally. The exception, of course, is the unusually firm virginal breast, which can have significant supine projection.

Some plastic surgeons believe that the concept of

breast manipulation somehow magically prevents constricting fibrosis of tissues around the implant, or capsular contracture. The major goal in all prosthetic breast surgery can be defined as the maintenance of the submammary anatomic space created for the prosthesis. Manipulation and maintenance can be done early, i.e., "prophylactically" after prosthetic surgery, or it can be attempted with some effectiveness secondarily by rupturing the fibrotic capsule surrounding the prosthesis. This is otherwise known as a manual release or closed capsulotomy.

Manipulation, therefore, can be done either in the form of immediate postoperative exercises or as a long-term process postoperatively in patients in whom significant constrictive fibrosis has already developed. In these latter patients this effort is an attempt to avoid secondary surgical dissection and release.

THE ANATOMIC SUBMAMMARY SPACE

The definition of the anatomic submammary space (Table 10–2) is a dissection either above or below the pectoral muscle that extends to within 2 to 4 cm of the infraclavicular border, to the parasternal border, to the midaxillary line, to a variable distance below the infra-

Table 10–2
Definition of Anatomic Submammary Space

Two to 4 cm below clavicle
Parasternal border
Midaxillary line
One to 3 cm below inframammary sulcus
Anterior axillary fold
Pectoral fascia or thoracic rib cage

mammary sulcus, and to the most anterior axillary fold (Figs. 10–8 and 10–9).

Dissection of this space should be done under direct vision, with meticulous hemostasis. When the prosthesis is placed subglandularly, the violation of the pectoral fascia or muscle, particularly superiorly or laterally, appears to stimulate space closure by fibrotic constriction. This probably involves the activity of myofibroblasts, which produce more active contracture of the collagenous healing process within the space. In the subpectoral position, the early, rapid tendency for spherical closure is greatly minimized, perhaps because of stabilization of the healing forces by the rib cage posteriorly. In our series, submuscular placement has shown significant lessening in fibrotic constrictions over placement in the submammary subcutaneous space.

THE SPECIFICS OF CLASSIFICATION

Manual compression of the implant to the limits of the anatomic space, whether subpectoral or submammary, determines encroachment upon the space by any

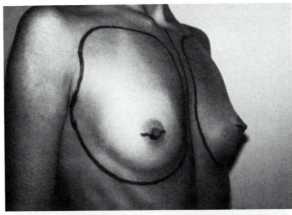

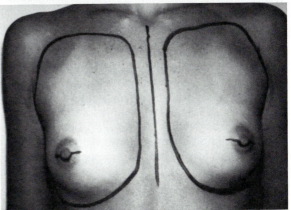

FIGURE 10–9
The defined limits of the submammary space dissection.

degree of capsular constrictive fibrosis. Since 1975 I have been classifying "capsule" formation into five distinct categories, or classes (Terino, 1982). These are specifically defined by detectable changes in the outlines of the anatomic submammary dissection space created during surgery. Any change in the configuration of this space is readily observable and palpable.

This classification is thought to be superior to the customary Baker classification because it involves more specific anatomic definitions that are readily reproducible. This can facilitate more objective dissemination of data among colleagues. Degrees of space closure or constricting fibrosis can be classified on a 0 to 4 basis, with relationship to both aesthetic contour and manual compressibility (Tables 10–3 and 10–4).

Class 0 is a space that has not closed substantially from the initial dissection. It will allow for two-hand compression, so that the fingers can almost touch through the breast tissue and prosthesis (Fig. 10–10).

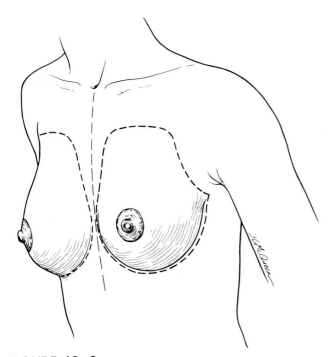

FIGURE 10–8
Schematic representation of the defined limits of the submammary space dissection.

TABLE 10–3
Classification of Anatomic Space Closure by Compressibility

0	Two-hand finger touch
1+	Slight space asymmetry
2+	One-hand finger touch
3+	Moderately compressible
4+	Minimal to no compressibility

TABLE 10–4
Classification of Anatomic Space Closure by Contour

0	Totally simulating normal anatomy
1+	Superior
2+	Excellent to slightly abnormal
3+	Possibly satisfactory
4+	Totally unacceptable deformity

Class 1 constitutes slight space closure with a detectable change in the shape and configuration, usually in the superior lateral or superior medial aspect. This alters the symmetry of the space but does not significantly alter ideal aesthetic breast contour or compressibility (Fig. 10–11). Class 2 indicates further closure or alteration of the space, which may produce a minor degree of artificiality in either contour or consistency. Now the implant begins to be palpably detectable by one-hand compression only (Fig. 10–12). The contour, however, remains excellent. Class 3 space closure indicates significant contracture from the original defined limits of the submammary space. Some compressibility and moderately satisfactory contour characteristics remain, but with severe limitation by the external capsule that has formed (Fig. 10–13). This is unacceptable to patients and surgeons. Class 4 is the severe form of capsule closure. There is no longer additional space for the prosthesis. This degree of fibrous contracture creates the well-known globular or spherical deformity of the breast, totally lacking natural contour and consistency (Figs. 10–14 and 10–15). Class 3 or 4 would be unac-

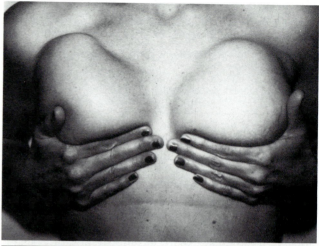

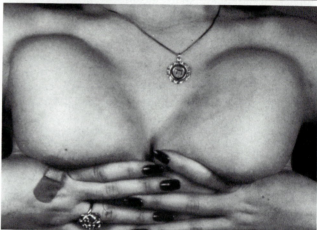

FIGURE 10–11
Minimal space closure.

ceptable to any patient or surgeon and would be considered a poor result. Classes 0 and 1 constitute superior results, and Class 2 is often very acceptable. Classes 0 through 2 should be achievable in over 95% of breast prostheses (Terino, 1982).

RESULTS: SCAR CONSIDERATIONS

The results of transareolar, intra-areolar, and circumthelial incisions are distinctly superior to inframammary incisions (Fig. 10–16). The scar in the inframammary location is quite unpredictable and at times can hypertrophy repeatedly and permanently despite meticulous surgical approximation. In addition, it can migrate upward or downward, depending on how the dynamics of spherical space contracture determine the final position of the prosthesis. Incisions just at or outside the areolar margins are less aesthetic than intra-areolar incisions because they tend to create a depigmented line of demarcation. The intra-areolar skin most often repigments within 6 to 18 months, resulting in an almost invisible scar.

As with all surgery, secondary dissections are approached with some trepidation. Re-entry through the

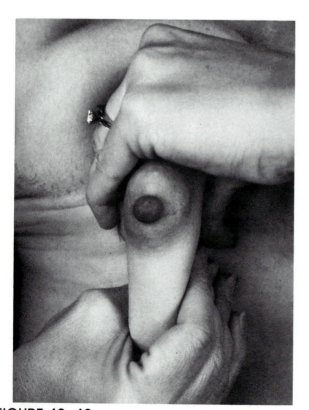

FIGURE 10–10
Class 0 spherical space closure.

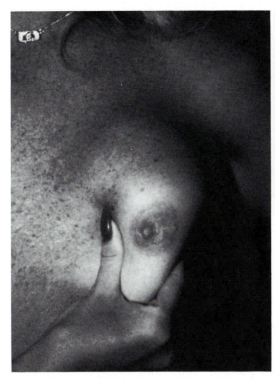

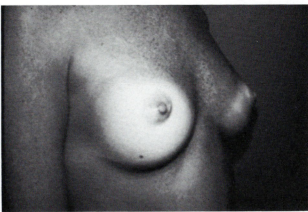

FIGURE 10–12
Class 2 space closure with one-hand compressibility only.

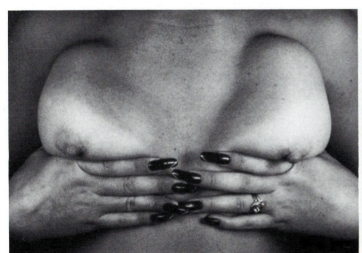

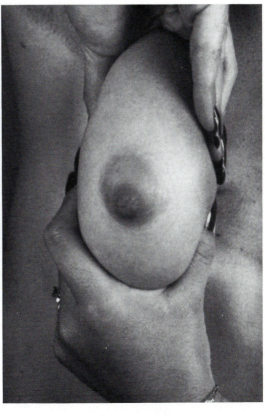

FIGURE 10–13
Significant space closure and minimal compressibility.

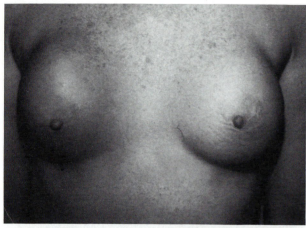

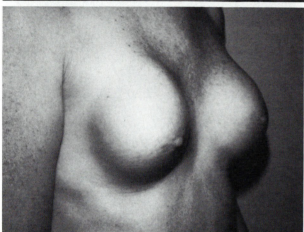

FIGURE 10–14
Class 4 total anatomic space contracture.

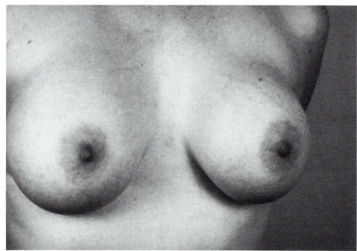

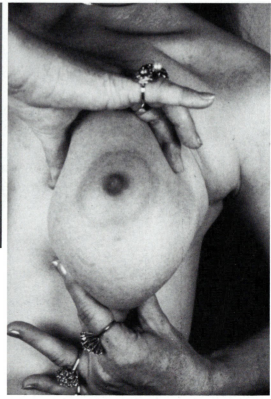

FIGURE 10–15
Class 4 spherical deformity.

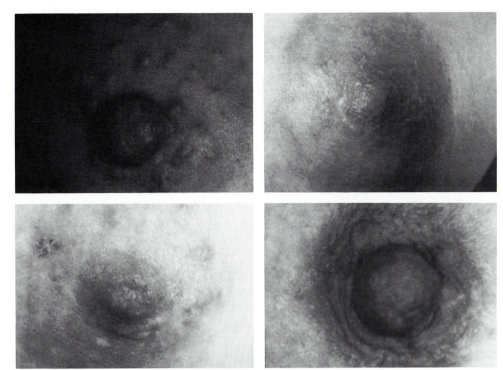

FIGURE 10–16
Excellent areolar scar results.

same intra-areolar perinipple scars is usually quite satisfactory and produces little, if any, additional scar deformity or disfiguration. On the other hand, depending on the areolar size and skin texture as well as the particular breast problem being addressed, shrinkage of the inferior aspect of the areolar hemisphere can occur. Retraction of the adjacent inferior breast tissue with ptosis of the nipple-areola complex is also possible, but extremely rare.

SUMMARY AND CONCLUSIONS

Transareolar, intra-areolar, transthelial, and perithelial incisional approaches for breast augmentation are quite superior in achieving a most inconspicuous result that is aesthetically pleasing. Limitations of this technique relate to problems with a small areola or the necessity of an unusually large prosthesis. This is particularly true of compressible, high-profile, or polyurethane prostheses. The basic principles of technique include complete visualization with fiberoptics, gentle meticulous sharp dissection, extended (5 to 7 days) transaxillary percutaneous Hemovac drainage, and careful layered anatomic closure. In a large series of patients, these factors appear to contribute significantly to success.

References

Courtiss, E. H., Webster, R. C., White, M. F.: Augmentation mammaplasty: Selection of alternatives. Plast. Reconstr. Surg. 54:552, 1974.

Davis, H. H.: Effects on the breast of removal of the nipple or severing of the ducts. Arch. Surg. 58:790, 1949.

Grossman, A. R.: The current status of augmentation mammaplasty. Plast. Reconstr. Surg. 52:1, 1973.

Jenny, H.: Areolar approach to augmentation mammoplasty. Heyer-Shulte Corp. (Data sheet).

Jones, F. R., Tauras, A. P.: Periareolar incision for augmentation mammaplasty. Plast. Reconstr. Surg. 51:641, 1973.

Lewis, J. R.: *Atlas of Aesthetic Plastic Surgery*. Boston, Little, Brown, 1973.

McKinney, P. J., Shedbalker, A. R.: Augmentation mammaplasty, using a non-inflatable prosthesis through circum-areolar incision. Br. J. Plast. Surg. 27:35, 1974.

Pitanguy, I., Carreirao, S. E., Garcia, L. C.: Transareolar incision for augmentation mammaplasty. Plast. Reconstr. Surg. 54:501, 1974.

Saad, M. N.: An extended circumareolar incision for breast augmentation and gynecomastia. Aesthetic Plast. Surg. 7:127, 1983.

Smith, S.: Breast augmentation: Periareolar approach. In: Regnault, P., Daniels, R. K. (eds.): *Aesthetic Plastic Surgery: Principles and Techniques*. Boston, Little, Brown, 1984, p. 569.

Terino, E. O.: Essential concepts in prosthetic breast surgery. Aesthetic Plast. Surg. 6:25, 1982.

Wilkinson, T. S.: Breast augmentation by periareolar incisions. In: Georgiade, N. G.: *Aesthetic Breast Surgery*. Baltimore, Williams & Wilkins, 1983, p. 71.

11

Jorge Fonseca Ely

Augmentation Mammaplasty— The Triple-V Approach

The lack of fully developed and well-shaped breasts may cause diminished self-esteem and frequently intervenes in personal relationships, often impairing sexual behavior.

Whenever excess skin and subcutaneous tissue are available, the redistribution of local tissues is favored by this author (Ely, 1972). Otherwise, the use of implanted prostheses is indicated.

A silicone gel prosthesis (Cronin and Gerow, 1964) is routinely employed. Volume and approach are discussed with the patient. The prosthesis was initially introduced through a submammary sulcus incision, leaving a slight scar.

The periareolar incision, initially described by Webster (1946) for gynecomastia, was employed as early as 1959 for mammary augmentation by J. Fernandez and M. Correa Iturraspe (1959) in Buenos Aires. At that time they used PolyStan strips. Subsequently, Maggiore (1970) and Jenny et al. (1972) presented a similar

approach, using an inflatable prosthesis. Whenever a well-sized areolar diameter is present, the periareolar incision is also suitable for the insertion of a Cronin prosthesis (Perras, 1965; Rees and Aston, 1980). It is best suited for patients with an areolar diameter greater than 35 mm (Bostwick, 1983).

A NEW APPROACH

Measuring an areola with a 30-mm diameter, we will find that the curved intra-areolar incision increases the opening to 45 mm (Fig. 11–1D). However, if we design three consecutive Vs, the access line will increase to 65 mm (Fig. 11–1E). Furthermore, due to skin elasticity, the seven angles of the triple-V incision "give" more than the two extremities of the curved incision.

Two lateral Vs are formed starting from lateral and medial sides of the areola (Fig. 11–1F and H), and a third one is tangential to the nipple (Fig. 11–1G). All

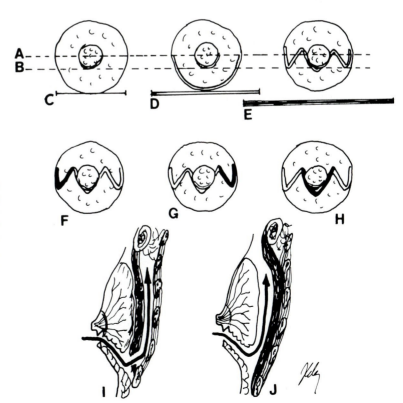

FIGURE 11–1

Guidelines to the triple V approach. A, Midareolar transverse line. B, Subareolar line. C, Areola diameter. D, Straight line corresponding to a semicircular incision. E, Line equivalent to the sum of the six sides of the triple V incision. F, The first V. G, The second V, a mirror image of the first one. H, The third V, tangential to the nipple. The pocket: I, Retropectoralis approach. J, Retromammary undermining.

113

the branches are approximately the same length, forming a staggered incision (Fig. 11–2A). This approach gives more room for the undermining, hemostasis, and prosthesis introduction maneuvers (Ely, 1972).

MARKING

Two transverse lines are traced, one crossing the center of the areola (A) and the second tangential to the lower end of the nipple (B) (Fig. 11–1). The first V runs along the areolar perimeter between lines A and B, returning to B. The second V is tangential to the nipple, and the third V is a mirror image of the first one (Ely, 1980).

SURGICAL TECHNIQUE

The surgery may be performed with the patient under general or local anesthesia. The incision is made 3 mm deep (Fig. 11–2A), and the dissection of the lower half of the areola is performed near the dermis, in order to preserve vessels and nerves of the nipple-areola complex (Schwarzmann's maneuver) (Fig. 11–2B). Beyond the areolar margin, the dissection continues at the subcutaneous plane, around the mammary tissue, down to the pectoral fascia at the level of the submammary sulcus (Fig. 11–2C). Cutting mammary tissue is carefully avoided, because the ductus may contain dermis. Contamination of the pocket increases the risk of thick capsule formation. Hemostasis is controlled with fiberoptic light and bipolar coagulation (Fig. 11–2D).

Undermining proceeds over the pectoral fascia if submammary insertion of the prosthesis is preferred (Fig. 11–2E). In most cases, the prosthesis is placed under the muscle (see Fig. 11–1I). The dissection is easier along the lateral border of pectoral muscle. Its distal insertions are bluntly detached from the sternum and lower ribs to prevent upward dislocation of the prosthesis. The subpectoral plane is practically avascular, but a careful inspection is carried out with fiberoptic light, and hemostasis is reviewed. The pocket is irrigated for removal of blood clots and loose fatty tissue.

The operating table is moved to the Trendelenburg position. With the head downward, the force of gravity works in favor of the prosthesis insertion. The prosthesis is carefully pushed into the pocket with two fingers, alternately advancing (Fig. 11–2G to I).

After the prosthesis is placed in the proper position and the mammary volume is satisfactory, suturing is done by layers, starting with the subcutaneous layer at the submammary sulcus level (Fig. 11–2J). A second suture line is made near the areolar perimeter (absorbable 5-0). Then the dermis is fastened together, beginning at the angles of the Vs (Fig. 11–2K). The breasts are checked for symmetry before final closure. Nylon suture (6-0) is employed for accurately finishing the skin closure. Drains, antibiotics, and steroids are not used routinely. Porous tape is applied to approximate the skin edges and keep the mammary shape in the correct position (Fig. 11–2N). A soft elastic brassiere completes the dressing.

POSTOPERATIVE CARE

Visual inspection and soft palpation are regularly carried out during the first 6 hours after surgery, and the patient is instructed to report any subsequent pain or swelling.

Two or 3 days after surgery, when the patient returns for a postoperative visit, the implant is moved gently throughout the extent of the capsule, upward, downward, to the left, and to the right. The patient is encouraged to gently repeat this maneuver three times a day. The idea is to allow the pocket to remain as large as possible during the healing phase.

After removal of the sutures (Fig. 11–2O), the porous tape is reapplied and replaced up to 30 days, to ensure the slightest possible scar tension. Heavy exercises are avoided during the first postoperative month. Direct exposure to sunlight is avoided for 3 months.

RESULTS

The scars are usually inconspicuous. Care must be taken in patients with very dark areolae. Greater risk of discoloration makes the areolar approach less enthusiastically indicated in those cases. The result of the case photographed step by step is shown in Figure 11–3. The triple-V approach is especially indicated in patients with very small areolae, as can be seen in Figure 11–4.

CONCLUSION

A new way to deal with small areolae is presented as an additional resource: the triple-V incision provides more space for dissection and prosthesis insertion, remaining within the limits of the areola.

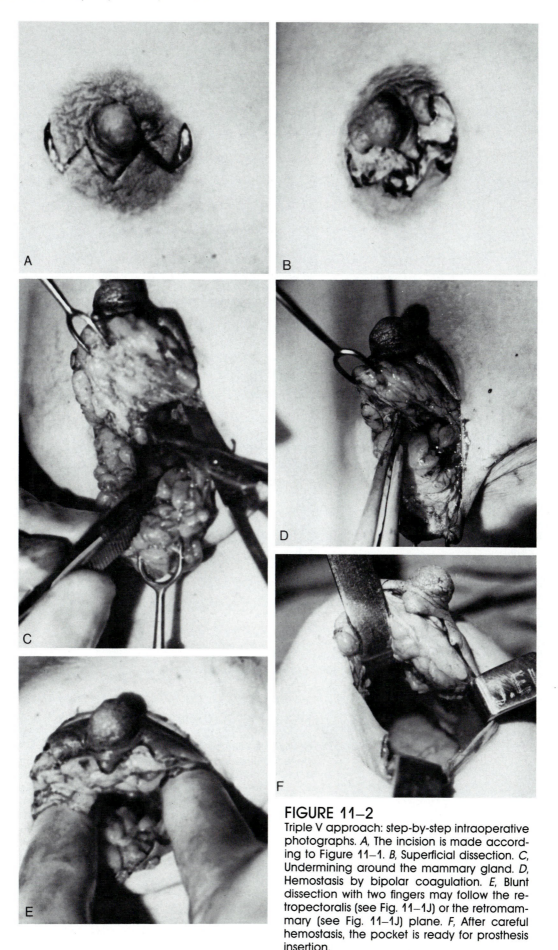

FIGURE 11–2

Triple V approach: step-by-step intraoperative photographs. *A,* The incision is made according to Figure 11–1. *B,* Superficial dissection. *C,* Undermining around the mammary gland. *D,* Hemostasis by bipolar coagulation. *E,* Blunt dissection with two fingers may follow the retropectoralis (see Fig. 11–1J) or the retromammary (see Fig. 11–1J) plane. *F,* After careful hemostasis, the pocket is ready for prosthesis insertion.

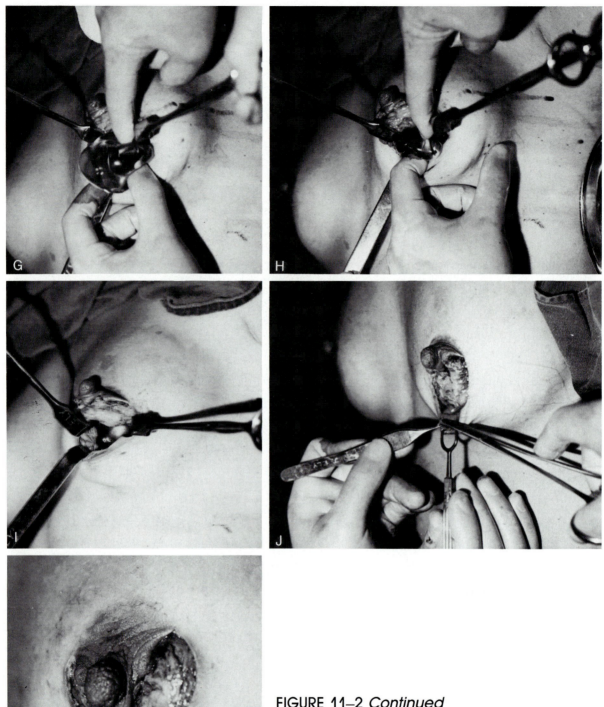

FIGURE 11–2 *Continued*
G and *H*, The silicone prosthesis is gently pushed into the pocket with two fingers. *I*, The insertion maneuver is completed. *J*, Subcutaneous suture at the level of the inferior rim of mammary gland. *K*, Beginning of dermal suture.

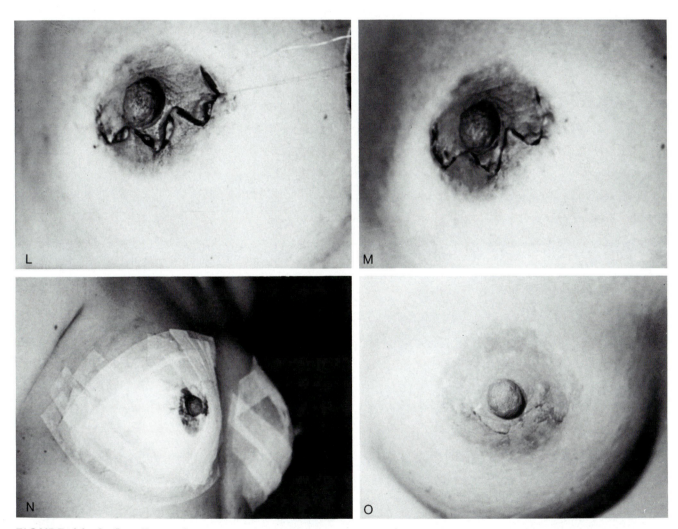

FIGURE 11–2 *Continued*
L and *M*, Absorbable sutures are placed in the dermal layer. *N*, Porous tape fixation. *O*, Two weeks after surgery.

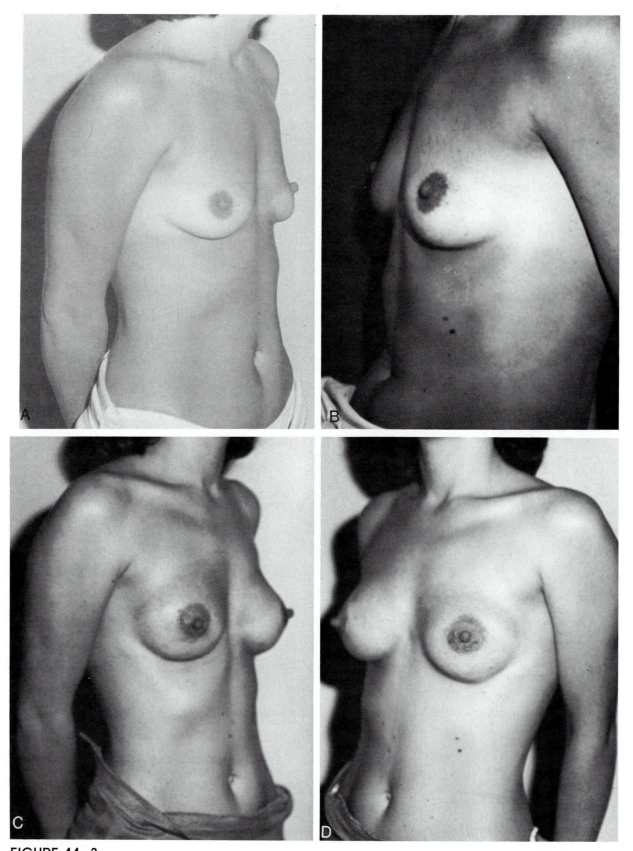

FIGURE 11–3
Case shown in Figure 11–2. *A* and *B*, Preoperative lateral views. *C* and *D*, Postoperative lateral views.

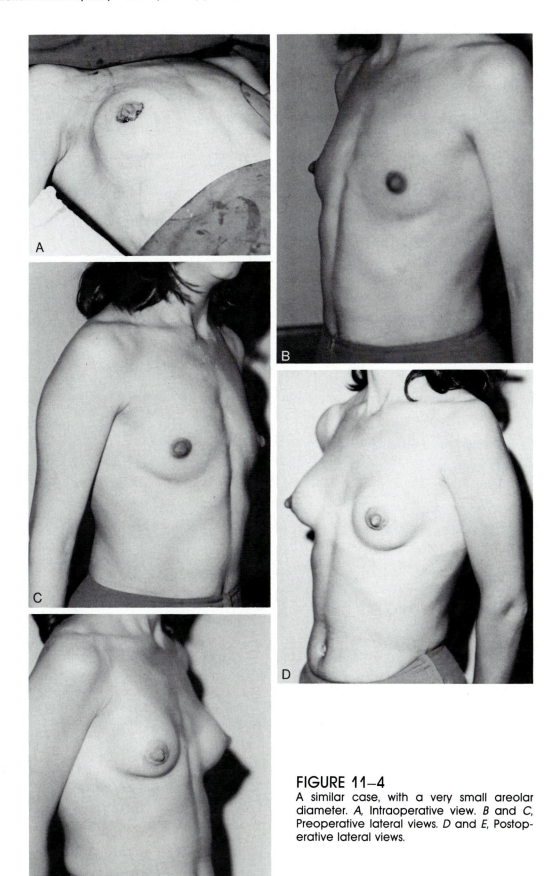

FIGURE 11–4
A similar case, with a very small areolar diameter. *A,* Intraoperative view. *B* and *C,* Preoperative lateral views. *D* and *E,* Postoperative lateral views.

References

Bostwick, J., II: *Aesthetic and Reconstructive Breast Surgery*. St. Louis, C.V. Mosby, 1983, p. 67.

Cronin, T. D., Gerow, F. J.: Augmentation mammaplasty: A new "natural feel" prosthesis. In: *Transactions of the Third International Congress of Plastic Surgery*. Amsterdam, Excerpta Medica Foundation, 1964, p. 41.

Ely, J. F.: Organic mammary augmentation. In: *Transactions of the First Congress of Aesthetic Plastic Surgery*. Madrid, Sanchez Pacheco, 1972, p. 31.

Ely, J. F.: *Cirurgia Plastica*. Rio de Janeiro, Guanabara Koogan, 1980a, p. 564.

Ely, J. F.: The triple "V" incision for augmentation mammaplasty. In: *Transactions of the Seventh International Congress of Plastic and Reconstructive Surgery*. Rio de Janeiro, Cartgraf, 1980b, p. 526.

Fernandez, J. C., Correa Iturraspe, M.: Correción de la hipomastia con viruta de polieno incluída por via areolar. El Dia Medico 75:1, 1959.

Jenny, H., Hartel, P., Vinas, J.: Mammaplasty. Microform J. Aesthetic Plast. Surg., Blue Header, 1972.

Maggiore, L. D. In: Lupo, G., Boggio, R. G.: *Chirurgia Plastica del Seno e Della Regione Mammaria*. Torino, Minerva Medica, 1970, p. 352.

Perras, C.: Plastic reconstruction of the small breast. J. Am. Med. Wom. Assoc. 20:951, 1965.

Rees, T. D., Aston, S. J.: Mammary augmentation, correction of asymmetry, and gynecomastia. In: Rees, T. D.: *Aesthetic Plastic Surgery*. Philadelphia, W. B. Saunders, 1980, p. 954.

Webster, J. P.: Mastectomy for gynecomastia through a semicircular intra-areolar incision. Ann. Surg. 124:557, 1946.

12

Boyd R. Burkhardt

Complications of Augmentation Mammaplasty

Prosthetic breast augmentation is one of the world's most popular aesthetic surgical operations. Like most aesthetic procedures, it is a completely elective undertaking designed to improve the patient's appearance and self-image, rather than to correct any true physical deformity. Well-controlled psychologic studies (Shipley et al., 1977, 1978) have shown that women seeking this operation are as stable psychologically as other women and that the operation has little effect on their basic personality characteristics but does make them happier with the way their clothing fits and with their body image.

Surgeons will generally agree that there should be a reasonable relationship between the potential benefits of a surgical operation and the incidence and severity of the complications that may accompany it. The perceived benefits of any operation should outweigh its potential risks. Unfortunately, this risk/benefit ratio is particularly difficult to define in breast augmentation because the potential benefits, as well as most of the complications, defy quantitative assessment. A classic example is the survey conducted by Hetter (1979), in which the patients appeared to have a high incidence of both capsular contracture and decreased nipple sensitivity; yet only 1% said they would not have the operation done again! We must be cautious, as physicians, before imposing any adverse judgments of our own on an operation that is pleasing to such a high percentage of patients.

Despite some admitted problems, breast augmentation is clearly both better and safer than it used to be. Most of this improvement, however, has come from trial-and-error changes in the implanted prostheses, rather than from a scientific understanding of the surgical complications. The synthetic sponge implants of the 1950s, although they consistently became hard and/or extruded (Broadbent and Woolf, 1967), were a welcome change from the earlier free fat grafts that frequently liquefied and drained and that produced only minimal enlargement even when successful. The Dacron-backed silicone gel implants of the early 1960s, growing out of the extensive biocompatibility investigations of silicone after World War II and out of the successful treatment of hydrocephalus using a shunt of silicone tubing, were clearly another major advancement. The Dacron backing eventually proved to be unnecessary for implant fixation, and the removal of this in the early 1970s was followed by a further reduction of complications (Williams, 1972).

The saline-inflatable implant was conceived to permit breast augmentation through a smaller, less conspicuous incision; and the double-lumen implant, to permit postoperative volume reduction by percutaneous needling (Hartley, 1976). More recently the polyurethane-covered implant, first introduced by Ashley in 1971, has enjoyed a remarkable new surge of popularity (Herman, 1984; Hester, 1988). A fascinating variety of additional implant variations and modifications have enjoyed their brief moment on stage but have not survived the marketplace.

Despite the progress that has been made, and despite the continued popularity and wide acceptance of this surgery, complications can and do occur. With the notable exception of capsular contracture, the incidence of problems is quite low. Although there is some overlap, I have for convenience separated the complications into various categories, depending on whether they are complications of surgery in general or of augmentation mammaplasty in particular or are related specifically to the prostheses. Fibrous capsular contracture, the most common and least understood complication of augmentation mammaplasty, has the dubious distinction of having earned a category of its own.

ORDINARY SURGICAL COMPLICATIONS

Hematoma incidence in reported series ranges from under 1% (Burkhardt et al., 1986) to almost 6% (Brownstein and Owsley, 1978). This differnce may be related to the dissection technique (blunt versus sharp), the prosthesis placement (retromammary versus retromuscular), the anesthesia (local versus general), or other technical variables. Drains have been advocated (Wiliams et al., 1975), but most surgeons today do not use them. Large hematomas may require evacuation, but most can simply be allowed to be absorbed. Hematomas have been suspected as a cause of contracture, but this relationship has never been proven (Burkhardt et al., 1986). In one case reported by Georgiade et al. (1979)

the use of intraluminal steroids was blamed for delayed vessel erosion and late postoperative hematoma.

Infection can occur around breast prostheses just as it can around any other implanted foreign material. Surprisingly, even breast implants that are clearly infected may not have to be removed. Although most infected implants inserted through inframammary incisions will become extruded, Courtiss et al. (1979) reported that about 75% of those inserted through a periareolar incision can be retained with vigorous antibiotic therapy. However, most, if not all, of the retained infected implants will develop significant capsular contracture.

As suggested by Marion (1984) and Pollock (1984), the polyurethane-covered implants might be expected to be associated with a higher incidence of infection, but conclusive data are lacking. If a polyurethane-covered implant does become infected, removal of all of the infected polyurethane foam can be a difficult technical problem (Umansky, 1985).

Hypertrophic scars may occur with the inframammary approach. Like hypertrophic scars following reduction mammaplasty, these may not always be corrected satisfactorily by either re-excision or steroid injection. The incidence of such scarring is not recorded and certainly is quite low, but it can be a major detraction from an otherwise excellent cosmetic result. I have not personally seen this problem in 15 years using the periareolar approach and do not know whether it occurs with the axillary approach.

Toxic shock syndrome has been documented (Barnett et al., 1983) from infection around breast implants. It is exceedingly rare.

COMPLICATIONS SPECIFIC TO AUGMENTATION MAMMAPLASTY

Nipple hyposensitivity is an obvious concern in an operation that has strong overtones of enhanced sexual attractiveness, and patients frequently ask about this preoperatively. The incidence of hyposensitivity has been reported as 15% (Courtiss et al., 1979) to 49% (Hetter, 1979), a rather wide range. Documentation is difficult, but as a practical matter, nipple hyposensitivity has not been a major source of patient dissatisfaction. The occasional patient who is unwilling to risk *any* loss of nipple sensitivity probably should not have the operation.

Surprisingly, the patients in Hetter's series experienced a higher incidence of sensory loss with the inframammary approach (49%) than with the periareolar approach (34%). Whether or not this difference is significant, there is certainly no evidence that the periareolar approach *increases* the risk of hyposensitivity. Some surgeons believe that retromuscular placement is less likely to produce sensory impairment, but this contention has never been documented.

Mondor's disease, a superficial cordlike thrombophlebitis, is occasionally palpable in the breast after augmentation mammaplasty and may even be recurrent (Fischl et al., 1975). It does not embolize and is not a serious problem.

Giant galactoceles (Luhan, 1979) and *aberrant lactation* through the surgical incision (Hartley and Schatten, 1971) have both been reported. These complications are very rare but are of interest because they demonstrate the potential for continuity between the ductal system of the breast and the periprosthetic space.

The double-bubble syndrome, or persistent postoperative mammary ptosis, can occur with either retromammary or retromuscular augmentation. The cause in retromammary augmentation is usually a ptotic breast augmented with too small an implant, which then becomes encapsulated and rides too high in relation to the nipple. The cause in retromuscular augmentation is simply retention of the normal inframammary fold behind a ptotic breast. Significant ptosis is a contraindication to retromuscular augmentation unless the patient is prepared to have a ptotic breast sitting in front of a retromuscular mound (Fig. 12–1).

IMPLANT-RELATED COMPLICATIONS

Deflation of the single-lumen inflatable prosthesis does occur. The incidence is unknown but increases with time. Published clinical series by Burkhardt et al. (1986) and McKinney and Tresley (1983) have documented an incidence of deflation ranging from 0% (24-month average follow-up) to 8% (32-month average follow-up). Early deflation may result from valve leakage or an unrecognized technical error like perforating the shell with a needle. Late deflation results from a perforation at the end of a fold in the shell, either because of material fatigue or because the inner surface of the shell

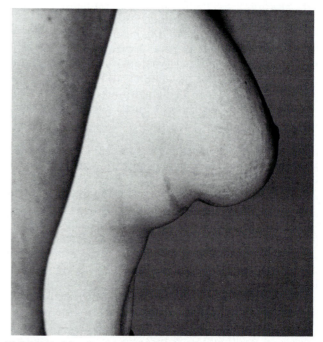

FIGURE 12–1

Breast contour distortion, without contracture, from retromuscular augmentation of a ptotic breast.

rubs against itself until it is abraded completely through (Worton et al., 1980). Late deflation may also occur because of implant rupture during closed compression capsulotomy. During the 1970s a "clear shell" inflatable implant was marketed that was made with a different polymerization process that produced a beautifully clear and much thinner shell. Although never recorded in our literature, its failure rate probably approached 100%, and it has been withdrawn from the market.

Although deflation of inflatable implants cannot be completely avoided, common sense suggests that it can be minimized by checking the valve and by filling the implants to the upper limit of the manufacturer's recommendations, thus reducing the number and severity of the surface folds. The occasional deflation is hardly a surgical disaster but does require replacement of the implant. Failure of the thin outer shell of the double-lumen implant is probably rather common but is rarely noticed by the patient because the volume loss is minimal.

Rippling of the augmented breast as reported by Clarendon (1980) is an uncommon but very distressing complication that is difficult to correct. It can occur with any type of implant, but is more common when an underfilled inflatable implant is placed in the retromammary position behind a very thin, ptotic breast; when there is no capsular contracture; and when intraluminal steroids are used in sufficient concentration to cause soft tissue atrophy. It is especially noticeable when the patient leans forward (Fig. 12–2).

This problem is less common with retromuscular placement, but retromuscular placement is often unsuitable for the ptotic breast (to be discussed later). Replacement with gel-filled implants may help, but a simpler solution is a push-up bra.

Irregularity of the breast and *fold flaw erosion* (Derman et al., 1983) can be considered together. A fold in the implant, whether inflatable or gel-filled, can produce

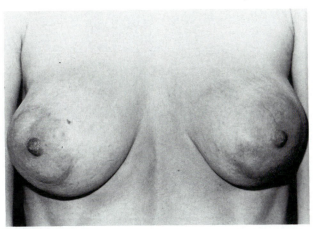

FIGURE 12–3
Distortion following closed capsulotomy. Note the visible irregularity behind the areola on both sides.

a palpable and visible irregularity in the breast (Fig. 12–3). This is particularly common after multiple closed capsulotomies in which an uncontrolled anterior tear in the capsule allows an irregularity in the implant to present in an abnormally superficial position. Although it may occur with any implant type, it is probably more common with the saline-filled implant because the shell is relatively thick and stiff, producing folds that are sharper and more pronounced. Occasionally a superficial fold will erode through the skin (Fig. 12–4). Because of this, I personally avoid performing closed capsulotomies whenever possible.

Gel leakage (from the gel-filled implants) occurs in two very different forms: the microscopic droplets of silicone gel that "bleed" through the intact silicone shell and the gross extrusion of gel that occurs following rupture of an implant, most commonly as a result of closed capsulotomy.

The initial recognition of gel "bleed" both *in vitro* (on filter paper) (Barker et al., 1978; Bergman and von der Ende, 1979) and *in vivo* (as droplets in the fibrotic capsule) was exciting because of its potential role as a cause of capsular contracture. In all other respects, and even though it has been shown by Hausner and associates (1978) to migrate to local lymph nodes, free gel in such small quantities seems to be harmless. Silicone in small quantities is ubiquitous in contemporary Western society: it enters the body as a coating for hypodermic needles and even as an anti-foaming agent in proprietary remedies for indigestion.

After an initial flush of optimistic enthusiasm, plastic surgeons had to recognize that gel bleed could not be the "cause" of capsular contracture, but might well be a contributing factor in the apparently higher incidence of contracture around gel-filled implants (see later).

Gel extrusion from a torn implant, most commonly the result of a vigorous closed capsulotomy, is another matter. Gel has been demonstrated to migrate along tissue planes into the axilla (Hueston and Hare, 1979) and the arm (Edmond and Versaci, 1980; Huang et al., 1978) and on at least one occasion has been extruded from the nipple via the ductal system of the breast (Zide, 1981). Under these circumstances, gel migration

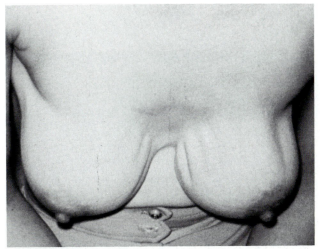

FIGURE 12–2
Rippling of a thin breast, without contracture, with an inflatable implant and possibly with steroids. (From Clarendon, C.: Breast thinning and streaking following the use of inflatable implants: A subjective clinical study. Ann. Plast. Surg. 5:436, 1980.)

124   BREAST AUGMENTATION

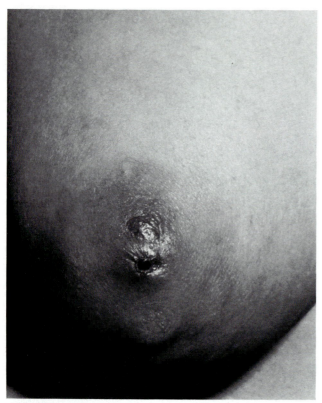

FIGURE 12–4
Exposure of the implant and a fold in the shell after closed capsulotomy.

has sometimes produced a granulomatous reaction requiring excision (Eisenberg and Bartels, 1977), but the etiology of this reaction remains obscure in the face of silicone's well-documented biocompatibility.

Human adjuvant disease is a hypothetical immunologic response to silicone gel that has attracted more legal attention than scientific support. Although experiments by Kossovsky et al. (1983) with guinea pigs have shown that silicone gel mixed with adjuvant can stimulate a cellular response to a later "challenge" with silicone gel, there is little or no scientific evidence that this occurs in humans. A single case report by Baldwin and Kaplan (1983) describes a patient in whom arthralgia, adenopathy, malaise, and weight loss developed 3 years after augmentation with gel-filled mammary implants, one of which was found to have ruptured. The symptoms improved after implant removal.

Sclerodoma after mammaplasty with gel-filled implants was reported in five patients in a retrospective study by Spiera (1988), with bibliographic reference to other papers relating silicone to connective tissue and autoimmune disease. Whether the association is one of cause and effect or simply coincidental remains to be seen, but the question is certainly valid.

CAPSULAR CONTRACTURE

There is, nonetheless, a pseudocapsule of fibrous tissue formed around the (silicone) implant. It will be necessary to

determine whether this, in time, will compress the implant and produce undesirable firmness or buckling (Broadbent and Woolf, 1967).

Capsular contracture is a particularly frustrating problem for everyone concerned with breast augmentation—the surgeon, the patient, and the manufacturer. It is the single most common complication of prosthetic use, yet has stubbornly resisted solution despite more than 25 years of persistent clinical and laboratory investigation. A summary of the best clinical information available suggests that the incidence of unacceptable contracture around retromammary silicone implants has been at least 50% (Burkhardt, 1983). Using sales figures from the implant industry, this means that over 50,000 women *annually* have had to accept surgical results less satisfactory than desired. Severity varies, but any significant degree of contracture detracts from the surgical result, and severe contracture can produce an "implant cripple," often defying even the most well-intentioned efforts at correction. Even more seriously, preliminary recent information (as yet inadequately substantiated) has suggested that contracture may so distort the breast as to interfere with proper mammographic examination, interfering with early diagnosis and treatment of carcinoma of the breast (Silverstein et al., 1988).

One cannot possibly understand the problems inherent in treating capsular contracture without briefly reviewing its history.

About 30 years ago, long before governmental regulatory restriction of implantable devices was even being considered, prosthetic augmentation with synthetic materials seemed a rational and welcome alternative to the problems of autologous fat transplants. Sponges of various chemical and physical configurations were manufactured and placed behind the breasts. The results were poor: 100% of these sponge implants either extruded because of infection or became severely contracted and hard (Broadbent and Woolf, 1967) (Fig. 12–5). The accepted explanation for the hardness was that the sponges became infiltrated with fibrous tissue. This was thought to be a sign of physiologic "rejection" of the

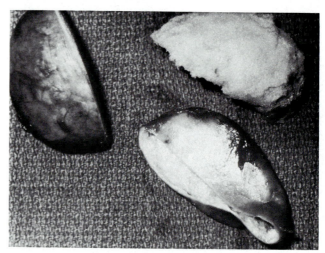

FIGURE 12–5
Contracture around a sponge implant.

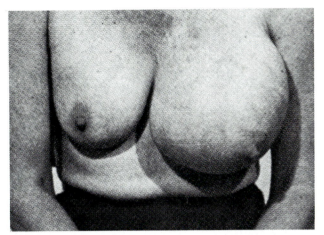

FIGURE 12–6
Seroma around a sponge implant. Cultures of the fluid frequently yielded *Staphylococcus albus*. (From Gurdin, M., Carlin, G. A.: Complications of breast augmentation. Plast. Reconstr. Surg. 50:530, 1967.)

foreign material, a perfectly rational assumption because the "rejection" was both universal and bilateral. Studies done more recently have shown, however, that the sponge was really not infiltrated at all, but was simply surrounded by a contracting fibrous capsule that was both histologically and clinically indistinguishable from the process we now recognize as circumferential capsular contracture (Peters and Smith, 1981) (see Fig. 12–5). It is interesting in retrospect to note that massive seroma formation was a common problem and that aspiration and culture often yielded *Staphylococcus albus* (Broadbent and Woolf, 1967; Gurdin and Carlin, 1967) (Fig. 12–6). Despite these problems, many patients remained happy with their sponge implants, and clinicians occasionally encounter these implants even today.

Introduction of the Dacron-backed natural feel silicone gel implants in the early 1960s was clearly a step forward. There were fewer extrusions, seromas were rare, and occasionally an implant would even remain soft—at least for a while! With this new implant, *unilateral* contracture made its initial appearance.

Although it was obviously difficult to understand why the body should react differently to two identical implants, the "foreign body rejection" theory still seemed so reasonable that it was never seriously challenged.

The Dacron backing was later found to be unnecessary for implant fixation and was eliminated in the late 1960s (Williams, 1972). The incidence of contracture dropped once again, and unilateral contracture became even more common. In the early 1970s, a single-lumen inflatable implant was introduced to facilitate insertion through a smaller incision around the areola. An unexpected fringe benefit was that once again the incidence of contracture dropped, and unilateral contracture now became as much the rule as the exception (Rees et al., 1973).

In broad perspective, there are two important threads running through this history that deserve special identi-

fication and attention. The first is that these trial-and-error modifications in implant technology have substantially reduced the incidence of capsular contracture. Although truly reliable data are not available, a preponderance of evidence suggests that the incidence of contracture with the most commonly used implants has been as noted in Table 12–1 (Burkhardt, 1983).

The second important historical thread is that the relative incidence of unilateral contracture has consistently increased as the overall incidence of contracture has diminished. With fewer contractures, more are one-sided. In fact, the relative probability of bilateral versus unilateral contracture seems to conform reasonably well to the mathematic projections for a random phenomenon (Burkhardt, 1984) (Table 12–2; Fig. 12–7). This is a terribly important clue. It indicates that contracture is breast-based and unrelated to the individual's particular systemic physiology. In other words, if we wish to identify the etiology of this problem, we should look at the breast itself, rather than at "wound healing" or other general physiologic mechanisms.

The next enigmatic clue to the cause of capsular contracture came not from augmentation mammaplasty, but from a quite different operation: subcutaneous mastectomy with immediate prosthetic reconstruction. Immediate insertion of a smooth silicone prosthesis into the subcutaneous pocket created by removal of the breast gland produced a very high incidence of contracture, whereas putting the same implant *behind* the muscles and their associated fascia achieved a predictably soft result (Jarrett et al., 1978; Woods et al., 1980). What could explain such a dramatic difference? Was it the size of the pocket? The nature of the surface? The massaging action of the muscle? Or did the muscle simply provide a fortuitous physical barrier between the smooth prosthetic surface and the bundle of freshly divided, contaminated breast ducts just behind the nipple?

No historical summary of capsular contracture would be complete without recognition of the remarkable resurrection of the foam-covered implant. This prosthetic modification was first introduced by Ashley (1971) nearly 20 years ago and was quickly buried by an avalanche of concerns about the physiologic response to polyurethane foam (Cocke et al., 1975; Slade and Peterson, 1982; Smahel, 1978). Improved versions of the original model have recently been the focus of multiple clinical reports claiming remarkable freedom from capsular contracture, both in elective augmentation mammaplasty (Herman, 1984) and in reconstructive procedures (Eyssen et al., 1984; Schatten, 1984; Hester, 1988).

TABLE 12–1
Estimated Incidence of Contracture for Commonly Used Implants

	%
Sponge implants	100
Patched gel-filled	70
Patchless gel-filled	55
Inflatable	35

TABLE 12–2
Actual Versus Predicted Bilateral Contracture Rates in Published Series

AUTHORS	IMPLANTS	CONTRACTURES AS PERCENTAGE OF IMPLANTS	BILATERAL CONTRACTURE AS PERCENTAGE OF PATIENTS	
			Actual	Predicted
Broadbent, 1967	Sponge	100*	100*	100
McKinney, 1983	Gel	31	26	9
Brownstein, 1978	Gel	29	17	9
Hipps, 1978	Gel	29	15	9
McKinney, 1983	Saline	16	7	2
Milojevic, 1983	Saline-gel	3	0	0

*Includes contracture and/or extrusion.
From Burkhardt, B. R.: Comparing contracture rates: Probability theory and the unilateral contracture. Plast. Reconstr. Surg. 74:527, 1984.

The addition of microtexturing of the outer shell of the Silastic prostheses appears to be another major step forward in disrupting the linear scar formation, as found with the smooth-walled prostheses (Ersek, 1989). Scar contracture is therefore decreased. The design of the microtexturing appears to be preferable to that of the polyurethane-covered prostheses. The polyurethane covering has been found to disintegrate over a period of years (Hester, 1988).

Etiologic Theories for Contracture

Because sound etiologic evidence has been lacking until recently, several different theories have been advanced to explain capsular contracture. Although there may be modest experimental and/or clinical support for some of these, I believe that most have now been abandoned at least as a *primary* cause.

A *physiologic response* (foreign body reaction, immune response, rejection phenomenon), discussed above, seems inconsistent with the prevalence of unilateral contracture.

Inadequate dissection, based on the observed pocket/implant disproportion, failed to explain why contractures usually showed up only after a prolonged postoperative delay instead of at the completion of surgery. *Hematoma,* obvious or occult, was theoretically an attractive etiology because it could explain unilateral contracture; but despite some supportive experimental work presented by Williams and associates (1975), the correlation between hematoma and contracture has not been consistent. *Gel bleed* may be a contributing or predisposing factor, but is not a primary cause of contracture. Some bleeding implants develop severe contracture, whereas other identical implants remain soft apparently forever (Gayon, 1979). Furthermore, saline-filled implants, which bleed little if at all, can still develop severe capsular contracture.

The evidence for a *bacterial etiology* falls into two general categories. The first is highly circumstantial. Fibrous sequestration is an acknowledged response to bacterial proliferation around any foreign body. *Staphylococcus epidermidis* is known to live in the ductal system of the breast: it may be cultured readily from nipple secretions (Courtiss et al., 1979), from breast milk (Boer et al., 1981), and from biopsy specimens of uninfected breast parenchyma (Argenta and Grabb, 1981). The ductal system of the breast may be contiguous with the periprosthetic space: we have reports of lactation around the implant and out of the incision (Hartley and Schatten, 1971), of periprosthetic galactoceles (Luhan, 1979), and of extrusion of free silicone gel from the nipple (Zide, 1981) (Fig. 12–8). Seromas around sponge implants frequently yielded *S. epidermidis* (Broadbent and Woolf, 1967). This organism is also present in retromammary pockets prior to insertion of implants and is present in established contractures (Burkhardt et al., 1981). Contracture following either subcutaneous mastectomy or elective augmentation is reduced by retromuscular placement of the implant (Jarrett et al., 1978; Mahler and Hauben, 1982; Woods et al., 1980). There is collateral clinical evidence that *S. epidermidis* produces contracture around penile implants, neurosurgical shunts, and cardiac pacemakers (Fig. 12–9). Finally, contamination of miniature mammary implants with *S. epidermidis* or *Staphylococcus aureus* causes capsular contracture in experimental animals (Kossovsky et al., 1984; Shah et al., 1981).

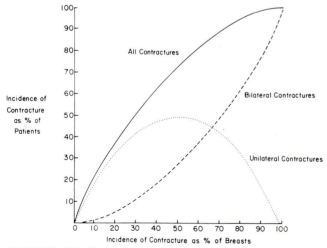

FIGURE 12–7
The predicted relationship between bilateral and unilateral contracture if contracture is a random, breast-based response. (From Burkhardt, B. R.: Comparing contracture rates: Probability theory and the unilateral contracture. Plast. Reconstr. Surg. 74:527, 1984.)

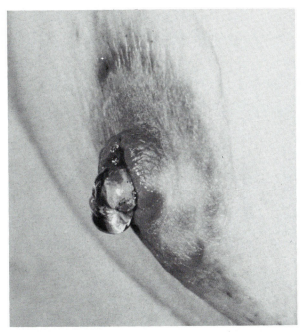

FIGURE 12–8
Silicone gel extruding from the nipple ducts after closed compression capsulotomy with implant rupture. (From Zide, B. M.: Complications of closed capsulotomy after augmentation (Letter). Plast. Reconstr. Surg. 67:697, 1981.)

The second category of evidence for an infectious etiology is more direct but consists of only one clinical study, which requires independent confirmation before it can be fully accepted. If bacterial contamination is suspect as the cause of contracture, an obvious question is whether local antibacterials can help. To answer this specific question, a prospective, blind, controlled clinical study was performed with the use of multiple independent judges and an internally consistent objective measuring system (Burkhardt et al., 1986). The results showed a dramatic and statistically significant reduction of contracture by means of any one of four antibacterial protocols. Intraoperative irrigation with 5% povidone-iodine solution (half-strength Betadine solution) was the most simple and reduced the incidence of contracture by 85% at 3 months and by 50% at 2 years (Fig. 12–10). Unless there was an experimental error that has remained undetected to date, these results are very difficult to reconcile with anything other than a bacterial etiology. Povidone-iodine irrigation is clearly *not* a definitive answer to the contracture problem, of course, but it does provide a modicum of welcome and long overdue relief.

What Rational Steps Can Be Taken to Reduce the Incidence of Contracture?

Even though surgeons may not yet fully understand the etiology of capsular contracture, there are still a number of things they can do to prevent it that are consistent with the evidence at hand. Most of these require a trade-off of some sort, which is why they are not universally adopted. On the other hand, some commonly used techniques lack significant clinical and experimental support.

Retromuscular implant placement reduces the incidence of contracture (Mahler and Hauben, 1982; Tebbetts, 1984). Although the best comparative figures are for reconstruction (Jarrett et al., 1978; Slade, 1984; Woods et al., 1980), as opposed to cosmetic augmentation, it is probable that the same general rules apply to both kinds of surgery. Those who still prefer the retromammary position will point out that with retromuscular placement local anesthesia is more difficult, postoperative pain is greater, asymmetry and displacement are more common, the inframammary fold may be poorly defined, the breast may develop significant contour abnormalities, and when contracture *does* occur it may be exceptionally difficult to treat (Fig. 12–11). Nevertheless, because retromuscular placement does reduce the incidence of contracture, it has become the preferred procedure of a growing number of surgeons.

Saline-filled implants have a reduced incidence of contracture. At least, this appears to be the case in every reported study offering a reasonable basis for comparison with gel-filled implants (Fig. 12–12). This reduced incidence is probably related to gel bleed, and the difficulty of reconciling this with a presumed bacterial etiology is one of the bacterial theory's major drawbacks. It is possible that the greatly increased surface area provided by the silicone droplets enhances susceptibility to bacterial growth, but this does seem to be stretching for an explanation.

Polyurethane foam–covered implants have a reduced incidence of contracture (Brand, 1984; Eyssen et al., 1984; Herman, 1984; Schatten, 1984; Hester, 1988). The

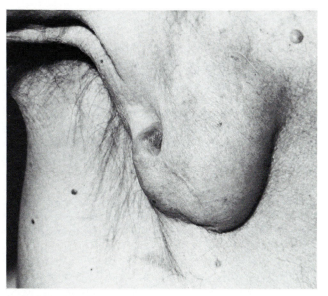

FIGURE 12–9
Capsular contracture around a cardiac pacemaker, with threatened exposure and extrusion. Culture yielded *Staphylococcus epidermidis.*

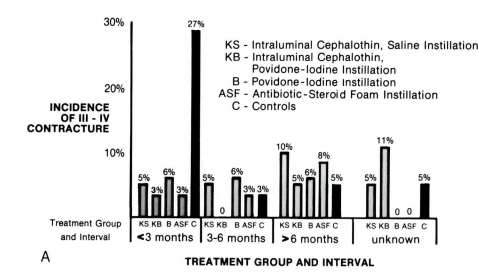

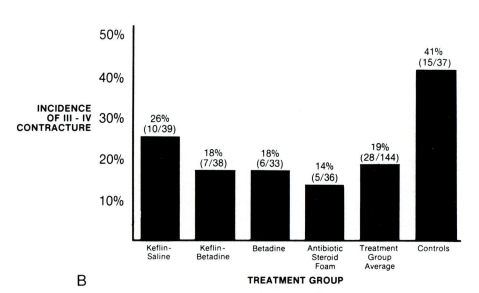

FIGURE 12–10

The incidence of contracture in a controlled study of local antibacterials by the time of onset *(A)* and at the end of the study *(B)*. (From Burkhardt, B. R., Dempsey, P. D., Schnur, P. L., Tofield, J. J.: Capsular contracture: A prospective study of the effect of local antibacterial agents. Plast. Reconstr. Surg. 77:919, 1986.)

effect of these implants is probably at least as significant as any of the other factors we have discussed. Despite this, their use remains cloaked in controversy. Their history is one of the most fascinating stories in the entire development of breast prostheses and certainly should be reviewed and understood by anyone planning to use them.

Much of the controversy surrounding the foam-covered implants arose, in retrospect, from our own 1970s preoccupation with "tissue reactivity" as a presumed cause of capsular contracture (it may actually have very little to do with the problem) and with the extraordinary claims that were made for an empirically designed foam-covered implant (Ashley, 1971) that clearly caused more "tissue reactivity" than anything else on the market (Cocke et al., 1975). Add to this the discouraging experiences with sponge implants in the 1950s, conflicting claims about polyurethane "inertness," a well-publicized instance of infection accompanied by implant extrusion and long-term drainage from embedded poly-

urethane (Umansky, 1985), claims of long-term polyurethane absorption (Slade and Peterson, 1982), and some natural cynicism from plastic surgeons jaded by previous experience with other implant failures (Fig. 12–13).

Although most clinical studies of the foam-covered implants have been retrospective, uncontrolled, nonblind, and apocryphal, the increasing number of favorable reports cannot fairly be ignored. There are at least two plausible explanations: (1) a physical interference with the contracting process (as suggested by the manufacturer and others) (Brand, 1984) and (2) elimination of the periprosthetic space by tissue adhesion, thereby reducing the likelihood of circumferential periprosthetic contamination and its stimulus to contracture. Unanswered residual concerns include the propensity for infection, the ultimate fate of the polyurethane, and how long protection against contracture will last.

Other recognized minor disadvantages of this particular implant include fragility during insertion and a tendency for the polyurethane to separate easily from

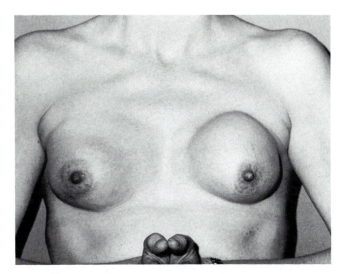

FIGURE 12–11
Capsular contracture following retromuscular augmentation. Note the lateral displacement of the right prosthesis with pectoralis contraction.

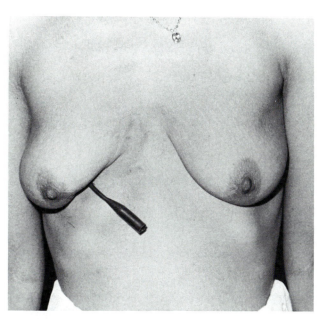

FIGURE 12–13
Elective removal of apparently uninfected polyurethane-covered prostheses 2 weeks after insertion was followed 2 months later by infection and persistent drainage from two small retained patches of polyurethane. The wound healed on a program of half-strength povidone iodine (Betadine) irrigations at home.

the silicone shell. It would seem prudent to at least consider some use of local antibacterials before inserting a foam-covered device into a soft tissue pocket that is known to have a significant incidence of bacterial contamination.

Local antibacterials reduce contracture (Burkhardt et al., 1986). As noted above, I use povidone-iodine irrigation as a matter of convenience: it is available, inexpensive, apparently harmless, and supported by blind, controlled data. Any one of a number of other agents might be equally effective, and in our study there was no significant difference between Betadine and various local antibiotics. Although the manufacturer of Betadine cannot at present label this substance for use in wound irrigation, there is ample surgical literature to support the concept (Kwaan and Connolly, 1981; Pollock et al.,

1978; Sindelar and Mason, 1979). The Food and Drug Administration (FDA) has recognized that approved drugs may be used legitimately for unlabeled indications (FDA Drug Bulletin, 1982).

Displacement exercises demand inclusion here, not because their effectiveness has been appropriately documented (it has not), but because they are mechanically appealing and enjoy the enthusiastic support of an overwhelming majority of plastic surgeons. The theory is that compressing and/or displacing the implants on a regular basis will keep the contracture from tightening down on the implant and will preserve a large space or "bursa," within which the implant will move. The exercises are prescribed with enthusiasm by most practitioners despite a complete lack of even a single appropriately controlled scientific study supporting their efficacy (Caffee, 1982; Terino, 1982; Vinnik, 1976).

The reasons for the continued clinical use of these exercises seem clear. With or without a personal conviction that they are effective, it is difficult as a practitioner to discontinue a program that other surgeons continue to use routinely and that you yourself have used routinely in the past, especially when it "makes sense" to patients. If you *do* stop, your patient (who has a reasonable chance of developing a contracture regardless) will undoubtedly blame any contracture on the lack of exercises, especially after talking with other patients and/or other surgeons. On the other hand, contracture occurrence in the *presence* of prescribed exercises can conveniently be blamed on either an act of God or an inadequate effort by the patient herself.

My personal opinion is that the use of these exercises is neither necessary nor helpful and that transferring

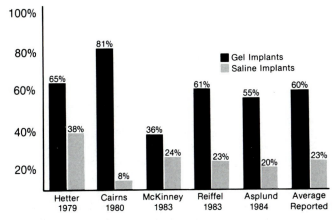

FIGURE 12–12
Reported comparisons between the contracture incidence of gel versus saline implants. (From Burkhardt, B. R., Dempsey, P. D., Schnur, P. L., Tofield, J. J.: Capsular contracture: A prospective study of the effect of local antibacterial agents. Plast. Reconstr. Surg. 77:919, 1986.)

this responsibility to patients in this manner is both pointless and unfair. The burden of proof, in any case, should fall upon those who claim the exercises are beneficial. All the clinical series on displacement exercises to date are retrospective, historically controlled, nonblind, and muddied by the random addition of such independent variables as steroids, antibiotics, and closed capsulotomies. Animal studies specifically designed to address the question have yielded equivocal results at best (Caffee, 1982). Since even constant postoperative compression with an elastic bandage was reported to be effective only until discontinued (Cronin et al., 1978), it is hard to rationally anticipate better results from intermittent squeezing or displacement. The only reasonably controlled clinical protocol I know was contained within our own study on local antibacterials, in which the two contributing surgeons used identical techniques except that one prescribed displacement exercises and the other did not. When the results were evaluated by independent judges, there was no significant difference in the incidence or severity of contracture between the two groups of patients (Burkhardt et al., 1986).

Local steroids were first introduced by Peterson and Burt (1974) and have now been used to try to suppress capsular contracture for over 15 years. The original concept of placing steroids directly into the pocket was supplanted by placing steroids within an inflatable or double-lumen implant (Perrin, 1976). Although there are still arguments about whether intraluminal steroids can be helpful (none of the studies to date have been prospective or properly controlled), there is no question at all that they can be disastrous! Three-quarters of a series of patients treated by the steroid technique that was recommended in 1976 later required removal or exchange of implants because of ptosis or severe soft tissue atrophy, and 13% of the same series *still* developed contracture despite the obviously toxic level of steroid administration (O'Neal and Argenta, 1982).

In my opinion, the use of intraluminal steroids lacks both an adequate rationale and a favorable risk/benefit ratio. Despite these personal reservations, it would be unfair to say flatly at this point that steroids are ineffective and should not be used.

It is important, however, to realize that the intensity of the steroid effect is related to multiple variables other than simply "dosage"—for example, concentration, length of exposure, thickness and permeability of the implant shell, two-way diffusion from the outer lumen of double-lumen devices. The potential steroid user should also question whether it is appropriate to use these drugs in prophylaxis of a relatively benign condition for which the etiology is probably infectious or at least unknown.

Correcting the Established Contracture

As pitifully little as surgeons know about preventing contracture, they know even less about correcting a contracture once it is established. In the absence of data, beautiful theories and favorable apocryphal re-

ports are a dime a dozen. Release of the constricting fibrous capsule, whether by forcible rupture, open incision, or complete excision, produces an immediate and gratifying return of the original softness. The problem is not one of physically correcting the contracture. That is easy. The problem is how to prevent recurrence.

What can one say about capsular correction that makes any sense at all? For starters, try not to hurt yourself! Rupture of the ulnar collateral ligament of the metacarpophalangeal joint of the thumb (gamekeeper's thumb) is a high price to pay, especially when it can be avoided by simply altering your compression technique (Tolhurst, 1978).

In addition, remember that closed capsulotomy is not a completely benign process for the patient. The potential problems include hematoma, asymmetry (Laughlin et al., 1977; Nelson, 1980, 1981), and implant rupture with deflation or gel extrusion (Edmond and Versaci, 1980; Eisenberg and Bartels, 1977; Feliberti et al., 1977; Hueston and Hare, 1979). Closed capsular rupture commonly requires frequent repetition to "maintain softness," and it is reasonable to expect the incidence of complications to increase as the procedure is repeated.

Open surgical capsulotomy is a better-controlled procedure because it is done under direct vision, but the estimates of recurrence once again range from the sublime (6%) (Freeman, 1972) to the ridiculous (89%) (Burkhardt et al., 1981). The only objectively documented study with which I am familiar suggests a discouraging recurrence rate of around 50% even with antibacterial irrigation (Burkhardt et al., 1986).

Fixing our attention on the fibrous capsule itself has led to capsulectomy, excising the entire capsule and theoretically recreating the original mammaplasty pocket and the original chance for a soft result. There are no supportive data. Finally, the multiple other ingenious "solutions" to contracture recurrence that have been reported in the literature simply do not have sufficient clinical or theoretic support to warrant further discussion.

Most instances of capsular contracture, even the moderately severe, are more of a personal inconvenience than a major surgical complication. Every experienced surgeon can tell of a few patients who have had a unilateral contracture and complained about the *soft* side, preferring the firmer breast because of better projection. In addition, even Hetter's 1979 study reporting a contracture incidence of around 60% indicated that a remarkably high percentage of patients would have the surgery done again given the same circumstances. I say this not to suggest that contracture is unimportant, but to try to place it in some perspective.

My personal approach is to encourage patients to simply accept moderate contractures, if possible, by explaining that we do not yet adequately understand this phenomenon, that correction often is not permanently successful, and that any attempt at correction carries with it some risk of complications. (It helps, of course, to have explained some of this *before* the original surgery.) If the patient still insists upon an attempted correction, I will try a closed capsulotomy after first demonstrating the process with an implant and a "capsule" of facial tissue.

For the severe problem that resists closed compression, I will do an open capsulotomy, irrigate the pocket with 5% povidone-iodine, and replace the existing implant with a polyurethane-covered model. I have used about two dozen of these implants strictly on a replacement basis, and the short-term results have been favorable, with the exception of the complication recorded in Figure 12–13. My own experience is too limited to be significant even if properly documented, but other authors, on the basis of much more extensive experience, have reported results that must be regarded as excellent. If the long-term results with the polyurethane-covered implants continue to be favorable, these devices may well prove to be the prosthesis of choice for primary augmentation as well as for the secondary correction of capsular contracture. Despite the theoretic problems of inducing adherence between the sponge and the smooth capsular wall, I have not found capsulectomy to be necessary. And despite my present unwillingness to adopt this prosthesis for general use, I do think that it is the best solution to date for the severe contracture.

WHAT NEXT?

Although any projections must be speculative, it seems obvious that surgeons will be unable to progress further without additional human study. By this I mean concurrently controlled, prospective, and, above all, *blind* evaluations of clinical series. Even if a satisfactory animal model were to appear (and this seems unlikely after 25 years), clinical confirmation of any laboratory advances would require proper studies in humans. Comparative human studies are not difficult to do and are well within the ability of every clinical practitioner who has a significant volume of augmentation patients. Clinical surgeons must realize that until they are willing to perform properly controlled human studies, they cannot expect further progress.

I believe that the most tantalizing challenge in augmentation mammaplasty today is to understand the physiologic basis for the good results reported with the polyurethane foam–covered implants.

As noted previously, I have very little personal experience with these. I have been concerned about infection, separation of the foam from the silicone shell, the unknown long-term results, and the technical difficulty of periareolar insertion. Still, it seems clear that the use of these implants is attended, at least in the short term, by a dramatic reduction in the incidence of severe contracture. Why?

One possibility is that the microfragmentation of the polyurethane foam does indeed physically interfere with the ability of the collagen fibers to interlock and contract, as suggested by Brand (1984). If this is the case, one must ask why the polyurethane sponge implants in the 1950s were such universal failures (Broadbent and Woolf, 1967).

A second possibility is that the growth of the surrounding tissues into the foam effectively eliminates the periprosthetic space that usually occurs around a smooth implant, consequently eliminating the potential for circumferential, periprosthetic spread of either ductal or hematogenous contamination. Various suppliers are now looking at the possibility of producing tissue adhesion to the silicone surface without this foam. One can only hope that marketing claims will be preceded by controlled human studies of effectiveness.

References

Argenta, L., Grabb, W. C.: Studies on the endogenous flora of the human breast and their surgical significance. Presented at the Annual Meeting of the American Society of Plastic and Reconstructive Surgeons, New York, October 20, 1981.

Ashley, F. L.: A new type of breast prosthesis: Preliminary report. Plast. Reconstr. Surg. 45:421, 1971.

Baldwin, C., Jr., Kaplan, E.: Silicone-induced human adjuvant disease? Ann. Plast. Surg. 10:270, 1983.

Barker, D. E., Ritsky, M. I., Schultz, S.: Bleeding of silicone from bag-gel breast implants and its clinical relation to fibrous capsule reaction. Plast. Reconstr. Surg. 61:836, 1978.

Barnett, A., Lavey, E., Peall, R. M., Vistnes, L. M.: Toxic shock syndrome from an infected breast prosthesis. Ann. Plast. Surg. 10:408, 1983.

Bergman, R. B., van der Ende, A. E.: Exudation of silicone through the envelope of gel-filled breast prostheses: An in-vitro study. Br. J. Plast. Surg. 32:31, 1979.

Boer, H. R., Anido, G., MacDonald, N.: Bacterial colonization of human milk. South. Med. J. 74:716, 1981.

Brand, K. G.: Polyurethane-coated silicone implants and the question of capsular contracture. Plast. Reconstr. Surg. 73:498, 1984.

Broadbent, T. R., Woolf, R. M.: Augmentation mammaplasty. Plast. Reconstr. Surg. 40:517, 1967.

Brownstein, M. L., Owsley, J. Q., Jr.: Augmentation mammaplasty: A survey of the major complications. In: Owsley, J. Q., Peterson, R. A. (eds.): *Symposium on Aesthetic Surgery of the Breast.* St. Louis, C.V. Mosby, 1978, p. 267.

Burkhardt, B. R.: Augmentation Mammaplasty and Capsular Contracture, 1963–1983. With supplements. Tucson, privately published, 1983.

Burkhardt, B. R.: Comparing contracture rates: Probability theory and the unilateral contracture. Plast. Reconstr. Surg. 74:527, 1984.

Burkhardt, B. R., Fried, M., Schnur, P. L., Tofield, J. J.: Capsules, infection and intraluminal antibiotics. Plast. Reconstr. Surg. 68:43, 1981.

Burkhardt, B. R., Dempsey, P. D., Schnur, P. L., Tofield, J. J.: Capsular contracture: A prospective study of the effect of local antibacterial agents. Plast. Reconstr. Surg. 77:919, 1986.

Caffee, H. H.: External compression for the prevention of scar capsule contracture: A preliminary report. Ann. Plast. Surg. 8:453, 1982.

Clarendon, C. C. D.: Breast thinning and streaking following the use of inflatable implants: A subjective clinical study. Ann. Plast. Surg. 5:436, 1980.

Cocke, W. M., Leathers, H. K., Lynch, J. B.: Foreign body reactions to polyurethane covers of some breast prostheses. Plast. Reconstr. Surg. 56:527, 1975.

Courtiss, E. H., Goldwyn, R. M., Anastasi, G. W.: The fate of breast implants with infections around them. Plast. Reconstr. Surg. 63:812, 1979.

Cronin, T., Persoff, M., Upton, J.: Augmentation mammaplasty: Complications and etiology. In: Owsley, J. Q., Peterson, R. A., (eds.): *Symposium on Aesthetic Surgery of the Breast.* St. Louis, C.V. Mosby, 1978, p. 276.

Derman, G. H., Argenta, L. C., Grabb, W. C.: Delayed extrusion of inflatable breast prostheses. Ann. Plast. Surg. 10:154, 1983.

Edmond, J., Versaci, A.: Late complication of closed capsulotomy of the breast. Plast. Reconstr. Surg. 66:478, 1980.

Eisenberg, H. V., Bartels, R. J.: Rupture of a silicone bag gel breast implant by closed compression capsulotomy. Plast. Reconstr. Surg. 59:849, 1977.

Ersek, R.: Progress in prostheses for breast augmentation. Travis County Med. Soc. J. 35:8, 1989.

Eyssen, J. E., von Werssowetz, A. J., Middleton, G. D.: Reconstruction of the breast using polyurethane-coated prostheses. Plast. Reconstr. Surg. 73:415, 1984.

Feliberti, M. C., Arrillaga, A., Colon, G. A.: Rupture of inflated breast implants in closed compression capsulotomy. Plast. Reconstr. Surg. 59:848, 1977.

Fischl, R. A., Kahn, S., Simon, B. E.: Mondor's disease: An unusual complication of mammaplasty. Plast. Reconstr. Surg. 56:319, 1975.

Freeman, B. S.: Successful treatment of some fibrous envelope contractures around breast implants. Plast. Reconstr. Surg. 50:107, 1972.

Gayon, R.: A histological comparison of contracted and noncontracted capsules around silicone breast implants. Plast. Reconstr. Surg. 63:700, 1979.

Georgiade, N. G., Serafin, D., Barwick, W.: Late development of hematoma around a breast implant, necessitating removal. Plast. Reconstr. Surg. 64:708, 1979.

Gurdin, M., Carlin, G. A.: Complications of breast augmentation. Plast. Reconstr. Surg. 40:530, 1967.

Hartley, J. H.: Specific applications of the double-lumen prostheses. Clin. Plast. Surg. 3:247, 1976.

Hartley, J. H., Schatten, W. E.: Postoperative complication of lactation after augmentation mammaplasty. Plast. Reconstr. Surg. 47:150, 1971.

Hausner, R. J., Schoen, F. J., Pierson, K. K.: Foreign body reaction to silicone gel in axillary lymph nodes after augmentation mammaplasty. Plast. Reconstr. Surg. 62:381, 1978.

Herman, S.: The Même implant. Plast. Reconstr. Surg. 73:411, 1984.

Hester, T. R.: The polyurethane covered mammary prosthesis: Facts and fiction. Perspect. Plast. Surg. 2:135, 1988.

Hetter, G. P.: Satisfactions and dissatisfactions of patients with augmentation mammaplasty. Plast. Reconstr. Surg. 64:151, 1979.

Huang, T. T., Blackwell, S. J., Lewis, S. R.: Migration of silicone gel after the "squeeze technique" to rupture a contracted breast capsule. Plast. Reconstr. Surg. 61:277, 1978.

Hueston, J. T., Hare, W. S. C.: Rupture of subpectoral prostheses during closed compression capsulotomy. Aust. J. Surg. 49:564, 1979.

Jarrett, J. R., Cutler, R. G., Teal, D. F.: Subcutaneous mastectomy in small, large, or ptotic breasts with immediate submuscular placement of implants. Plast. Reconstr. Surg. 62:702, 1978.

Kossovsky, N., Heggers, J. P., Parsons, R. W., Robson, M. C.: Acceleration of capsule formation around silicone implants by infection in a guinea pig model. Plast. Reconstr. Surg. 73:91, 1984.

Kwaan, J. H. M., Connolly, J. E.: Successful management of prosthetic graft infection with continuous povidone-iodine irrigation. Arch. Surg. 116:716, 1981.

Laughlin, R. A., Raynor, A. C., Habal, M. B.: Complications of closed capsulotomies after augmentation mammaplasty. Plast. Reconstr. Surg. 60:362, 1977.

Luhan, J. E.: Giant galactoceles, 1 month after bilateral augmentation mammaplasty, abdominoplasty and tubal ligation. Aesthetic Plast. Surg. 3:161, 1979.

Mahler, D., Hauben, D. J.: Retromammary versus retro-pectoral breast augmentation: A comparative study. Ann. Plast. Surg. 8:370, 1982.

Marion, R. B.: Polyurethane-covered breast implant. Plast. Reconstr. Surg. 74:728, 1984.

McKinney, P., Tresley, G.: Long-term comparison of patients with gel and saline mammary implants. Plast. Reconstr. Surg. 72:27, 1983.

Nelson, G. D.: Complications of closed compression after augmentation mammaplasty. Plast. Reconstr. Surg. 68:71, 1980.

Nelson, G. D.: Complications from the treatment of fibrous capsular contracture of the breast. Plast. Reconstr. Surg. 68:969, 1981.

O'Neal, R. M., Argenta, L. C.: Late side effects related to inflatable breast prostheses containing soluble steroids. Plast. Reconstr. Surg. 69:641, 1982.

Perrin, E. R.: The use of soluble steroids within inflatable breast prostheses. Plast. Reconstr. Surg. 57:163, 1976.

Peters, W. J., Smith, D. C.: Ivalon breast prostheses: Evaluation 19 years after implantation. Plast. Reconstr. Surg. 67:514, 1981.

Peterson, H., Burt, G.: The role of steroids in prevention of circumferential capsular scarring in augmentation mammaplasty. Plast. Reconstr. Surg. 54:28, 1974.

Pollock, A. V., Froome, K., Evans, M.: The bacteriology of primary wound sepsis in potentially contaminated abdominal operations: The effect of irrigation, povidone-iodine and cephaloridine on the sepsis rate assessed in a clinical trial. Br. J. Surg. 65:76, 1978.

Pollock, H.: Polyurethane-covered breast implant. Plast. Reconstr. Surg. 74:729, 1984.

Rees, T. D., Guy, C. L., Coburn, R. J.: The use of inflatable breast implants. Plast. Reconstr. Surg. 52:609, 1973.

Schatten, W. E.: Reconstruction of breasts following mastectomy with polyurethane-covered, gel-filled prostheses. Ann. Plast. Surg. 12:147, 1984.

Shah, Z., Lehman, J. A., Tan, J.: Does infection play a role in breast capsular contracture? Plast. Reconstr. Surg. 68:34, 1981.

Shipley, R. H., O'Donnell, J. M., Bader, K. F.: Personality characteristics of women seeking breast augmentation: Comparison to small-busted and average-busted controls. Plast. Reconstr. Surg. 60:369, 1977.

Shipley, R. H., O'Donnell, J. M., Bader, K. F.: Psychosocial effects of cosmetic augmentation mammaplasty. Aesthetic Plast. Surg. 2:429, 1978.

Silverstein, M. J., Handel, N., Gamagami, P., et al.: Breast cancer in women after augmentation mammaplasty. Arch. Surg. 123:681, 1988.

Sindelar, W. F., Mason, G. R.: Irrigation of subcutaneous tissue with povidone-iodine solution for prevention of surgical wound infections. Surg. Gynecol. Obstet. 148:227, 1979.

Slade, C. L.: Subcutaneous mastectomy: Acute complications and long term followup. Plast. Reconstr. Surg. 73:84, 1984.

Slade, C. L., Peterson, H. D.: Disappearance of the polyurethane cover of the Ashley natural-Y prostheses. Plast. Reconstr. Surg. 70:379, 1982.

Smahel, J.: Tissue reactions to breast implants coated with polyurethane. Plast. Reconstr. Surg. 61:80, 1978.

Spiera, H.: Scleroderma after silicone augmentation mammaplasty. J.A.M.A. 260:236, 1988.

Tebbetts, J. B.: Transaxillary subpectoral augmentation mammaplasty: Long-term follow-up and refinements. Plast. Reconstr. Surg. 74:636, 1984.

Terino, E.: Essential concepts in prosthetic breast surgery. Aesthetic Plast. Surg. 6:25, 1982.

Tolhurst, D. E.: "Nutcracker" technique for compression rupture of capsules around breast implants. Plast. Reconstr. Surg. 61:795, 1978.

Umansky, C.: Infection with polyurethane-coated implants. Plast. Reconstr. Surg. 75:925, 1985.

Vinnik, C. A.: Spherical contracture of fibrous capsules around breast implants. Plast. Reconstr. Surg. 58:555, 1976.

Williams, C., Aston, S., Rees, T. D.: The effect of hematoma on the thickness of pseudosheaths around silicone implants. Plast. Reconstr. Surg. 56:194, 1975.

Williams, J. E.: Experiences with a large series of Silastic breast implants. Plast. Reconstr. Surg. 49:253, 1972.

Woods, J. E., Irons, G. B., Arnold, P. G.: The case for submuscular implantation of prostheses in reconstructive breast surgery. Ann. Plast. Surg. 5:115, 1980.

Worton, E. W., Seifert, L. N., Sherwood, R.: Late leakage of inflatable silicone breast prostheses. Plast. Reconstr. Surg. 65:302, 1980.

Zide, B. M.: Complications of closed capsulotomy after augmentation (Letter). Plast. Reconstr. Surg. 67:697, 1981.

CONGENITAL AND DEVELOPMENTAL BREAST ABNORMALITIES

13

Ray A. Elliott, Jr.

Asymmetric Breasts

The minor asymmetry of body halves and paired structures that is common to most of us (Gorney and Harries, 1974) tends to go unnoticed. Less subtle variations, on the other hand, are readily identified and may cause significant concern. Accordingly, subtle differences in breast appearance are usually accepted by the patient and doctor alike, whereas gross asymmetry may produce significant physical and psychologic problems (Corso, 1972; Elliott et al., 1975; Simon, 1975).

Pitanguy (1967) reported noticeable asymmetry in 4% of a total breast treatment population of 1400 patients seen for the gamut of breast procedures. As a practical observation, Hueston (1976) noted that a volume asymmetry greater than one-third was difficult to conceal with everyday attire.

The patient seeking correction of breast asymmetry presents a unique challenge. Accurate analysis of the problem, sensitivity to the desires of the patient, and a thorough understanding of the treatment options are needed to guide both the physician and the patient on a proper course of management. Surgical judgment and technique must be at their best so that there is no disappointment with the results.

CLASSIFICATION

Attempts to classify asymmetries tend to be unwieldy or incomplete. These efforts fail largely because both the etiology and the nature of the defect are potentially important. A simple anatomic classification that ignores etiology can be used to categorize treatment (Smith et al., 1986).

NORMAL GROWTH AND DEVELOPMENT

Although much about the etiology of breast asymmetry remains elusive, some known facts are relevant to understanding the variety of such deformities. There are genetic factors and errors that guide early development, hormones add their influence at puberty, and mechanical and environmental factors may alter the mature breast or breast development. To understand the subtleties of pathology and pathophysiology, one must have some familiarity with normal growth and development (Arey, 1958; Chatterton, 1978; Pers, 1968).

Breast Embryology

The primordia of the human breast appear between the ventral limb buds of the 4-month embryo as two ectodermal ridges, known as the mammary ridges or milk lines. Projected onto the fetus, these ridges would extend from the axilla to the ipsilateral groin. The coalescence of cells that persists in the cranial third of each ridge as minute elevations becomes the breast anlagen; their loci determine the position of the fully developed breasts.

The breast anlagen develop with a proliferation of milk ducts; their common termini form a nipple, the elevation of which may be evident at birth or await infancy. The areola and its glands (of Montgomery) can be identified in the 5-month embryo.

Chest Wall Embryology

The configuration of the chest wall deep to the breasts is dependent upon the development of the ribs and sternum and, to a lesser degree, the vertebral column (Pers, 1968).

Ribs arise from processes on the vertebral mass of the embryo. In the thoracic and upper lumbar regions, costal processes of varying length follow the developing body curvatures and encircle the thoracic and upper portion of the abdominal cavities. Most join the midline ventral mesenchymal bands, which are destined to become the sternum, uniting in a cephalocaudal direction to complete the thoracic cage. The normal breast anlagen are evident on the anterior musculature of the developing chest wall.

Hormonal Influence

After fetal development is complete, the normal breast awaits the hormonal stimulation of puberty to achieve volume and shape. In the female, perhaps as many as ten hormones under pituitary and ovarian control determine breast growth during the second decade of life (Gerow, 1972). Breast volume is determined by the finite number of cells in the developing primordia and by the vigor of the cellular response to this hormone stimulation. In the male, androgen-estrogen balance seldom permits significant breast enlargement. Enlargement of the male breast is discussed in Chapter 47.

ERRORS IN GROWTH AND DEVELOPMENT

It is not likely that circulating hormones can act selectively on totally comparable breast primordia to create asymmetry. Theoretically, perhaps, if the vascular supply were sufficiently asymmetric to cause unequal transport of hormones, the latter could become a factor. Genetic defects and errors in the primordia and embryologic development of the breast and thoracic cage account for a wide spectrum of asymmetries.

Absence of Structures

Total absence of a structure may be caused by total absence of the anlage (agenesis), or developmental failure of a normal anlage (aplasia). If symmetric nipples are present in the infant, asymmetry created by aplasia will not be evident until puberty. Although an injured gland (e.g., by x-ray) may fail to develop and a congenital absence of the gland (amazia) with a nipple present has been seen (Fig. 13–1), to my knowledge, congenital absence of the nipple and areola (athelia) with normal gland development has not been reported. Total absence of the breast (amastia), therefore, is usually diagnosed in the newborn.

True congenital amastia is a rare deformity, with only 44 cases reported between 1886 and 1965 (Trier, 1965). Nearly one-half of these were unilateral, and most had an absence of the ipsilateral pectoral muscles and were in females.

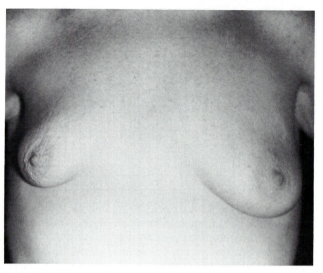

FIGURE 13–2
Congenital asymmetry: Most variations in the location of asymmetric breasts are related to volume differences and the effect of gravity.

Variations in Location

The location of the developing breast will depend upon the loci of the primordial cells. Although ectopic cells occasionally result in supernumerary structures, variations in location of two asymmetric breasts are quite common (see Fig. 13–1). However, most are related to volume differences (Fig. 13–2) and can, therefore, be corrected readily by matching the breasts.

Excess Structures

An ectopic cluster of primordial breast cells retained along the milk line can produce a supernumerary nipple complex (polythelia) of varying sophistication (Fig. 13–3) and occasionally even an ectopic extra breast (polymastia). Polythelia is seen most often on the anterior chest and upper abdomen (Fig. 13–4) but may occur in the axilla or groin as well. An extra nipple and areola on a breast has been seen, and fully developed breasts have been reported in the axilla (Kaye, 1974) and even on the back (Castano, 1969).

Variations in Size

The sizes of the "normal" nipple, areola, and gland structures vary greatly from patient to patient. These variations are most disturbing when they are asymmetric.

As stated above, the volume of the breast will vary with the vigor of the cellular respose to hormone stimulation and the finite number of cells in the primordia. Thus, in breast enlargement there may be an increase in cellular number (hyperplasia) and/or cellular size (hypertrophy). A decrease in the number of primordia cells (hypoplasia) or a weak response should usually

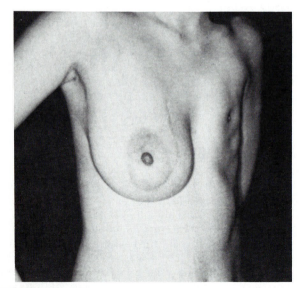

FIGURE 13–1
Congenital asymmetry: Unilateral absence of the gland (amazia) and underlying muscles with a rudimentary nipple and areola.

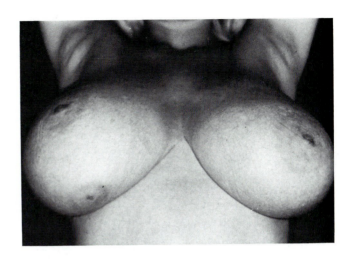

FIGURE 13–3
Congenital asymmetry: Asymmetric hypermastia. There is a well-developed, nonfunctional, extra nipple-areola complex (polythelia) on the right breast.

produce a smaller breast (Figs. 13–5 and 13–6). A difference in the number of cells in the primordia probably sets the stage for most congenital asymmetries. However, when cell numbers are equal and the transport systems for hormones are equal, differences in breast size must depend on differences in cell response. The quality of the cell, hormone circulation, and total cell number can all be altered by trauma (e.g., surgery and radiation), drugs, infection, and neoplasms.

Variations in Shape

The shape of the breast will vary with the arrangement of glandular tissue and the integrity of the skin envelope (Fig. 13–7). Lower quadrant deficiencies are more commonly related to the pattern of cellular distribution within the anlage, while upper quadrant deficiencies are more often related to a loss of the skin envelope tone and elasticity.

The tuberous breast deformity has been attributed to aberrations in the spacial relationships between the skin and the gland, with the circumference of the skin attachment to the chest wall remaining constant during puberty, while the skin distal to this attachment expands to accommodate the developing breast gland (Rees and Aston, 1976). I believe, as do others (Dinner and Dowden, 1987; Elliott, 1988), that in this deformity there are deficiencies of breast gland and skin envelope in the inferior quadrants. When there is an associated weakness of the dermal support of the areola, glandular tissue can herniate into the areola, guided by its attachment to the nipple. Further compounded by micromastia and upward displacement of the inframammary crease, the deformity can be quite grotesque (Fig. 13–8).

The effect of gravity on the breast mass and the quality and relative size of the skin envelope influence breast shape. Significant sagging of the breast (ptosis) may be an isolated defect, or it may complicate another asymmetry. In older women and some postpartum younger women, a decrease in glandular mass (atrophy) and an atonic or stretched skin envelope can be quite deforming. This deformity is troublesome enough when bilateral and equal; it can be very distressing when unilateral (Fig. 13–9).

Text continued on page 143

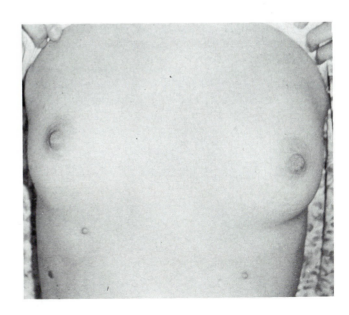

FIGURE 13–4
Congenital asymmetry: Symmetric hypomastia. Asymmetric rudimentary polythelia.

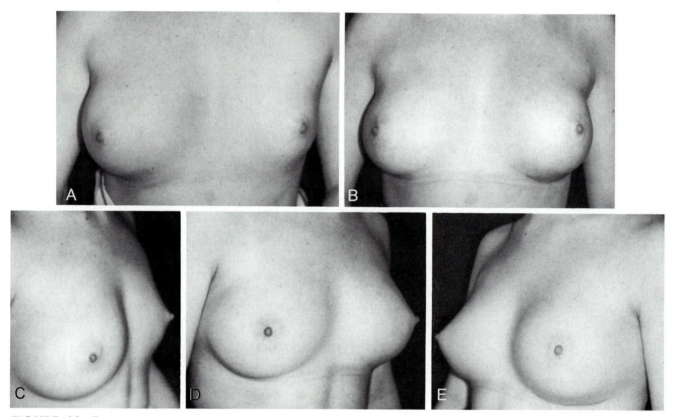

FIGURE 13–5
Congenital asymmetry: Unilateral hypomastia. *Treatment:* Unilateral augmentation. *A*, Preoperative front view. *B*, Postoperative volume match. *C*, Preoperative oblique profile of hypomastia. *D*, Augmented profile. *E*, Profile of right breast, not operated upon.

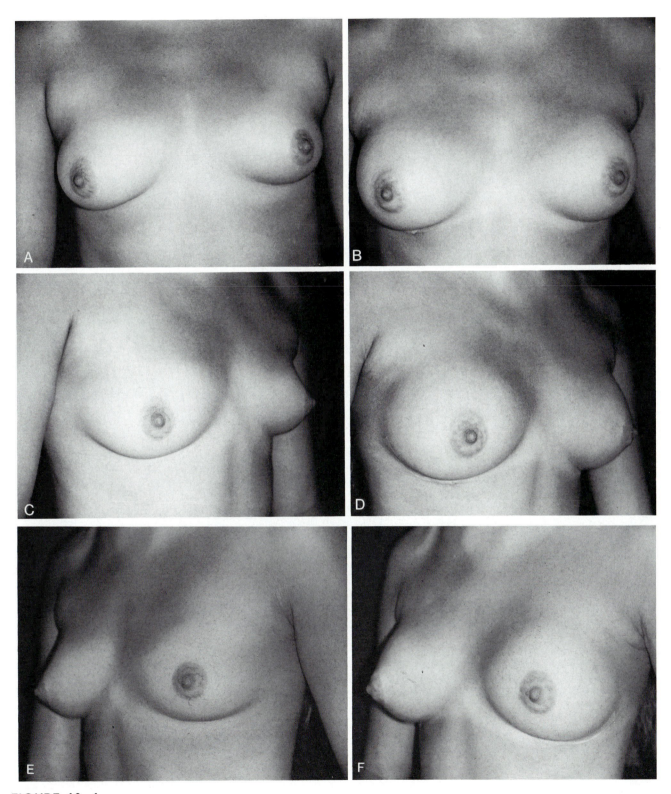

FIGURE 13–6

Congenital asymmetry: Asymmetric hypomastia. *Treatment:* Asymmetric augmentation. *A,* Preoperative front view. *B,* Postoperative volume match. *C,* Preoperative oblique profile. *D,* Augmented profile. *E,* Preoperative oblique profile. *F,* Augmented profile.

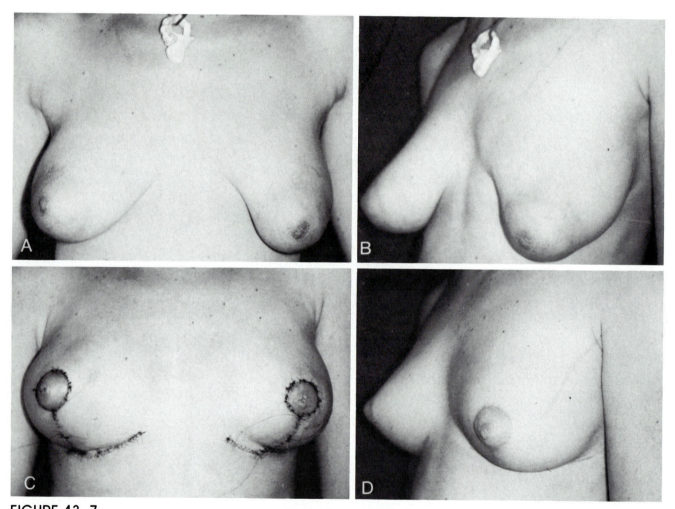

FIGURE 13–7

Congenital asymmetry: Asymmetric breast shape and volume. *Treatment:* Asymmetric mastopexy; unilateral augmentation. *A,* Asymmetric ptosis and left tubular micromastia. *B,* Oblique view showing the abnormal shape of the left breast. *C,* Asymmetric mastopexy (see Fig. 13–23) with left augmentation. *D,* Result.

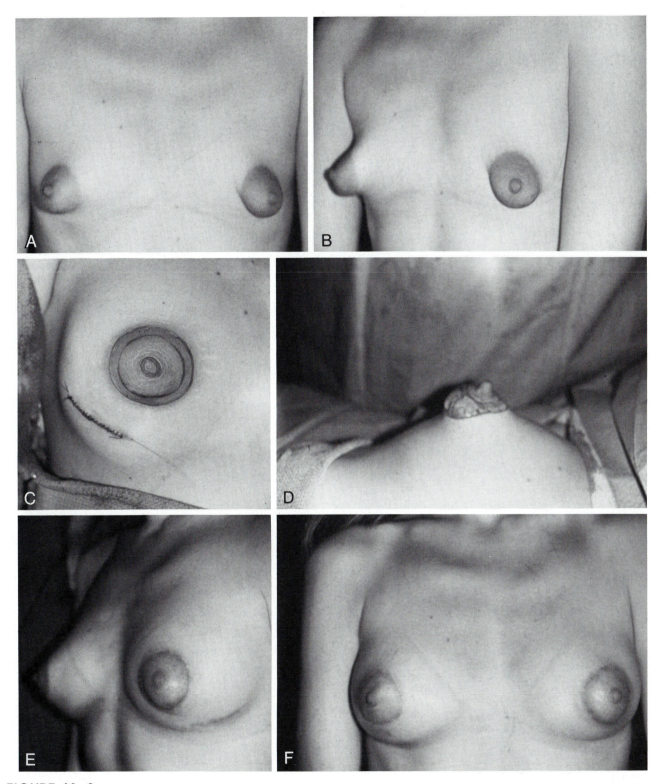

FIGURE 13–8

Congenital asymmetry: Tuberous breasts; asymmetric micromastia. *Treatment:* Bilateral areolaplasty; symmetric breast augmentation. *A,* Preoperative front view. *B,* Preoperative oblique view. *C,* Right breast augmentation with plan for areolar reduction and herniorrhaphy. *D,* Gland herniation prior to repair. *E,* Postoperative front view. *F,* Postoperative oblique profile.

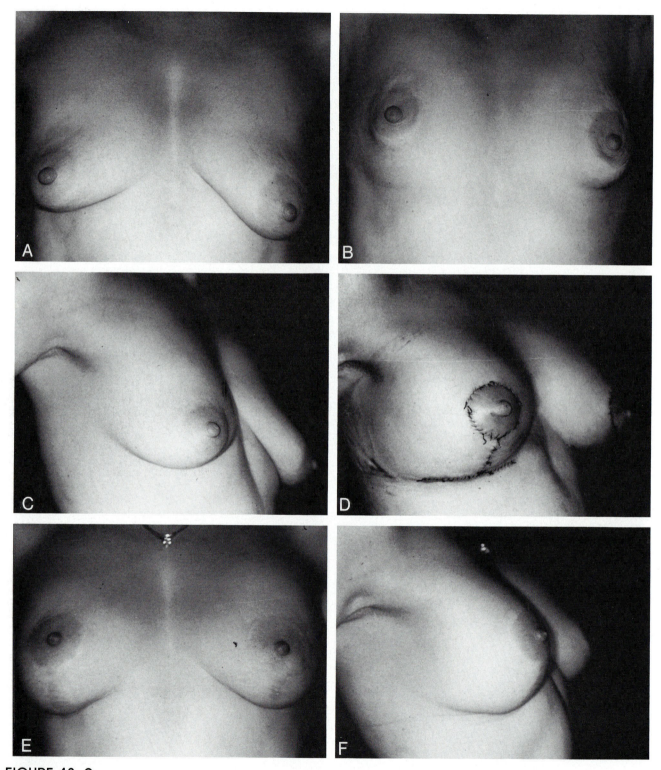

FIGURE 13–9

Congenital asymmetry: Asymmetric ptosis; symmetric micromastia. *Treatment:* Bilateral mastopexy; bilateral augmentation, symmetric. *A,* Asymmetry of shape and location. *B,* View with arms raised, emphasizing the difference in the skin envelopes. *C,* Preoperative oblique contour. *D,* Early postoperative contour. *E* and *F,* Result after 5 years.

ACQUIRED ASYMMETRY

The breast may be altered by a variety of acquired insults, including injury (Fig. 13–10), surgery (Fig. 13–11), infection (Fig. 13–12), or neoplasm (Fig. 13–13). The resulting distortion is frequently unilateral. The surgical removal of a prepubertal subareolar mass, childhood irradiation of the breast area, and burn scar contractures that distort the breast are examples of preventable acquired asymmetry.

Neoplasms account for a number of acquired asymmetries. For example, the benign giant fibroadenoma seen in young adults is capable of producing a gross enlargement of the involved breast (Fig. 13–14). Malignant tumors of the breast can also cause significant unilateral distortion, and the asymmetric deformities associated with their treatment are well known.

All elective breast surgery includes symmetry as a goal, but complications do occur (Cholnoky, 1972). Today there is still an incidence of encapsulation (Fig. 13–15) and occasional malposition (Fig. 13–16) of a prosthesis to compromise the otherwise pleasing results of augmentation. Unfortunately, these problems may cause asymmetry (Fig. 13–17). The debates about the benefit of subpectoral placement, antibiotics, vitamin E, massage, and the new generation of prostheses in the prevention of encapsulation have not been conclusive (Burkhardt, 1988). On the other hand, the incrimination of hematoma and infection seems more certain.

Woods et al. (1978) reported a significant incidence of asymmetry of the size and position of the areola after breast reduction at the Mayo Clinic. Many of these complications should be preventable (Peterson, 1983; Pitanguy, 1983).

PATIENT EVALUATION AND CONSULTATION

The clinical evaluation of asymmetrical breasts requires a detailed patient history, psychosocial evalua-

tion, and physical examination. This complete information is needed for development of proper treatment recommendations for the individual case.

History

Securing a history of breast development is basic; but as with all surgical candidates, a complete history of present and past illness, a family history, and a review of systems is beneficial. This information may, for example, explain an acquired asymmetry, indicate a genetic predisposition, or improve the safety of the anesthesia and surgery.

Psychosocial Evaluation

Evaluation of the motivation and stability of any person seeking elective cosmetic surgery has a recognized importance. The patient with a gross asymmetry has usually been subjected to prolonged psychosocial pressure while attempting to mask the deformity. The motivation for correction of an asymmetry may far exceed that strong motivation seen in the average patient requesting symmetric augmentation or reduction (Gifford, 1976).

Psychologic stability must be weighed against the severity of the deformity and the potential for obtaining a significant uncomplicated improvement. Years ago, in the early days of elective cosmetic mammaplasty, a psychiatric consultation was frequent, particularly before an augmentation procedure (Edgerton et al., 1961; Grossman, 1976). Today, although occasionally a second opinion is requested, the experienced cosmetic surgeon familiar with the preoperative stress and postoperative gratitude of these patients will be able to offer corrective surgery to even borderline persons without a psychiatric consultation. The obviously unstable patient should still have a formal psychiatric consultation; an anatomic correction may not be beneficial, with or without professional support.

Text continued on page 149

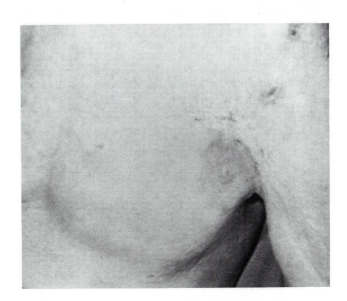

FIGURE 13–10

Acquired asymmetry: Burn scar contracture with a displaced nipple areola complex.

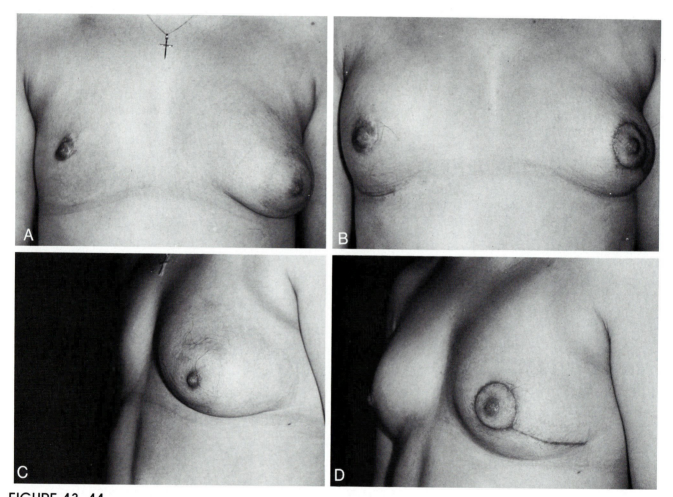

FIGURE 13–11

Acquired asymmetry: Surgical excision of a tender mass in infancy. *Treatment:* Unilateral (staged) staged augmentation; contralateral mastopexy and areolar reduction. *A,* Absent right gland and asymmetric areolar stretch. *B,* Right first-stage augmentation (before tissue expansion) and left balancing mastopexy. *C,* Preoperative oblique contours. *D,* After final augmentation of the right breast and lateral mastopexy and areolar reduction of the left breast.

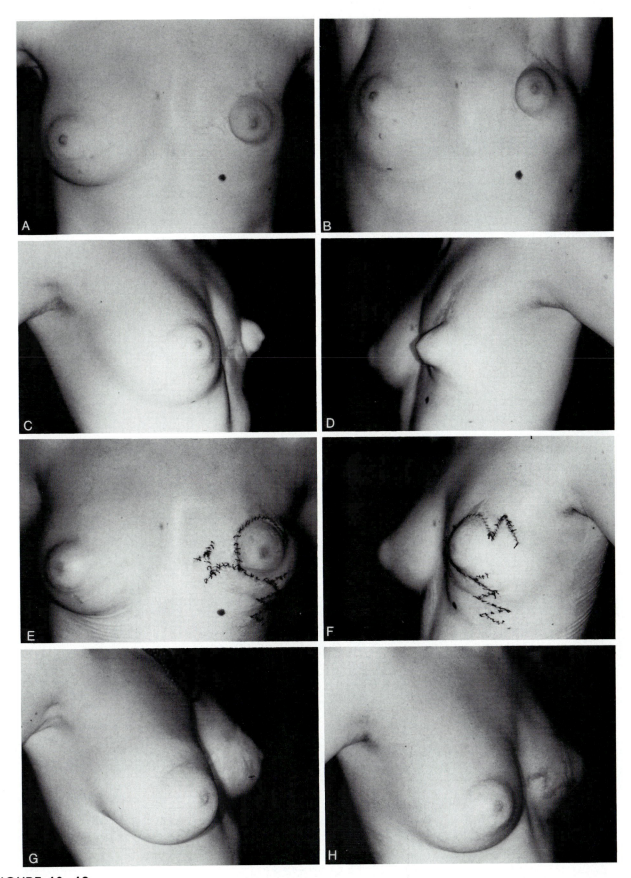

FIGURE 13–12

Acquired asymmetry: A 15-year-old girl who had a severe staphylococcal infection at 10 days of age. *Treatment:* Multiple local flap expansion of skin envelope and relocation of areola; areolaplasty and unilateral augmentation. *A,* Severe hypomastia with contracture around the areola. *B,* Elevated arms emphasizing medial displacement of the areola. *C* and *D,* Oblique views showing severity and herniation. *E,* Subpectoral augmentation with flaps to relocate the areola and incision for herniorrhaphy. *F,* Author's infra-areolar W-V-Y skin expansion (see Surgical Technique). *G,* Oblique contours and scars after 1 year. *H,* After 5 years.

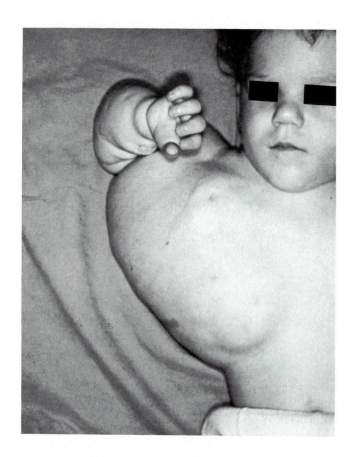

FIGURE 13–13
Acquired asymmetry: Massive distortion by a unilateral hemangioma.

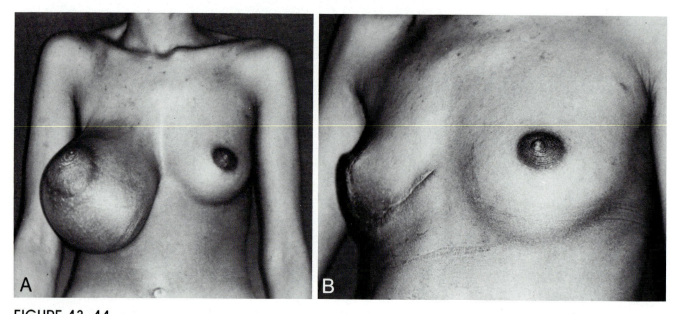

FIGURE 13–14
Acquired asymmetry: Massive unilateral fibroadenoma (teenage). *Treatment:* Tumor enucleation; mastopexy. *A,* Gross unilateral deformity. *B,* Contour and volume match obtained.

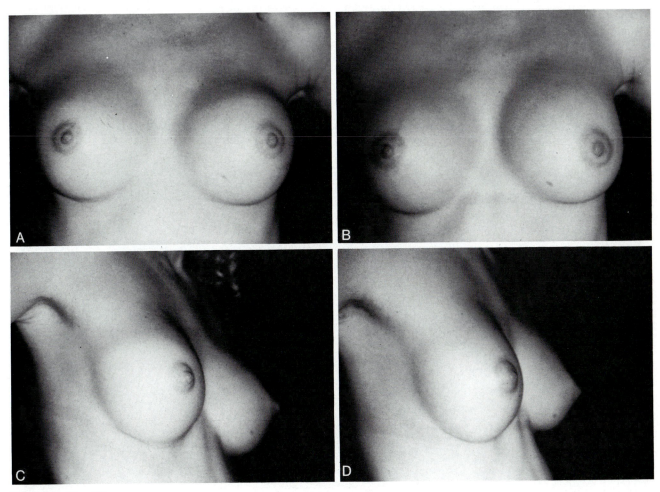

FIGURE 13–15

Acquired asymmetry: Recurrent unilateral encapsulation; history of submammary augmentation for symmetric micromastia and failed closed capsulotomy. *Treatment:* Unilateral subpectoral replacement of prosthesis (old pocket preserved). *A,* Encapsulation of the left subglandular prosthesis. *B,* Two years after subpectoral replacement. *C,* Preoperative oblique view of the encapsulated left breast prosthesis. *D,* Result after 2 years.

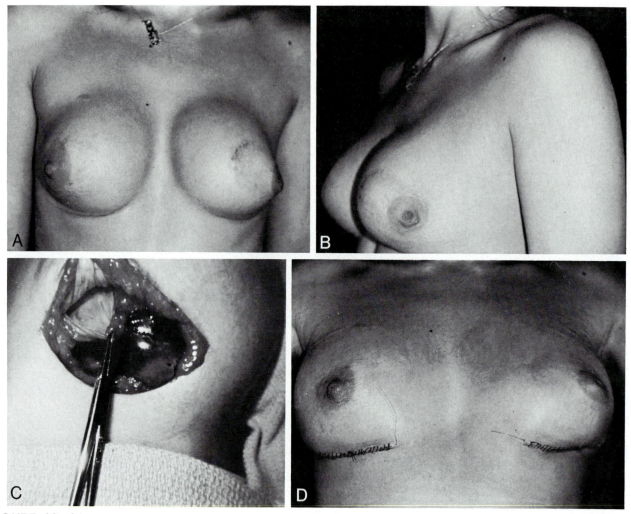

FIGURE 13–16

Acquired asymmetry: Migrant nude dancer with a history of symmetric augmentation and a later attempt to reposition prostheses using the same pockets. *Treatment:* Repositioned prostheses. *A,* Encapsulation and medial malposition of prostheses. Note irritation on the left breast from taping the areola into the anterior position. *B,* Severe lateral position of the nipple and areola. *C,* Operative view of the smooth medial pocket (abandoned) and prosthesis in a new, deeper, more lateral pocket. *D,* Postoperative breast contour and nipple-areola position. Note old scar used for exposure and revised.

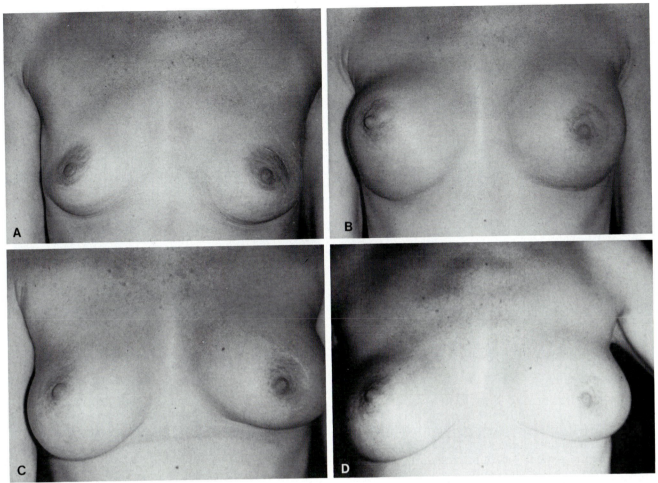

FIGURE 13–17
Congenital and acquired asymmetry: Asymmetric micromastia diagnosed as congenital malposition of the right breast. *Treatment:* History of symmetric augmentation with intentional relocation of the right breast mound. *A,* Preoperative asymmetric micromastia. *B,* Equal volume subglandular prostheses with low placement on the right, after 3 months. *C,* After 4 years. *D,* After 12 years.

Physical Examination

The physical examination may confirm or deny suspicions gained from the history and from the clothed body posture. Our initial consultation is usually limited to the upper torso, but a complete physical examination is done routinely before surgery.

An examination of the thorax and breasts with the arms both by the sides and elevated over the head and a breast examination in the supine position with the arms slightly abducted will reveal most pathologic conditions. A circumferential examination of the muscular and bony thorax is essential in all cases. The halves of the thorax are compared, and the vertical alignment of the thorax is noted, along with any differences in muscle mass or shoulder position (Fig. 13–18).

A comparison of the breasts and their relationship to the chest wall is needed to define the type of asymmetry. The relative volume, shape, and position of the breasts, and the size, color, and location of the nipples and areolae are compared and recorded. Breast volume can

be measured (Bouman, 1970; Kirianoff, 1974), but we have not found a clinical need for this information. Mammography is requested only when a neoplasm is suspected.

Photographs

Preoperative photographs should be routine. We take four standard photographs: anterior views with the arms by the sides and elevated above the head and bilateral oblique views to reveal the breasts in profile. Zarem (1988) recommends that these views include the shoulders and thorax. Special views are added as required.

Recommendations

The consultation is completed with a discussion regarding breast size, a review of expectations, and reinforcement of the realistic goals of surgical treatment.

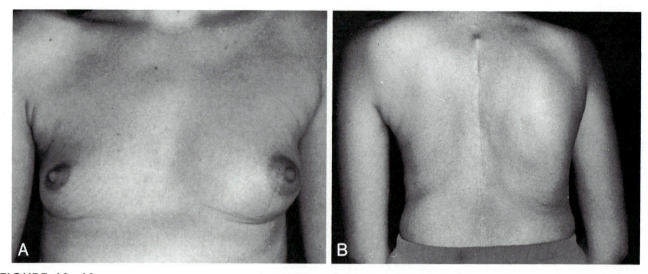

FIGURE 13–18

Congenital asymmetry: Combined deformities of the thorax, vertebral column, and breast. *A,* Asymmetric micromastia with deficient pectoral musculature on right thorax. *B,* Associated scoliosis (corrected) and a prominent (wing deformity) right scapula. (From Elliott, R., Hoehn, J.: Asymmetrical breasts. In: Georgiade, N.: *Reconstructive Breast Surgery.* St. Louis, C.V. Mosby, 1976, p. 89.)

The operative scars and their location are described along with a lay synopsis of the recommended procedure. The usual postoperative course is outlined, and the more common potential complications are discussed. Only after the patient is well informed about the proposed treatment will the stage be properly set for cooperation and satisfaction (Cole, 1988).

SURGICAL PLANNING

The individualized treatment plan can usually be determined during the patient evaluation. Any unusual problem or special technical requirements are noted. The selection of established and familiar techniques is favored. Good surgical principles and technique tend to minimize difficulties in execution and enhance the result.

Glandular Asymmetry

If an appropriate breast exists on one side, ideally that breast is matched, e.g., by augmentation (see Fig. 13–5) or reduction (Fig. 13–19), to produce symmetry (Elliott and Hoehn, 1976). When a greater volume is desired in both breasts, an unequal augmentation is recommended (see Fig. 13–6). Because in specific gravity and weight a gel prosthesis closely approximates breast tissue, the rate of physiologic descent of matched breast mounds is likely to be equal after asymmetric augmentation if the tensions of the skin envelopes are reasonably matched. When both breasts are larger than desired, the amount of gland excision can be different for each. Combinations of augmentation and reduction will require even more complex planning (Simon et al., 1975).

Volume is more easily matched than breast position and shape. It is difficult to balance micromastia and macromastia corrections exactly, because the required scars are quite different, and the attainable breast shape can vary considerably (Fig. 13–20). Both a reduced breast and an augmented breast will gradually descend as would a normal maturing breast of the same size (see Fig. 13–19). However, symmetry can be difficult to obtain when skin tension of the envelope varies greatly. When ptosis correction, with or without augmentation, is needed to balance a reduction, the technique and scars are similar (Elbaz and Werheecke, 1972; Marchac and Sagher, 1988) and the result tends to be more symmetric (Fig. 13–21).

Nipple and Areolar Asymmetry

Good symmetry of the nipple and areola is more important than an exact match of breast volume, but both should be routine goals of aesthetic breast surgery. The classification and treatment of nipple and areolar anomalies are discussed in a separate chapter.

Nipples may be asymmetric in their prominence and direction. Sometimes a simple reduction or redirection procedure will gain symmetry (Fig. 13–22). Correction of nipple inversion, commonly a unilateral deformity, is more complex, and a match cannot always be attained.

The size of the areola will usually vary proportionally with breast volume; hence significant differences can be seen with glandular asymmetry (see Figs. 13–11, 13–14, 13–18, and 13–21). Bilateral areolar reductions, with or without repositioning, can be matched for size. The scar of a unilateral reduction is more noticeable (see Fig. 13–19). Procedures for enlargement are not likely to be very aesthetic because of the unpredictable pigmentation

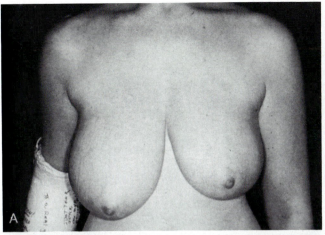

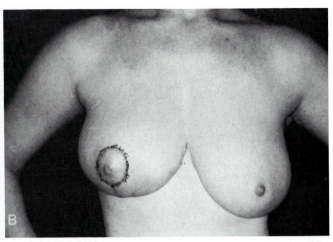

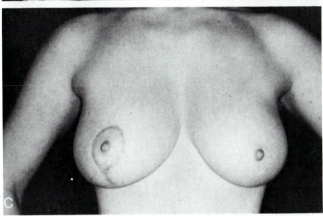

FIGURE 13–19

Congenital asymmetry: Unilateral hypermastia; bilateral ptosis. The patient wanted to match the left breast. *Treatment:* Unilateral breast reduction A, Right hypermastia. Patient is satisfied with the ptotic left breast. B, Reduction with the author's extended superior pedicle technique (see Surgical Technique and Fig. 13–23). C, Descent of breast operated upon, after 8 months, without any upward migration of the nipple and areola. (From Elliott, R., Hoehn, J., Greminger, R.: Correction of asymmetrical breasts. Plast. Reconstr. Surg. 56:260, 1975.)

associated with free grafts. Physiologic areolar enlargement will follow a significant augmentation. This is, of course, a very slow process, but free of telltale encircling scars.

For total reconstruction of the nipple and areola, areolar sharing (Millard, 1972; Wexler, 1973), saving (Millard et al., 1971), and tattooing (Little and Spear, 1988) have had their advocates. These procedures require an informed understanding of the cosmetic limitations of even the best results. The labia minora (dark brown), high anteromedial thigh (light brown), and oral mucosa (light pink) have been reliable donor sites for free grafts in selected cases (Brent, 1979).

After mastopexy and reduction procedures, the physiologic descent of the breast mass is accompanied by a tendency for upward migration of the nipple and areola (see Figs. 13–20 and 13–21), a phenomenon that requires operative allowance or prevention. The author's extended dermal pedicle technique obviates this problem (see Figs. 13–7, 13–9, and 13–19).

Physiologic descent of the breast mass after augmentation can result in the nipple and areola pointing downward if the prosthesis cannot descend with the breast. The modern generation of the prostheses, which are free of patches that adhere to the chest wall, tend to avoid this deformity.

Chest Wall Asymmetry

Reconstruction of a chest wall deformity is relatively complex. A decision to alter the thorax should, there-

fore, depend upon the severity and location of the defect. Minor deformities are often masked simply by altering the breast (Krause et al., 1969; Hartrampf, 1988). More severe deformities may require a custom-made prosthesis created from moulage models (Baker et al., 1975) or a muscle flap. The use of a custom prosthesis (Fig. 13–22) has been advocated for pectoral muscle deficiency (Poland, 1841) and for correction of pectus excavatum (Masson et al., 1970). The latissimus dorsi (Bostwick, 1983) and rectus abdominus (Hartrampf, 1988) muscles offer useful flaps. Reconstruction of sternal and rib cage deformities with bone is usually reserved for patients requiring greater rigidity, for an associated cardiac or pulmonary dysfunction. Transfer of the insertion of the latissimus dorsi muscle can substitute for the pectoral muscle mass at the anterior axillary fold in the selected case.

Acquired Asymmetry

Much of the surgical planning for congenital and acquired deformities is similar. However, the cause of the deformity may change some treatment options.

Posttraumatic and postoperative deformities are potentially the most unusual, and their treatment is highly individual. Severe infection may also limit breast development or distort existing structures. Treatment may require resurfacing, repositioning of structures (see Fig. 13–12), or tissue expansion and augmentation (Buchman et al., 1974; Guan et al., 1988; Neale et al., 1982;

Text continued on page 157

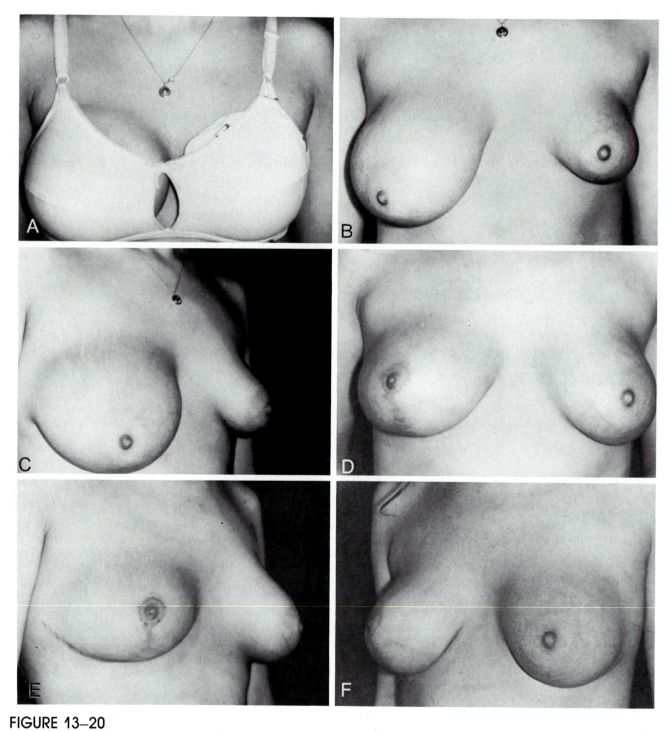

FIGURE 13–20

Congenital asymmetry: Unilateral hypermastia; contralateral micromastia. *Treatment:* Unilateral reduction; contralateral augmentation (prior to extended superior pedicle reduction [see Fig. 13–23] and tissue expansion). *A,* Attempt to mask severe asymmetry in clothing. *B* and *C,* Preoperative deformity. *D* to *F,* Postoperative result. Note the preventable mismatch of areolar size and upward migration of the right nipple and areola.

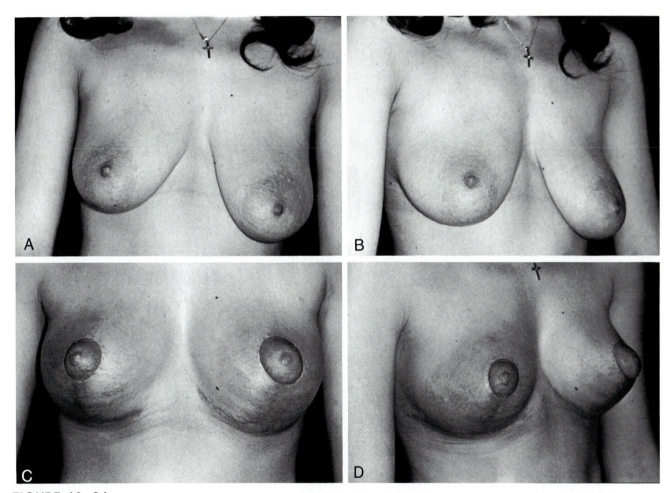

FIGURE 13–21

Congenital asymmetry: Asymmetric ptosis; unilateral hypermastia. *Treatment:* Unilateral mastopexy; contralateral reduction mammaplasty. *A* and *B,* Asymmetric ptosis and left hypermastia. Note the difference in areolar size (related to volume). *C* and *D,* Similar scars and volume match after right mastopexy and left reduction with the vertical bipedicle technique. Note overreduction of areola and later elevation of the nipple and areola position as the breasts settled. (From Elliott, R., Hoehn, J.: Asymmetrical breasts. In: Georgiade, N.: *Reconstructive Breast Surgery.* St. Louis, C. V. Mosby, 1976, p. 89.)

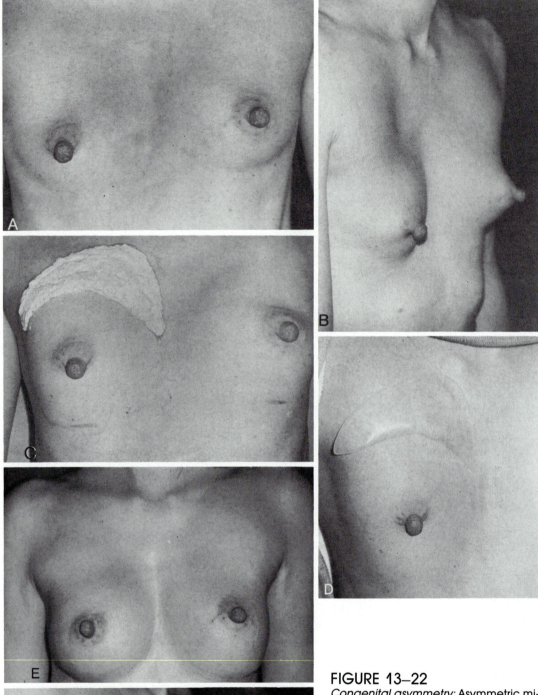

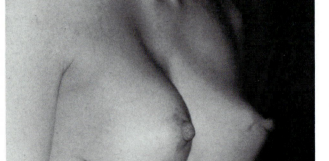

FIGURE 13–22

Congenital asymmetry: Asymmetric micromastia; unilateral nipple ptosis; pectoralis muscle deficiency. *Treatment:* Unilateal custom implant and nipple suspension; asymmetric breast augmentation. *A* and *B*, Preoperative chest wall, breast, and nipple asymmetry. *C*, Moulage for a custom prosthesis. *D*, Silastic gel prosthesis for muscle defect. *E* and *F*, Result with a right subpectoral custom prosthesis and asymmetric (right, 180 cc; left, 210 cc) subglandular augmentation.

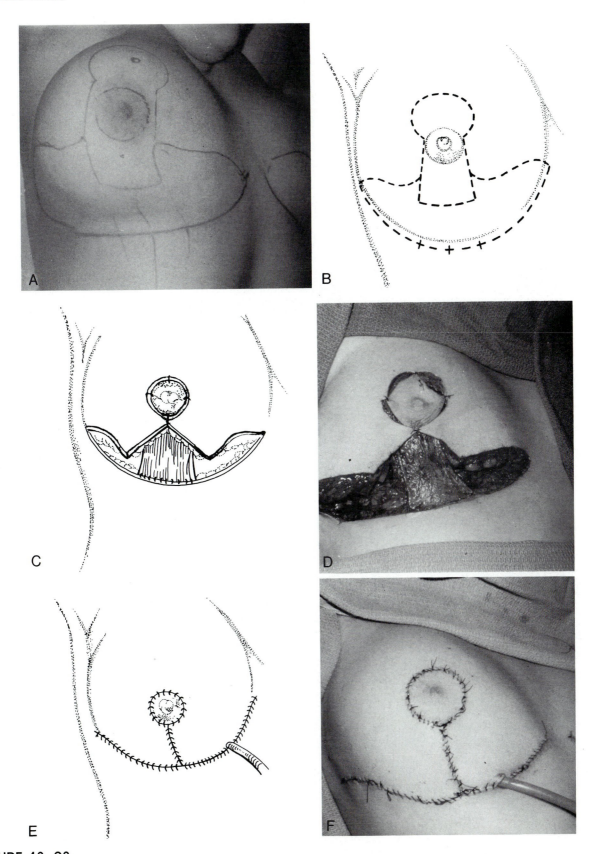

FIGURE 13-23

Surgical technique: The author's extended superior pedicle technique for mastopexy and breast reduction. *A* and *B,* Superior-based pedicle with a 5.5-cm dermal extension inferior to the areola. *C* and *D,* Dermal pedicle sutured to the dermis of the inframammary fold fixes the areola inframammary fold and prevents upward migration of the nipple and areola as the breast settles. *E* and *F,* Final closure and drainage. Contrast the results in Figures 13-7, 13-9, and 13-19, in which the extended superior pedicle technique was used, with Figures 13-20 and 13-21, in which the vertical bipedicle technique was used.

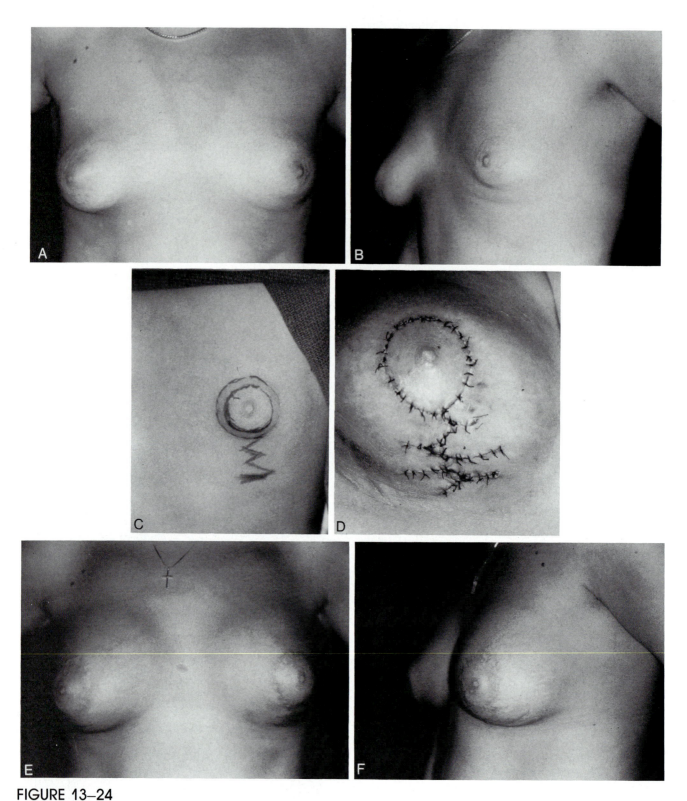

FIGURE 13–24

Surgical technique: The author's W-V-Y technique for expanding the inferior quadrants of the breast. *A* and *B,* Preoperative views. Inferior quadrant deficiency is more noticeable on the left breast. *C* and *D,* Plan for areolaplasty and lower quadrant expansion. Note that the running W is longer than the desired areola inframammary distance to allow for the shortening that results from the V-Y closure. *E* and *F,* The expanded inferior quadrant envelope and areolar herniorrhaphy permit smooth augmentation contours.

Versaci et al., 1986). Pontis (1973) described breast sharing, but myocutaneous flaps have obviated this technique (Bostwick, 1983; Hartrampf, 1988).

Mastectomy for cancer creates a variety of asymmetric defects, including those in the axilla and subclavicular areas where node-bearing fat and muscle are excised. The current, less radical procedures and the explosion of knowledge regarding surgical reconstruction have improved the symmetry of the average result (Lejour et al., 1988). Large benign tumors are another potential cause of asymmetry (see Fig. 13–14).

OPERATIVE SEQUENCE

When similar corrective procedures are done bilaterally, I have found it advantageous to operate first on the breast that is nearest the desired volume. However, when an augmentation and a reduction are required on the same patient, the reduction is usually done first. If an inadequate skin envelope might be a factor, it is better, however, to do the augmentation first.

SURGICAL TECHNIQUE

The technical challenges and options for breast augmentation, breast reduction, and mastopexy are well known to the trained cosmetic surgeon. With experience, favorite techniques evolve from familiarity and patient satisfaction. The relative merit of the various techniques will not be debated here, because they are detailed in other chapters. However, I will offer three personal techniques that evolved to improve my results.

When the nipple/areolar complex is moved 10 centimeters or less in a breast reduction or mastopexy, for over 10 years I have used a superior-based pedicle with a 5.5-cm dermal extension (Fig. 13–23). Elevation of the dermal extension facilitates total excision of both lower quadrants and tailoring of the lateral breast flap as a single specimen. Fixing the dermal extension to the inframammary fold dramatically prevents the late upward migration of the nipple and areola seen with other reduction techniques and adds support to the three-point juncture of the inverted-T–patterned flaps. Complications have been very few; and in contrast to the negative experience others have reported with the basic superior pedicle technique (Courtiss and Goldwyn, 1976), for me the procedure has been both rapid and safe. This may be related to several key points: I avoid a narrow waist on the keyhole design, open only into the lower third of the new areolar site, and preserve the breast attachment to muscle beneath the areola. Using this technique, nipple sensation is preserved, and the areola to inframammary crease distance remains fixed. Delayed healing and indentation at the three-point closure of the inverted T are no longer seen.

Another technical improvement has evolved for the correction of the severe tuberous breast deformity which is not corrected by simple rearrangement of the glandular tissue and augmentation (Rees and Aston, 1976). During the past decade, I have combined W-V-Y hori-

zontal expansion of the infra-areolar skin envelope, repair of the areolar hernia, and breast augmentation to gain improved results (Fig. 13–24). As others (Dinner and Dowden, 1987; Elliott, 1988) have reported, surgical scars to increase the infra-areolar envelope are an acceptable tradeoff for better contour and patient satisfaction. An effective differential tissue expander could, perhaps, render all of these techniques obsolete.

I tried the published methods for correction of the inverted nipple before discovering that separation of the shortened ducts and the interpositioning of bilateral dermal flaps of areloa tunneled above the breast mound gave more lasting results. This procedure was independently discovered and subsequently reported to others (Elsahy, 1976; Teimourian and Adham, 1980). Kami et al. (1988) recently reported a technique for preserving the lactiferous ducts. They release to the fibrous tissue around the ducts and maintain eversion with a bolster and milk suction pump.

Malposition of a mammary prosthesis may require reoperation. Enlargement of a mature pocket is not usually successful. Preservation of the old pocket and development of a properly located, deeper pocket is recommended (see Fig. 13–16). Deforming encapsulation that does not respond to closed capsulotomy (Baker et al., 1976) is treated similarly (see Fig. 13–15). A subpectoral pocket (Biggs and Yarish, 1988) and the use of a polyurethane-covered prosthesis (Brand, 1988; Hester et al., 1988) are favored today.

CONCLUSION

Asymmetry of the breast remains a troublesome deformity, but technical modifications and experience continue to improve the surgical results. Progress will usually follow when the surgeon remains critical of his accomplishments. Good results can be obtained with a wide variety of techniques when chosen well and performed with care.

References

Arey, I.: *Developmental Anatomy*. Philadelphia, W. B. Saunders, 1958, pp. 409, 449.

Baker, J., Bartles, R., Douglas, W.: Closed compression technique for rupturing a contracted capsule around a breast implant. Plast. Reconstr. Surg. 58:137, 1976.

Baker, J., Mara, J., Douglas, W.: Repair of concavity of thoracic wall with silicone elastomer implant. Plast. Reconstr. Surg. 56:212, 1975.

Biggs, T., Yarish, R.: Augmentation mammaplasty: Retropectoral versus retromammary implantation. Clin. Plast. Surg. 15:549, 1988.

Bostwick, J.: Correction of breast asymmetries. In: *Aesthetic and Reconstructive Breast Surgery*. St. Louis, C. V. Mosby, 1983, p. 103.

Bouman, F.: Volumetric measurement of the human breast and breast tissue before and during mammaplasty. Br. J. Plast. Surg. 23:263, 1970.

Brand, G.: Foam-covered mammary implants. Clin. Plast. Surg. 15:533, 1988.

Brent, B.: Nipple-areolar reconstruction following mastectomy: An alternative to the use of labial and contralateral nipple-areolar tissues. Clin. Plast. Surg. 6:95, 1979.

Buchman, H., Larson, D., Huang, T., et al.: Nipple and areola reconstruction in the burned breast. Plast. Reconstr. Surg. 54:531, 1974.

Burkhardt, P.: Capsular contracture: Hard breasts, soft data. Clin. Plast. Surg. 15:521, 1988.

Castano, M.: Dorsal scapular supernumerary breast in a woman. Plast. Reconstr. Surg. 43:536, 1969.

Chatterton, R.: Mammary gland: Development and secretion. Obstet. Gynecol. Annu. 7:303, 1978.

Cholnoky, T.: Augmentation mammaplasty: Survey of complications in 10,941 patients by 265 surgeons. Plast. Reconstr. Surg. 45:573, 1972.

Cole, N.: Informed consent: Considerations in aesthetic and reconstructive surgery of the breast. Clin. Plast. Surg. 15:541, 1988.

Corso, P.: Plastic surgery of the unilateral hypoplastic breast: A report of eight cases. Plast. Reconstr. Surg. 50:134, 1972.

Courtiss, E. Goldwyn, R.: Comments on the superior pedicle. In: Goldwyn, R. *Plastic and Reconstructive Surgery of the Breast.* Boston, Little, Brown, 1976, p. 264.

Dinnen, M., Dowden, R.: The tubular/tuberous breast syndrome. Ann. Plast. Surg. 19:414, 1987.

Edgerton, M., Meyer, E., Jacobson, W.: Augmentation mammaplasty: Further surgical and psychiatric evaluation. Plast. Reconst. Surg. 27:279, 1961.

Elbaz, J., Werheecke, G.: La ciatrice en L dans les plasties mammaires. Ann. Clin. Plast. 17:283, 1972.

Elliott, M.: A musculocutaneous transposition flap mammaplasty for correction of the tuberous breast. Ann. Plast. Surg. 20:2, 1988.

Elliott, R., Hoehn, J., Greminger, R.: Correction of asymmetrical breasts. Plast. Reconstr. Surg. 56:260, 1975.

Elliott, R., Hoehn, J.: Asymmetrical breasts. In: Georgiade, N.: *Reconstructive Breast Surgery.* St. Louis, C. V. Mosby, 1976, p. 89.

Elsahy, N.: An alternative operation for inverted nipples. Plast. Reconst. Surg. 57:436, 1976.

Gerow, F.: Surgical management of micromastia. In: Masters, F., Lewis, J.: *Symposium on Aesthetic Surgery of the Face, Eyelid and Breast.* St. Louis, C. V. Mosby, 1972, p. 152.

Gifford, S.: Emotional attitudes toward cosmetic breast surgery: Loss and restitution of the "ideal self." In: Goldwyn, R. M.: *Plastic and Reconstructive Surgery of the Breast.* Boston, Little, Brown, 1976, p. 103.

Gorney, M., Harries, T.: The preoperative and postoperative consideration of natural facial asymmetry. Plast Reconstr. Surg. 54:187, 1974.

Grossman, A.: Psychologic and psychosexual aspect of augmentation mammaplasty. Clin. Plast. Surg. 3:167, 1976.

Guan, W., Jin, Y., Cao, H.: Reconstruction of postburn female breast deformity. Ann. Plast. Surg. 21:65, 1988.

Hartrampf, C.: The transverse abdominal island flap for breast reconstruction: A 7-year-experience. Clin. Plast. Surg. 15:703, 1988.

Hawtoff, D., Ram, S., Alani, H.: Reconstruction of mammary hypoplasia associated with chest wall deformities. Plast. Reconstr. Surg. 57:172, 1976.

Hester, T.: Nahai, F., Bostwick, J., Cubic, J.: A 5-year experience with polyurethane-covered mammary prostheses for treatment of capsular contracture, primary augmentation mammaplasty, and breast reconstructions. Clin. Plast. Surg. 15:569, 1988.

Hueston, J.: Unilateral agenesis and hypoplasia: Difficulties and suggestions. In: Goldwyn, R. M.: *Plastic and Reconstructive Surgery of the Breast.* Boston, Little, Brown, 1976, p. 361.

Kami, T., Wong, A., Kim, I.: A simple method for the treatment of the inverted nipple. Ann. Plast. Surg. 21:316, 1988.

Kaye, B.: Axillary breasts. Plast. Reconstr. Surg. 53:61, 1974.

Kirianoff, T.: Volume measurements of unequal breasts. Plast. Reconstr. Surg. 54:616, 1974.

Krause, J., Crikelair, G., Cosman, B.: The Cronin implant in the treatment of combined chest wall and breast deformities. Plast. Reconstr. Surg. 44:536, 1969.

Lejour, M., Jabri, M., Deralmaecker, R.: Analysis and long-term results of 326 breast reconstructions. Clin. Plast. Surg. 15:689, 1988.

Little, J., Spear, S.: The finishing touches in nipple areolar reconstruction. Perspect. Plast. Surg. 2:1, 1988.

Marchac, D., Sagher, U.: Mammaplasty with a short horizontal scar evaluation and results after 9 years. Clin. Plast. Surg. 15:627, 1988.

Masson, J., Payne, W., Gonzales, J.: Pectus excavatum use of preformed prostheses for correction in adults. Plast. Reconstr. Surg. 46:399, 1970.

Millard, D.: Nipple and areola reconstruction by split skin graft from the normal side. Plast. Reconstr. Surg. 50:350, 1972.

Millard, D., Devine, J., Warren, D.: Breast reconstruction: A plea for saving the uninvolved nipple. Am. J. Surg. 122:763, 1971.

Neale, H., Smith, G., Gregory, R., MacMillan, B.: Breast reconstruction in the burned adolescent female. Plast. Reconstr. Surg. 70:718, 1982.

Pers, M.: Aplasias of the anterior thoracic wall, the pectoral muscles and the breast. Scand. J. Plast. Reconstr. Surg. 2:125, 1968.

Peterson, R.: The McKissock dermal pedicle. In: Georgiade, N.: *Aesthetic Breast Surgery.* Baltimore, Williams & Wilkins, 1983, p. 195.

Pitanguy, I.: Surgical treatment of breast hypertrophy. Br. J. Plast. Surg. 20:78, 1967.

Pitanguy, I.: Breast reduction and ptosis. In: Georgiade, N. (Ed.): *Aesthetic Breast Surgery.* Baltimore, Williams & Wilkins, 1983, p. 256.

Poland, A.: Deficiency of the pectoralis muscle. Guy's Hosp. Rep. 6:191, 1841.

Pontes, R.: Single stage reconstruction of the missing breast. Br. J. Plast. Surg. 24:396, 1973.

Rees, T., Aston, S.: The tuberous breast. Clin. Plast. Surg. 3:339, 1976.

Simon, B., Hoffman, S., Kahn, S.: Treatment of asymmetry of the breasts. Clin. Plast. Surg. 2:375, 1975.

Smith, D., Palin, W., Katch, V., Bennett, J.: Surgical treatment of congenital breast asymmetry. Ann. Plast. Surg. 17:92, 1986.

Teimourian, B., Adham, M.: Simple technique for correction of inverted nipple. Plast. Reconstr. Surg. 65:504, 1980.

Trier, W.: Complete breast absence. Plast. Reconstr. Surg. 36:430, 1965.

Versaci, A., Balkovich, M., Goldstein, S.: Breast reconstruction by tissue expansion for congenital and burn deformities. Ann. Plast. Surg. 16:20, 1986.

Wexler, R.: Areolar sharing to reconstruct the absent nipple. Plast. Reconstr. Surg. 51:176, 1973.

Woods, J., Borkowski, J., Masson, J., Irons, G.: Experience with and comparison of methods of reduction mammaplasty. Mayo Clin. Proc. 53:487, 1978.

Zarem, H.: Standards of medical photography. In: Nelson, G., and Krause: *Clinical Photography in Plastic Surgery.* Boston, Little Brown, 1988, p. 73.

MAMMARY HYPERTROPHY

14

Gordon Letterman
Maxine Schurter

A History of Reduction Mammaplasty

BEGINNINGS

Ablation of the female breast was performed in antiquity for religious or utilitarian reasons. St. Agatha's sacrifice of her breasts to avoid the attentions of Quintianus is legendary. Hippocrates described amputation by cauterization as practiced by the Scythians.

But who did the first reduction mammaplasty for female hypertrophy? That it was not Durston, as is so often claimed, was shown by Letterman and Schurter (1974). Biesenberger (1931) stated that Hans Schaller, a barber surgeon of Augsburg, was the first to attempt the removal of a hypertrophied breast by operation. It is reasonable to assume that before the advent of anesthesia, and before the first aesthetic breast surgery was described in the twentieth century, Hans Schaller could not have done much more than an ablation or, at the very most, an amputation.

There is some historical evidence that reduction was done for hypertrophy in 1890, but with sacrifice of the nipples and areolae. Kelly (1899), of Baltimore, Maryland, did an historically significant abdominal reduction on a 32-year-old woman. Peters (1901) reported that the same patient had previously undergone bilateral breast reduction in 1890 at the age of 23 by J. W. Chambers, also of Baltimore.

A similar case of reduction without salvage of the nipples was reported by Lexer (1912). He, of course, was later to become a pioneer in nipple transpositions.

It is difficult to give credit to one surgeon in the early 1900s. This is partly due to the fact that medical writing was not as extensive as it is today. In addition, operations on the breasts were demonstrated to surgeons in training, but they were not recorded until the student performed them. For this reason, there are some hyphenated eponyms for certain operations.

Thorek (1942) wrote that in 1926 Mornard described the operation of separation of the skin from the gland, transposition of the nipple upward, and inferior quadrant resection of the gland. Mornard had learned it from Morestin. However, Dufourmentel said that he had performed the same operation in 1916, and Dartigues saw Villandre perform it in 1911 (Fig. 14–1).

Lexer (1921) published a paper describing his breast reduction in detail. This was lost in the literature because of the obscure journal in which it was published and the misleading title of the paper and because it was in Spanish. Kraske (1923) published a paper describing the procedure again and in German. From that time, it became known as the Lexer-Kraske operation.

LATERAL OR OBLIQUE?

Holländer (1924), of Berlin, described a lateral glandular resection with an L-shaped oblique closure (Fig. 14–2). Gläsmer (1927), of Heidelberg, published a report of a technique of lateral breast excision and lateral closure.

In 1952 Helene Marc wrote her book on the oblique method of breast reduction. The procedure was basically that of Biesenberger. The gland to be resected, however, was removed from the lateral inferior part of the breast. Skin also was taken laterally, and the final scar was lateral to the nipple and areola. She did not mention Holländer or Gläsmer, and she attributed the origin of her procedure to Aubert (1923) of Marseille.

Dufourmentel and Mouly (1961) adopted the lateral skin and glandular excision of Marc, added their own special techniques, and abandoned Biesenberger's method of wide separation of skin and gland. This operation became the procedure of choice for many plastic surgeons in France. Furthermore, many surgeons who had French connections by virtue of training or language adopted the procedure. Two methods that have branched off from the oblique reduction are the B technique of Regnault (1974) and the L-shaped suture line of Meyer and Kesselring (1975). A nice modification of the lateral method is that of Nicolle (1982). He uses a modified Strömbeck pattern rotated laterally, a laterally based breast pedicle for retained gland, and an inverted-T closure located on the lateral aspect of the breast.

In the United States Shatten (1971) has used, described, and taught the Dufourmentel and Mouly procedure extensively.

FREE NIPPLE-AREOLA GRAFTS

The first succinct description of a successful transplantation of a free nipple-areola graft has been ascribed to Thorek (1922). In the spring of 1921 he presented a paper entitled "Possibilities in the Reconstruction of the Human Form" at a meeting of the Chicago Medical Society. In the course of this presentation he described his operation of reduction mammaplasty. The following year the paper was published with photographs in the *New York Medical Journal.*

Thorek wrote: "In a careful search of the available literature no record is found of the deliberate attempt to transplant the nipple. This experimental study proves

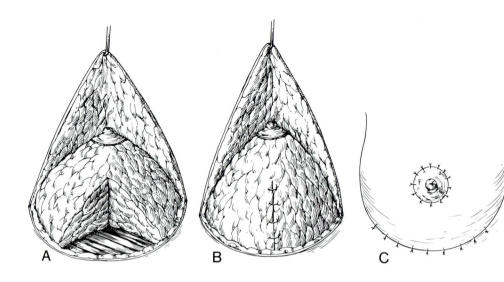

FIGURE 14–1
A to *C,* Operation described by Mornard. The skin is widely separated from the gland, the inferior quadrant of the breast is excised, and the nipple is transposed.

that that may be accomplished for cosmetic reasons." The breasts were amputated and remodeled. The nipples were then transplanted to their new locations (Fig. 14–3).

During the ensuing 25 years numerous papers on free grafting of the nipple and areola were written by Thorek (1930, 1931, 1936, 1939, 1945, 1946). His comprehensive book on plastic surgery of the breast and abdomen (1942) contains a detailed description of the preoperative preparation, measurements, patient's position, anesthesia, and ten steps of the operative procedure. Thorek's "Twenty-five Years' Experience with Plastic Reconstruction of the Breast and Transplantation of the Nipple" was summarized in 1945.

Dartigues (1928) challenged Thorek's claim of priority in the successful use of the free nipple graft. Thorek (1930) promptly disputed Dartigues' claim on the basis of a historical review of the correction of third-degree ptosis that Dartigues (1925) himself had written. Speaking of free nipple grafts, he said "En 1922 Max Thorek (de Chicago) représentait ce procédé (New York Medical Journal and Medical Record, 15 Novembre 1922)."

Maliniac (1944) wrote that "under no circumstances can the nipple itself, in the anatomical sense of the word, be successfully transplanted free." However, Thorek (1931) published photomicrographs of biopsy specimens of free nipple grafts, and Adams (1944) demonstrated the survival of the smooth musculature within the free grafts.

Maliniac (1950) described his procedure for reconstruction after mammectomy. His indication for mammectomy was any advanced hyperplasia. Because the gland was completely removed, he was not opposed to the use of free nipple grafts. He prepared a large inferiorly based dermofat flap, which he folded under the anterior skin fat flap to give bulk and shape to the breast (Fig. 14–4).

It is a lengthy and tedious task to remove the epithelium from such a large flap. The procedure, therefore, could not compete with other methods of reduction. It remains, however, a very good tool for reconstruction after subcutaneous mastectomy, with or without a silicone prosthesis. Letterman and Schurter (1955, 1967, 1975, 1977) have modified it for this purpose.

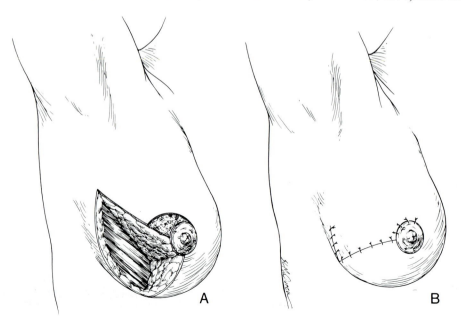

FIGURE 14–2
A and *B,* Method of Holländer, with lateral breast resection, partial transposition of nipple, and lateral skin closure.

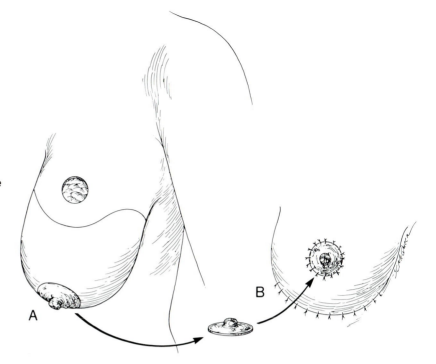

FIGURE 14-3
A and B, Thorek's reduction, with free nipple and areola transplantation.

Adams (1944) indeed did much to popularize nipple transplantation, and he described his own variations of Thorek's technique. Adams' untimely death followed his last paper (1957), entitled "Mammaplasty with free transplantation of the nipples and areolae," which he presented at the First Congress of the International Society of Plastic Surgeons meeting in Stockholm in 1955.

Bames (1949), long an advocate of a two-stage procedure for the correction of gigantomastia, realized that

essentially nothing was lost in the use of the free nipple-areola grafts and concluded that it was time to abolish a two-stage reduction in favor of a single procedure using free grafts.

Hans May (1950), once Lexer's assistant, stated that the procedure of amputation and reconstruction using free nipple-areola grafts is the procedure of choice for excessively hypertrophic breasts.

Amputation mammaplasty with free nipple-areola grafts continues today to be a very satisfying and satis-

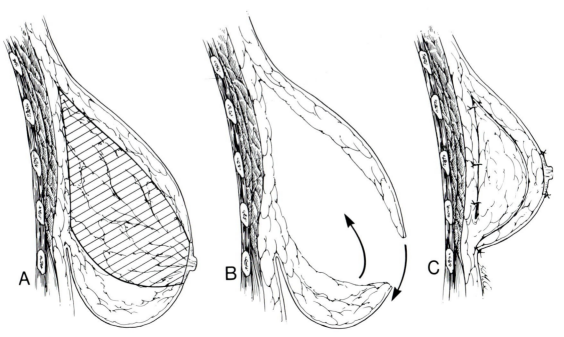

FIGURE 14-4
A to C, Subcutaneous mastectomy with reconstruction by dermofat flap, after the method of Maliniac.

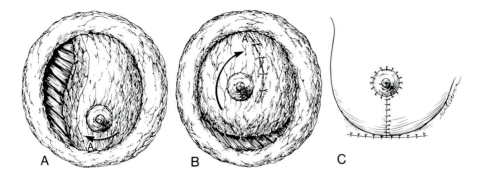

FIGURE 14—5

A to *C,* Biesenberger's technique of wide separation of the skin from the gland, excision of the lateral half of the gland, and nipple transposition. (Note the movement of point A.)

factory operation. Schurter and Letterman (1961) have used it often for patients who are beyond the nursing age, those who do not feel that erotic sensitivity is important, and those patients in whom for medical reasons the procedure should be performed quickly.

Letterman and Schurter (1984) presented a 25-year follow-up on free nipple-areola grafts in reduction mammaplasty at the annual meeting of the American Society of Aesthetic Plastic Surgery in Washington, D.C.

BIESENBERGER'S METHOD

Biesenberger (1928) studied all of the methods of plastic surgery of the breast reported prior to 1927. He was cognizant of both their good and their bad features. Furthermore, he was a serious student of the anatomy of the breast. Based on these studies, Biesenberger set forth a list of requirements for the ideal breast reduction:

1. That the breast be lifted to a youthful and natural form in proportion to other parts of the upper body.
2. That the breasts have symmetry.
3. That the nipple and areola be transplanted to an appropriate location.
4. That there be no jeopardy of blood supply to the nipple and areola.
5. That there be no interference with the function of the organ.
6. That the scars not be visible through clothing or above the areola.
7. That the operation be applicable to all forms of deformity.
8. That the procedure be a one-stage operation.

When he published a report of his own procedure, he felt it fulfilled all of these requirements. His operation became the most popular worldwide for the next 30 years.

The areola is incised, and the skin is elevated from the entire gland. The outer half of the breast parenchyma is removed. The two cut edges of the gland are then sutured together. The skin is draped over the new form, and the excess skin is trimmed away. The nipple and areola are brought out in the proper location. The final skin closure is in the shape of an inverted T.

Nipple transposition had previously been performed by numerous surgeons: Lexer (1921), Aubert (1923), Lotsch (1923), Passot (1923), Kraske (1923), Dufour-

mentel (1925), and Axhausen (1926). A few surgeons had elevated the skin from the gland: Mornard, as described by Thorek (1942), and Axhausen (1926). A lateral glandular resection was done by Gläsmer (1927) and Höllander (1924). However, the combination of the three elements—(1) separation of skin and gland, (2) resection of the lateral half of the gland, and (3) transposition of the nipple on the retained gland—was original with Biesenberger and was the outcome of his concept of the anatomy of the breast (Fig. 14–5).

Through the years many modifications were proposed, primarily involving the location of the glandular element to be resected. Gillies and McIndoe (1939) removed breast tissue above the nipple and areola and approximated the cut edges. Aufricht (1949) resected a wedge from the upper quadrant, the upper and lateral quadrants, or the entire upper half. Ragnell (1957) removed a large upper segment and a smaller lower segment of breast tissue. Penn (1960) removed the lateral and medial sectors, leaving a central, vertically oriented segment of breast to carry the nipple and areola. His skin closure also included a flap below the areola that was based on the inframammary fold. Kaplan (1978) resected up to three of the quadrants, depending on the areas of maximum hypertrophy.

Wise (1956, 1963) used a modified Biesenberger operation, but his papers are especially noteworthy for his patterns and mechanical aids to make the operation safer and to produce a more aesthetic breast. His skin pattern has been the basis of marking for many different procedures, including the pattern of Strömbeck (1960). Wise's original paper continues to be of value to the surgeon in estimating the size of the reduced breast. His pattern was derived from a brassiere, and he showed the relationship between brassiere cup size and chest circumference.

Even after all of the many new procedures introduced, Hester in 1985 revived the Biesenberger operation, leaving a central core of breast to carry the nipple and areola. The branches of the main blood supply to the breast are preserved during this dissection.

FLAPS

In 1960 plastic surgeons of the world were performing breast reductions by either some form of Biesenberger's operation or a resection and free nipple grafts. At that time the *British Journal of Plastic Surgery* was one of two plastic surgery journals generally available. It was in this journal that Strömbeck (1960) published his article describing a pattern and reduction technique with transposition of the nipple and areola on a transverse bipedicle flap of glandular tissue.

Plastic surgeons greeted this new operation with either great enthusiasm or disinterest. But those who tried it found that the results were good. As time went by, however, it was realized that when the pedicles were very short, upward rotation was restrictive and nipple inversion or necrosis could result. Later, Strömbeck (1971) showed that the bipedicle flap could be converted into a unipedicle flap without danger. This unipedicle breast flap carrying the nipple and the areola, particularly if it was medially based, was not unlike the Schwarzmann (1930) procedure. Schwarzmann was ahead of his time; he had reported performing the operation on 150 patients without complications. A medially based breast flap with its dermis intact was rotated upward to a new nipple site. Unfortunately, this operation, of great historical interest, had long been lost in the literature (Fig. 14–6).

Several years after Strömbeck's operation was recorded, Skoog (1963) presented another bold concept of transposition of the nipple. He stated that for 15 years, or since 1948, he had used some form of Biesenberger's operation. After Strömbeck's publication, he had used that procedure for 3 years. Like other plastic surgeons, he was striving for a better operation, and he based his new procedure on the assumption that the nipple could be carried on cutaneous vessels alone. He created a lateral cutaneous pedicle for the nipple and the areola and resected gland and fat where necessary. Skin closure was in the usual inverted-T form. He also stated that the nipple and the areola could be carried on a bipedicle flap (transverse). Skoog's description of

the operation was published in *Acta Chirurgica Scandinavica,* which was not widely read by plastic surgeons at that time. The markings in that original paper were somewhat difficult to follow, and meticulous technique was required to prepare the dermal pedicle. For these reasons the operation did not achieve great popularity.

The history of breast reduction is reminiscent of that of abdominal reduction, which began with transverse resections, followed by vertical resections, and then a combination of the two. Just 12 years after Strömbeck reported on the transverse pedicle, McKissock (1972) described a vertically oriented bipedicle flap of breast for transposition of the nipple. He resected glandular tissue both medially and laterally. He also modified existing patterns to shape a wire marker for location of the new nipple site together with skin and glandular resection. This method of breast reduction quickly became the most popular method in the United States and remained so for a number of years.

In the natural progression of events, it was inevitable that someone would convert this bipedicle breast flap to a unipedicle flap; this was done by Weiner (1973), who based the flap superiorly.

Just as inevitably, the unipedicle flap was to be based inferiorly. Ribeiro (1973, 1975) carried the nipple on a wide inferior pedicle from which the epithelium had been removed. Glandular tissue is resected from above the areola. The upper skin flap is elevated as in Biesenberger's procedure. The medial and lateral cut edges of the gland are approximated. There is no vertical scar.

Among the early contributors to the use of the inferiorly based pedicle were Robbins (1977), Courtiss and Goldwyn (1977), Georgiade (1979, 1983), and Reich (1979). It is one of the most commonly used methods of breast reduction in the United States at the present time (Fig. 14–7).

FIGURE 14–6
A and *B,* Schwarzmann's method of carrying the nipple on a dermoglandular pedicle.

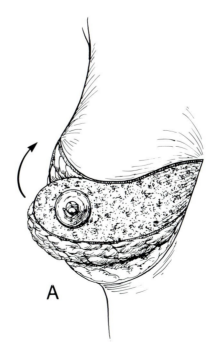
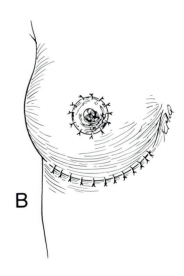

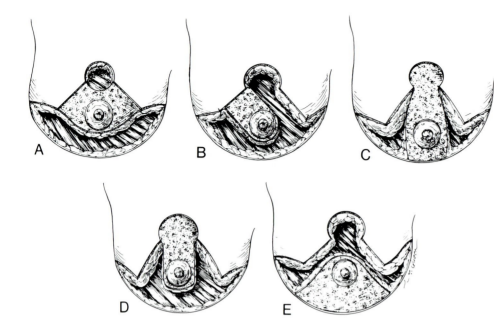

FIGURE 14-7

Flaps. *A*, Transverse bipedicle dermoglandular flap. *B*, Dermal flap of Skoog. *C*, Vertical bipedicle dermoglandular flap. *D*, Superior unipedicle dermoglandular flap. *E*, Inferior unipedicle dermoglandular flap.

KEEL RESECTION

It is not really possible to place keel resection in one of the other categories, since it has little in common with any of them. Pitanguy (1964) presented his own operation at the First Latin American Congress of Plastic Surgeons in Bogota in 1962, and it was published in Spanish 2 years later. He described it in English several years later (1967).

Pitanguy's operation for breast reduction consists of the following:

1. Preservation of a dermal triangle around the nipple and areola. He feels that it is not so much the dermis that is important, but the vascular channels just beneath it. Although the concept stemmed from the work of Schwarzmann, the reasons for its use were different.
2. Resection of glandular tissue in a keel shape. The first time this method of parenchymal excision was found in the literature was in the work of Arié (1957).

He was a breast surgeon at the Institute of Cancer in Sao Paulo and obviously had great influence on Pitanguy's thinking.

3. Elevation of nipple and areola on underlying gland without separation of skin from the gland. Although this had been done by surgeons during the earlier part of the century, the manner of carrying the nipple and areola appears to be original.
4. Inverted-T skin closure. This had been common for decades, but it was a departure from Arié's procedure (Fig. 14-8).

Pitanguy believes "the keel" operation is applicable to any size or form of reduction. Letterman and Schurter (1976, 1981), however, after using the procedure extensively, found that occasionally elevation of the nipple may be difficult. When this is the case, minimal sectioning of the lower parts of the dermal triangle will usually facilitate delivery of the nipple and areola at the higher level without tension. This maneuver may impair sensation; in a way, it converts the operation to a superior pedicle procedure.

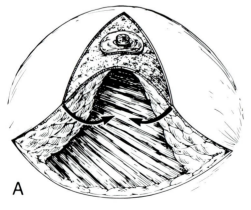

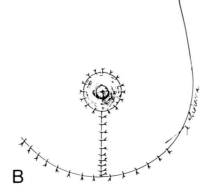

FIGURE 14-8

A and *B*, Keel resection (*A* and *B*) with the nipple on a triangular dermoglandular base.

FIGURE 14-9
A to *C,* Peixoto's method of reduction for minimal transverse scars.

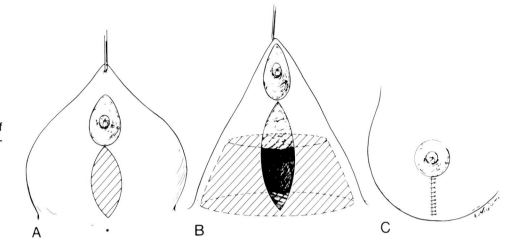

This operation has had a tremendous influence on Brazilian plastic surgeons, many of whom have been trained by Pitanguy. Although it is in common use in Brazil and many other South American countries, it has never been widely practiced in the United States.

SHORT SCARS

All through the history of breast reduction, surgeons have been especially concerned with adequate blood supply of the nipple and areola, skin, and gland. They have also wanted to preserve sensation of the nipple and lactation of the gland. Contour and symmetry are always important.

Now the trend is to accomplish the preceding goals with short inframammary scars. This concept is not really new. Arié (1957) used a vertical closure only, but the scar passed well below the inframammary field, and this was never popular with patients. Lassus (1970) revived reduction with a vertical closure and continues to use it (1988). Stark (1977), referring to his modification of the Biesenberger technique, states: "A horizontal incision 6 to 8 cm long is made slightly above the submammary crease. The submammary wound—and, hence, scar—is short."

Peixoto (1980) presented his personal technique, which he believed was applicable to reduction of any size. The object was to keep the transverse scars of minimum length (Fig. 14-9).

The glandular resection is patterned after Pitanguy's operation. The skin resection is the key to the short inframammary scars. Pitanguy (1980) commented on this procedure, stating that contour was more important than scars, particularly those that are hidden in the inframammary crease.

Marchac (1982) has written about reduction and mastopexy with short inframammary scars. Skin excision is primarily vertical. Glandular resection is as in Pitanguy's operation. Skin closure results in an upper and lower dog-ear. The upper is taken up in the new areolar site, while the lower is excised as a transverse ellipse. The latter elevates the inframammary crease.

Maillard (1983) describes a Z mammaplasty in *Plastic*

Reconstructive Breast Surgery. It is not applicable to large resections nor to procedures performed on older women whose breasts have lost elasticity. Postoperative results depend on settling of the remaining skin to the newly fashioned breast. The entire gland is elevated off the pectoralis major muscle to facilitate upward advancement. The Z closure retains some of the elements of the L and B techniques of Meyer and Regnault. Maillard (1987) gave a teaching course at the meeting of the International Society of Aesthetic Plastic Surgery in New York City. His skin markings were more explicit, and the original technique was somewhat modified.

SUMMARY

This chapter began with the predecessors of true reduction mammaplasty and ends with present-day trends. There are many authors who have contributed to this historical procession who are not included because of lack of space. If the reader wishes to find other diagrams, references, and concepts, he can refer to Stephenson (1972), Lalardrie and Jouglard (1974), and Letterman and Schurter (1976, 1978).

References

Adams, W. M.: Free Transplantation of the nipples and areolae. Surgery 15:186, 1944.

Adams, W. M.: Mammaplasty with free transplantation of the nipples and areolae: A thirteen-year follow-up report. In: Skoog, T. (ed.): *Transactions of the First Congress of the International Society of Plastic Surgeons, Stockholm and Uppsala.* Baltimore, Williams & Wilkins, 1957.

Arié, G.: Una nueva técnica de mastoplastia. Rev. Lat. Am. Cir. Plast. 3:23, 1957.

Aubert, V.: Hypertrophie mammaire de la puberté: Résection partielle restauratrice. Arch. Franco-Belg. Chir. 26:284, 1923.

Aufricht, G.: Mammaplasty for pendulous breasts: Empiric and geometric planning. Plast. Reconstr. Surg. 4:13, 1949.

Axhausen, G.: Über Mammaplastik. Med. Klin. 22:1437, 1926.

Bames, H. O.: Gigantomastia: Two-stage operation for reduction of extremely large breasts versus one-stage technic. Plast. Reconstr. Surg. 4:352, 1949.

Biesenberger, H.: Eine neue Methode der Mammaplastik. Zentralbl. Chir. 55:2382, 1928.

Biesenberger, H.: *Deformitäten und Kosmetische Operationen der Weiblichen Brust.* Vienna, Maudrich, 1931.

Courtiss, E., Goldwyn, R.: Reduction mammaplasty by the inferior pedicle technique. Plast. Reconstr. Surg. 59:500, 1977.

Dartigues, L.: Traitement chirurgical du prolapsus mammaire. Arch. Franco-Belg. Chir. 28:313, 1925.

Dartigues, L.: Mammectomie totale et autogreffe libre areolo-mamelonnaire: Mammectomie bilaterale esthetique. Bull. Mem. Soc. Chir. Paris 20:729, 1928.

Dufourmentel, C., Mouly, R.: Plastie mammaire par la méthode oblique. Ann. Chir. Plast. 6:45, 1961.

Dufourmentel, L.: La mastopexie par déplacement sous-cutane avec transposition du mamelon. Bull. Mem. Soc. Chir. Paris 20:20, 1925.

Georgiade, N. G., Serafin, D., Riefkohl, R., Georgiade, G. S.: Is there a reduction mammaplasty for all seasons? Plast. Reconstr. Surg. 63:765, 1979.

Georgiade, N. G., Serafin, D., Morris, R., Georgiade, G.: Reduction mammaplasty utilizing an inferior pedicle nipple-areolar flap. Ann. Plast. Surg. 3:211, 1979.

Georgiade, N. G., Georgiade, G. S.: Reduction mammoplasty utilizing the inferior pyramidal dermal pedicle flap. In: Georgiade, N. G. (ed.): Aesthetic Breast Surgery. Baltimore, Williams & Wilkins, 1983.

Gillies, H., McIndoe, A.: The technique of mammaplasty in conditions of hypertrophy of the breast. Surg. Gynecol. Obstet. 68:658, 1939.

Gläsmer, E.: Die Formfehler und Die Plastischen Operationen der Weiblichen Brust. Stuttgart, Ferd. Enke, 1930.

Hester, T. R., Bostwick, J., III, Miller, L., Cunningham, S. J.: Breast reduction utilizing the maximally vascularized central breast pedicle. Plast. Reconstr. Surg. 76:890, 1985.

Holländer, E.: Die Operation der Mammahypertrophie und der Hängebrust. Dtsch. Med. Wochenschr. 50:1400, 1924.

Kaplan, I.: Reduction mammaplasty: Nipple-areola survival on a single breast quadrant. Plast. Reconstr. Surg. 61:27, 1978.

Kelly, H.: Report of gynecological cases. Bull. J. Hopkins. Hosp. 10:197, 1899.

Kraske, H.: Die Operation der Atrophischen und Hypertrophischen Hängebrust. Münch. Med. Wochenschr. 70:672, 1923.

Lalardrie, J-P., Jouglard, J. P.: Chirurgie Plastique de Sein. Paris, Masson, 1974.

Lassus, C.: A technic for breast reduction. Int. J. Surg. 53:69, 1970.

Lassus, C.: The short scar in reduction mammoplasty. Presented at the PSEF/ASAPS Symposium Plastic Surgery of the Breast, Santa Fe, N.M., 1988.

Letterman, G. S., Schurter, M.: Total mammary gland excision with immediate breast reconstruction. Am. Surg. 21:835, 1955.

Letterman, G., Schurter, M.: Reduction mammaplasty with preservation of nipple-glandular continuity. J. Am. Med. Wom. Assoc. 20:942, 1965.

Letterman, G. S., Schurter, M. S.: Experiences with adenomammectomy and immediate breast reconstruction. In: Broadbent, T. R. (ed.): Transactions of the Fourth International Congress of Plastic Surgery. Amsterdam, Excerpta Medica Foundation, 1967.

Letterman, G., Schurter, M.: Will Durston's "Mammaplasty." Plast. Reconstr. Surg. 53:48, 1974.

Letterman, G., Schurter, M.: Inframammary-based dermofat flaps in reconstruction following a subcutaneous mastectomy. Plast. Reconstr. Surg. 55:156, 1975.

Letterman, G., Schurter, M. A.: A history of mammaplasty with emphasis on correction of ptosis and macromastia. In: Goldwyn, R. M. (ed.): Plastic and reconstructive surgery of the breast. Boston, Little, Brown, 1976.

Letterman, G., Schurter, M.: A comparison of modern methods of reduction mammaplasty. South. Med. J. 69:1367, 1976.

Letterman, G., Schurter, M.: Adenomammectomy. Surg. Clin. North Am. 57:1035, 1977.

Letterman, G., Schurter, M.: History of reduction mammaplasty. In: Owsley, J. Q., Peterson, R. A. (eds.): Symposium on Aesthetic Surgery of the Breast. St. Louis, C. V. Mosby, 1978.

Letterman, G., Schurter, M.: Free nipple-areolar grafts in reduction mammaplasty. Presented at the Seventeenth Annual Meeting of the American Society for Aesthetic Plastic Surgery, Washington, D. C., March 29, 1984.

Lexer, E.: Hypertrophie bei der Mammae. Münch. Med. Wochenschr. 59:2702, 1912.

Lexer, E.: Correcion de los pechos pendulos (mastoptose) por medio de la implantacion de grasa. Guipuzcoa Medica 6:210, 1921.

Lotsch, F.: Uber Hängebrustplastik. Zentralbl. Chir. 50:1241, 1923.

Maillard, G. F.: Refinements of the Z-mammoplasty with minimal scarring. Presented at the meeting of the ninth Congress of the ISAPS, New York, 1987.

Maillard, G. F., Montandon, D., Goin, J.: Plastic Reconstructive Breast Surgery. New York, Masson, 1983.

Maliniac, J. W.: Critical analysis of mammectomy and free transplantation of the nipple in mammaplasty. Am. J. Surg. 65:364, 1944.

Maliniac, J. W.: Breast Deformities and Their Repair. New York, Grune & Stratton, 1950.

Marc, H.: La Plastie Mammaire par la "Méthode Oblique." Paris, G. Doin, Paris, 1952.

Marchac, C. D., DeOlarte, G.: Reduction mammaplasty and correction of ptosis with a short inframammary scar. Plast. Reconstr. Surg. 69:45, 1982.

May, H.: Mammaplastic procedures in the female. Pa. Med. 53:609, 1950.

McKissock, P.: Reduction mammaplasty with a vertical dermal flap. Plast. Reconstr. Surg. 49:245, 1972.

Meyer, R., Kesselring, U.: Reduction mammaplasty with an L-shaped suture line. Plast. Reconstr. Surg. 55:139, 1975.

Nicolle, F.: Improved standards in reduction mammaplasty and mastopexy. Plast. Reconstr. Surg. 69:453, 1982.

Passot, R.: La Chirurgie Esthétique Pure. Hôpital (Paris) 11:184, 1923.

Peixoto, G.: Reduction mammaplasty: A personal technique. Plast. Reconstr. Surg. 65:217, 1980.

Penn, J.: Breast reduction II. In: Wallace, A. B. (ed.): Transactions of the International Society of Plastic Surgeons, Second Congress. Edinburgh, E. & S. Livingstone, 1960, p. 502.

Peters, L.: Resection of the pendulous, fat abdominal wall in cases of extreme obesity. Ann. Surg. 34:229, 1901.

Pitanguy, I.: Hipertrofias mamarias. Trib. Med. 4:3, 1964.

Pitanguy, I.: Surgical treatment of breast hypertrophy. Br. J. Plast. Surg. 20:78, 1967.

Pitanguy, I.: Discussion: Reduction mammaplasty: A personal technique by Gerardo Peixoto. Plast. Reconstr. Surg. 65:226, 1980.

Ragnell, A.: Further experience of preservation of lactation capacity and nipple sensitivity in breast reduction. In: Skoog, T. (ed.): Transactions of the First Congress of the International Society of Plastic Surgeons, Stockholm and Uppsala. Baltimore, Williams & Wilkins, 1957.

Regnault, P.: Reduction mammaplasty by the "B" technique. Plast. Reconstr. Surg. 53:19, 1974.

Reich, J.: The advantages of a lower central breast segment in reduction mammaplasty. Aesthetic Plast. Surg. 3:47, 1979.

Ribeiro, L.: A new technique for reduction mammaplasty. Plast. Reconstr. Surg. 55:330, 1975.

Ribeiro, L., Backer, E.: Mastoplastia con pediculo de seguridad. Rev. Esp. Cir. Plast. 6:223, 1973.

Robbins, T. H.: A reduction mammaplasty with the areola-nipple based on an inferior dermal pedicle. Plast. Reconstr. Surg. 59:64, 1977.

Schatten, W. E., Hartley, J. H.: Reduction mammaplasty by the Dufourmentel-Mouly method. Plast. Reconstr. Surg. 48:306, 1971.

Schurter, M., Letterman, G.: Comment. Personal Preferences for Reduction Mammaplasty, Ivo Pitanguy. In: Goldwyn, R. M. (ed.): Plastic and Reconstructive Surgery of the Breast. Boston, Little, Brown, 1976.

Schurter, M., Letterman, G.: Amputation mammaplasty with free nipple grafts. J. Am. Med. Wom. Assoc. 16:854, 1961.

Schwarzmann, E.: Die Technik der Mammaplastik. Chirurg 2:932, 1930.

Skoog, T.: A technique for breast reduction: Transposition of the nipple on a cutaneous vascular pedicle. Acta Chir. Scand. 126:453, 1963.

Stark, R. B.: A procedure for mammary reduction and mastopexy: Summary of 100 personally performed operations. Aesthetic Plast. Surg. 1:145, 1977.

Stephenson, K. L.: A history of mammaplasty. In: Masters, F. W., Lewis, J. R. (ed.): Symposium on Aesthetic Surgery of the Face, Eyelid, and Breast. St. Louis, C. V. Mosby, 1972.

Strömbeck, J. O.: Mammaplasty: Report of a new technique based on the two-pedicle procedure. Br. J. Plast. Surg. 13:79, 1960.

Strömbeck, J. O.: Reduction mammaplasty. Surg. Clin. North Am. 51:453, 1971.

Thorek, M.: Possibilities in the reconstruction of the human form. N. Y. Med. J. 116:572, 1922.

Thorek, M.: Esthetic surgery of the pendulous breast, abdomen and arms in the female. I. M. J. 58:48, 1930.

Thorek, M.: The possibilities of surgical esthetic remodeling of the human form. Tri-State Medical Journal 3:621, 1931.

Thorek, M.: Histological verification of the efficacy of free transplantation of the nipple. N. Y. Med. J. Med. Rec. 134:474, 1931.

Thorek, M.: Simplicity versus complicated methods in the reconstruction of pendulous breasts. I. M. J. 69:338, 1936.

Thorek, M.: Plastic reconstruction of the female breasts and abdomen. Am. J. Surg. 43:268, 1939.

Thorek, M.: *Plastic Surgery of the Breast and Abdominal Wall.* Springfield, Ill., Charles C Thomas, 1942.

Thorek, M.: Twenty-five years' experience with plastic reconstruction of the breast and transplantation of the nipple. Am. J. Surg. 67:445, 1945.

Thorek, M.: Plastic reconstruction of the breasts and free transplantation of the nipple. Int. Surg. 9:194, 1946.

Weiner, D. L., Aiache, A. E., Silver, L., Tittiranonda, T.: A single dermal pedicle for nipple transposition in subcutaneous mastectomy, reduction mammaplasty, or mastopexy. Plast. Reconstr. Surg. 51:115, 1973.

Wise, R. J.: A preliminary report on a method of planning the mammaplasty. Plast. Reconstr. Surg. 17:367, 1956.

Wise, R. J., Gannon, J. P., Hill, J. R.: Further experience with reduction mammaplasty. 32:12, 1963.

15

Jaime Planas

Hints for Improving Shape and Symmetry in Reduction Mammaplasty

In plastic surgery artistic feeling and improvisation are basic elements in surgical success. However, there are few procedures in which geometric planning is as important as in mammary reduction. Operating without making measurements first, as was formerly done, frequently leads to unsatisfactory aesthetic results. Correct marking before the operation is as important as the surgical act itself. Wise's pattern (Wise, 1956, 1976) and others based on the same principles are of immeasurable value in this regard. Moreover, experience has shown that the best way to prevent necrosis is by avoiding extensive undermining of the skin. Arié (1957) and Strömbeck (1960, 1968) were pioneers of the modern techniques of removing the tissues *en bloc* without previously undermining the skin. Most of the necrosis and other poor results at that time occurred because the concepts were unknown.

I began performing mammary reductions in 1949, using Biesenberger's technique (Biesenberger, 1928). The skin was totally undermined, and the gland was left hanging from the pectoral aponeurosis, unstable and movable, exactly like jelly wobbling on a plate. One had the feeling that at any moment the breast could fall to the floor. Such great surgeons as Harold Gillies and Archibald McIndoe (Gillies, 1939; McIndoe, 1958) recommended the separation of the breast tissue from the skin by stripping it with gauze, the dissection being "carried out bluntly in the same manner as one would skin a rabbit." Understandably, the traction and tearing of the skin resulted in vascular lesions. Skin and gland necrosis was frequent. Fitting this skin to the preshaped gland was an endless struggle. There were so many problems that some surgeons did the operation in two stages, reducing one breast in each surgical act.

Other technical improvements have contributed to increasing possibilities of success. Thus, the extensive mobilization of the areola allows the surgeon to displace it out through the hole of its new placement without tension on the tissues. A loose breast is the best guarantee of success. Hollowing out the tissues in the shape of a Gothic cupola (Pitanguy, 1962, 1967), extensive undermining of the retromammary space, and propelling the nipple with a flat flap (Planas, and Mosely, 1980) or with a dermis flap (Ribeiro and Backer, 1973) are, to my mind, the key to the good results we are obtaining today.

The technique that is described here can be applied to all cases of mammary hypertrophy and mammary ptosis with no hypertrophy, the only difference being that in simple ptosis no tissues are resected.

Our technique is the result of many years of observation, application of new maneuvers, and failures and difficulties that have been overcome little by little. The procedure is based on borrowed techniques and our own ideas, which we have been changing and introducing at the same time as we were acquiring a better understanding of the reasons for our failures. We firmly believe that these changes have improved symmetry; avoided nipple inversion; and, especially, established guidelines for the surgeon so that he knows beforehand the exact length of the residual scars and the shape of the breast. The resulting scar is the typical inverted-T scar.

SURGICAL TECHNIQUE

Step 1: Marking

It is very important that the surgeon draw the incision lines preoperatively with the patient either standing or seated opposite him.

The midline is drawn, as well as the two meridians, which run from the midclavicle to the nipples (Fig. 15–1). Wise's pattern is used.

It has been recommended that one plan the entire marking by first choosing the level of the new nipple. Many designs and measures have been recommended, but by using any of them the surgeon ignores the length of the resulting scars. The problem arises at the end of the suturing when a surplus of tissues cannot be adjusted and no major changes can be made (Fig. 15–2). We recommend, instead, that one plan the reduction by first choosing the length of the submammary incision. The nipple is then automatically placed at a precise point, which may change by 1 cm, higher or lower (which is not important); however the surgeon will know beforehand the length of the submammary scar.

Experience has taught us that a scar that extends from the anterior axillary line laterally to 1.5 or 2 cm from the midline medially will be a hidden scar (Fig. 15–3).

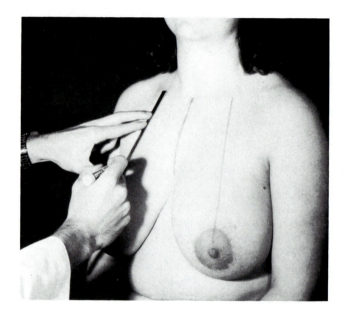

FIGURE 15–1
Marking the references with the patient standing.

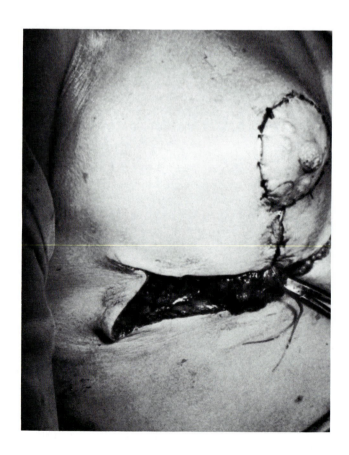

FIGURE 15–2
Incorrect marking may end in dog-ears and longer scars.

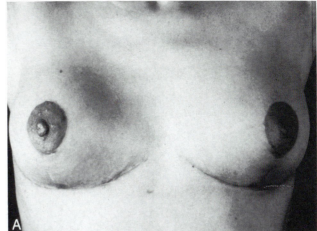

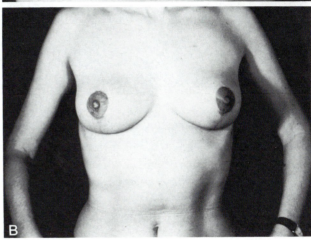

FIGURE 15–3
Submammary scars *(A)*, which will not be visible in normal view *(B)*.

If the two edges of a wound are equal, the adjustment will be smooth, and no dog-ears will remain (Fig. 15–4). Therefore, it is important that the sum of the two pedicles equal the length of the submammary incision.

By placing Wise's pattern over the meridian and moving it up and down, the correct length of the pedicles may be obtained (Fig. 15–5).

It is important when one is drawing the lines that the skin be maintained stretched if exact measures are to be obtained.

Step 2: De-epithelialization

Under general anesthesia, with the patient appropriately prepared and draped, both the nipple keyhole and the horizontal bipedicle nipple flap are de-epithelialized (Fig. 15–6).

To facilitate this maneuver, it is helpful to wrap around the base of the mamma a rubber band (Fig. 15–7).

Step 3: Excision

Holding the mamma with a strong forceps, the upper horizontal incision is made inferior to the nipple pedicle (Fig. 15–8). There are two important components to this portion of the operation. A "keel resection" of the

proximal flap is done as advocated by Pitanguy (Pitanguy, 1967; Planas, 1980), and the extra tissue carved out of the proximal breast flap is left attached to the inferior dermal flap (Fig. 15–9). The inferior flap is left attached or hanging by its base until a decision is made as to how much, if any, of this flap will be used to give extra tissue support to the breast.

The angles of the lower flap are cut in about 3 or 4 cm to allow the flap to hang away from the field (Fig. 15–10).

Step 4: Undermining

The upper flap is undermined to the level of the second or third rib (Fig. 15–11). This undermining makes possible a tensionless molding of the breast and creates a pocket to receive a fat or dermofat flap should this be necessary to push out the nipple or fill the breast. It is useful in this stage to leave two long stitches inserted in the pectoral muscle at the level of the third rib to hold the mentioned flap should this be necessary, as already explained (Fig. 15–12).

Step 5: Nipple Transposition

The nipple-areola complex is mobilized fully by cutting through the dermis and part of the subcutaneous
Text continued on page 178

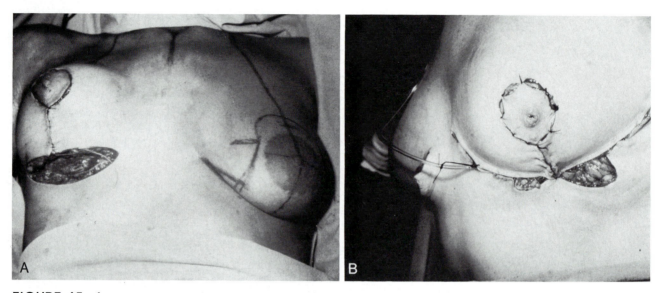

FIGURE 15–4
A, Both edges of the wound have equal length. *B,* Excess of tissues in the longer edge.

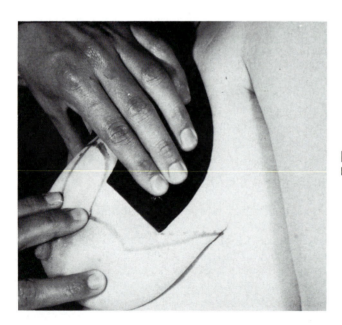

FIGURE 15–5
Determining the right length of the pedicles.

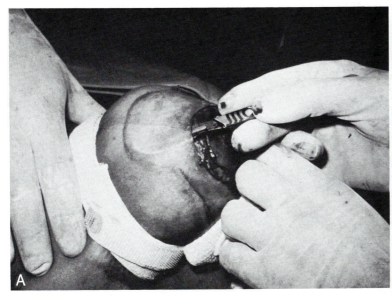

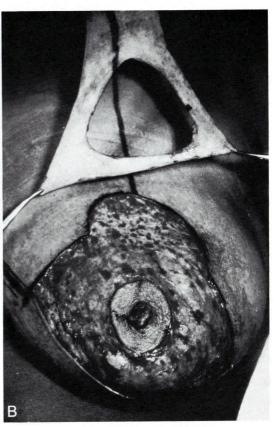

FIGURE 15–6
A and *B*, De-epithelialization of the nipple keyhole.

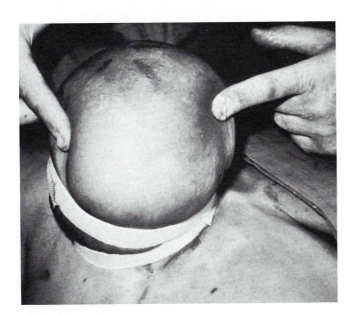

FIGURE 15–7
Use of a compression band to facilitate de-epithelialization.

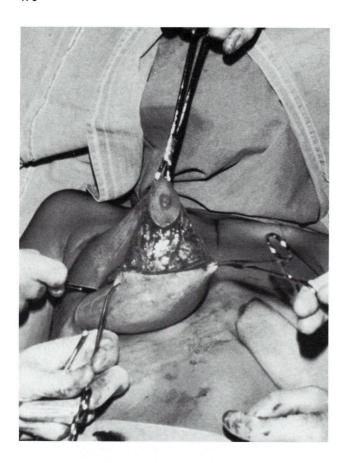

FIGURE 15–8
Holding the mamma with a forceps.

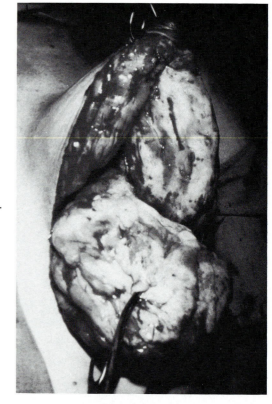

FIGURE 15–9
Keel resection of the proximal flap.

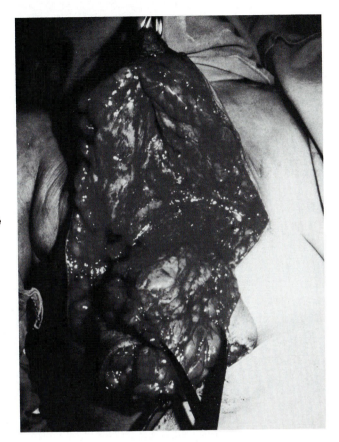

FIGURE 15-10
The angles of the lower flap are cut to allow the flap to be held away from the field.

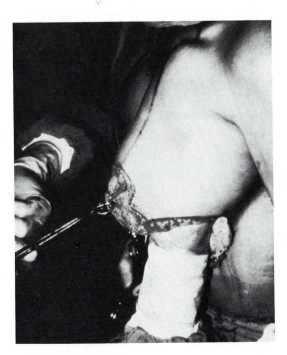

FIGURE 15-11
The upper flap is undermined to the level of the second or third rib.

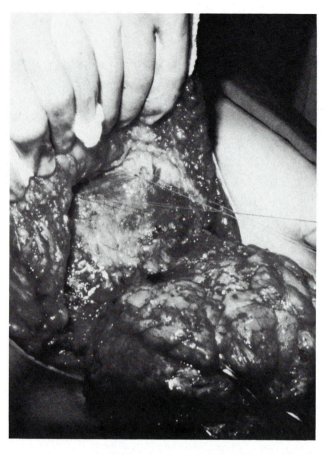

FIGURE 15–12
Two provisional stitches of polyglactin 910 are attached to the uppermost part of the undermining to be used later.

tissue to allow a tensionless advancement of the nipple to its new site. But if such mobilization is presumed to be difficult, the whole dermis around the areola and the pedicles may be cut in a more liberal manner (Fig. 15–13). When the distance of the nipple to its new location is great and the transposition is difficult by a central pedicle, a medial or lateral pedicle may be designed similar to that described by Skoog (1976). It should be rotated about 90 degrees (Fig. 15–14).

Step 6: Nipple Positioning

The areola is fixed to its new location, and the two pedicles are sutured together subcutaneously with long-term absorbable sutures (polyglactin 910). This vertical suture is very important because it supports the tension of the newly built mamma (Fig. 15–15).

Step 7: Dermofat Flap

At this point a decision is made as to whether or not to excise the entire inferior dermofat flap or to use part of it to augment the subareolar area and the upper pole of the breast. We use in almost all cases a gland and fat flap, which is tied to the long sutures we have left attached to the pectoral muscle during step 4 (see Fig. 15–12). This flap projects the nipple (Fig. 15–16) and fills the upper pole of the breast (Fig. 15–17). Based in the submammary region, these flaps are well vascular-

ized and can be tailored as long as necessary. Fat breasts with scarce glandular tissue need stronger support; in these cases it is better to use a dermal flap, as recommended by Ribeiro (1973), instead of a fat flap.

Tissues to be discarded are now excised (Fig. 15–18).

As has been shown, the entire procedure is performed without discarding any of the tissues until the very last step of the operation.

Step 8: Wound Closure

The wounds are closed with 4-0 polyglactin 910 intradermic sutures. No drains are used. A light compression dressing is used.

The postoperative results have generally been very pleasing, with improvement in breast symmetry and nipple projection (Figs. 15–19 to 15–21).

PITFALLS AND HOW TO PREVENT THEM

Uneven Nipple Location

The best way to avoid asymmetric location of the nipple is for the surgeon to perform a correct demarcation previous to the operation with the patient seated opposite him. Marking the incisions on the operating table and with the patient sleeping is a fight in which the enemy always wins. First, a vertical line is made

Text continued on page 185

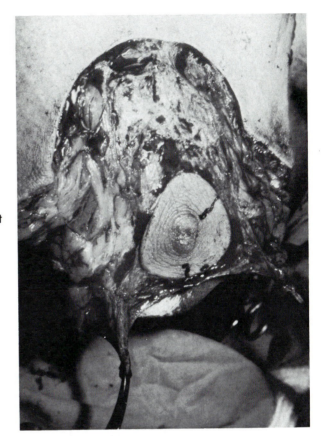

FIGURE 15–13
Liberation of the periareolar dermis and the pedicles in difficult cases.

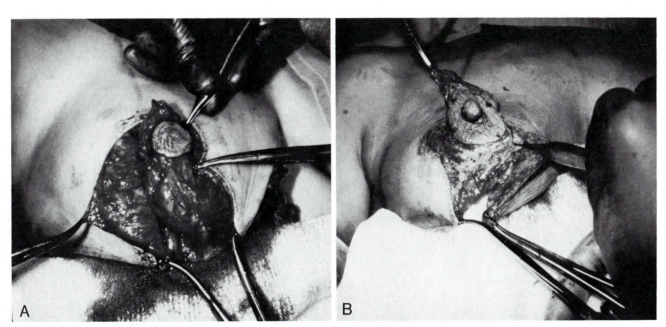

FIGURE 15–14
A, Rotation of a medial pedicle. *B,* Rotation of a lateral pedicle.

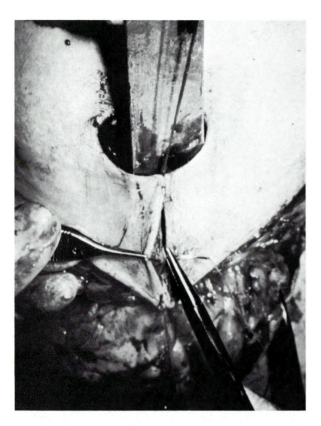

FIGURE 15–15
Suture of the two pedicles with reabsorbable subcutaneous sutures.

FIGURE 15–16
A, Depression of the nipple due to lack of support. *B,* Projection of the nipple after filling the space with dermofat flap.

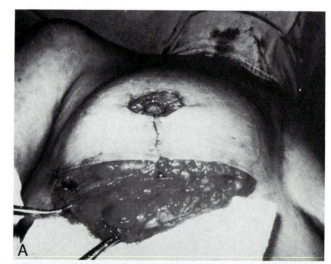

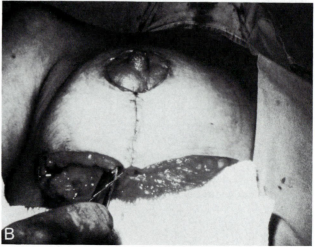

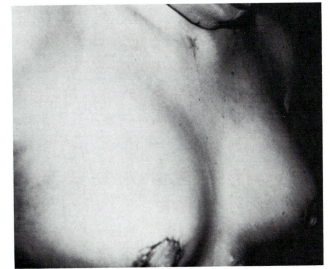

FIGURE 15-17
The fat flap fills the upper pole of the breast.

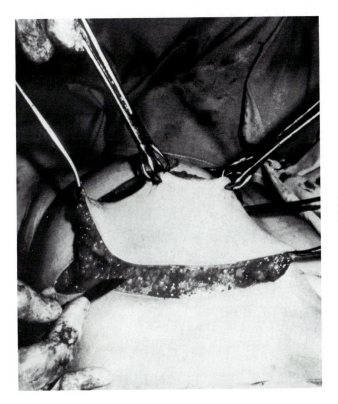

FIGURE 15-18
Resection of the excess tissues.

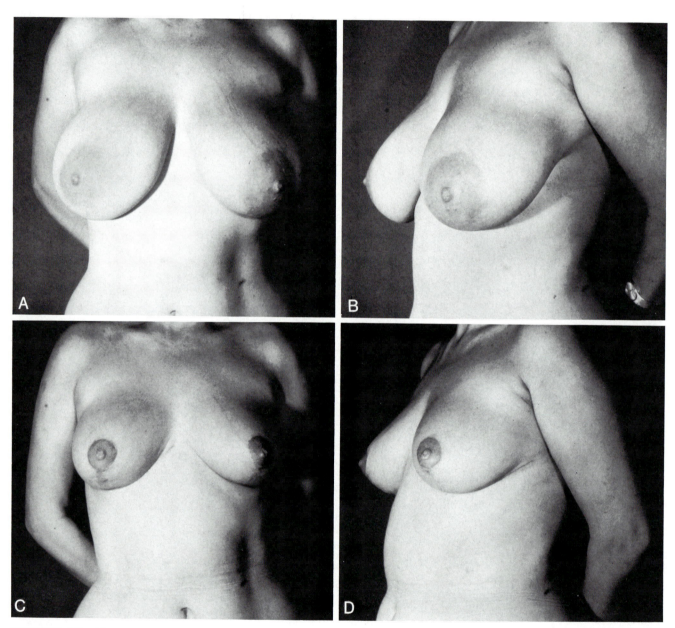

FIGURE 15–19
A and *B*, Preoperative views of a 34-year-old patient with hypertrophy of the breasts. *C* and *D*, Three months postoperatively.

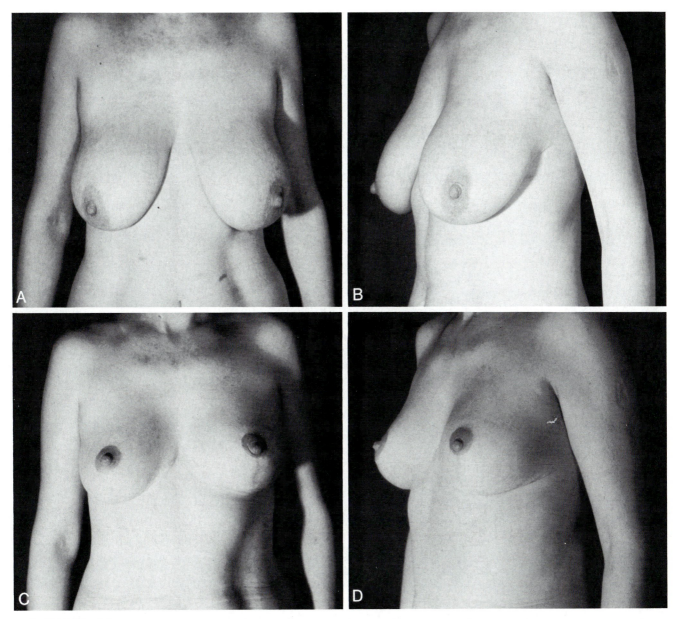

FIGURE 15–20
A and *B*, Preoperative views of a 37-year-old patient with hypertrophy and ptosis of breasts. *C* and *D*, One year postoperatively.

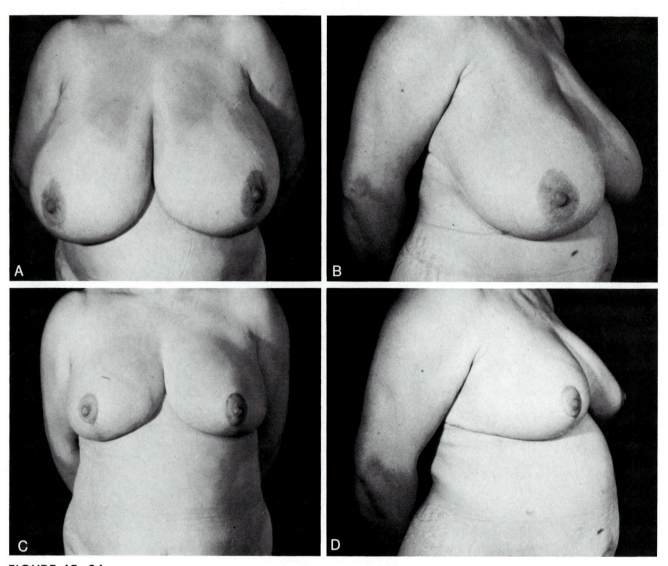

FIGURE 15–21
A and B, Preoperative views of a 39-year-old patient with gigantomastia. C and D, Four months postoperatively.

from the sternal notch down. The two meridians are now marked by two lines, which run from the midclavicle to the nipples. The nipples may already be asymmetric, and measurements must also be taken from the midline to the meridians for better control.

Sagging of the Lower Pole

It is a general belief that the breast operated upon will hang after some time due to the weight of the tissues; as a result, the lower pole increases in size and the areola becomes less vertical and more horizontal. This is what we call the upper gaze deformity (Fig. 15–22). When observing a breast with such a deformity, one can see that the distance from the submammary sulcus to the areola has increased. In our experience this deformity is due to incorrect measurement of this distance when marking the incision lines. This happens often when one is marking soft ptotic breasts. Applying the template over flaccid skin is misleading. When the skin is later stretched, the distance becomes longer (Fig. 15–23). A scar may shrink but never elongates (this is a basic principle of plastic surgery). If the distance is correct, the breast may soften but will not swing (Figs. 15–24 and 15–25). The best advice in avoiding postoperative sagging is to be sure that the length of the vertical scar is no longer than 5 to 6 cm.

Asymmetry of Volume

Excision of tissues to make both sides equal is not easy. Leaving the inferior dermofat flap until the end of the procedure allows us to add more or less of the flap until symmetry and projection are obtained (Fig. 15–26). This is in accord with the maxim of Sir Harold Gillies: "In plastic surgery never throw anything away" (and "It is well to have a lifeboat to get you home").

Unequal Contour

Because templates are used for marking the incisions, it is not usual to have different contour on both sides. But it is good to know that by closing or opening the angle of the template, different shapes can be given to the mammae. This technique is useful when correcting asymmetric breasts and in tuberous breasts.

Horizontal Scar above the Submammary Sulcus

A horizontal scar on the lower pole of the mamma is more visible (Fig. 15–27) and should be prevented by carefully placing the incision precisely in the submammary sulcus. There are data affirming that the submammary sulcus is not displaced by neighboring traction. Misplacing the incision occurs more often when one makes the markings with the patient on the operating table. With the patient lying down, it is more difficult to find the proper placement.

Some surgeons place the incision purposely above the submammary crease with the aim of elevating the sulcus, but the submammary sulcus must be considered as a fixed, unchangeable line with a memory.

Sinking of the Nipple

If the nipple-areola complex needs to be forced to arrive at its new location because the pedicles are short, the areola will sink. It will also sink if a loose nipple has no back support. Support may be given by adding a fat flap from the lower pedicle as described in step 7 (see Fig. 15–16). Stretched pedicles can be elongated by freeing more of the areola, with care taken to preserve enough circulation.

Vascular Failure of the Nipple-Areola Complex

We believe that a blue areola is more often due to tightness of the tissues than to excessive cutting of the vessels. A blue areola may sometimes become normal when the surgeon decides to remove all the stitches and excise more tissue to allow a looser closure. There is an excessive fear of cutting the dermis or leaving the pedicles too thin. It must be remembered that the important vessels run *under* the dermis and not *through* it.

Sloughing of the Suture Line

Sloughing of the suture line is often due to too much tension of the suture at the central crossing of the T incision. We try to diminish tension at this point by a few relaxing stitches in each side of the vertical suture. Because it is said that helium-neon laser speeds open wound healing, we have used five sessions of helium-neon infrared laser treatment in the early postoperative period in our last 65 cases, and this complication has been reduced dramatically.

Hypertrophic Scars

We all know that scars in the thorax are often unsightly. Pressure is perhaps the best preventive of hypertrophic scars. Pressure can be applied either by an elastic device or by simply covering the scars with tape for two months or so.

Acknowledgments

The author would like to thank Dr. Jose M. Palacin, Ms. Montserrat Bretcha, and Ms. Laura Vinas for their help in preparation of the manuscript.

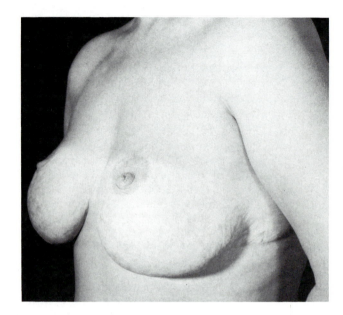

FIGURE 15–22
Sagging of the breast is a very common complication.

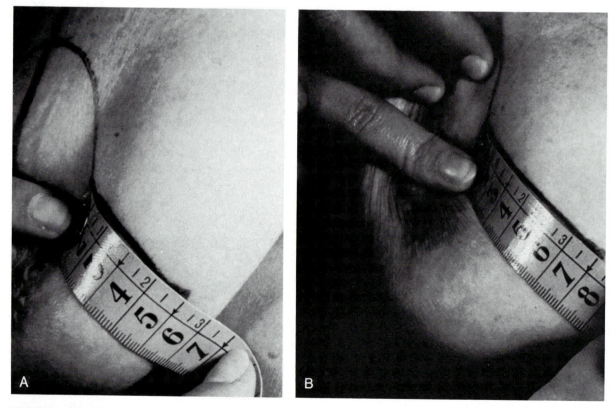

FIGURE 15–23
A, Taking measurements with the skin relaxed. *B,* After the skin is stretched, the length of the line has increased.

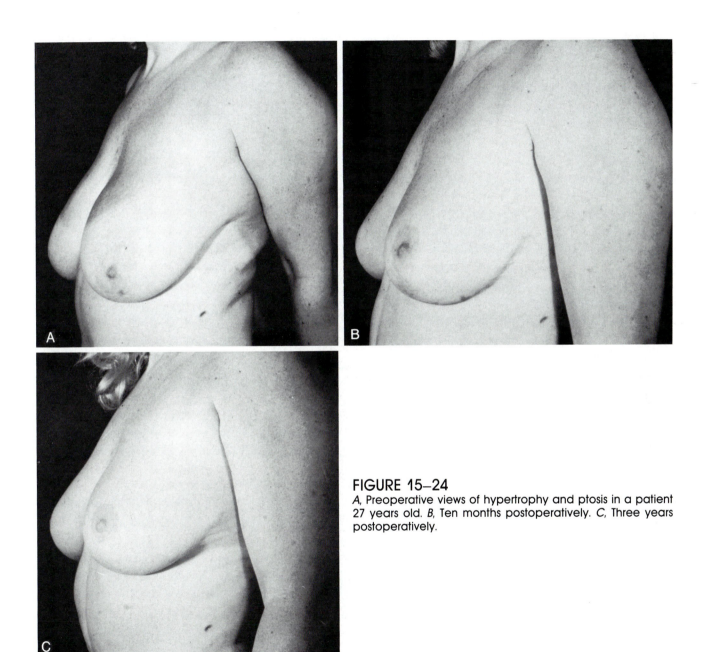

FIGURE 15–24

A, Preoperative views of hypertrophy and ptosis in a patient 27 years old. *B,* Ten months postoperatively. *C,* Three years postoperatively.

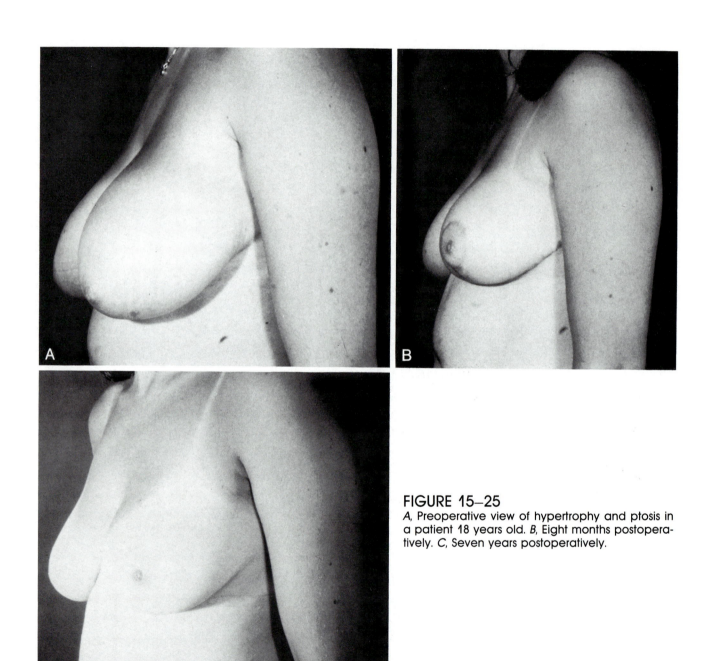

FIGURE 15–25
A, Preoperative view of hypertrophy and ptosis in a patient 18 years old. *B,* Eight months postoperatively. *C,* Seven years postoperatively.

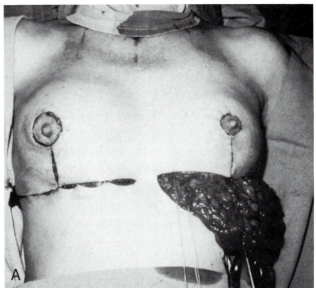

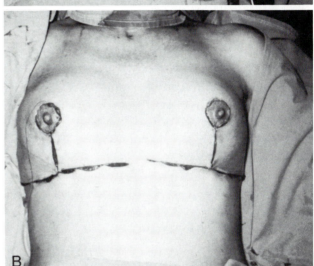

FIGURE 15–26
The hanging lower flap is of great help in obtaining symmetry. *A*, Before finishing the second side. *B*, Symmetry obtained after introduction of a fat or dermofat flap.

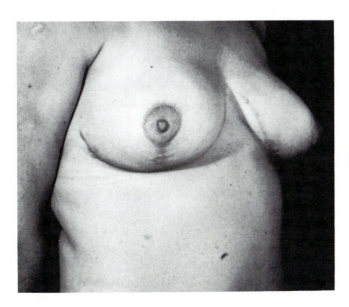

FIGURE 15–27
Displaced inframammary incision.

References

Arié, G.: Una nueva técnica de mastoplastia. Rev. Lat. Am. Cir. Plast. 3:23, 1957.

Biesenberger, H.: Eine neue Methode der Mammaplastik. Zentralbl. Chir. 38:2382, 1928.

Gillies, H., McIndoe, A. H.: The technique of mammaplasty in conditions of hypertrophy of the breast. Surg. Gynecol. Obstet. 68:658, 1939.

McIndoe, A. H., Rees, T. D.: Mammaplasty: Indications, technique and complications. Br. J. Plast. Surg. 10:307, 1958.

Pitanguy, I.: Mamaplastias: Estudio de 245 casos consecutivos e apresentacao da tecnica pessoal. Rev. Bras. Chir. 42:201, 1961.

Pitanguy, I.: Une nouvelle technique de plastie mammaire. Ann. Chir. Plast. 7:199, 1962.

Pitanguy, I.: Surgical treatment of breast hypertrophy. Br. J. Plast. Surg. 20:78, 1967.

Planas, J., Mosely, L. H.: Improving breast shape and symmetry in reduction mammaplasty. Ann. Plast. Surg. 4:297, 1980.

Ribeiro, L., Backer, E.: Mastoplastia con pediculo de seguridad. Rev. Esp. Cir. Plast. 6:223, 1973.

Schwarzmann, E.: Über eine neue Methode der Mammaplastik. Wien Med. Wochenschr. 86:100, 1936.

Skoog, T.: A technique of breast reduction: Transposition of the nipple on a cutaneous vascular pedicle. Acta Chir. Scand. 126:453, 1963.

Skoog, T.: Atlas de Cirugia Plastica Salvat. Barcelona, 1976.

Strömbeck, J. G.: Mammaplasty, report of a new technique based on the two pedicle procedure. Br. J. Plast. Surg. 13:79, 1960.

Strömbeck, J. G.: Reduction mammaplasty. In Grabb, W. C., Smith, J. W. (eds.): *Plastic Surgery.* Boston, Little, Brown, 1968, p. 821.

Thorek, M.: *Plastic Surgery of the Breast and Abdominal Wall.* Springfield, Ill., Charles C Thomas, 1942.

Wise, R. J.: Preliminary report on a method of planning the mammaplasty. Plast. Reconstr. Surg. 17:367, 1956.

Wise, R. J.: Treatment of breast hypertrophy. Clin. Plast. Surg. 3:289, 1976.

16

Ivo Pitanguy

Principles of Reduction Mammaplasty

We live in a constantly changing world that intermixes races, cultural ideals, and concepts of beauty. Affected by the media, fashion, and social norms of the time, women are strongly influenced in their appreciation of body contour. We have seen the full-breasted, voluptuous figures of three decades ago slowly fade away, giving way to the smaller-breasted, slimmer bodies of the health- and exercise-conscious women of today.

These patients have often experienced much physical and psychologic trauma by the time they come to us for a corrective procedure, and so one must not misinterpret this as a form of vanity. Rather, it is an opportunity to relieve their physical discomfort and produce an aesthetically pleasing result that will allow them to readapt to social habits that were forfeited because of embarrassment in revealing their large breasts.

EVOLUTION OF PERSONAL TECHNIQUE

The first description of reduction mammaplasty dates back to the nineteenth century, when Durston (1869) partially amputated a ptotic breast. Since then, several techniques have been developed by Pousson (1897), Guinard (1903), Morestin (1909), Lexer (1912), Kraske (1921), Biesenberger (1931), Gillies (1939), and Dufourmentel (1939).

Procedures in which large portions of the gland were resected medially and superiorly risked interrupting the blood supply and innervation to the nipple-areola complex, as well as leaving large dead spaces that produced hematomas or seromas. Techniques that had set patterns and nipple placement inhibited the surgeon's ability to make alterations during the procedure.

Other techniques required wide skin undermining, which essentially separated the gland from the skin. The skin acts like a pseudosuspensory ligament to the breast; and when the proportional separation of the "contents" from the "container" is too great, the embryologic continuity is disrupted. Consequently, these breasts often flattened superiorly and sagged inferiorly, and the nipple rotated upward instead of outward.

Prudente and Arié (1957), from Sao Paulo, Brazil, developed a technique in which an almond-shaped piece of skin was resected through a subareolar incision. Although the principles were good, the shape was not always consistent. In 1959, the author presented a mod-

ification of this technique at the International Society of Plastic Surgeons Meeting in London. This modification extended the incision above the areola to the place where the new nipple would be naturally located (point A), at the level of the projection of the inframammary sulcus on the midclavicular line. The advantage was that it allowed for resection of tissue from the lower pole while gaining skin from the upper pole. This afforded a nice shape to the breast while minimizing the scarring with one vertical incision. However, second- and third-degree hypertrophies required larger resections; and later that year, the classic Pitanguy reduction mammaplasty was developed.

This procedure evolved from point A of the Arié-Pitanguy technique and worked through a triangle, points A, B, and C, resulting in an inverted-T scar. The resection was located at the breast's lower pole, usually done in a shape similar to a ship's keel, its length being determined according to the deformity and pathologic condition to be corrected. It was performed in a stepladder fashion and preserved two columns of the breast tissue that, when reapproximated, moved the nipple-areola complex upward to its natural position while avoiding any dead space formation. Most importantly, there were no fixed patterns, and the attachment of the skin to the gland was maintained, allowing the breast to support itself in a brassiere-like fashion.

Over the past 28 years, these two techniques have been used for 2822 personally performed operations with excellent long-term outcomes and minimal complications. One of their main advantages is the ease of execution, without previous demarcation of the future site of the nipple-areola complex and without dissection of the gland from its natural envelope. They afford the surgeon the possibility of correction of different types of breast deformities, resulting in harmonious breasts with scars at the natural creases and preservation of physiology, in lactation as well as in sensitivity. Due to their simplicity, these techniques are as easily understood by beginners as by well-trained surgeons.

INDICATIONS FOR SURGERY

Age

The ideal age of the patient is between 16 and 20 years, virginal hypertrophy being the sole indication for

TABLE 16–1
Breast Hypertrophy: 1959 to 1987

AGE GROUP (years)	%
10–19	6.8
20–29	25.1
30–39	32.2
40–49	19.5
50–59	13.6
60 +	2.8

Total: 2822 cases

surgery before the age of 16. There are no upper age limits, provided the potential benefits and medical risks of the surgery are equally considered (Table 16–1).

Main Complaints

More than half of our patients presented with a physical complaint of back pain, anterior thoracic pain, or mastodynia (Table 16–2). The weight of pendulous breasts produces changes in posture that can result in kyphosis with compensating lordosis and osteoarthrosis of the vertebral bodies (Fig. 16–1).

During inspiration the muscles elevate the chest wall, raising the mammary glands by third-degree leverage. The weight of the large ptotic breasts increases the effort of respiration during thoracic expansion. If this condition persists through the years, the patient may develop pulmonary problems that in turn may lead to emphysema and ultimately to cardiovascular problems. Large brassieres, necessary for support, may cut deep permanent grooves into the shoulders. In tropical climates and summer months, the moisture that collects in the submammary sulcus often leads to intertrigo.

Psychologic suffering is perhaps the most insidious problem experienced by patients with hypertrophic breasts. During adolescence style of clothing, social habits, and identity are strongly influenced by the rapid changes in the size and shape of their breasts. This deformity may cause an inferiority complex, preventing the woman from fully developing her personality, because she does not identify with her body image. These psychologic problems should not be regarded as a contraindication for surgery. In the immediate postoperative period a positive behavioral change can be observed. The patient presents a better posture, the style

TABLE 16–2
Breast Hypertrophy: 1959 to 1987

MAIN COMPLAINTS	%
Physical discomfort	45.1
Poor posture	35.2
Premenstrual pain	35.0
Psychologic problems	28.2
Clavicular achromic region deformity	26.8
Backache	26.6

Total: 2822 cases

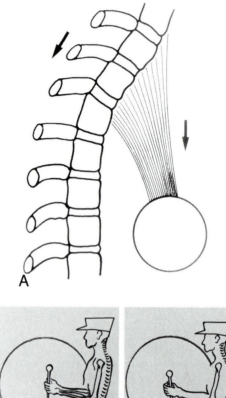

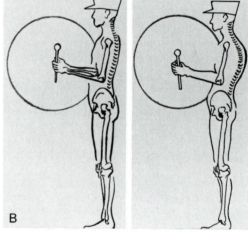

FIGURE 16–1
A and B, The effects of pendulous breasts on the vertebral column are similar to the postural changes experienced by a bass drummer during a long parade.

of clothing changes, and her social lifestyle seems to improve almost immediately.

PREOPERATIVE EVALUATION

All patients should undergo a thorough physical examination and if over 35 years of age, should have a full radiologic workup. Breast disease, if present, must be cared for before any elective surgical procedure is attempted.

Pathologic examinations of 1975 consecutive cases, performed by the same pathologist, revealed 21 incidental malignancies that were found in the specimens after surgery (Table 16–3). Papillary carcinoma was the most common lesion identified. The majority of the malignancies were identified in the upper outer portion of the gland and in the central portion of the specimens. For

TABLE 16–3
Breast Hypertrophy: 1959 to 1987

HISTOPATHOLOGIC FINDINGS	NO. CASES
Benign tumors	
Fibroadiposity	1011
Mammary dysplasia	645
Mammary atrophy	196
Steatonecrosis	6
Siliconosis	5
Total	1863
Malignant tumors	
Papilliferous carcinoma	14
Adenocarcinoma	5
Fibrosarcoma	1
Paget's disease	1
Total	21
Disease-free	91
Total cases	1975

this reason, we always carefully palpate the remaining portion of the reduced breast to identify the presence of any missed disease (Fig. 16–2).

PATIENT SELECTION

Many times the patient's expectations are beyond what the surgery can offer. Therefore, during consultation, the physician should make every effort to explain clearly the real possibilities and limitations of the procedure and discuss the resulting scars.

Patients most suitable for the classic Pitanguy technique are those with second- or third-degree hypertrophy and those with virginal hypertrophy or gigantomastia. Before 1961, 8% of our patients underwent free nipple grafting. Since then, no patients have required this procedure; nevertheless, we do not wish to invali-

date this procedure as a viable alternative when necessary.

The patients most suitable for the Arié-Pitanguy technique are those with mild ptosis and first-degree hypertrophy. Patients with second-degree hypertrophy may also be candidates, provided the shape of the breast is not sacrificed to accommodate the scar. If the incision extends more than 1.5 to 2 cm below the inframammary sulcus, it may need to be converted to a small L- or T-shaped incision (case 1, Fig. 16–3). After rotation of the gland and contraction of the wound, most scars below the sulcus have a tendency to move upward 1.5 to 2 cm within the first few postoperative months (case 2, Fig. 16–4).

SPECIAL CONSIDERATION

One often encounters a patient who may be suitable for both the classic Pitanguy and Arié-Pitanguy techniques. The decision whether to use one or the other can be difficult for the inexperienced surgeon. One must bear in mind two important factors: shape and skin quality.

Those patients with heavy glandular lower poles will often be best suited for the Arié-Pitanguy technique, provided the skin texture is good. One may find it easier to resect a large portion of the gland through one vertical incision, by basing the resection on the middle and centralizing the gland.

However, for those patients with poor elasticity and much skin excess, the classic Pitanguy technique may afford more consistent and better long-term results. One may try to use the Arié-Pitanguy technique with these cases but will often have to convert the vertical scar into an L, which extends beyond the anterior axillary line or into a T having one long arm and one short arm (case 3, Fig. 16–5).

It is important not to have any fixed measures in mind when approaching the problem of asymmetric breasts. Both techniques may be applied, depending on the proportion of one side in relation to the other. It may be better in some patients to reduce only one side and not touch the other (case 4, Fig. 16–6). Other patients may require a classic Pitanguy reduction on both sides to accommodate one very large breast and a smaller contralateral breast (case 5, Fig. 16–7).

The correction of asymmetric breasts with or without a prosthesis can be a difficult problem as well. When one breast is well shaped, the author's philosophy has been to model the poor side to the nicely shaped one, avoiding the use of a prosthesis altogether (case 6, Fig. 16–8). However, in cases of asymmetry where one breast is much smaller, transareolar or submammary inclusion of a prosthesis with reduction of the contralateral breast may offer the best results (case 7, Fig. 16–9).

We have encountered an occasional case in which the nipple-areola complexes were in a good position but the lower pole required reduction. This could be corrected by beginning the incision below the areola and not touching the nipple area at all. Other cases have required exactly the opposite, with movement of the nipple-areola complex and no infra-areolar reduction.

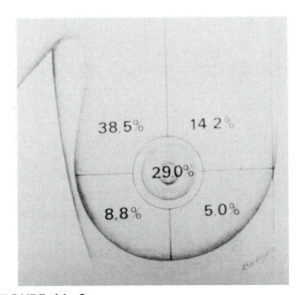

FIGURE 16–2
Locations of occult carcinomas in mammary specimens.

Text continued on page 201

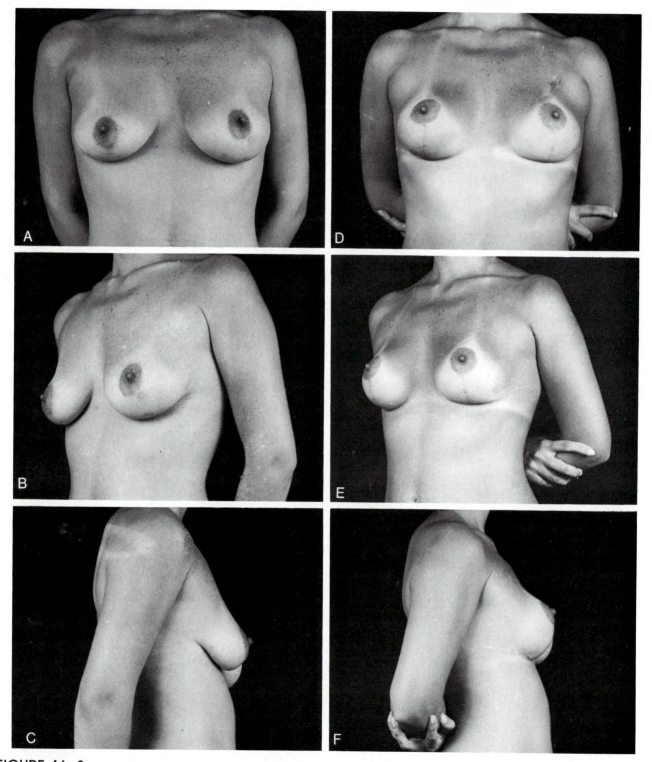

FIGURE 16–3
Case 1. A 34-year-old woman with ptosis, corrected with the Arié-Pitanguy technique, with conversion of the scar to a small L. *A* to *C*, Preoperative appearance. *D* to *F*, Appearance 10 months postoperatively.

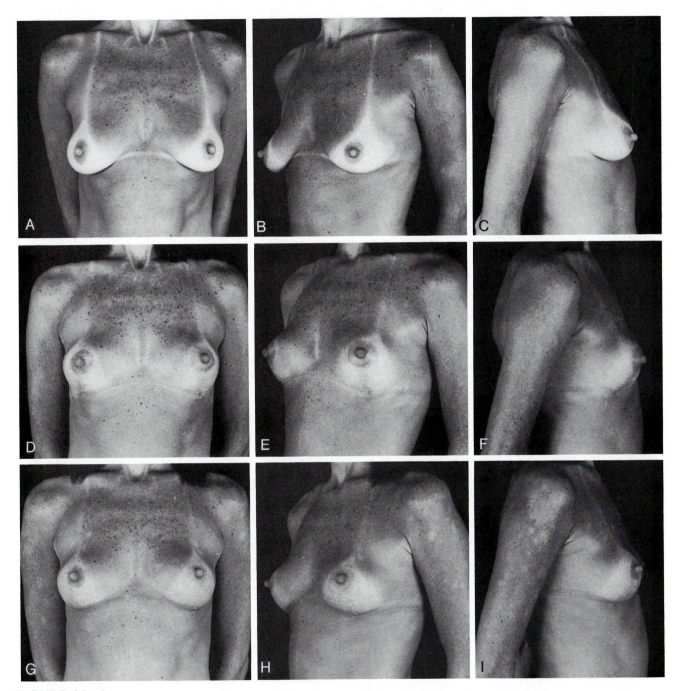

FIGURE 16–4

Case 2. A 31-year-old woman with ptosis, corrected with the Arié-Pitanguy technique. At 5 weeks postoperatively, the scar that had extended below the submammary sulcus was beginning to contract upward with rotation of the gland. By 13 months, the scar ascended and was well concealed in the sulcus. *A* to *C*, Preoperative appearance. *D* to *F*, Appearance 5 weeks postoperatively. *G* to *I*, Appearance 13 months postoperatively.

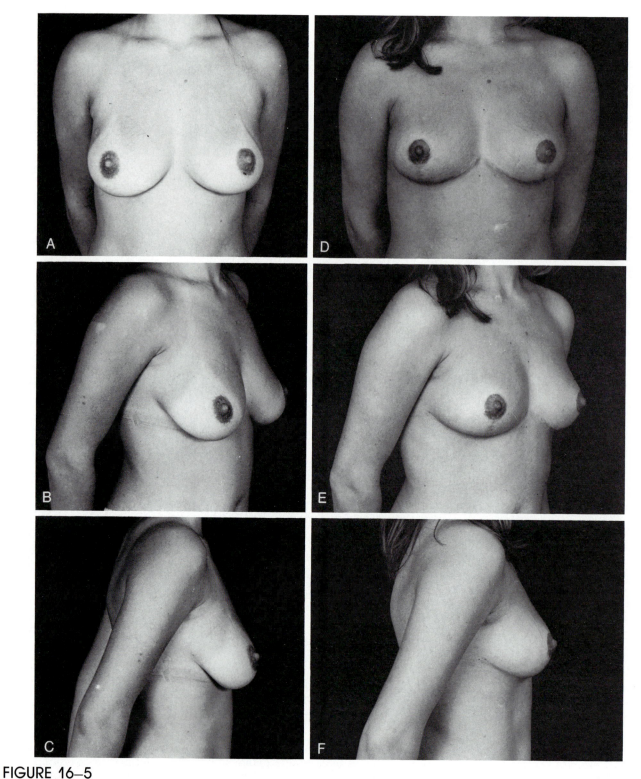

FIGURE 16–5

Case 3. A 29-year-old woman with second-degree hypertrophy and ptosis, corrected with the classic Pitanguy technique. Note that in this case the Arié-Pitanguy technique could have been used; however, because of the excess skin in the lower pole, we thought the result would be better and more consistent with the classic Pitanguy technique. *A to C,* Preoperative appearance. *D to F,* Appearance 12 months postoperatively.

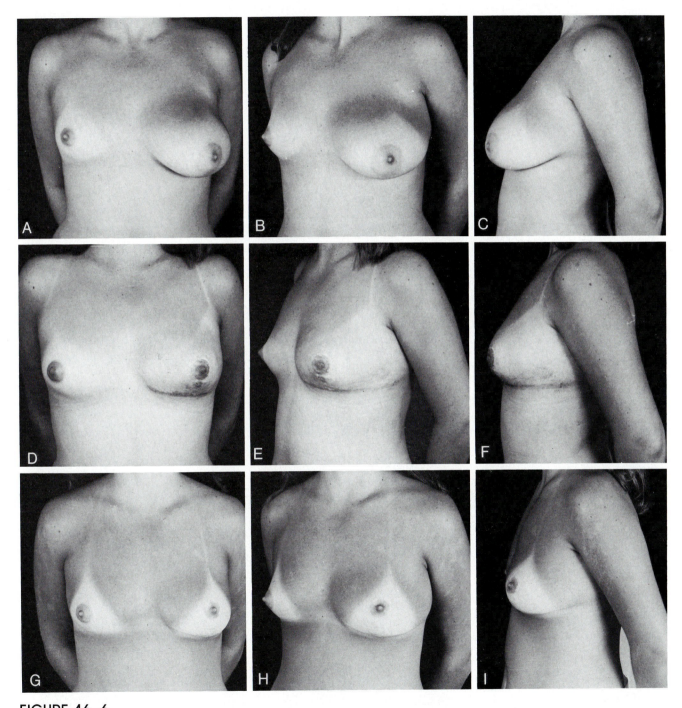

FIGURE 16–6

Case 4. A 17-year-old girl with marked asymmetry and second-degree hypertrophy of the left side, but a small, nicely shaped breast on the right. Only one side required reduction. *A* to *C*, Preoperative appearance. *D* to *F*, Appearance 3 months postoperatively. *G* to *I*, Appearance 2 years postoperatively.

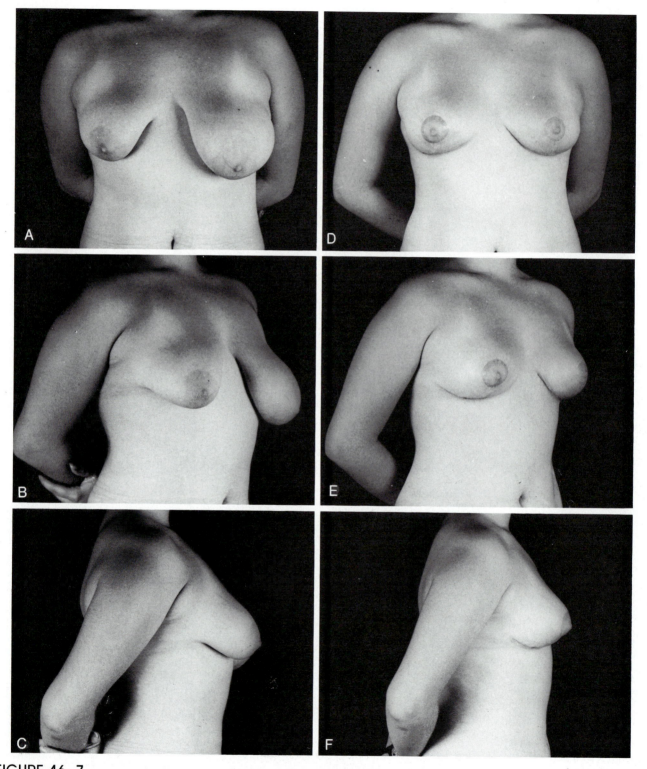

FIGURE 16–7

Case 5. A 28-year-old woman with marked asymmetry and ptosis. Such cases require reduction of both breasts with the classic Pitanguy technique for a good result with symmetric scars. *A* to *C*, Preoperative appearance. *D* to *F*, Appearance 8 months postoperatively.

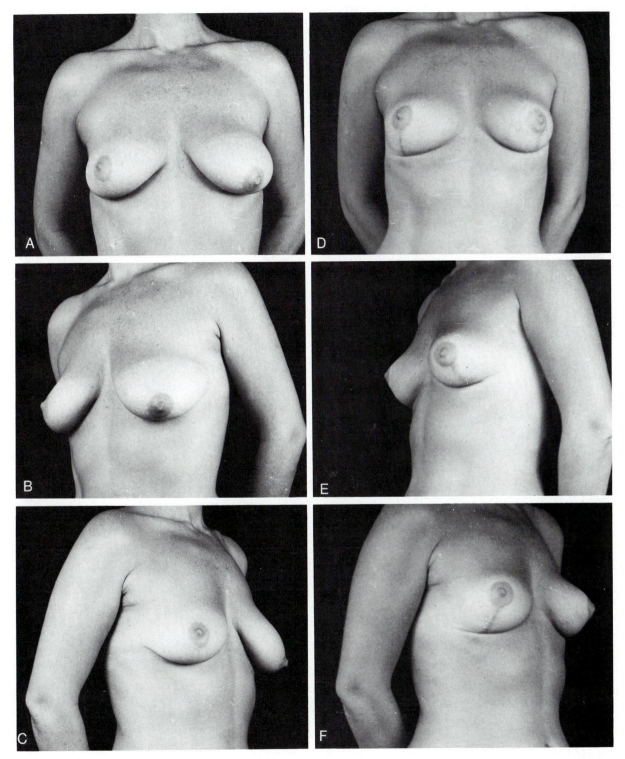

FIGURE 16–8

Case 6. A 21-year-old woman with asymmetric ptosis. The right breast has a good shape, allowing the reduction of the left breast to be adapted to the right with the Arié-Pitanguy technique. *A* to *C*, Preoperative appearance. *D* to *F*, Appearance 8 months postoperatively.

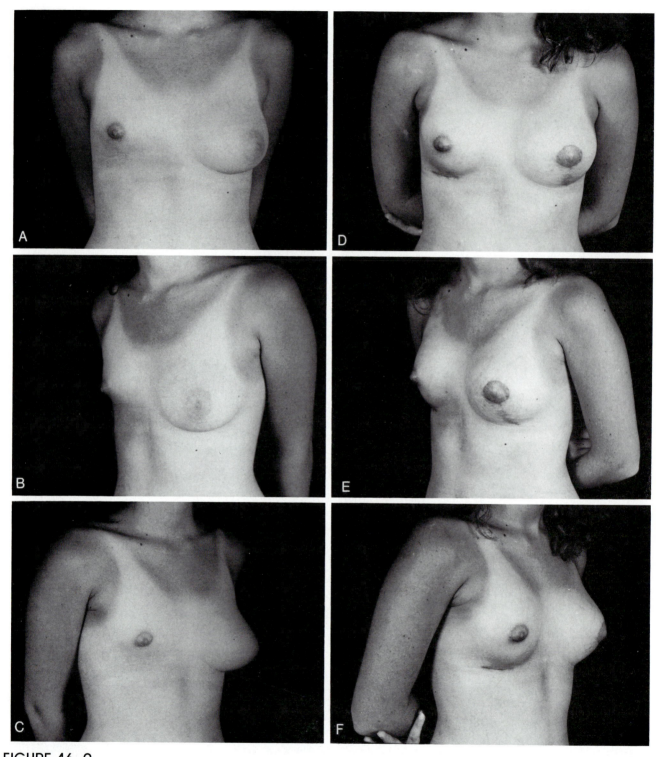

FIGURE 16–9

Case 7. A 16-year-old girl with marked asymmetry and hypoplasia of the right breast. Reduction of the left breast and inclusion of a prosthesis on the right for symmetry were performed with the Arié-Pitanguy technique for minimizing scarring. *A* to *C*, Preoperative appearance. *D* to *F*, Appearance 7 months postoperatively.

SURGICAL TECHNIQUE: CLASSIC PITANGUY REDUCTION MAMMAPLASTY

Step 1: Preparation

The patient is placed on the operating room table with arms extended at 90 degrees to the axilla, shoulders perfectly centered, and head elevated to 15 degrees. The back of the table should be elevated to 45 degrees. Demarcation of the skin is begun. Two sutures are placed for assistance in marking the skin, one at the suprasternal notch and a second in the midxyphoid area.

Step 2: Demarcation

The midclavicular line is used as the first point of reference. With the use of a hemostat, the upper suture is placed in the supraclavicular groove and extended through the nipple to arrive below the submammary sulcus. This line is then marked (Fig. 16–10).

Placing the fingertips of the dominant hand below the submammary sulcus and pressing slightly upward, one can establish the exact point of the sulcus and mark it (point A). Point A is placed along the midclavicular line (Fig. 16–11).

To establish points B and C, one must first look at both breasts to establish whether or not they are symmetric. If one breast is larger, the initial markings should be done on the smaller breast first so that the larger breast can be adapted to the smaller; but if the shape of the smaller breast is not good, it should be adapted to the larger breast.

With the first two fingers of each hand, the surgeon

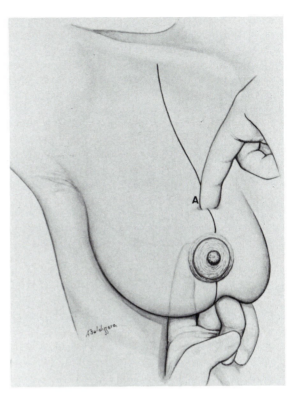

FIGURE 16–11

grasps the breast, below the horizontal line drawn through the nipple, at points where the tissue will be resected. The assistant depresses the midline inferior pole while the surgeon folds the skin in his fingers over the clamp. This will allow one to establish points B and C, as well as determine the amount of potential resection. Points B and C should be equidistant from the nipple on both sides (Fig. 16–12).

Points D and E demarcate the limits of the inframammary sulcus. One places point D medially, being sure not to extend beyond the sulcus, and point E laterally, without extending beyond the anterior axillary line. One should try to keep the two points equidistant from points B and C, while attempting to keep points B and E as short as possible. Points B and E and C and D are connected with a line, which should be contoured to the type of resection necessary. With excess skin, the line should be more concave to the sulcus; with more gland and less skin, it should be more convex.

Points D and E are connected. From this stage on, one should try to limit the amount of manipulation of the gland by using instruments only (Fig. 16–13).

With a compass and marking the suture, the exact measurements are transferred to the opposite side. The nipple and areola are then marked on both sides. If the areola is excessively hypertrophic with small breasts, it will be safer to make the areola marking slightly larger so that the closure can be done without tension (Fig. 16–14).

Step 3: Schwarzmann's Maneuver

With the assistant grasping the breast from the axillary base and the medial base, the skin over the areola will

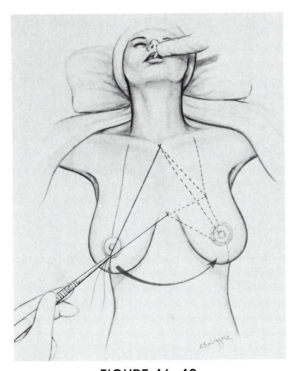

FIGURE 16–10

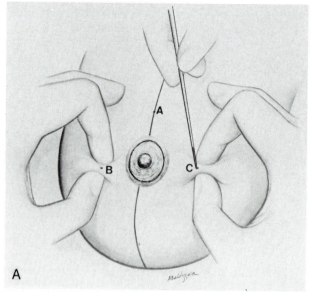

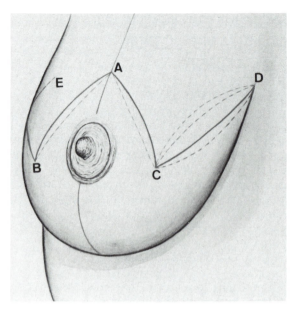

FIGURE 16–13

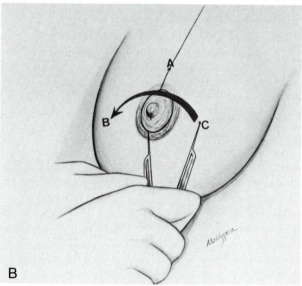

FIGURE 16–12

Using a No. 15 scalpel, a deep incision is made into the gland along the line between C and D. A compress is placed into the wound, and a similar incision is made along the line from B to E. The breast is then elevated, and an incision is made between D and E, at the inframammary sulcus. One must be sure to bevel the incision upward to leave enough tissue to support the inferior border during closure (Fig. 16–17B).

The gland is again elevated at 90 degrees to the chest wall, and resection is commenced, according to the form of the deformity, commonly in a keel-like fashion (which is more like the inner nave of a church) or in straight amputation fashion. If a keel is desired, the resection is begun from the level of the areola, making incisions first medially, then laterally, and then medially and again laterally, to create a stepladder type of resection that

become taut and expedite Schwarzmann's maneuver. This is done within the confines of the triangle ABC, extending 1 to 2 cm below the areola. Once the proper plane is established here, the dissection will proceed smoothly without injury to the dermis (Fig. 16–15).

The skin is then incised from point A to the areola, and two flaps of tissue are created to aid in retraction, once the incisions are extended to points B and C (Fig. 16–16).

Step 4: Resection of Gland

A Kocher clamp is placed on the skin at point A, and the first assistant elevates the breast, perpendicular to the chest wall. The second assistant prepares the cautery to control any major bleeding vessels. This may prevent any break in the surgeon's concentration or avoid disruption of the flow of resection (Fig. 16–17A).

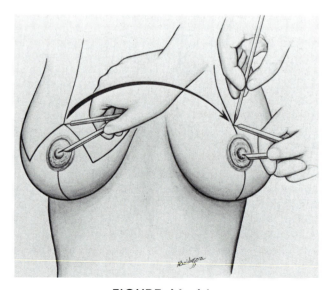

FIGURE 16–14

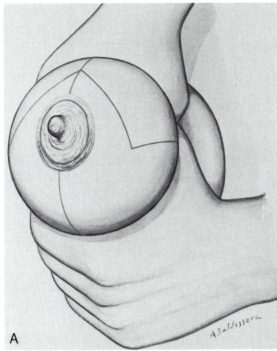

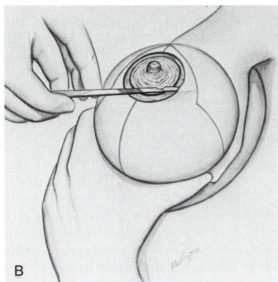

FIGURE 16–15

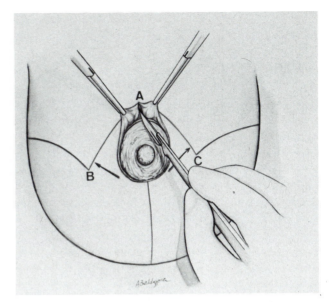

FIGURE 16–16

surgeon is satisfied with the outcome, the breasts are closed in three layers. The dermis is approximated carefully; 4-0 absorbable sutures are used for both the horizontal and vertical incisions, in an inverted fashion. One should always suture toward the T, from the medial and lateral edges of the wound. This will help to relieve much of the tension that often develops in this area. The skin is then reapproximated in a running subcuticular fashion with 3-0 monofilament.

Step 6: Nipple-Areola Placement

One should not suture the skin over the potential nipple-areola site before marking, because when the skin is removed, the areola tends to open, and there may be too much tension when closing it. Using the same marker, the surgeon determines the new location of the areola, which should be placed slightly below the optimal site. In almost all cases, there is some degree of rotation upward, with the nipple moving into its proper location within the first 4 to 6 months.

After marking the first side, the surgeon transfers the exact location to the opposite side using the marking suture. The areola is sutured in a Gillies fashion, starting at the four quadrants and then circumferentially (Fig. 16–19).

Step 7: Dressing

Micropore is placed on the skin in a triangular fashion around the areola, perpendicularly over the vertical incision, and obliquely directed toward the T over the horizontal incision, to relieve as much tension as possible. A fluff dressing and plaster cast are applied with a wraparound, stretchable cling.

will reapproximate easily and project the nipple upward. The gland is then amputated, weighed, and sent for pathologic sectioning (Fig. 16–17C to G).

One should not attempt to close the breast before going to the opposite side first. When the incisions and Schwartzmann's maneuver are completed on the other side, the second assistant will raise the first breast for the surgeon to view the necessary amount of tissue to be resected for symmetry.

Step 5: Closure

The breasts are temporarily closed with a few sutures and compared for size and shape (Fig. 16–18). Once the

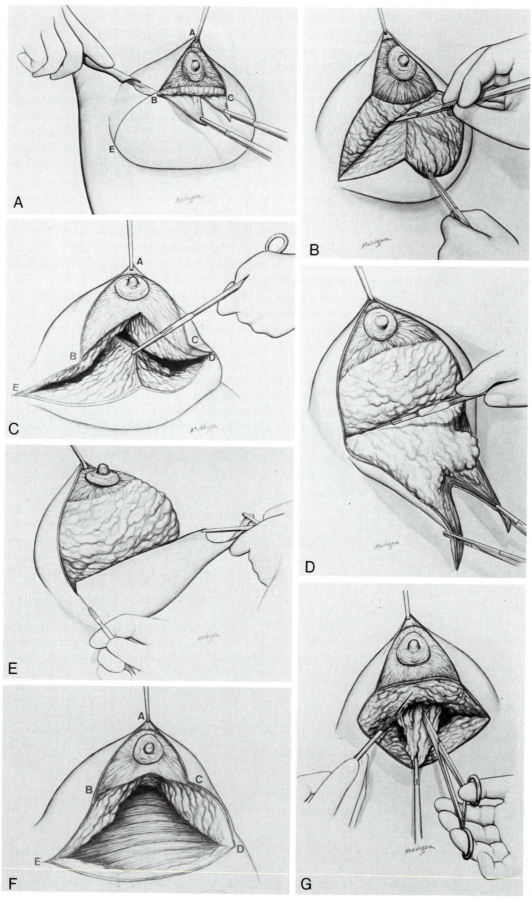

FIGURE 16–17

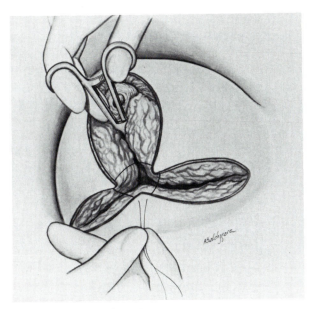

FIGURE 16–18

ARIÉ-PITANGUY TECHNIQUE

Step 1: Preparation

The preparation of the patient is similar to that described earlier.

Step 2: Demarcation

Two marking sutures are placed at the suprasternal notch and midsubxyphoid area. A similar midclavicular line is drawn, as in the classic Pitanguy technique.

Point A is established in a similar way, as in the classic Pitanguy technique, and marked. Point D is placed at the submammary sulcus at or just lateral to the midclavicular line.

Points B and C are placed at opposite sides of the areola. The lines are connected to form a losangular or rhomboid incision (Figs. 16–20 and 16–21).

The nipple-areola complexes are marked in a fashion similar to that in step 2 of the classic Pitanguy technique. If the breasts are quite small and the areola is hypertrophic, it may be safer to choose a larger template, because there may not be enough skin to close the breast without tension.

One may start with the intention of performing the Arié-Pitanguy technique through a losangular incision but find that this extends below the inframammary sulcus more than 2 cm and will require conversion to a small L- or T-shaped incision. In other cases, an adequate resection may not be possible with a central wedge of tissue, and one then has the option of converting to the classic Pitanguy technique by creating points D and E. Therefore, it is best to mark the submammary sulcus

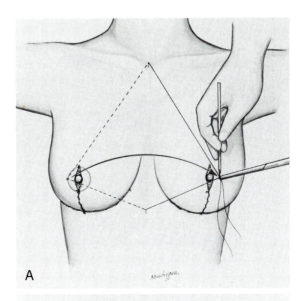

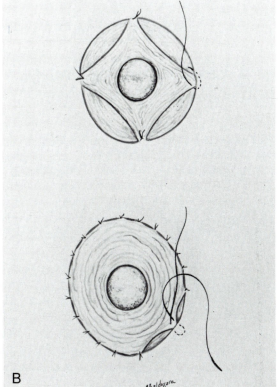

FIGURE 16–19

before beginning if there is any uncertainty as to the final creation of the inframammary sulcus.

Step 3: Schwarzmann's Maneuver

The skin is de-epithelialized within the confines of points A, B, C, and D.

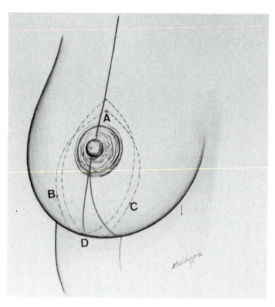

FIGURE 16–20

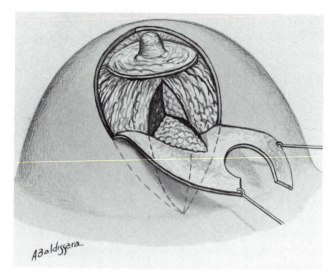

FIGURE 16–22

Step 4: Resection of Skin and Gland

Depending on the case, an appropriate wedge of gland may be resected from the central portion of gland. Unlike the "keel-like" resection, the excision does not reach the lateral edges of the incision (Fig. 16–22).

If only skin resection is sufficient (Fig. 16–23), the inferior pole of the gland may be mobilized off the pectoralis fascia by a slight undermining to allow the gland to ride upward, freely.

Step 5: Closure

After glandular resection, the two columns of tissue are reapproximated with several 3-0 long-acting, absorbable sutures. In some cases, the inferior pole will require more bulk. By mobilizing the axillary tail and fixing it to the inferomedial portion of the gland, one can fill this area nicely (Fig. 16–24).

When the skin is excessively flaccid, it is often necessary to perform an additional resection of the skin to tighten the skin envelope over the gland. One can

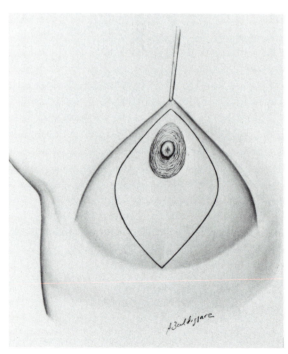

FIGURE 16–21

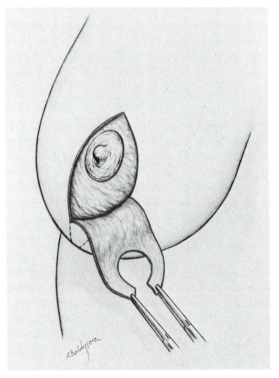

FIGURE 16–23

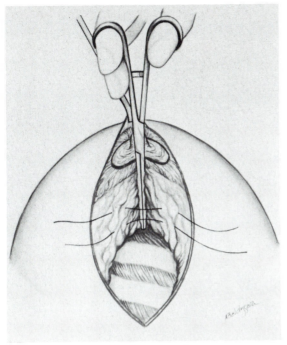

FIGURE 16–24

undermine and resect the excess skin, taking care not to extend beyond the margins of the resection and avoid the formation of any dead space (Fig. 16–25).

At this point, the incision may extend below the sulcus. If *greater* than 1.5 to 2 cm, it should be converted to a small L or T. If *less than* 1.5 to 2 cm, the incisions have a tendency to move upward and give shape to the lower pole through the rotation of the gland in the first 3 to 4 months (Fig. 16–26).

Step 6: Nipple-Areola Placement

The nipple is placed in a fashion similar to that in step 6 of the classic Pitanguy technique. When the areola is excessively hypertrophic and the breasts are small, choosing a larger areola template is safer and will provide better long-term results. For, in attempting to make the areola too small, one may not have enough skin to close without tension on the periareolar area.

Step 7: Dressing

A similar dressing is applied as previously described.

POSTOPERATIVE CARE

Antibiotics are routinely given for 5 to 7 days with parenteral or oral analgesia when necessary. Significant

pain in the first 24 hours may be an indication of hematoma formation and warrants removal of the dressing for checking the wound. Otherwise, dressings are changed on the first postoperative day and replaced with a soft, elastic, well-fitted brassiere. The following day, the patient is discharged with strict instructions to limit all activity during the first week.

Alternate sutures are removed on the seventh postoperative day and the remainder on the tenth day. The running subcuticular sutures are removed in 14 days with replacement of the micropore dressing. New Micropore dressing is used for 7 to 10 more days.

During the first 2 months, the patient is advised to limit all heavy activity and continue the compressive brassiere for 6 months. Follow-up checks are done at 3 months and 6 months when possible. Sunlight to the scar is avoided for 3 to 6 months, depending on the case. Breast-feeding has been commenced as early as 12 to 14 months after surgery.

COMPLICATIONS

There are no specific complications referable to these two techniques. A comparison of the results achieved using several different procedures *before 1961* with those using the described techniques *after 1961* reveals an overall lower rate of complications (Table 16–4).

TABLE 16–4
Breast Hypertrophy

COMPLICATIONS	PERCENT 1955 to 1961	PERCENT 1962 to 1987
Cutaneous problems	3.6	3.8
Areolar problems	1.2	0.9
Hematoma	1.2	0.4
Hypertrophic scar	10.3	1.4
Total	16.3	6.5

Hypertrophic scarring has occasionally been a problem, especially with the horizontal incision; but it may be minimized by handling the tissues with care, especially in the region of the T, which is particularly susceptible to ischemia.

The areola is another area that requires special concern. It has a tendency to widen if closed under tension and may be extremely difficult to correct. For this reason, when treating patients with small ptotic breasts and hypertrophic areolae, one will have better results using a larger areola template, because there may not be enough skin to close the breast without tension.

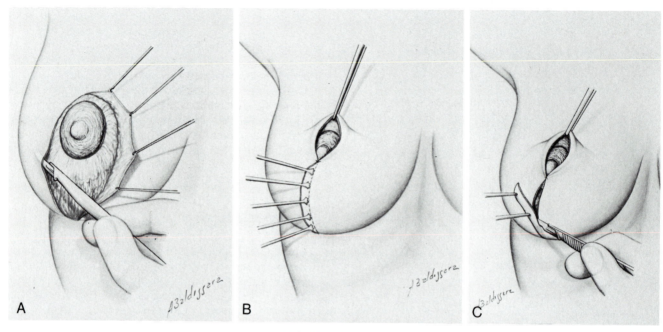

FIGURE 16–25

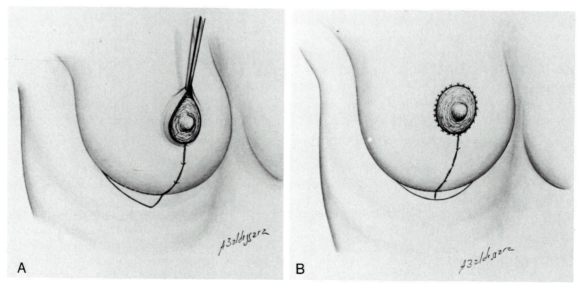

FIGURE 16–26

CONCLUSION

These two techniques have enabled us to treat various types of breast morphology with ease and without separating the gland from its natural skin envelope. This allows the breast to maintain its own support, with scars that lie in the natural submammary crease. Preservation of function and sensitivity are maintained, and the complications are very few.

Analyzing our personal results with these techniques and those obtained by the several young surgeons at our university plastic surgery service during the last 27 years, we have found a homogeneity regarding the parameters we studied, even in relation to complications, which confirmed their applicability, versatility, and social importance (cases 8 to 13, Figs. 16–27 to 16–32).

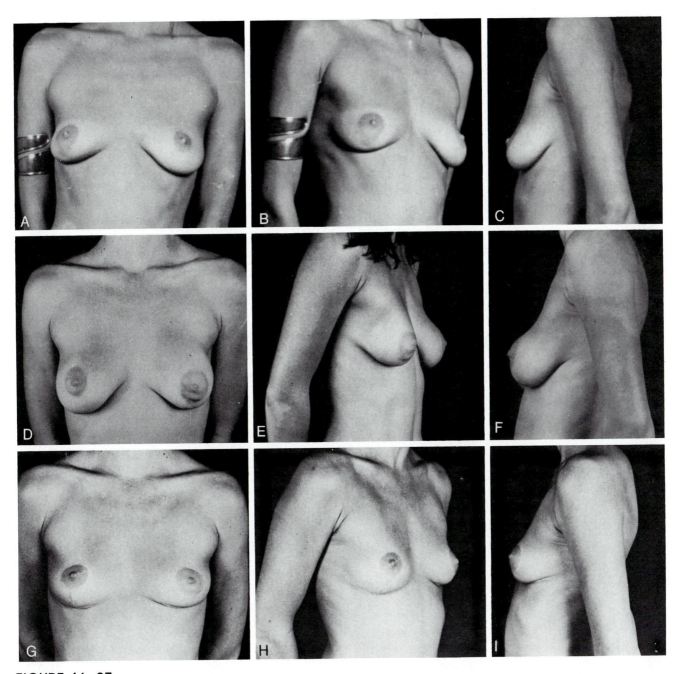

FIGURE 16–27

Case 8. A 42-year-old woman with small asymmetric ptosis who had inclusion of a prosthesis that subsequently ptosed further. Removal of the prosthesis and reduction with the Arié-Pitanguy technique were performed without use of any prosthesis. *A* to *C*, Preoperative appearance. *D* to *F*, Appearance 3 months postoperatively. *G* to *I*, Appearance 15 months postoperatively.

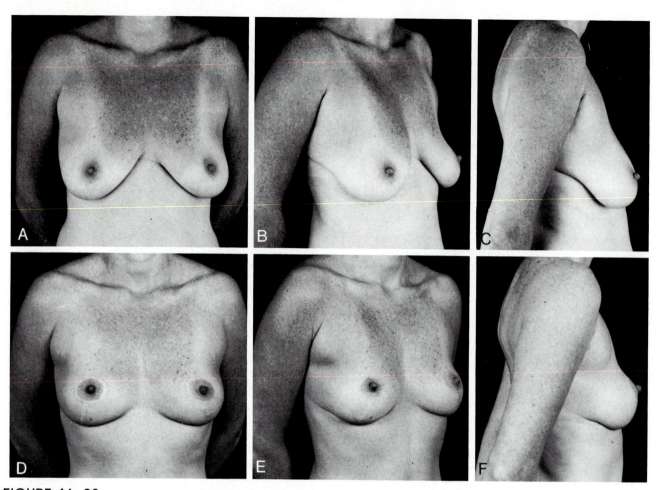

FIGURE 16–28

Case 9. A 37-year-old woman with ptosis and lipodystrophy, corrected with the Arié-Pitanguy technique and liposuction of the abdominal lipodystrophy. *A* to *C*, Preoperative appearance. *D* to *F*, Appearance 14 months postoperatively.

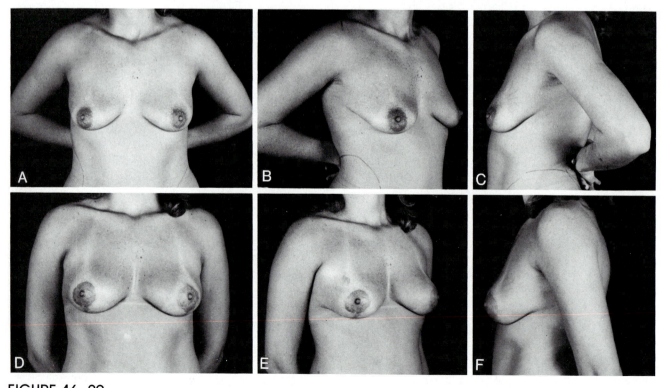

FIGURE 16–29

Case 10. A 37-year-old woman with ptosis and lipodystrophy, corrected with the Arié-Pitanguy technique and liposuction. *A* to *C*, Preoperative appearance. *D* to *F*, Appearance 12 months postoperatively.

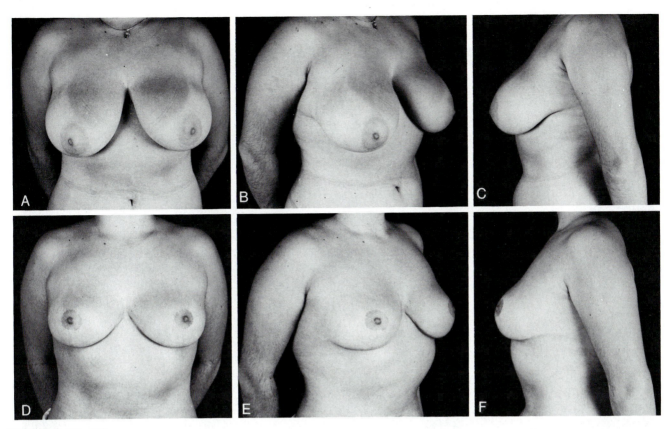

FIGURE 16–30
Case 11. A 21-year-old woman with third-degree hypertrophy, reduced with the classic Pitanguy technique. *A* to *C*, Preoperative appearance. *D* to *F*, Appearance 6 months postoperatively.

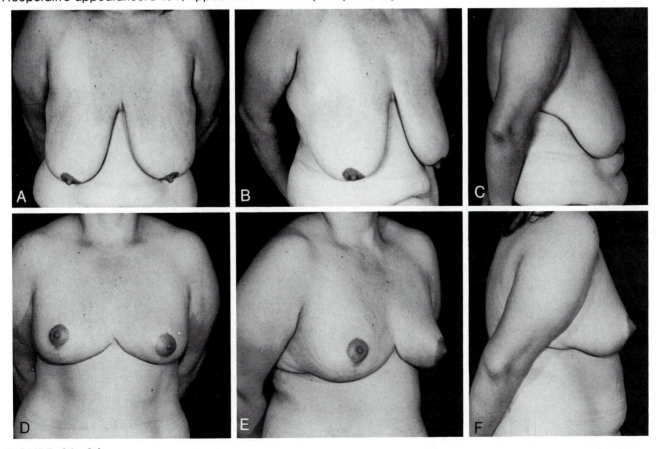

FIGURE 16–31
Case 12. A 52-year-old female with extreme ptosis and excess skin of the lower pole, which required reduction by means of classic Pitanguy reduction mammaplasty. *A* to *C*, Preoperative appearance. *D* to *F*, Appearance 6 months postoperatively.

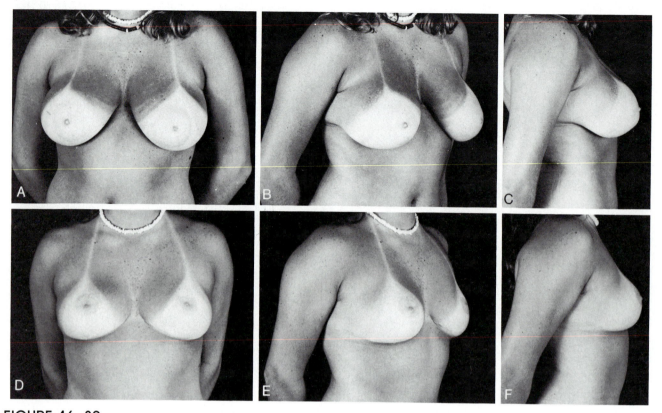

FIGURE 16–32
Case 13. A 17-year-old woman with third-degree hypertrophy, corrected with the classic Pitanguy technique. Note the postoperative change in posture. *A* to *C,* Preoperative appearance. *D* to *F,* Appearance 14 months postoperatively.

References

Ashley, F. L., Braley, S., Rees, T. D., Braley, S. Goulian, O., Ballantyne, D. L., Jr.: The present status of silicone fluid in soft tissue augmentation. Plast. Reconstr. Surg. 39:411, 1967.

Arié, G.: Una nueva técnica de mastoplastia. Rev. Latinoam. Cir. Plast. 3:23, 1957.

Biesenberger, H.: *Deformitäten und kosmetische Operationen der weiblichen Brust.* Vienna, Maudrich, 1931.

Converse, J. M.: *Reconstructive Plastic Surgery.* Philadelphia, W.B. Saunders, 1964.

Conway, H.: Weight of the breasts as a handicap to respiration. Am. J. Surg. 103:674, 1962.

Crikelair, G. F., Malton, S. D.: Mammaplasty and occult breast malignancy: Case report. Plast. Reconstr. Surg. 23:601, 1959.

Dartigues, L.: Les anomalies du sein en dehors des hypertrophies et du prolapsus. Bull. Mem. Soc. Med. Paris 139:569, 1935.

Dufourmentel, C.: *Chirurgie Reparatrice et Correctrice des Formes.* Paris, Masson, 1939.

Durston, W.: Sudden and excessive swelling of a woman's breast. Phil. Trans. Roy. Soc. 4th ed. London, 1869.

Gillies, H., McIndoe, A. H.: The technique of mammaplasty in conditions of hypertrophy of the breast. Surg. Gynecol. Obstet. 68:658, 1939.

Goldwyn, R. M.: Pulmonary function and bilateral reduction mammaplasty. Plast. Recontr. Surg. 53:84, 1974.

Goldwyn, R. M.: *Plastic and Reconstructive Surgery of the Breast.* Boston, Little, Brown, 1976.

Guinard, M.: Comment on: Rapport de l'ablation esthetique des tumeurs du sein par M. H. Morestin. Bull. Mem. Soc. Chir. Paris 29:568, 1903.

Kraske, M.: Die Operation der atrophischen und hypertrophischen Hängebrust. Münch. Med. Wochenschr. 70:672, 1923.

Lexer, E.: Hypertrophie bei der Mammae. Münch. Med. Wochenschr. 59:2702, 1912.

Morestin, H.: Hypertrophie mammaire traitée par la resection discoide. Bull. Mem. Soc. Chir. Paris 33:649, 1907.

Penn, J.: Breast reduction. II. In: Wallace, A. B. (ed.): *Transactions of the International Society of Plastic Surgeons, Second Congress,* Edinburgh, E. & S. Livingstone, 1960, p. 502.

Pitanguy, I.: Breast hypertrophy. In: Wallace, A. B. (ed.): *Transactions of the International Society of Plastic Surgeons, Second Congress,* Edinburgh, E. & S. Livingstone, 1960, p. 509.

Pitanguy, I.: Aproximação eclética ao problema das mamaplastias. Rev. Bras. Cir. 41:179, 1961.

Pitanguy, I.: Mamaplastias. Estudo de 245 Casos Consecutivos e Apresentação de Técnica Pessoal. Rev. Bras. Cir. 42:201, 1961.

Pitanguy, I.: Beitrag zur Technik der Hautüberpflanzung zwecks Verbesserung der Hypertrophie der Brüste. Aesthet. Med. 11:65, 1962.

Pitanguy, I.: Une nouvelle technique de plastie mammaire: Étude de 245 cas consécutifs et présentation d'une technique personelle. Ann. Chir. Plast. 7:199, 1962.

Pitanguy, I., Torres, E.: Estudo histopatoológico de tecido mamário retirado para fins de plástica. Rev. Bras. Cir. 43:162, 1962.

Pitanguy, I. Contribuição à Técnica de Enxerto Livre para a Correção das Grandes Hipertrofias Mamárias. Rev. Latinoam. Cir. Plast. 7:75, 1963.

Pitanguy, I.: Hipertrofias mamárias. Trib. Med. 6:3, 1964.

Pitanguy, I.: Transareolar incision for gynecomastia. Plast. Reconstr. Surg. 38:414, 1966.

Pitanguy, I.: Surgical treatment of breast hypertrophy. Br. J. Plast. Surg. 20:78, 1967.

Pitanguy, I.: Hipertrofias mamárias. Cuad. Hosp. Clin. Bolivia, 1969, p. 14.

Pitanguy, I.: Mamaplastias: Estudo comparativo de evolução técnica em torno de 1196 casos pessoais. Rev. Bras. Cir. 61:227, 1971.

Pitanguy, I.: Personal preferences for reduction mammaplasty. In: Goldwyn, R. M. (ed.): *Plastic and Reconstructive Surgery of the Breast.* Boston, Little, Brown, 1976, p. 167.

Pitanguy, I.: *Aesthetic Plastic Surgery of Head and Body.* Berlin, Springer-Verlag, 1981.

Pousson, M.: De la mastopexie. Bull. Mem. Soc. Chir. Paris 23:507, 1897.

Schwarzmann, E.: Über eine neue Methode der Mammaplastik. Wien Med. Wochenschr. 86:100, 1936.

Skoog, T.: A technique of breast reduction transposition of the nipple on a cutaneous vascular pedicle. Acta Chir. Scand. 126:453, 1963.

Snyderman, R. K., Lizardo, J. G.: Statistical study of malignancies found before, during, or after routine breast plasty operations. Plast. Reconstr. Surg. 25:253, 1960.

Strömbeck, J. O.: Mammaplasty: Report of a new technique based on the two pedicle procedure. Br. J. Plast. Surg. 13:79, 1960.

Thorek, M.: *Plastic Surgery of the Breast and Abdominal Wall.* Springfield, Ill., Charles C Thomas, 1942.

Some Methods for Improving the Results of Reduction Mammaplasty and Mastopexy: The Lateral Pedicle Technique

Surgical correction of excessively large or pendulous breasts is now an operation that is performed with increasing frequency, in a population in which a youthful and athletic figure is universally desired. This surgery originated mainly for the reduction of large, heavy, and painful breasts; and surgical success was measured in terms of symptomatic relief and primary healing. Changing fashions in women's clothes now emphasize a slender, firm figure with minimal foundation garments. This has led to a considerable increase in demand for mastopexy and minor breast reduction. Previously acceptable standards of the end result for gross breast reduction are no longer sufficient. We now have a new generation of patients who seek restoration of a firm, youthful breast contour but also expect from the plastic surgeon a cosmetic result where scars are sufficiently fine and well concealed that they can confidently sunbathe "topless" on the beach.

Most current techniques for such breast surgery are based on variations of the Strömbeck (1961) dermal breast pedicle and Wise (1956) skin pattern. Such methods give reliable primary healing and few complications such as hematoma, which previously were relatively common. Modifications such as McKissock's (1972) and Skoog's (1974) have improved the breast shape, giving a rounder contour and better nipple projection, but produce a higher incidence of diminished nipple sensitivity.

The author's technique is based on a laterally based dermal breast pedicle that is designed to concentrate also on preservation of nipple sensation, good long-term maintenance of breast shape with greater projection, and improved quality of the scars.

It would be unrealistic to suppose that all results could be consistently of an equally high standard. Adverse factors such as a flat nipple, a broad breast with large axillary tail, marked skin striae, frequent fluctuation in body weight, and an unathletic physique will all tend to contribute to a less favorable final result. Variation in the dominant sensory nerve supply to the nipple from the fourth intercostal lateral cutaneous branch can oc- casionally affect the normally expected result, and patients should be advised of this risk.

TECHNIQUE: GENERAL PRINCIPLES

The technique to be described is applicable to all degrees of breast reduction and mastopexy with or without augmentation but will be described separately for the two conditions so that important details might be stressed. However, for both conditions the technique has the same three principles.

First, a laterally based dermal breast-nipple-areola pedicle containing the full thickness of breast tissue is used, in contrast to the Skoog technique, in which much of the breast thickness is trimmed away, inevitably including some sensory nerve branches and blood supply.

Second, a widely overlapping or "wraparound" closure of soft tissues inferior to the nipple-areola is used, in contrast to the Strömbeck or Pitanguy (1967) method of inverting the breast from below, after which the tissues may later tend to unfold as the scar softens.

Third, the skin is closed obliquely below the nipple, a method that creates a better quality scar and a more rounded form to the breast than the more widely practiced vertical skin closure, which may give a somewhat square or inverted contour to the lower breast outline.

The breasts are marked preoperatively with the patient standing. The meridian line is normally drawn from the suprasternal notch, so that the horizontal distance between the elevated nipples is also proportionately reduced. This meridian line may, however, be varied, depending on whether the nipples are judged to be more medially located or excessively divergent.

A modified Strömbeck-Wise pattern creates instead an oblique radial skin closure (Fig. 17–1), with average length of 5.5 cm. This again must be adjusted to suit the patient's size and should also be kept somewhat shorter when the breasts are noted to be too broad or disproportionately wide in their lateral quadrants. The

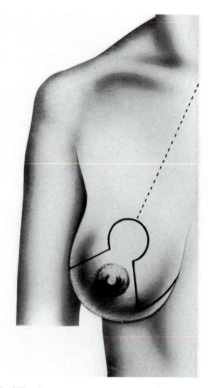

FIGURE 17–1
A modified Strömbeck-Wise pattern gives the desired obliquity of skin closure.

inframammary skin marking is placed 2 cm above the existing inframammary crease.

The areola is marked separately with a stencil and averages 4.5 cm in diameter. Hypotensive anesthesia is routinely employed, so that blood loss is minimal and the duration of surgery shortened.

The upper skin areas within the pattern are de-epithelialized at the deep dermal level, and the redundant transverse ellipse of breast and skin tissue is excised (Figs. 17–2 and 17–3).

A crescent-shaped strip of full thickness breast tissue is then excised medial and superior to the nipple, and the remaining breast tissue is partly mobilized off the pectoral muscle (Fig. 17–4). A laterally based breast pedicle is thereby formed that is freely mobile, as is also the remaining breast tissue superiorly and medially. Much of this undermining can be done by blunt dissection, without needing to divide those vessels or nerves entering the deep surface of the breast lateral to the nipple meridian. The medial breast skin, together with the subcutaneous tissue, is undermined for approximately 3 cm to allow the breast tissue to migrate upward and medially when the skin flaps are approximated. A superficial relaxing incision is then made through the dermis at the lateral edge of the nipple pedicle, thus allowing the nipple to rotate upward and medially. Hemostasis is obtained with the use of electrocautery.

The skin is now closed below the nipple with interrupted subcuticular 4-0 PDS sutures at approximately 2-cm intervals, and the nipple pedicle then rotates upward into its new location (Fig. 17–5).

The remaining de-epithelialized breast tissue at the apex of the keyhole pattern is retained in order to add to the breast volume behind the newly located nipple (Fig. 17–6). This tissue is incised at its margin through the dermis and subcutaneous fat and is then lightly sutured at its inferior margin to the underlying pectoral muscle. This gives added forward thrust to the nipple-areolar complex when it is rotated upward and superficial to it.

When required, the excess breast tissue in the lateral quadrant or axillary tail is trimmed away superficially but without extending the skin incision (Fig. 17–7). The lateral quadrant usually needs to be positioned more medially to give the breast a more youthful and graceful form. Usually three PDS sutures (2-0) are placed between the lateral quadrant and the border of the pectoralis major muscle. These must be tied lightly for avoidance of strangulation of the tissues.

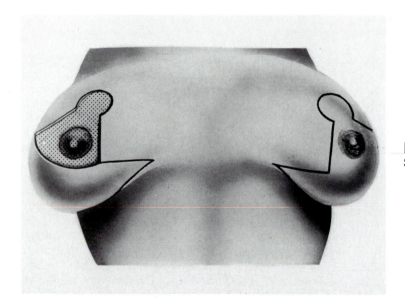

FIGURE 17–2
Skin areas are de-epithelialized.

2

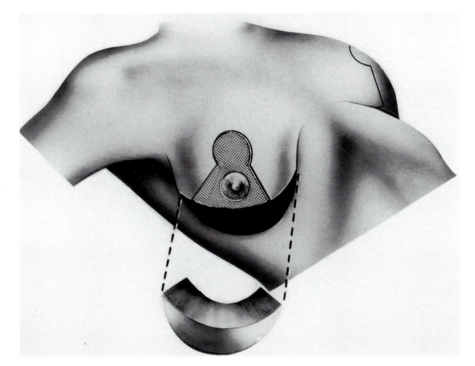

FIGURE 17–3
Area of de-epithelialization and medial area of breast excised.

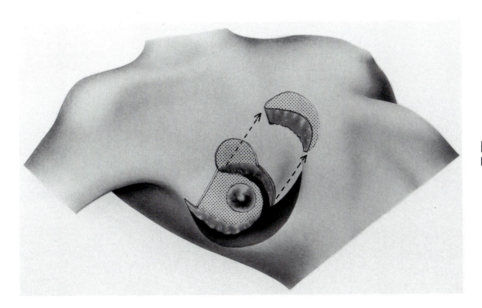

FIGURE 17–4
Excised crescent of breast.

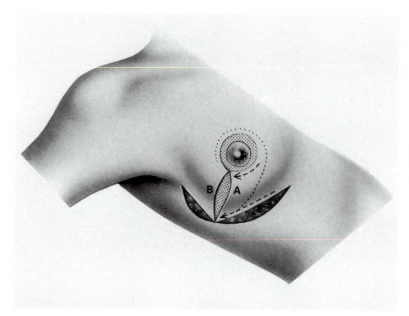

FIGURE 17–5
Closure of skin below the nipple-areola complex with subcuticular, interrupted sutures.

FIGURE 17–6
Remaining portion of de-epithelialized breast tissue shown at the apex of the keyhole pattern for increased breast volume behind nipple.

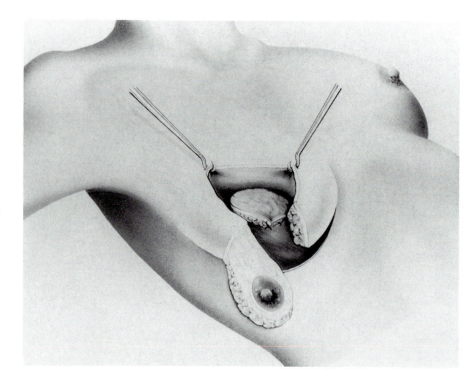

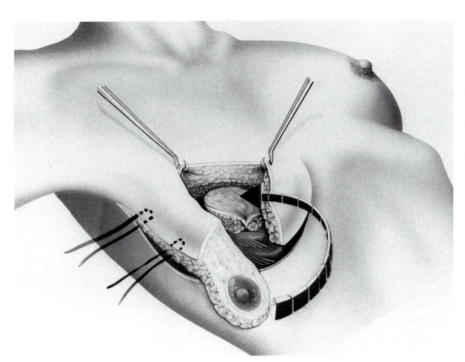

FIGURE 17–7
Excess tissue in lateral and axillary tail is excised as needed.

All skin closure is now completed with running 5-0 PDS sutures, inserted in a spiral fashion so as to produce good skin eversion and tension on the skin 3 to 4 mm away from the skin margins (Figs. 17–8 to 17–10). The technique (Straith, 1961), avoids the problem of sutures discharging through the wound, which may be encountered when the suture is placed more superficially at the dermal-epidermal junction.

Jackson-Pratt suction drains are inserted in each breast and 1-inch Steri-Strips splint the suture lines. Postoperatively the drains are removed after 48 hours, and the Elastoplast dressing after 7 to 9 days. The patient then wears a soft brassiere for daytime support and continues to change the 1-inch Micropore dressing every 4 to 6 days during the subsequent 6 weeks. Excessive stress on all scars is avoided for the initial 6 weeks, after which full activity is progressively resumed.

In the long term, breast scars tend to become paler than the adjacent skin. After 6 weeks patients can safely tan the breast skin, promoting some migration of melanin pigment into the scar, which is retained, giving the scar a much more natural skin color. Contrary to popular belief, this has not resulted in hyperpigmentation, but patients are cautioned and advised to apply protective cream or lotion initially until a tan has developed.

OPERATIVE TECHNIQUE FOR MASTOPEXY

Skin markings are the same as for a reduction mammaplasty, and the entire enclosed area is de-epithelialized around the areola (Fig. 17–11). In cases of severe or moderately severe ptosis, the medial skin and sub-

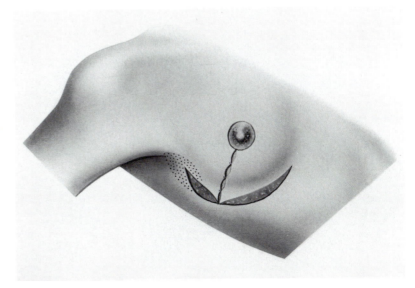

FIGURE 17–8
Skin closure with running spiral sutures.

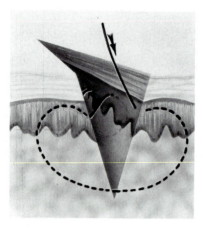
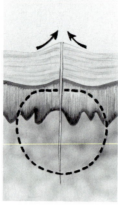

FIGURE 17-9
Running subcuticular suture on cross section, emphasizing good skin eversion.

cutaneous tissue are dissected off the whole of the medial breast tissue and for approximately 3 cm superiorly (Fig. 17–12). The medial skin flap is progressively thicker toward its base, where it contains only subcutaneous fat and no breast tissue, and is also well supplied by the internal mammary vessels. With mainly blunt dissection, the breast is freed from the pectoral muscle, so that the entire breast now becomes a laterally based pedicle containing the nipple and dermis superficially.

Skin closure is performed as for reduction mammaplasty, which shifts the breast tissue in an upward and medial direction and at the same time achieves wide overlapping of the medial and lateral pedicles. Aftercare is as has already been described for breast reduction.

In mild cases of ptosis where nipple elevation of approximately 4 cm or less is required, a less radical mobilization of the breast pedicle is often sufficient.

RESULTS

The technique described evolved gradually in what appeared to be a logical modification of Strömbeck's original method, and I have now practiced the currently described method during the past 15 years and in a very

large number of cases. Early complications of hematoma, delayed healing, and fat necrosis have been minimal.

For breast reduction (Figs. 17–13 to 17–16), preservation of the full thickness of the breast tissue beneath the areola ensures a good forward projection of the nipple, and this effect can also be augmented by retaining the desired amount of breast tissue in the de-epithelialized area at the apex of the key pattern. This technique should be distinguished from that described by Skoog (1974), in which the laterally based areolar pedicle is thinned of all or most of the underlying breast tissue. This was done to improve the mobility of the pedicle but leads to diminished nipple sensitivity and a weakened vascular supply. I have found that on occasion the lateral pedicle, particularly in the obese patient, is insufficiently mobile. A small superficial relaxing incision at the lateral margin of the de-epithelialized pedicle gives the desired mobility.

In cases of mastopexy (Figs. 17–17 to 17–21) the same laterally based pedicle is employed, but no breast tissue is removed superior to the pedicle. Instead, the de-epithelialized key pattern area above the areola is incised around its margins and undermined superiorly in

Text continued on page 226

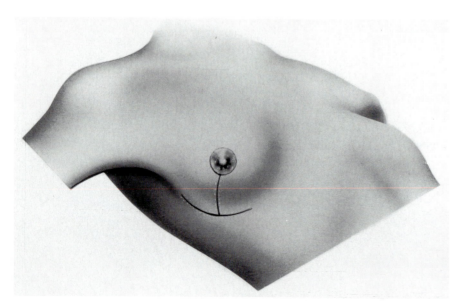

FIGURE 17-10
Completion of skin closure.

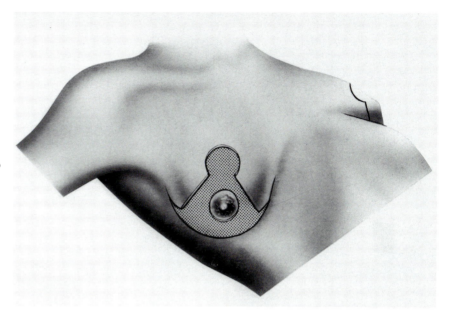

FIGURE 17-11
Mastopexy skin markings, undermining, and the area of de-epithelialization.

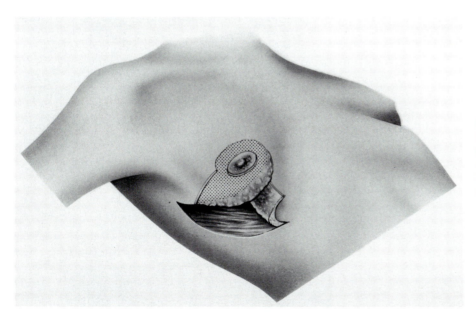

FIGURE 17-12
The medial skin and subcutaneous tissue are dissected from the medial breast tissue for approximately 3 cm in patients with moderate to severe ptosis.

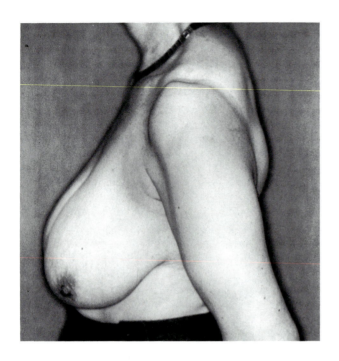

FIGURE 17–13
Preoperative view of large ptotic breasts with laterally rotated nipples.

FIGURE 17–14
The patient shown in Figure 17–13, 2 years postoperatively.

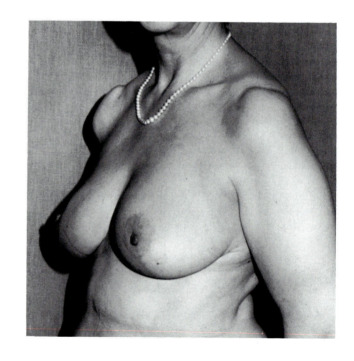

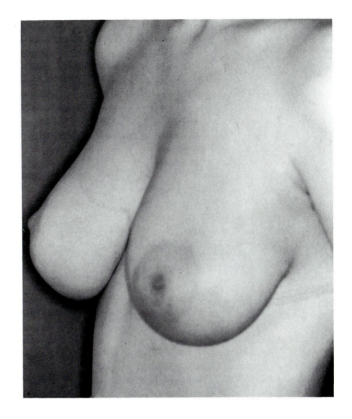

FIGURE 17–15
Moderate breast hypertrophy (resection 300 right, 250 left).

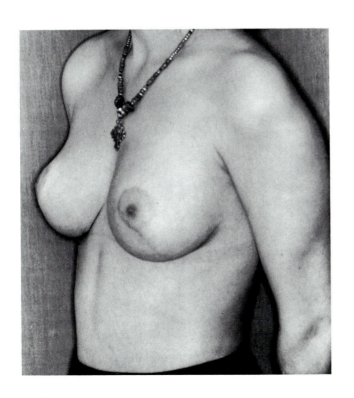

FIGURE 17–16
The same patient in Figure 17–15, 2 years postoperatively. The contour is well maintained, and the scars are acceptable.

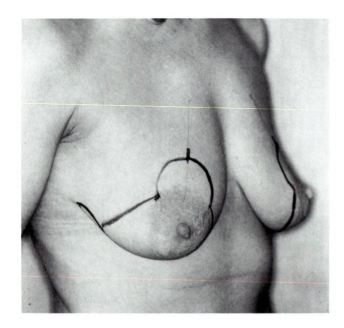

FIGURE 17–17
Ptotic scaphoid breasts after two pregnancies.

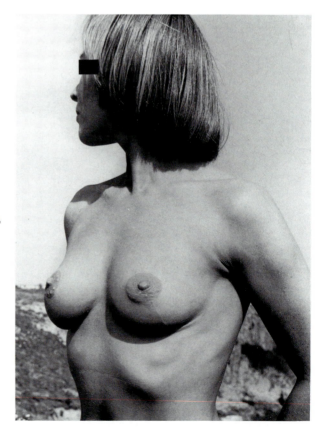

FIGURE 17–18
The patient shown in Figure 17–17, 3 years postoperatively,
photographed on the beach.

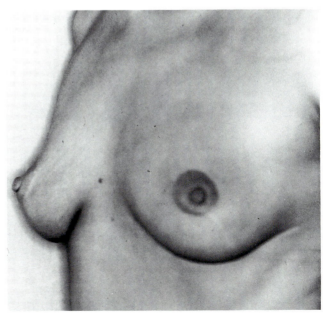

FIGURE 17–19
Mild ptosis after one pregnancy in a professional dancer.

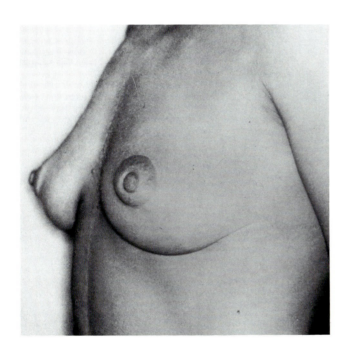

FIGURE 17–20
The patient shown in Figure 17–19, 1 year postoperatively.

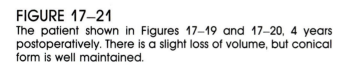

FIGURE 17–21
The patient shown in Figures 17–19 and 17–20, 4 years postoperatively. There is a slight loss of volume, but conical form is well maintained.

order to allow upward displacement of this tissue, which adds fullness to the superior quadrants of the breast as well as adding to the forward projection of the nipple.

Skin closure of the oblique incision line below the areola produces wide overlapping of the breast tissues and dermis, which gives strong support to the newly fashioned breast tissue, as well as assisting in forming and maintaining a desired conical breast contour. The elevated and newly fashioned breast tissue with wraparound skin closure is designed to temporarily produce an exaggerated degree of superior fullness. Gradually over the next 6 months, as the scar tissue softens, the lower quadrants of the breast fill out, producing an attractive breast form. As already stated earlier, the final long-term result is influenced by a number of physical factors, some of which will have contributed to an overstretching or thinning of the dermis. In such adverse conditions, secondary tightening of the lower breast scars may be necessary 6 months or more later.

The oblique radial closure extending downward and laterally from the areola has produced a much finer scar than the more conventional vertical skin closure. Its obliquity approximates more closely the lines of elective incision, and its greater length reduces tension on the skin edges.

In order to minimize stretching of the breast scars, patients are instructed to wear 1-inch Micropore to splint the scars for 6 to 8 weeks after surgery. It should be changed every 4 to 5 days but will tolerate bathing and does not usually cause skin irritation.

SUMMARY

Changing fashions and popular demand are forcing us to adopt higher standards in breast surgery. A surgical technique for breast reduction and mastopexy is presented that has been employed for many years by the author, giving improved long-term results when judged after 2 or more years. Detailed consideration is given to the placement of incisions, the techniques of skin closure, and postoperative scar management, as well as techniques to improve nipple projection and reduce fullness of the lateral quadrant, which all contribute to a more aesthetic breast form.

References

McKissock, P. K.: Reduction mammoplasty with a vertical dermal flap. Plast. Reconstr. Surg. 49:245, 1972.

Pitanguy, I.: Surgical treatment of breast hypertrophy. Br J. Plast. Surg. 20:78, 1967.

Skoog, T.: *Plastic Surgery: New Methods and Refinements*. Philadelphia, W. B. Saunders, 1974, p. 350.

Straith, R. E.: The subcuticular suture. Postgrad. Med. 196:16, 1961.

Strömbeck, J. O.: Mammoplasty: Report on a new technique based on the two-pedicle procedure. Br. J. Plast. Surg. 13:79, 1961.

Wise, R. J.: A preliminary report on a method of planning the mammoplasty. Plast. Reconstr. Surg. 17:367, 1956.

Reduction Mammaplasty: The Strömbeck Method

A woman's reason for seeking reduction mammaplasty is either that the size and heaviness of her breasts trouble her or that they have become loose and ptotic. An enlarged bosom, subsequent to weight problems or otherwise, results in such problems as discomfort from the bands of the brassiere and even direct pressure on the brachial plexus. Pain in the shoulders and back is common, and intertrigo may occur in the submammary region. Large breasts have a restrictive influence on athletic activities. Certainly, aesthetic considerations are an important factor.

A ptotic breast can result from pregnancy or excessive weight loss. The problem is cosmetic when the breasts are otherwise of normal size. Large breasts always become ptotic with time and, apart from genuine breast hypertrophy, may be part of a general adiposity.

The disadvantages of the operation must be considered in addition to the indications. Scars, the risk of disturbance of the sensitivity of the nipple-areola region, and even postoperative sagging must be discussed in detail with the patient.

Contraindications range from the psychologic (e.g., dysmorphophobia and an unrealistic view of the surgical result) to the somatic (e.g., poor operative risk, where the operation endangers the life of the patient). Reduction mammaplasty is generally a rewarding operation that most patients judge very positively. But even under ideal circumstances, in which a plastic surgeon had had optimal results in all patients, there would be some who still would not be satisfied.

With most older techniques, the skin of the breast was first dissected free from the gland. Then the gland was reduced, and the skin was tailored to fit the gland. With the technique I use now, the skin and the gland are resected in one piece, and the forming is made without, or with very limited, undermining of the skin. The size of the skin flaps is exactly determined before the reduction is done.

The nipple and areola are transposed on a pedicle consisting of dermis and gland. I described the technique in 1960 and have then modified it, so that the principle can be applied to all breast sizes and mastopexy (Strömbeck, 1960, 1964, 1976, 1986). The two disadvantages of this method are the relatively long horizontal scar in the submammary fold. The less experienced surgeon might find it difficult to achieve a perfect transposition of the nipple region, because it must be approximated without any tension whatsoever.

THE AUTHOR'S STANDARD PROCEDURE

Preoperative Planning

Careful preoperative planning is imperative in order to achieve good symmetry and natural shape. This planning is carried out with the patient in a sitting position and starts with marking the breast meridian and the new position of the areola. This position should correspond with the projection of the submammary fold on the breast skin, that is, at a level through the breast from the submammary fold at a right angle to the skin (Fig. 18–1). Note that the most common error in doing reduction mammaplasties is placing the areola too high.

To determine the size of the skin flaps, I use a pattern (Fig. 18–2), not because all breasts should be of the same size, but because I have found it to be an easy way to achieve symmetric results. The length of the incision in the submammary fold is marked and made as short as possible so that it does not extend too far medially or laterally and will be within the newly shaped breast (Fig. 18–3). By testing where the lower corner of the pattern reaches the submammary fold (Figs. 18–4 and 18–5), one can check whether the skin flaps are of sufficient size or whether it is necessary to elongate them (Fig. 18–5). The lower borderline of the flaps is determined and may be somewhat longer than the corresponding length of the submammary incision (Fig. 18–6). It is important to check for symmetry, and possible size differences must be judged preoperatively (Fig. 18–7).

Operation

The operation is performed with the patient under general anesthesia and in a supine position. In addition, a local anesthetic (0.25% lidocaine with epinephrine, 1:400,000) is infiltrated under the incision lines and above the pectoral fascia (Fig. 18–8). This will reduce

Text continued on page 232

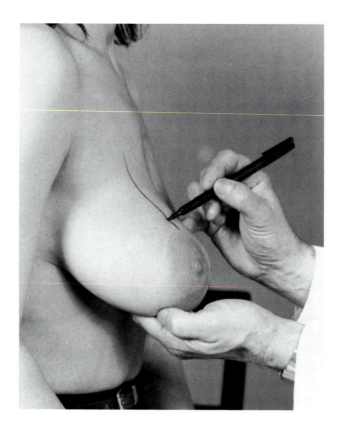

FIGURE 18–1

Preoperative markings. The breast meridian is marked. The tip of the finger is in the inframammary fold; and the point of its projection on the breast surface, the new nipple position, is being marked.

FIGURE 18–2

Pattern applied to the breast with the border of the pattern approximately 1 cm above the marking of the inframammary fold.

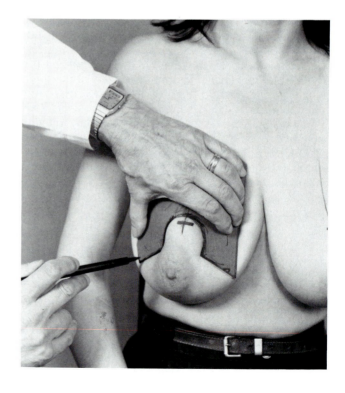

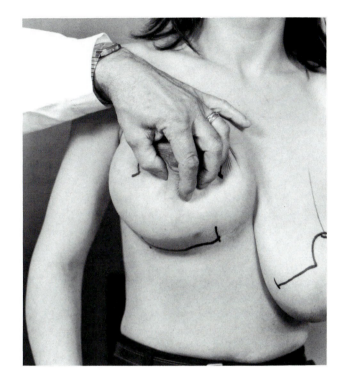

FIGURE 18–3
The inframammary fold is marked. The length of this incision should be as short as possible so that the incision does not extend outside the newly shaped breast.

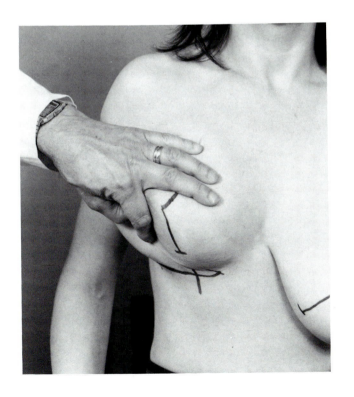

FIGURE 18–4
By moving the breast laterally, the lower corner of the medial skin flap is approximated to the inframammary fold. This point is marked on the skin of the inframammary fold.

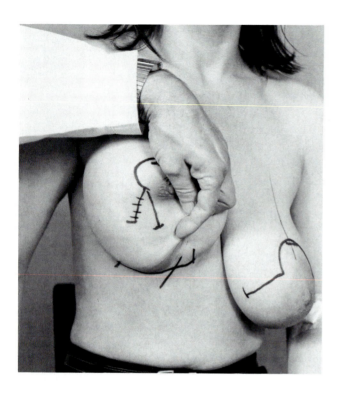

FIGURE 18–5
The breast is moved medially and folded so that the lower corner of the lateral skin flap hits the inframammary fold. It is in this case evident that this corner will not reach the same point as the medial skin flap did. The lateral corner has been moved medially so that the lateral skin flap will have adequate length.

FIGURE 18–6
The lower part of the skin flaps is designed. The length of these incisions will sometimes have to exceed the corresponding length in the submammary fold to keep the horizontal scar line as short as possible.

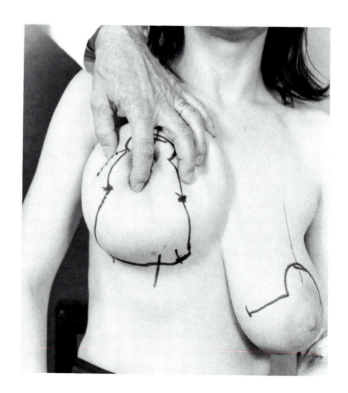

FIGURE 18–7
The postoperative planning is completed. Note that good symmetry should be achieved.

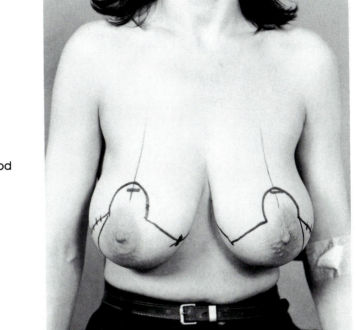

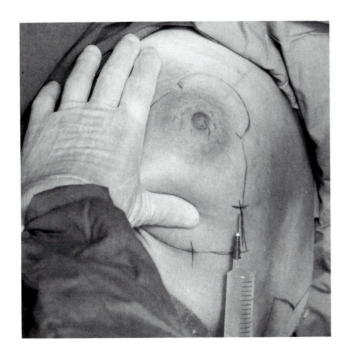

FIGURE 18–8
Local anesthesia with epinephrine is infiltrated to reduce bleeding.

the bleeding considerably (total bleeding never exceeds 200 gm) and also allows a more superficial general anesthesia.

The breast is maximally extended with a tourniquet around the base of the breast, and the areola-carrying glandular pedicle is designed (Fig. 18–9). When I first described this technique in 1960 (Strömbeck, 1960) as a bipedicle procedure, the areola was in the middle of a horizontal bridge between the skin flaps. Because difficulties sometimes arose in folding this bridge, I started to divide the lateral pedicle completely when necessary in order to get a good rotation of the areola into its new position. Over the years I have been doing this more and more often, and now I plan the operation from the start with only one medial pedicle. I made the base broad, extending into the "keyhole" for the areola and in larger breasts also below the lower corner of the medial skin flap. The epithelium over the nipple-carrying glandular flap is removed (Fig. 18–10).

The resection starts with an incision from the lateral corner of the pedicle along the skin marking to the lateral corner of the submammary incision all the way through skin and gland to the pectoral fascia (Fig. 18–11). The glandular resection is then completed (Figs. 18–12 and 18–13).

The skin edges can now be adapted and the nipple transposed to its new position. *It is important that the areola be sutured without any tension* (Figs. 18–14 to 18–16).

In cases where the pedicle is very short, the dermal part of the pedicle does not stretch enough to allow the areola to be transposed without tension. Dermis has then to be incised where the tension is.

Postoperative Care

The drains can usually be removed the day after surgery but are kept in place for another day or more if the bleeding has been more than 60 ml. The patient is kept hospitalized for 1 or 2 days after surgery. The sutures are removed after 1 to 2 weeks. For young patients I recommend that the scar lines be taped with paper tape for at least 3 months.

Complications

The following data are based on a personal series of 670 patients, which was reviewed in 1976 (Strömbeck), and a series of 323 patients who underwent surgery with medial pedicles; some of these patients were included in the earlier series.

Hematoma

Postoperative bleeding is usually minor. Small hematomas with a slight swelling do not demand any special measures; however, larger hematomas have to be evacuated. The frequency of hematomas needing evacuation in the first series was 2.7%; and in the second, 0.6%.

Glandular Complications

Circulatory disturbances in the fat can cause fat necrosis. The risk of this complication is greater in overweight patients. Smaller areas of fat necrosis are noted as a small lump, which the patient might believe is malignant. In these cases, needle biopsy or extirpation of the lump might be performed. In larger fat necroses, there is usually a temperature rise up to 39°C, and these must be drained. The spontaneous sloughing of necrotic tissue may take a long time; therefore, surgical revision, which considerably shortens the healing time, is performed.

The frequency of fat necrosis in the first series was 2.1% of 1306 breasts (670 patients); and in the second series, 1.1% of 581 breasts (323 patients). If the patients

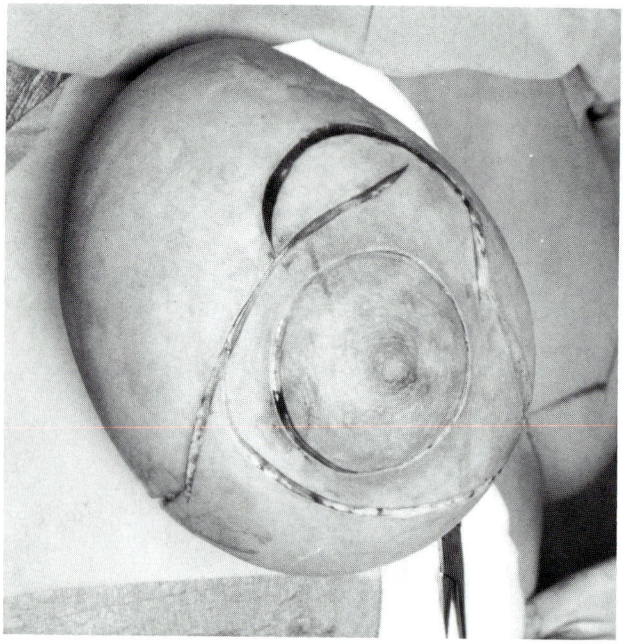

FIGURE 18–9
The tourniquet on the base of the breast keeps the breast extended. The areola has been circumsized superficially with a diameter of 4.5 cm, and the medially based glandular flap has been designed.

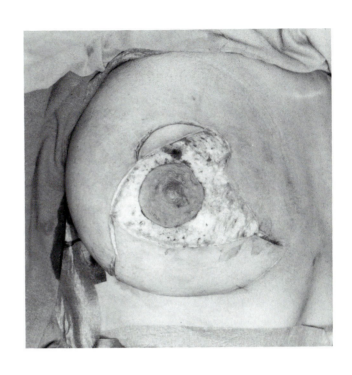

FIGURE 18–10
The epithelium of the areola-carrying glandular flap is removed. The base is broad and extends into the "keyhole" for the areola.

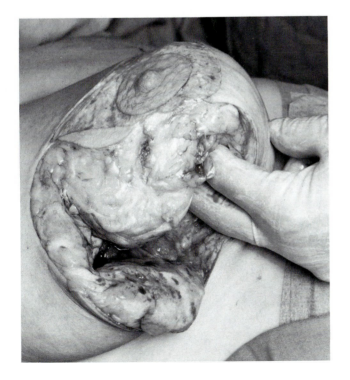

FIGURE 18–11
Incision all the way through the breast along the skin-marking line from the upper lateral corner of the pedicle to the lateral corner of the submammary incision.

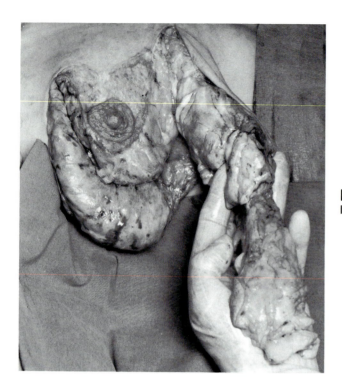

FIGURE 18–12
Incision along the borders of the pedicle is made.

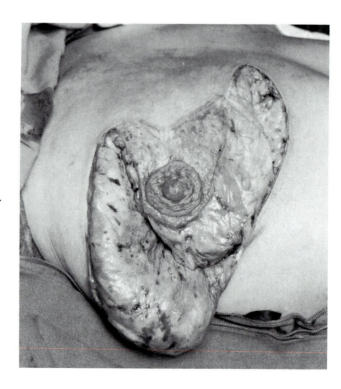

FIGURE 18–13
The resection is completed.

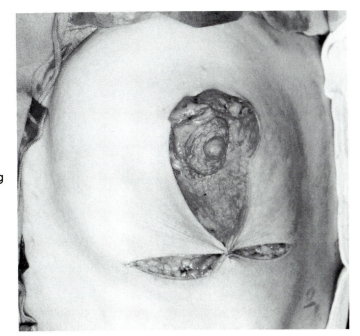

FIGURE 18–14
By joining the lower corners of the skin flaps, the folding of the breasts starts.

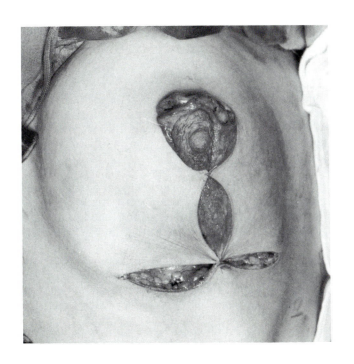

FIGURE 18–15
The transposition of the areola should be without any tension. If necessary, dermis could be cut to release the tension.

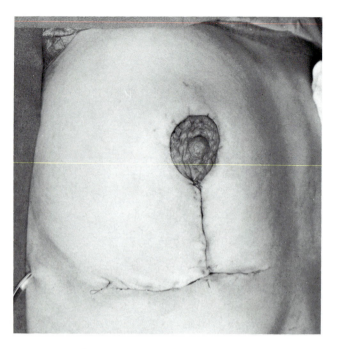

FIGURE 18–16
Suturing of the skin is completed. A suction drain is inserted laterally through a separate incision.

are grouped according to their degree of obesity, the frequency of fat necrosis in patients of normal weight was in the two series 0.4% and 0%, respectively, whereas in very obese patients it was 9% and 4.7%, respectively. A large area of fat necrosis prolongs healing time and could also result in a greater reduction of the breast volume than was planned, which could be visible, because this complication most often occurs only on one side.

Nipple-Areola Necrosis

Necrosis of the nipple-areola complex is rare. In the previously mentioned series of 670 patients, total necrosis occurred in 3 patients, all of whom were extremely obese. In these three cases, the patients were less concerned about the necrosis than I was, and none of them wanted any nipple reconstruction. In the second series of 323 patients, partial areola necrosis occurred in three breasts, all in greatly overweight women. The necrotic areas healed spontaneously, leaving somewhat depigmented areas.

Skin Complications

Skin necrosis does not occur, but there might be a separation in the T part of the scar. This usually heals by secondary intention.

Late Complications

Because the deep dermis is left in the pedicle, it is possible that epithelial cysts might develop. In practice, however, this is extremely rare. The frequency lies on a few milia and is probably due to the fact that a small epithelial island has been left behind. Hypertrophy of the scars occurs and happens unfortunately most often in very young patients. Most cases of hypertrophy occur in the medial and lateral parts of the horizontal scar line. When the hypertrophy has subsided after 1 or more

years, it leaves a broad, atrophic scar, which then could be revised with some hope of success.

Advantages of This Technique

The operation is a simple one. It provides good symmetry, and the breasts have a natural shape. It can be applied to all types of breasts. In addition, the complications are few.

Disadvantages of This Technique

The length of the horizontal scar is a weak point. But as has been stated in the previous description of the technique, the scar could and should be kept within the newly shaped breast and not extend too far medially or laterally. Sometimes a gathering of the skin flaps is necessary.

The entire areola region might have a tendency to sink during the first postoperative year. This sinking occurs in cases in which the areola-carrying flap is made rather thin, so that it does not have enough support from underneath. It is also essential that at operation the areola be sutured without any tension.

Branches coming from the intercostal nerves are damaged when one excises the lower segment of the breast, which makes for a somewhat higher frequency of sensitivity disturbances in the areola than that of methods that leave the lower part of the breast intact.

LATERAL RESECTION WITH AN L-SHAPED SCAR

In young patients I used another technique in which the resection is done above and lateral to the areola,

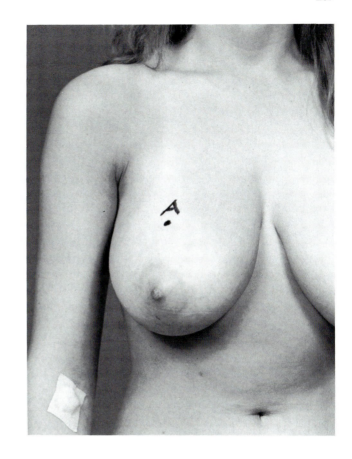

FIGURE 18–17
The projection of the inframammary fold on the middle line of the breast skin is marked, point A.

after which the upper part of the breast is moved laterally and caudally, which results in an L-shaped scar, as described in 1977 (Strömbeck, 1977). Because this technique is not based on a geometric calculation, the shape of the breast to begin with is more rounded medially and flatter laterally. The shape is improved by gravity, and after some weeks the breast looks very natural. The results could be compared with those achieved by the modified skin excision and L-shaped scar technique of Dufourmentel and Mouly (1976) and Paule Regnault's B technique (1976). This procedure is used for younger patients with breasts only moderately hypertrophic and not too ptotic or lax. It is also used for mastopexy in moderate cases at all ages.

Preoperative Planning

With the patient in the sitting position, the projection of the inframammary fold on the midline is marked (point A) (Fig. 18–17). Then the breast is moved laterally so that the skin above the inframammary fold becomes flat and tense. From the midpoint of the inframammary fold a vertical line is drawn 6 to 8 cm in length. The upper point of this line is point B (Fig. 18–18). The lateral part of the submammary fold is marked as shown in Figure 18–19. With the breast hanging down, a line from the lateral corner of the submammary fold is drawn horizontally in the direction of the areola. A point 7 to 10 cm from the lateral corner of the

inframammary fold is marked (point C) (Fig. 18–20). The distance from the lateral corner of the submammary fold to point C should be equal to the distance from the medial corner of the submammary fold to point B. Points B, A, and C are joined with a curved line (Fig. 18–21). This line should represent the skin circumference around the areola in its new position (Figs. 18–22 and 18–23).

Operation

The operation starts with the determination of the areola-carrying glandular flap with the pedicle medial and caudal (Fig. 18–24). With the breast distended, the areola is circumcised superficially in a diameter of 5 cm. The part of the pedicle lying outside the medial skin incision is de-epithelialized (Fig. 18–25). Pressing the breast in a caudal direction, the surgeon incises the skin along the upper marking all the way through the gland down to the pectoral fascia (Fig. 18–26). After blunt dissection downward over the fascia, it is possible to stabilize the breast and to cut along the borders of the areola-carrying flap down to the muscle all the way out to the lateral corner of the submammary fold (Figs. 18–27 and 18–28). The lateral skin border is stabilized with two Gillies hooks, and the skin is undermined in a superficial layer in the medial part of the breast up to 3 cm above point C (Fig. 18–29). The undermined skin is folded up, and the resection is completed (Figs. 18–30

Text continued on page 243

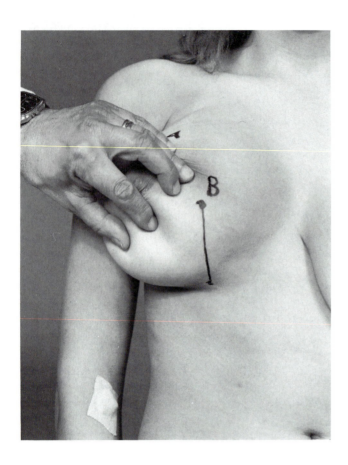

FIGURE 18–18
With the breast pressed laterally, a vertical line is drawn from the midpoint of the inframammary fold 7 cm long. The upper end of this line is point B.

FIGURE 18–19
The lateral part of the submammary fold is marked.

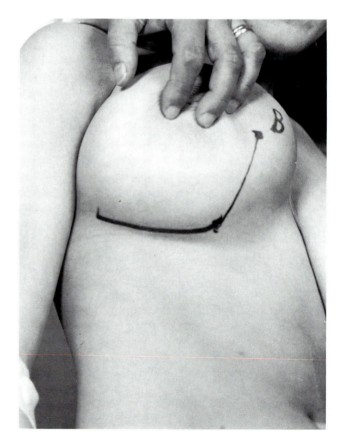

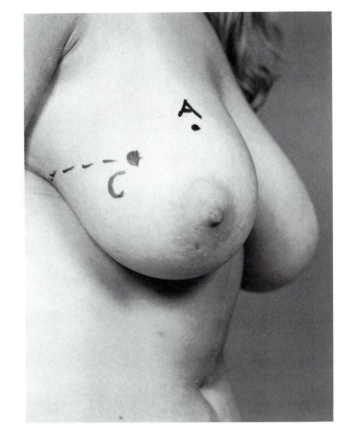

FIGURE 18–20
With the breast hanging down, a horizontal line is marked from the lateral corner of the inframammary fold. A point on this line 9 cm from the lateral corner of the inframammary fold is marked, point C.

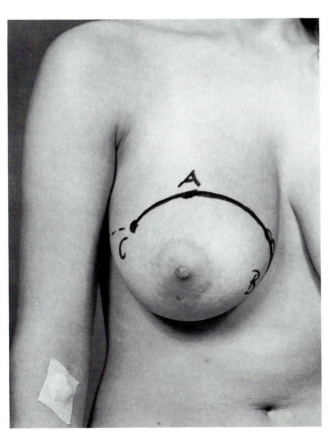

FIGURE 18–21
Points B, A, and C are joined with a curved incision.

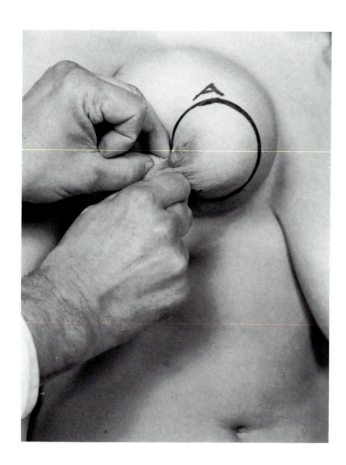

FIGURE 18–22
This curved line should represent the skin line surrounding the areola.

FIGURE 18–23
The preoperative marking is completed.

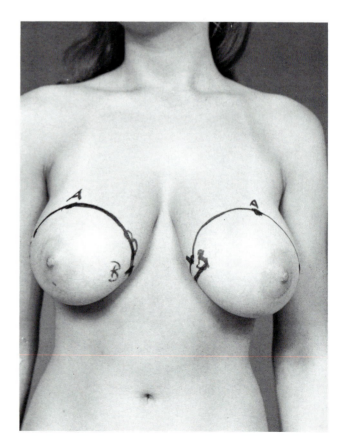

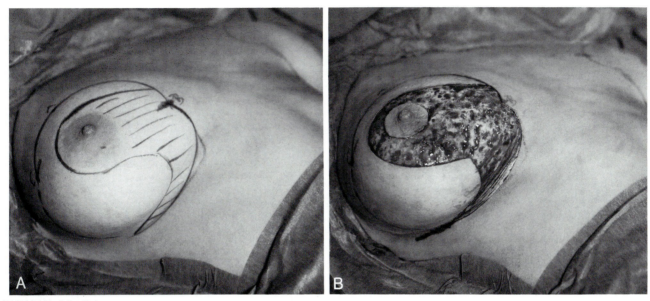

FIGURE 18–24
A, The shape of the glandular pedicle is marked before the operation. *B*, The epithelium in the pedicle area has been removed.

FIGURE 18–25
An incision along the upper borderline of the skin markings has been made all the way to the fascia of the muscle.

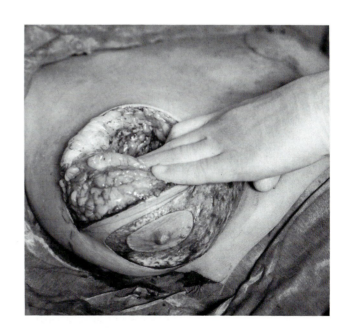

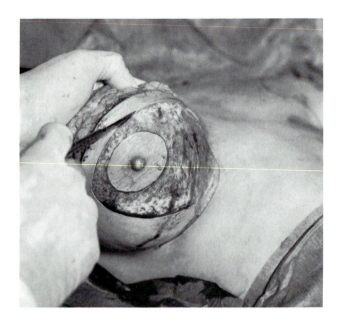

FIGURE 18–26
The breast is lifted forward. The incision along the borderline of the pedicle is being made.

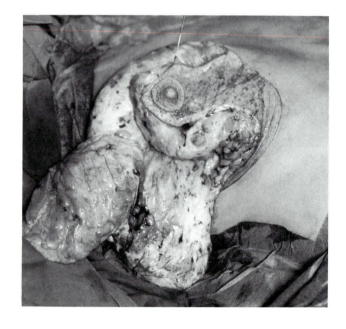

FIGURE 18–27
The incision is completed.

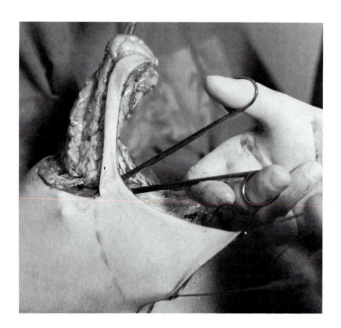

FIGURE 18–28
The skin in the lateral part of the breast is dissected off to some 3 cm above point C.

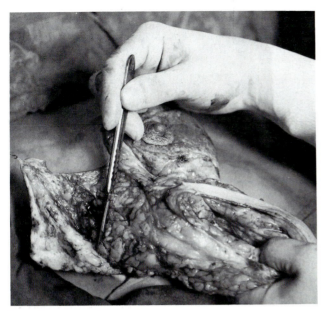

FIGURE 18–29
The skin is folded up, and the resection of the gland is completed.

and 18–31). The lateral borderlines of the gland may be sutured approximating each other (Fig. 18–32), although I no longer put any sutures in the gland.

With suturing of point B against point C, the shaping of the breast starts. As the distance C to A to B is frequently considerably longer than the circumference of the areola, it may be an advantage to suture some centimeters above point C and, thus, reduce the discrepancy in length between the skin and the areola (Fig. 18–33). The skin surplus can then be reduced so that good contouring of the breast is achieved, which results in an L-shaped scar (Fig. 18–34). The skin around the areola is then dispersed so that any skin surplus is equally divided (Fig. 18–35; see Fig. 18–36).

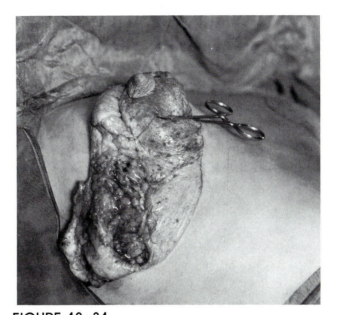

FIGURE 18–31
The lateral cut surfaces of the gland are sutured together, a procedure that is not necessary and sometimes even makes the shaping more difficult. I prefer not to put any stitches at all in the gland.

RESULTS

The result of mammaplasty must be considered good if the patient is satisfied and happy. The patient's judgment depends on whether or not the problems she had, somatic or psychologic, have disappeared and whether or not the shape of the breasts and the scars are acceptable to her. This judgment is highly individual, and the importance of parameters such as size, shape,

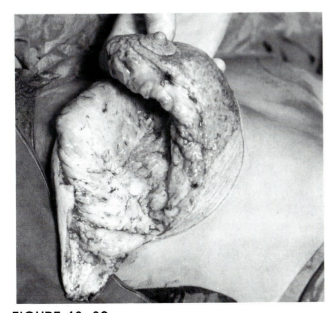

FIGURE 18–30
The patient after resection.

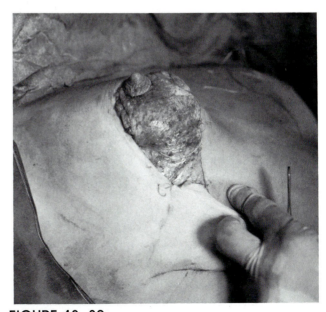

FIGURE 18–32
Points B and C being joined with a suture. In this case, it was possible to go about 3 cm above point C. This procedure makes the skin circumference around the areola shorter.

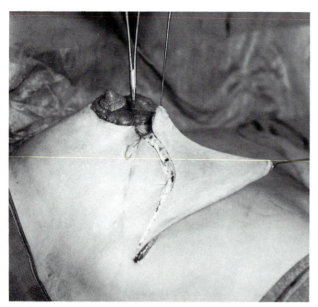

FIGURE 18–33
The surplus skin is now "tailored" off to give a smooth undersurface of the breast.

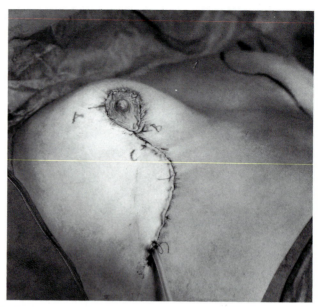

FIGURE 18–35
The skin closure is completed.

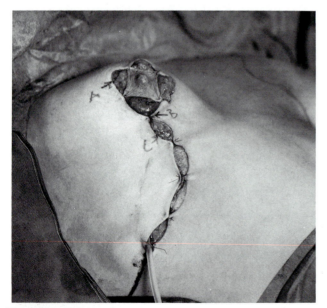

FIGURE 18–34
The areola circumference is evenly divided in the skin opening.

ptosis, scars, and sensitivity differs from patient to patient. There is usually no opportunity for the patient to compare her result with the result in other women.

The surgeon's judgment is founded on his assessment of the appearance of the breasts. They should look natural in comparison with the total body and not look operated on, but it is impossible not to be influenced by a comparison with the preoperative condition. Having operated on many patients, the surgeon also has a much more extensive frame of reference, where such factors as the turgor of the tissue, the body constitution, age, and so forth, automatically must be considered. This

means that the opinion of the surgeon concerning the result often differs from that of the patient.

My previously published findings were based on asking patients to evaluate the results of their surgery by completing a questionnaire (Strömbeck, 1964, 1980). This has been followed by personal follow-up.

In one follow-up study (Strömbeck, 1980), I asked 250 patients whether they thought that the results were in correspondence with the expectations they had before the operation. Eighty-three percent thought that they were. Asked whether they would have the same operation again if they had the opportunity to make a second choice, 92% answered yes.

Only 46% of the patients under 25 years old were very satisfied with the results, whereas 66% in the group 25 years and older were very satisfied. The degree of satisfaction was also related to the amount of tissue resected. Only 38% of the patients who had less than 250 gm of tissue resected were very satisfied, whereas 60% of the patients who had more than 250 gm resected were very satisfied.

Because of the greater dissatisfaction among younger patients, for a follow-up study, I chose patients whose upper age was 39 years and who had been operated on between 1976 and 1980. Of the 112 patients who answered the questionnaire, 51 had undergone surgery with the Strömbeck technique (Strömbeck, 1960), and 61 had had lateral resection with the L-shaped scar (Strömbeck, 1977) (L-L). I operated on all patients.

Because the younger patients and those with smaller resections were overrepresented in the L-L group, direct comparison between the groups was impossible. Thus, the results of the follow-up do not specifically separate patients in terms of which technique was used.

Patients' expectations were met in 81% of the cases, whereas 10% thought their expectations were not met and 9% were doubtful. Ninety-one percent of the patients would have the same surgery again, whereas 6%

were doubtful and 3% would not have it again. Ninety-three percent of the group were very satisfied or satisfied with the surgery, whereas 4.5% and 2.5% were rather satisfied or dissatisfied, respectively.

Although 74% of the patients thought that the shape of their breasts was good, 21.5% thought they were ptotic and 4.5% thought that the shape was unnatural. Size was rated as adequate by 80% of the sample, too big by 18%, and too small by 2%.

With regard to nipple-areola sensitivity, a pronounced difference was found between the two operative techniques, a difference that is clearly significant and demonstrates that the lateral resection spared more of the nerves coming from the chest wall. The percent distribution is calculated on the number of nipples, with 96 operations according to the Strömbeck procedure and 114 using the L-L technique. Fifty-two percent of the patients, as opposed to 65%, found sensitivity to be the

same as before the operation, 26% versus 24% found sensitivity to be somewhat reduced in comparison with the preoperative condition, 15% versus 4% thought it to be poor, and 6% versus 5% had a feeling of discomfort in the nipple.

Of all patients, 53% regarded the scars to be almost invisible, 42% found them somewhat disturbing, and 5% thought them to be ugly. I had expected a difference to the advantage of the L-L technique. Such a difference was found. Fifty percent versus 55% regarded the scars as almost invisible, but the difference is not very significant.

The position of the nipple was thought to be satisfactory in 84% of those having undergone the Strömbeck procedure and in 76% of those having undergone the L-L procedure.

The appearance of the areola was thought to be good by 70% of patients experiencing both procedures.

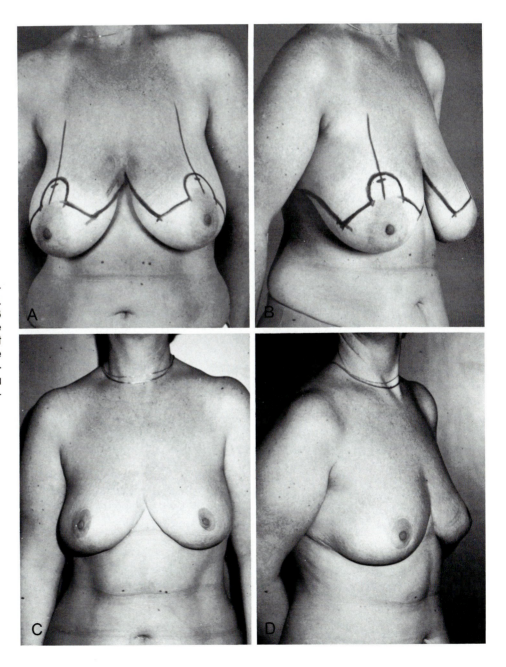

FIGURE 18–36

A and *B*, Preoperative photographs of a 33-year-old patient. *C* and *D*, The same patient 3 years after surgery; 460 gm were removed from the right breast and 510 gm from the left. The patient is satisfied with the results. On the left side, there is a tendency toward inward traction of the areola.

Photographs were taken of the 59 patients who came for follow-up examination (27 had undergone the Strömbeck procedure, and 32 had undergone the L-L procedure), and five plastic surgeons were asked to rate them as to the appearance of the breasts. The judges, who rated the photographs independently, did not know which patient had had which operation and had no access to preoperative photographs. They rated the success of the surgery somewhat more favorable than the patients had (Figs. 18–36 to 18–39).

Among the patients in this follow-up study, only 41 have had a child after the operation. Of these, 14 nursed 3 months or more, 5 nursed 1 to 2 months, and 22 nursed less than 1 month or not all. Of 8 patients who had nursed both before and after surgery, 2 nursed better after the operation than before and 2 had less success than before the operation, whereas 4 had the same nursing capacity before and after surgery.

A reduction mammaplasty is a beneficial operation in which the advantages in very large breast hypertrophies are quite evident. In the more cosmetic reduction mammaplasties, the disadvantages must be clearly explained to the patients with a careful discussion regarding size, scars, sensitivity, and postoperative sagging. The patient's motives for seeking the operation should be explored; and in those cases in which there is a pronounced discrepancy between the patient's concern and the real deformity, surgery should not be performed. These patients in all likelihood have problems that are not suitable for surgical treatment, e.g., personal problems or psychologic disturbances. Although such patients could be in great need of help, a plastic surgeon is unlikely to be appropriate, even when the patient herself is convinced that reduction mammaplasty offers the best solution to her problems.

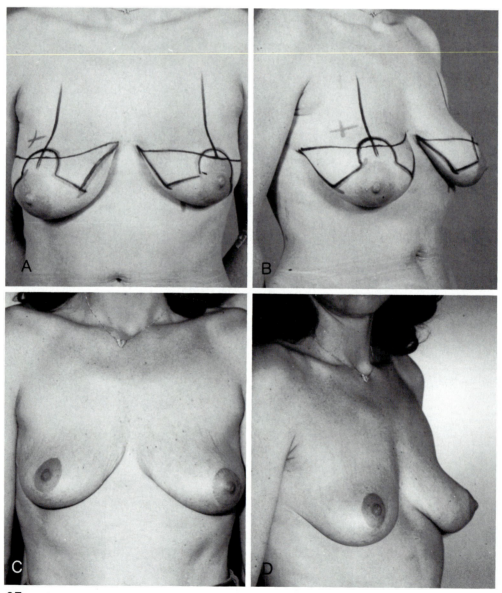

FIGURE 18–37

A and B, Preoperative photographs of a 28-year-old patient. C and D, The same patient 3 years after resection of 185 and 75 gm.

FIGURE 18–38
A and *B*, Preoperative photographs of a 17-year-old patient. *C* and *D*, The same patient 5 years after reduction with the L-L technique; 530 and 525 gm were removed. The patient thought the results were rather good but that they did not correspond to her preoperative expectations, and she was hesitant when asked whether she would have the operation if given a second chance. The surgeons judge the results as good.

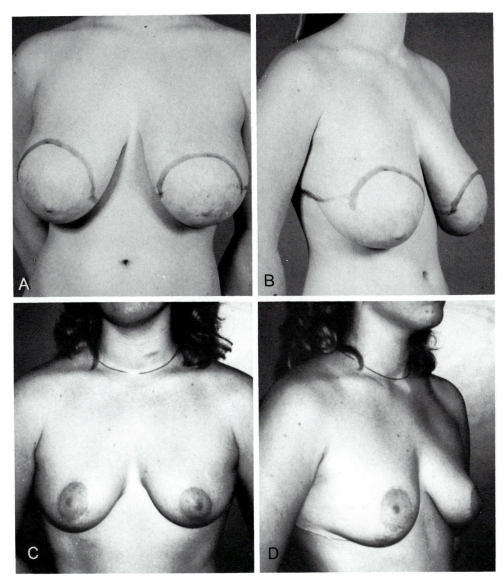

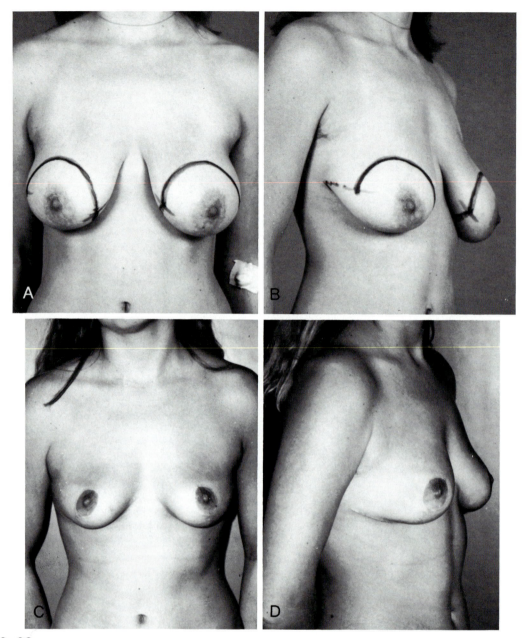

FIGURE 18–39
A and *B*, Preoperative view of an 18-year-old patient. *C* and *D*, The same patient 2 years after the L-L technique was performed, with 310 and 335 gm removed. The patient is satisfied with the results.

References

Dufourmentel, C., Mouly, R.: Reduction mammaplasty by lateral approach. In: Goldwyn, R. M. (ed): *Plastic and Reconstructive Surgery of the Breast.* Boston, Little, Brown, 1976, p. 233.

Regnault, P. C. L.: Reduction mammaplasty by the "B" technique. In: Goldwyn, R. M. (ed.): *Plastic and Reconstructive Surgery of the Breast.* Boston, Little, Brown, 1976, p. 269.

Strömbeck, J. O.: Mammaplasty: Report of a new technique based on the two-pedicle procedure. Br. J. Plast. Surg. 13:79, 1960.

Strömbeck, J. O.: Macromastia in women and its surgical treatment. Acta Chir Scand Suppl 341, 1964.

Strömbeck, J. O.: Reduction mammaplasty by upper and lower resection. In: Goldwyn, R. M. (ed.): *Plastic and Reconstructive Surgery of the Breast.* Boston, Little, Brown, 1976, p. 195.

Strömbeck, J. O.: Benign diseases of the female breast: Surgical treatment and cosmetic aspects. In: Exerpta Medica International Congress Series No. 412, *Proceedings of the VIII International Congress of Gynecology and Obstetrics,* Mexico City 17–22 October 1976. Amsterdam, Exerpta Medica, 1977, p. 184.

Strömbeck, J. O.: Late results after reduction mammaplasty. In: Goldwyn, R. M. (ed.): *Long-Term Results in Plastic and Reconstructive Surgery.* Boston, Little, Brown, 1980, p. 722.

Strömbeck, J. O.: Reduction mammaplasty. In: Strömbeck, J. O., Rosato, F. E. (eds.): *Surgery of the Breast.* Stutgart, New York, Georg Thieme Verlag, 1986, p. 277.

Reduction Mammaplasty: The Dermal Vault Technique

The dermal vault technique for reduction mammaplasty has evolved in a way that parallels the fascinating history of this branch of plastic surgery (Lalardrie, 1974). Originally, Biesenberger's technique (1928) was used. Its salient feature was its reliance on the false unity between the gland and the nipple-areola complex and on the vascularization provided by the internal mammary artery. In practice it involved the following

1. A small area of de-epithelialization around the nipple-areola complex, as proposed by Schwarzmann (1930).
2. Undermining between the gland and skin, which was extensive except in the internal part.
3. External and inferior resection of the gland, which was problematic, because in 20% of cases the internal mammary vascularization was anatomically insufficient. Glandular resection was necessarily limited and, in some cases, left too voluminous a breast.
4. Skin remodeling, adapting the container to the contents. My personal preference was for the curved clamp; others resorted to preoperative markings.
5. Exteriorizing the nipple-areola complex.
6. Dressing the reduced breast.

The following morning, with some trepidation, we lifted the dressing to examine the nipple-areola complex with the fear of seeing it white or blue. Fortunately, because we were careful, it was practically always pink. But no one can live with such anxiety forever.

Then Pitanguy (1960), Strömbeck (1960), and Skoog (1963) came to the rescue and totally transformed the outlook for mammary reduction by introducing the new concept of skin-glandular unity. With them, mammaplasty became safer and more reliable. They rediscovered a truth: the mammary gland is a skin gland.

For some 10 years they performed their techniques. But I remained dissatisfied in the case of large breasts, where in some cases I resorted to Thorek's (1942) technique, mammary amputation with free graft of the nipple-areola complex.

At the same time I had occasion to perform subcutaneous mastectomies, and in 1970 I carried out a subcutaneous mastectomy on a ptotic breast (Lalardrie, 1970). I had the idea of remodeling the skin through an extensive de-epithelialization; this was the confirmation that vascularization of the nipple-areola complex could

be purely cutaneous. From then on, I adapted this technique to reduction mammaplasty.

This involved, in successive stages, the following:

1. De-epithelialization, the extent of which depended on the degree of ptosis of the breast to be reduced.
2. An unlimited glandular resection, which in some cases went as far as subcutaneous mastectomy.
3. Adaptation of the skin to the glandular stump, using the curved clamp with which we were already familiar through Biesenberger's (1928) technique.

At this time, attempts were being made to reduce the length of scars, a sword of Damocles hanging over every type of mammaplasty, and we observed that a balance had to be struck between inferior skin resection and possible periareolar resection. For a while we were happy to obtain short, submammary scars, but soon we observed that the "ruse" involved therein led to poor scar quality, and we sought once again to obtain a better balance between the two resections: areolar and submammary. This was the beginning of the dermal vault technique (Lalardrie, 1972).

APPLICATION OF THE TECHNIQUE

We now have over 18 years' experience with this technique and have performed it on 2500 patients with hypertrophic or ptotic breasts and on 200 patients requiring remodeling of the opposite breast in cases of reconstruction after amputation. We can therefore say that this technique is suitable for all cases of mammary hypertrophy and ptosis.

In cases of hypertrophy, there is no limit to the glandular resection, and the reduction can be perfectly adapted to the patient's body shape. The only contraindication could be a rigid gland where there is the risk of concavity in the nipple-areola complex. This problem could be avoided by reducing the thickness of the glandular flap carrying the nipple-areola complex, because a thinner flap is more supple.

The technique is eminently suited to cases of ptosis because thanks to extensive de-epithelialization, the nipple-areola complex may be raised by as much as 15 cm.

ADVANTAGES OF THE TECHNIQUE

The technique provides absolute vascular security, because it respects the subcutaneous vascularization, preserving a large superior pedicle. The technique ensures excellent vascularization of the glandular stump and the nipple-areola complex. With 5200 breasts operated on to date, we have had only one case of partial areolar necrosis, where 2.3 kg was resected. Since 1970 we have carried out anatomic studies that have confirmed the existence and consistency of subdermal vascularization from the acromiothoracic artery, the internal mammary artery, and the external mammary artery.

The technique allows unlimited glandular resection (Fig. 19–1). This is a major advantage, because many techniques do not allow a sufficient reduction of large breasts. Some surgeons exculpate themselves by claiming that the patients themselves wanted this, but for me

this is a poor excuse: the breast must be perfectly adapted to the patient's build; and if she is obese, she should first be encouraged to lose weight.

The technique provides for a pleasing form, more like an apple than like a pear (Fig. 19–2). Using the curved clamp makes it possible to achieve a perfect match between the skin (the container) and the glandular stump (the contents). The fact that this technique ensures such a perfect match makes it eminently suitable for correcting mammary asymmetry. One other consequence of this adjustment is the remarkable stability of the breast; we have established that if the breast is to remain stable, the forward projection should never exceed one-third of the diameter of the mammary base. If the breast meets this requirement, a brassiere is unnecessary (provided the breast is not subject to variations in volume as a result of pregnancy, slimming, and so forth).

The surgeon's hands are free right up to the end of the operation. As we shall see in the description of the

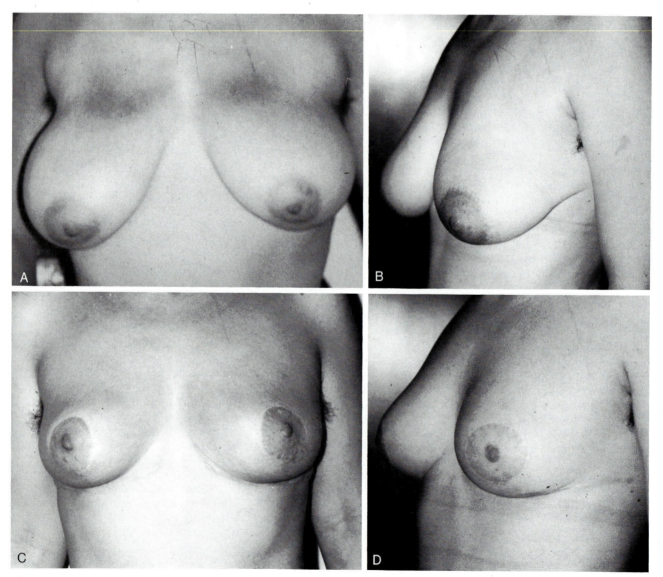

FIGURE 19–1

A and *B*, Mammary hypertrophy. *C* and *D*, Same patient 10 years after surgery.

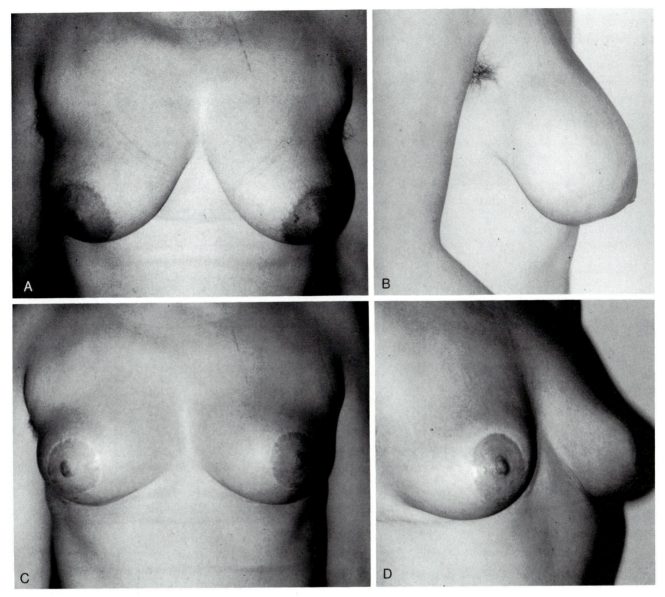

FIGURE 19–2
A and *B*, Mammary ptosis. *C* and *D*, Same patient 8 years after surgery.

technique, there are no preoperative markings that would tie the surgeon's hands from the outset. The initial marking—which is that of the first de-epithelialization—is no more than a guideline and may be corrected at the stage of the periareolar de-epithelialization. This being so, the need for a step-by-step approach should be stressed, avoiding any resection, whether glandular or cutaneous, that would irrevocably compromise the outcome. The dermal vault technique can hence be said to be a truly "plastic" technique.

The scars are relatively short and well-positioned. What long worried us with other mammaplasties was the length of the submammary scar and, above all, the fact that it extended too far and too high into the intermammary cleft and into the axillary area. In our technique, we endeavor to create a true inverted-T scar, with the internal branch as short as possible.

DISADVANTAGES OF THE TECHNIQUE

It would be wrong to say that this technique has no drawbacks. These may be summarized as follows:

The very simplicity of this technique can make it difficult to execute in practice, especially for the novice. It is necessary to have seen many such operations performed and to have performed many oneself in order to achieve a perfect result.

The poor quality of the scars, in particular the periareolar scar, is another drawback. In my early surgical experience I endeavored to greatly reduce the length of the submammary scar through extensive secondary de-epithelialization. This resulted in many cases in a wide periareolar scar. I have conquered this drawback by reducing the extent of secondary de-epithelialization, but the submammary scar is necessarily longer. In severe cases of ptosis, the two scars may join to give a single horizontal scar. I know that in saying this I lay myself open to criticism, but I prefer this result to scars rising into the mammary cleft.

On the question of scar quality, I would like to point out that the ingestion of estrogens, especially through the oral contraceptives, can cause a hypertrophic reaction in the scars. I ask my patients to stop taking oral contraceptives 2 months before the operation and not to take them again until 6 to 12 months afterward.

Another problem is the risk of hypoesthesia or anesthesia of the nipple. While I have observed no problems in lactation (a reduced breast lactates better than a hypertrophic breast), in some 5% of cases I have observed temporary or permanent anesthesia of specific nipple sensation. In most cases of anesthesia the phenomenon was unilateral, and I am at a loss to explain why.

DESCRIPTION OF THE TECHNIQUE

No preoperative markings are made. The patient is placed in the three-quarters sitting position, and we draw the following:

1. The breast meridian (which may not necessarily pass through the nipple if it is off center).
2. An areolar circle (radius, 2 to 2.2 cm).
3. A circle of de-epithelialization (radius, 5 to 7 cm); this radius is determined by a procedure identical to that used in determining the vertical excision in Biesenberger's technique (Fig. 19–3).

In the cases of marked ptosis, the upper part of the external circle is extended upward into an ellipse in order to bring the upper pole to a point 14 to 16 cm from the midclavicle. The skin between the two circles is de-epithelialized. The breast is raised by a retracting suture placed above the areola. The skin is cut on the breast meridian between the lower pole of the external circle and the inframammary fold. On each side of the incision the skin is separated from the gland to a sufficient extent to free the lower part of the gland. This cut is prolonged along the semicircumference of the external circle (Fig. 19–4).

Glandular Resection

The gland is cut horizontally 1 cm below the lower pole of the areola, over the whole width of the area freed. When the depth of the incision has reached 1 to 1.5 cm, the upper lip is raised by a suture. The surgeon holds this lip between the index and forefinger of his left hand and puts his other two fingers on the surface of the breast; he then turns his hand so that his palm is toward him. The scalpel is placed in the existing incision and now cuts the gland parallel to its surface; we thus have a slice whose thickness is controlled by the surgeon's left hand and the gland to be resected falls progressively (Fig. 19–5).

The remaining cutaneoglandular thickness must be homogeneous, but thicker at the center than at the periphery. The scalpel approaches the surface of the gland, at first laterally, then at the level of the upper pole; but on reaching the fatty tissue, care must be taken not to come too near the skin. With practice, the surgeon can use his left hand to gauge the thickness of the cut and its homogeneity. This is important in that it allows an equal resection of the two breasts; when these

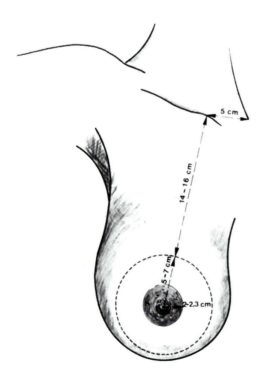

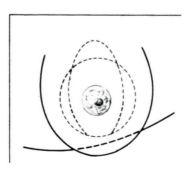

FIGURE 19–3
Preoperative markings showing the extent of de-epithelialization. The circle of de-epithelialization is made oval in cases of serious ptosis.

remains only in the central area because in cases of marked hypertrophy, there is no gland at the periphery because the volume of the glandular stump determines the residual mammary volume. In cases of moderate hypertrophy, however, it is necessary to leave some gland over the whole surface of the cut and more especially at the upper pole. It is also necessary to effect a complete undermining between the gland and the pectoral muscle. This is achieved automatically in the type of glandular resection performed for cases of major hypertrophy.

The glandular stump and the nipple remain vascularized by the subdermal blood supply from the cutaneous vessels of the external mammary, acromiothoracic, and internal mammary arteries. This technique respects the subdermal vascularization and is hence completely safe.

Remodeling of the Skin

The upper edge of the areola is then brought to the top of the de-epithelialized area at point A (Fig. 19–6). Two points situated 6 to 8 cm from this point on the edges of this area are brought together by a temporary suture at point B (Fig. 19–7). Should the skin edges immediately under point B be invaginated, this must be corrected by de-epithelialization of the invaginated area. The lower vertical skin flaps are then brought forward

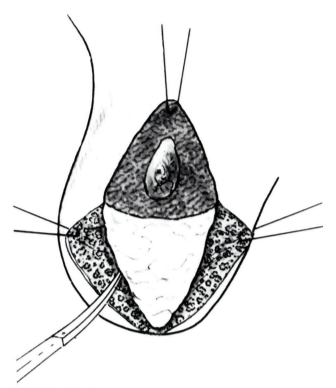

FIGURE 19–4
Dissection of the lower part of the gland.

are not identical it is possible to obtain symmetry without weighing the cut gland or operating simultaneously on the two breasts.

This type of resection is, in a sense, a subtotal mastectomy; the new breast is formed from a dermal and fat thickness and a glandular stump. This latter

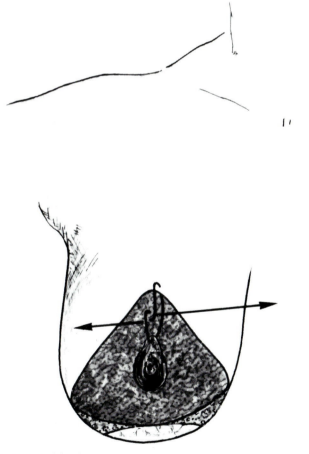

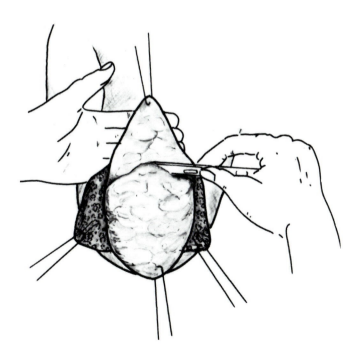

FIGURE 19–5
Glandular cut of homogeneous thickness leaving a control disk.

FIGURE 19–6
Elevation of the nipple. Folding of the upper zone of de-epithelialization.

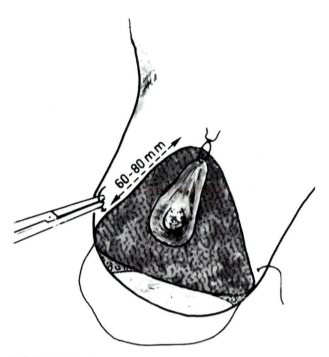

FIGURE 19–7
The edges of the circle of de-epithelialization are brought together at a point determined by the surgeon.

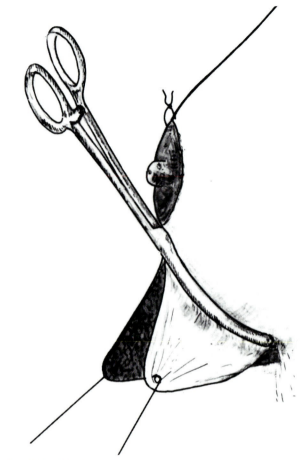

FIGURE 19–8
A curved clamp is applied. Vertical cutaneous resection.

and pulled toward the front and side. A curved clamp, similar to that used in McIndoe's (1958) operation, is then applied (Fig. 19–8). The skin of the two flaps is cut along the line of the clamp; it is preferable not to cut all the skin thickness but to keep the dermis. This procedure allows a better suture by dermodermal adhesion because the glandular suture is not possible (because no gland is left at the level of the lower pole).

The horizontal skin resection is performed in the usual way. However, the central part of the lower edge must be precisely situated in the submammary fold. The skin excision should be horizontal and not curved upward; this will make it invisible under a brassiere and obviate keloid scarring at the extremities. The internal parts of the skin resection must be reduced to a minimum.

The final step involves a complementary circular de-epithelialization (Fig. 19–9) in order to bring down the lower edge of the areola to a point 4 to 5 cm from the inframammary fold. This has both an *advantage*—skin tension is brought to bear on the areola, probably a contributory factor in breast stability—and a *disadvantage*—in major reductions the outer edge of the areolar suture is puckered; though this phenomenon normally disappears in a few weeks, it sometimes leaves a scar, which may widen.

Exteriorization of the Dermal Cylinder

At this stage, the suture at point A is cut, and a dermoglandular cylinder comes forward; the greater the breast ptosis, the longer it is (Fig. 19–10). This cylinder constitutes the whole volume of the remaining breast,

and its invagination will create the "dermal vault" (Fig. 19–11), which, although it is not the sole feature of this operation, has given its name to this technique. This vault is formed by a dermodermal adhesion and serves to create the breast mound. Drainage is normal practice in this operation, and the drain may be left in place for 48 hours.

Elastic adhesive bandages or Steri-Drape are used as a dressing and are changed a week later. Two to 3 weeks after the operation, the intradermal sutures are removed.

DISCUSSION

The dermal vault technique, as we have seen, holds a number of pitfalls for the novice. Therefore, I would like to discuss some of the specific problems it presents:

1. In the preoperative markings, the line of the external circle will depend on the degree of hypertrophy and ptosis, and one must be wary of removing too much skin at the outset. Furthermore, the external circle provides a way of repositioning the nipple-areola complex when this is initially too medial on the breast relief.
2. The undermining between the mammary gland and the pectoral muscle is one of the crucial aspects of

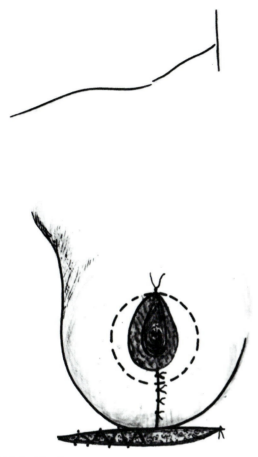

FIGURE 19–9
Secondary de-epithelialization for final positioning of the "keyhole" of the areolar vault. Horizontal cutaneous suture with external line of the lower edge.

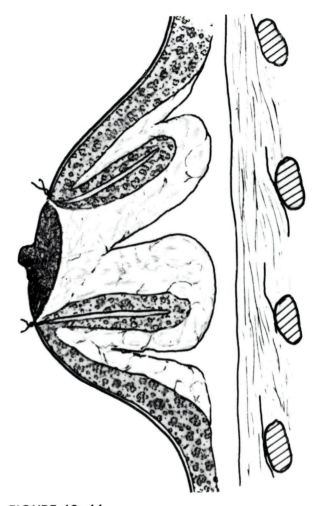

FIGURE 19–11
Cross section. The dermoglandular cylinder constituting the dermal vault is reinvaginated.

the technique. One should not be afraid of prolonging it as far as possible superiorly and laterally.

3. It is often difficult to gauge the volume of glandular resection of the second breast, especially where there is initial asymmetry. It is not by weighing what is removed that we can solve the problem, because the important thing here is not so much what is resected as what remains. If the volume of the second breast is insufficient at the end of the operation, it is easy to provide extra volume by using a dermofat flap taken from the mammary and thoracic skin, as proposed some years ago by Longacre (1954).

4. The technique cannot correct a supermammary preaxillary adipose cushion, but should one be present, it may be removed directly by excision, leaving a scar in the natural preaxillary skin fold. In most cases the scar is invisible.

5. The most delicate act for the inexperienced surgeon is the placing of the curved clamp. It is extremely difficult to give an indication valid for all breasts, except for the following guidelines:

   a. Excessive tension on the skin edges should be avoided, because this would impair the quality of the vertical scar.

   b. It is also important to avoid taking too much skin in the clamp, because the end of the clamp will determine the site of the future submammary sulcus, and it is this inframammary sulcus that will determine the new site of the nipple-areola complex.

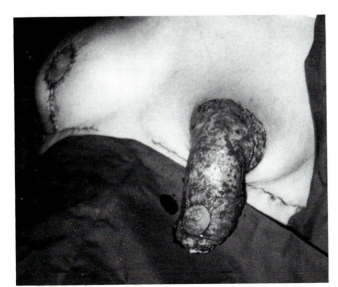

FIGURE 19–10
Exteriorization of the dermoglandular cylinder.

c. The curved clamp should not be too horizontal, because this would lead to an excessive reduction of the mammary base and the risk of secondary ptosis.

d. The curved clamp should not be too vertical, because the mammary base would be insufficiently reduced and the distance between the areola and the inframammary sulcus would be too great.

6. It is necessary to secure the superior edge of the submammary sulcus to the underlying musculature in order to avoid glandular laxity in the postoperative phase.

7. *And* it must be borne in mind that the complementary areolar de-epithelialization must not be too extensive, because this could result in excessive skin tension and a poor quality periareolar scar.

CONCLUSION

The dermal vault technique is a synthesis of modern techniques, respecting the unity of skin and gland and using a subdermal superior vascular pedicle. It affords absolute vascular security, allows unlimited glandular resection and shorter scars, and is simple in its conception. It must also be recognized that it may be difficult in execution.

References

Biesenberger, H.: Eine neue Methode der Mammaplastik. Zentrailbl. Chir. 55:2382, 1928.

Georgiade, N. G., Serafin, D., Morris, R., Georgiade, G.: Reduction mammaplasty utilizing an inferior pedicle nipple-areolar flap. Ann. Plast. Surg. 3:211, 1979a.

Georgiade, N. G., Serafin, D., Riefkohl, R., Georgiade, G.: Is there a reduction mammaplasty for "all seasons"? Plast. Reconstr. Surg. 63:765, 1979b.

Georgiade, N. G. (ed.): *Aesthetic Breast Surgery.* Baltimore, Williams & Wilkins, 1983, p. 408.

Lalardrie, J. P.: The "dermal vault" technique: Reduction mammaplasty for hypertrophy with ptosis. *Transacta der III Tagung der Vereinigung der Deutschen Plastichent Chirurgen.* Koln, 1972, p. 105.

Lalardrie, J. P.: Reduction mammaplasty by "dermal vault" technique after 425 cases. *Transactions of the Sixth International Congress of Plastic and Reconstructive Surgery.* Paris, Masson, 1976, p. 519.

Lalardrie, J. P., Jouglard, J. P.: *Chirurgie Plastique du Sein.* Paris, Masson, 1974, p. 290.

Lalardrie, J. P., Morel-Fatio, D.: Mammectomie totale souscutaneé suivie de reconstruction immediate ou secondaire. Mem. Acad. Chir. 96:651, 1970.

Longacre, J. J.: Correction of hypoplastic breast: Reconstruction of "nipple type breast" with local dermo-fat pedicle flaps. Plast. Reconstr. Surg. 14:431, 1954.

McIndoe, A., Rees, T.: Mammaplasty: Indications, techniques and complications. Br. J. Plast. Surg. 10:307, 1958.

McKissock, P. K.: Reduction mammaplasty with a vertical dermal flap. Plast. Reconstr. Surg. 49:245, 1972.

Pitanguy, I.: Breast hypertrophy. *Transactions of the Second International Congress of Plastic and Reconstructive Surgery, London, 1960.* Edinburgh, Livingstone, 1960, p. 509.

Schwarzmann, E.: Die Technik der Mammaplastik. Chirurg 2:932, 1930.

Skoog, T.: A technique of breast reduction. Acta Chir. Scand. 126:453, 1963.

Strömbeck, J. O.: Mammaplasty: Report of a new technique based on the two pedicle procedure. Br. J. Plast. Surg. 13:79, 1960.

Thorek, M.: *Plastic Surgery of the Breast and Abdominal Wall.* Springfield, Ill., Charles C Thomas, 1942.

20

Norman E. Hugo
Michael C. Stalnecker

Reduction Mammaplasty: Single Superiorly Based Pedicle

Reduction mammaplasty is sought by women of any age group who suffer from enlarged breasts that give rise to either emotional difficulties or physical symptoms. Included among emotional difficulties are profound social embarrassment at being large, restrictions on the type of clothing that can be worn, and a matronly appearance. Shoulder grooving by brassiere straps, neck, shoulder, and back pain, intertrigo, mammary drag or pain, and ulnar paresthesia are some of the physical symptoms. The physical symptoms are often of paramount concern in the older age group, whereas the younger age group is more concerned with the emotional symptoms.

The etiology of increased breast size to the point of disability remains obscure (Mayl et al., 1974), occurring in some women shortly after menarche; whereas in others, it is manifested in later life, after chronic enlargement.

Reduction of breast size was recorded in antiquity (Aegineta, 1847), and a brief and cogent review was published by Letterman and Schurter (1974).

The modern era of breast reduction is characterized by minimal undermining of skin flaps (Penn, 1955; Strömbeck, 1960), preoperative marking (Bames, 1948; Aufricht, 1949), form determined by the skin brassiere (Aufricht, 1949; Wise, 1956), and increased attention to nipple vascularity and innervation (Courtiss and Goldwyn, 1976; Mathes et al., 1981). Schwarzmann's (1930) observations on the subdermal blood supply of the nipple-areola complex led to the concepts of de-epithelialized pedicles. Strömbeck's (1960) operation utilized a horizontal bipedicle dermal flap that was modified in certain circumstances to a medially based pedicle (Strömbeck, 1971). Skoog's (1963) technique created a laterally based dermal pedicle. Both methods demonstrated that nipples based on unilateral dermal pedicles would survive; however, transposition of the areolar complex was often difficult and resulted in retraction, inversion, or vascular compromise. Bipedicle techniques tended to produce a boxy, stuffed look with lateral fullness.

Better aesthetic results were sought, and to that end the single superiorly based dermal pedicle offered straightforward migration of the nipple-areola complex and rapid resection of the skin and parenchymal elements. Since Weiner's initial description (Weiner et al.,

1973) and Hugo and McClellan's report (1979), there have been numerous modifications; but none offers advantages in reliability and speed (Tanski, 1980; Arufe, 1977; Conroy, 1979; Hauben, 1984).

METHOD

The Wise-Strömbeck pattern was modified to decrease tension on the vertical line of closure, which allows for a more conical, less boxy breast with less tendency for the infra-areolar portion to descend, causing the nipple to ride high. The patient is always marked out in the erect position with indelible ink and then prepared and draped in routine fashion (Fig. 20–1A). Patients are cautioned against aspirin ingestion preoperatively and checked preoperatively with a bleeding time. The enlarged nipple-areola complex is reduced to 4.5 cm in diameter, and the superior dermal pedicle is constructed (Fig. 20–1B). The entire pedicle is then elevated with at least a 1.5-cm thickness. After the skin incisions are made, the inferior aspect of the breast is amputated by means of electrocautery (Fig. 20–1C and D). This minimizes blood loss. Hemostasis is obtained throughout with electrocautery. The wounds are closed with 3-0 intradermal and 4-0 subcuticular absorbable suture. Several points should be remembered. The superiorly based pedicle may be thinned to 1.5 cm and may be as long as 18 cm, but no thinner or longer. After infolding of the pedicle, the nipple-areola complex may sag or be indented superiorly. This is self-correcting after a few days. Closure is begun at the vertical segment and then medially and laterally to avoid dog-ears. The excess is then accounted for by halving the remaining circumference as the midline is approached. Suction drains are infrequently used. Resilient gauze dressings and a surgical brassiere are applied. The patient is usually discharged within 1 or 2 days.

RESULTS

One hundred seventy-eight enlarged breasts of 89 women have been reduced by this method. The objectives of reduction include setting of the nipple-areola complex at the level of the inframammary fold, conical

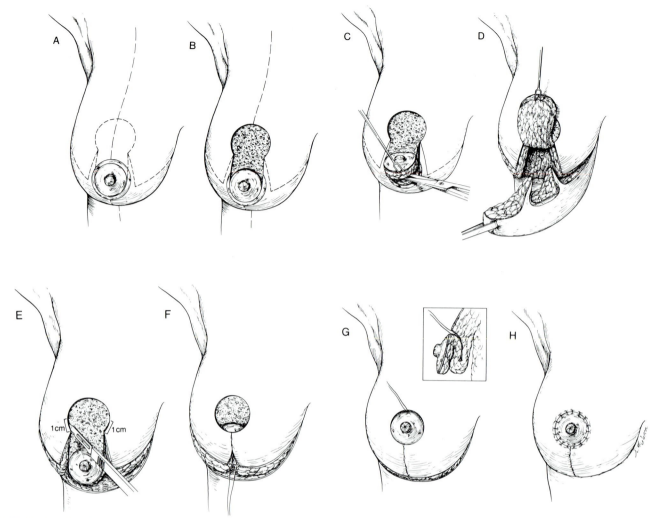

FIGURE 20–1

A, Patient marked in the upright position. The standardized Strömbeck pattern is modified by extending its length by 1 cm and narrowing the keyhole by 2 cm. The superior pedicle is de-epithelialized *(B),* and the flap is raised *(C),* before the inferior portion of the breast is amputated by electrocautery. To facilitate insetting of the pedicle *(D),* the superior portion is incised for 1 cm on each side *(E).* The vertical incisions are then closed and the nipple-areola complex set in *(F).* To facilitate superior fullness, several 5-0 nylon sutures are used to pull up the pedicle *(G).* The inferior portion is then closed *(H).*

adolescent-appearing breasts, minimal scars, the ability to breast feed, consistent viability of nipple-areola sensation, ease and speed of surgery, durability of the results, and minimal complications such as infection and hematoma. The long-term aesthetic results can be ascertained by the accompanying photographs (Figs. 20–2 to 20–7). The average weight reduction per breast was 741 gm, or 1482 gm per patient. The average duration of operation was 136 minutes (as calculated on the last 55 consecutive patients). All operations were teamed with a resident surgeon.

The complication rate is 3.9% overall and may be compared with those of other series (Table 20–1). Complete loss of the nipple-areola complex did not occur. Partial loss followed by spontaneous healing occurred in four breasts, or 2.2%. Infection occurred in three breasts, or 1.7%.

Sensation of the nipple-areola complex was not measured quantitatively; but on questioning, patients volunteered that postoperative sensation was approximately the same as preoperative sensation. Weiner's review found that after 6 months 80% of patients said sensitivity was normal or "not a problem" and that nipple erectility was always present. Nevertheless, Weiner now uses a dermoparenchymal flap in most cases to improve postoperative sensitivity (Weiner et al., 1982). In our institution we now employ the inferior wedge technique for patients with large breasts because of its advantages in circulation and sensation to the nipple-areola complex. However, the single superior pedicle is still applicable in some patients with minimal hypertrophy. It should be noted that patients with larger breasts have less sensation before reduction mammaplasty than their counterparts with small breasts having augmentations (Courtiss and Goldwyn, 1976) and that objective postoperative tests show sensation to be more diminished than thought after patient questioning alone (Hauben, 1984).

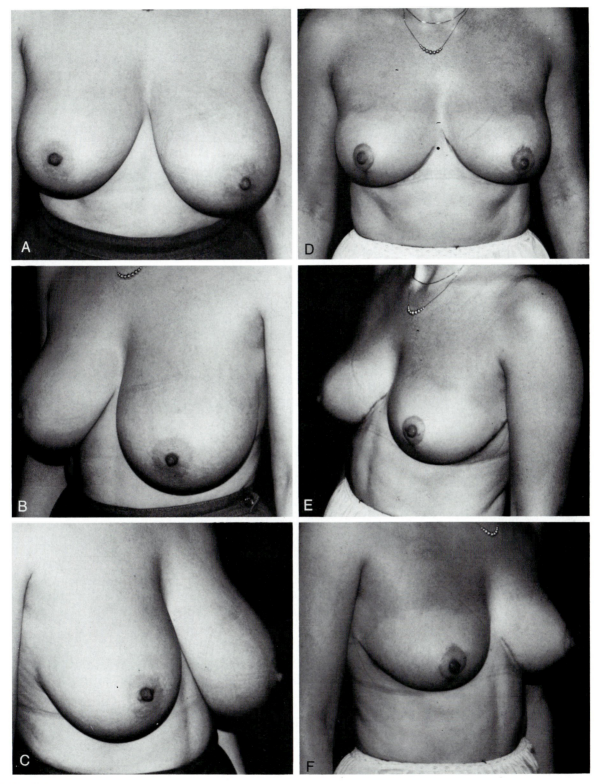

FIGURE 20–2
A to *C*, A 29-year-old woman with asymmetrically enlarged breasts. *D* to *F*, Three months after resection of 370 gm on the right and 607 gm on the left.

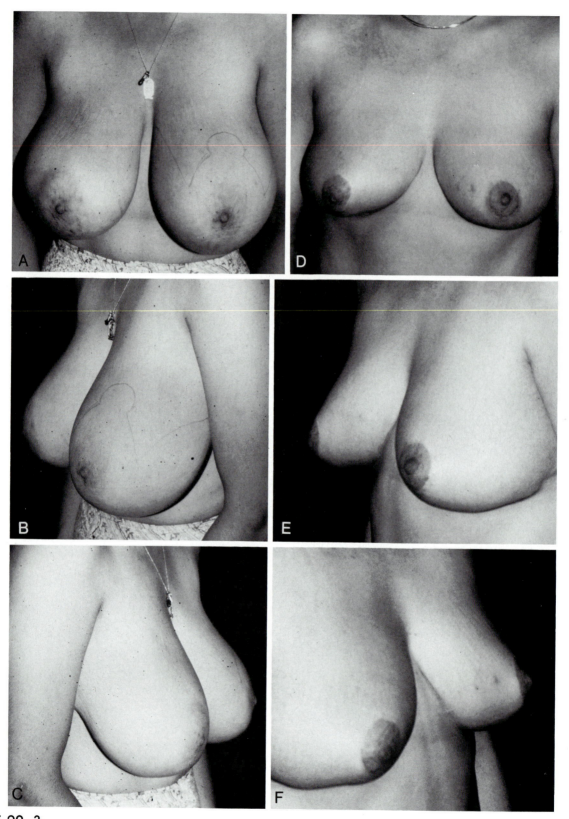

FIGURE 20–3

A to *C*, A 20-year-old woman with emotional and physical distress from large breasts. *D* to *F*, One year after resection of 952 gm on the right and 1050 gm on the left.

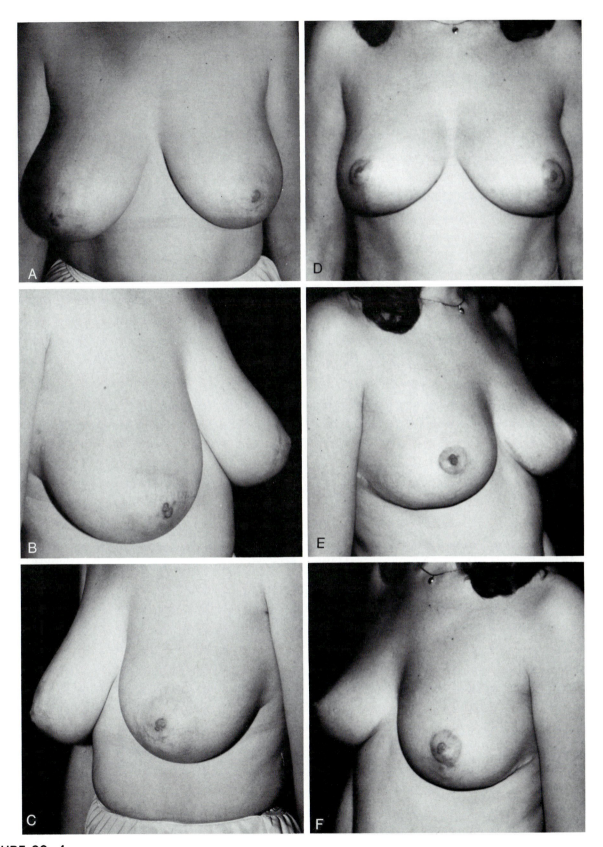

FIGURE 20–4
A to *C*, A 22-year-old with ptotic, enlarged breasts. *D* to *F*, Two and one-half years after resection of 375 gm on each side.

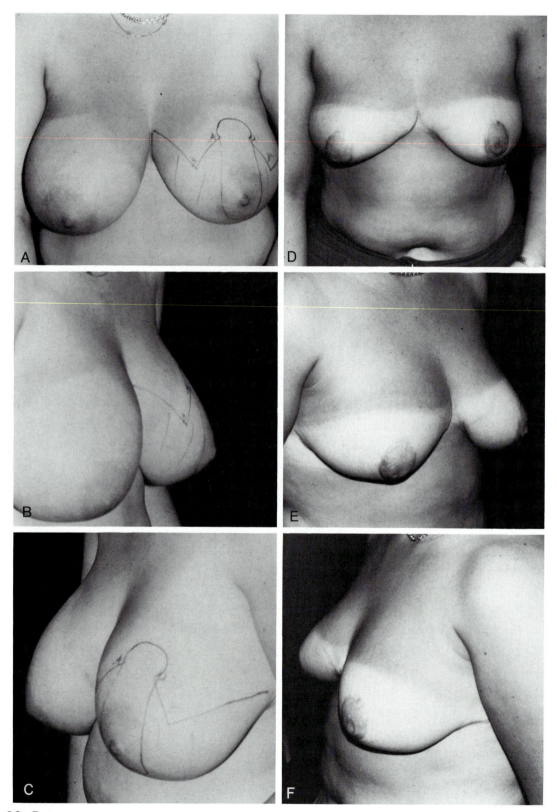

FIGURE 20–5
Before *(A to C)* and 1 year after *(D to F)* views of a 19-year-old woman. Resection of 703 gm on the left and 862 gm on the right.

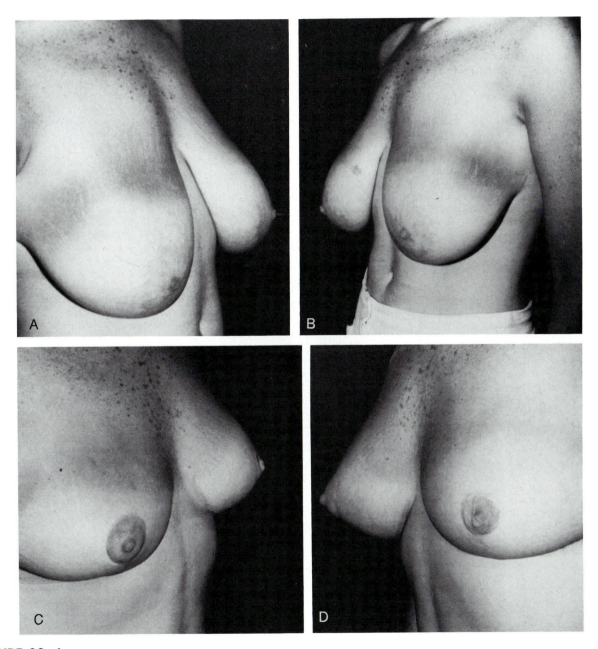

‹FIGURE 20–6
Nineteen-year-old woman before *(A* and *B)* and 1 year after *(C* and *D)* resection of 540 gm on the right and 480 gm on the left.

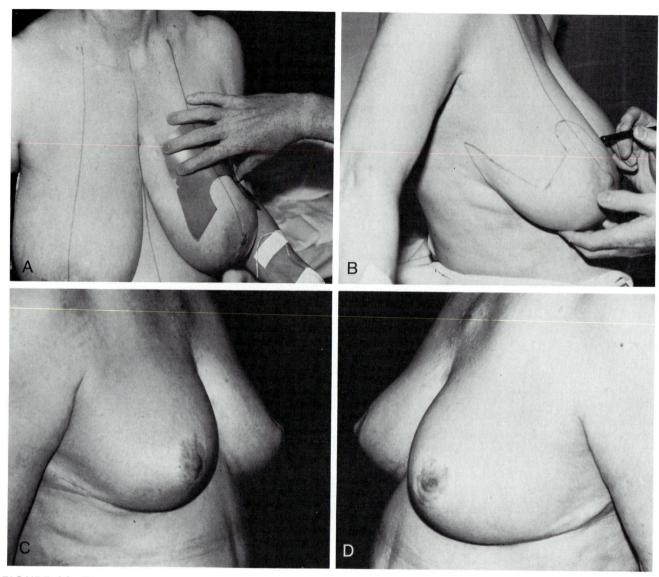

FIGURE 20–7
A and *B*, Marking a 48-year-old woman with a modified pattern in the erect position. *C* and *D*, Three and one-half years after resection of 1200 gm on the right and 930 gm on the left.

TABLE 20–1
Comparison of Complications Following Reduction Mammaplasty

AUTHORS	METHOD	NO. BREASTS	PARTIAL AREOLAR LOSS	COMPLETE NIPPLE-AREOLA LOSS
Strömbeck (1964)	Horizontal bipedicle	219	7 (3.2%)	0
McKissock (1972)	Vertical bipedicle	125	1 (0.8%)	0
Cramer and Chong (1976)	Superior pedicle	180	1 (0.6%)	0
Courtiss and Goldwyn (1977)	Inferior pedicle	24	1 (4.1%)	0
Hugo (1979)	Superior pedicle	178	4 (2.2%)	0
Stark (1981)	Wedge resection	202	7 (3.5%)	2 (1%)
Weiner (1982)*	Superior pedicle†	360	1 (0.3%)	0

*Includes mastopexies and subcutaneous mastectomies.
†Both dermal and dermoparenchymal.

References

Aegineta, P.: The Seven Books of Paulus Aegineta, Vol. 2, Book 6, Trans. F. Adams. London, London Syndenham Society, 1847, Sect. 46, p. 334.

Arufe, H. N., Erenfryd, A., Saubidet, M.: Mammaplasty with a single, verticle, superiorly-based pedicle to support the nipple-areola. Plast. Reconstr. Surg. 60:221, 1977.

Aufricht, G.: Mammaplasty for pendulous breasts: Empiric and geometric planning. Plast. Reconstr. Surg. 4:13, 1949.

Bames, H. O.: Reduction of massive breast hypertrophy. Plast. Reconstr. Surg. 3:560, 1948.

Conroy, W. C.: Reduction mammaplasty with maximum superior subdermal vascular pedicle. Ann. Plast. Surg. 2:189, 1979.

Courtiss, E. H., Goldwyn, R. M.: Reduction mammaplasty by the inferior pedicle technique. Plast. Reconstr. Surg. 59:500, 1977.

Courtiss, E. H., Goldwyn, R. M.: Breast sensation before and after plastic surgery. Plast. Reconstr. Surg. 58:1, 1976.

Cramer, L. M., Chong, J. K.: Unipedicle cutaneous flap: Areolar-nipple transposition on an end-bearing superiorly based flap. In Georgiade, N. G.: *Reconstructive Breast Surgery*. St. Louis, C. V. Mosby, 1976.

Hauben, D. J.: Experience and refinements with supero-medial dermal pedicle for nipple-areola transposition in reduction mammaplasty. Aesthetic Plast. Surg. 8:189, 1984.

Hugo, N. E., McClellan, R. M.: Reduction mammaplasty with a single superiorly based pedicle. Plast. Reconstr. Surg. 63:230, 1979.

Letterman, G., Schurter, M.: Will Durston's "mammaplasty." Plast. Reconstr. Surg. 58:48, 1974.

Mathes, S. J., Wang, T. N., Vasconez, L. O.: Vascular anatomy of the breast: Experimental and clinical considerations. Presented at American Society Aesthetic Plastic Surgery, Houston, Texas, April 1981.

Mayl, N., Vasconez, L., Jurkiewicz, M.: Treatment of macromastia in the actively enlarging breast. Plast. Reconstr. Surg. 54:6, 1974.

McKissock, P.: Reduction mammaplasty with a verticle dermal flap. Plast. Reconstr. Surg. 49:245, 1972.

Penn, J.: Breast reduction. Br. J. Plast. Surg. 7:357, 1955.

Schwarzmann, E.: Die Technik der Mammaplastik. Chirurg 2:932, 1930.

Skoog, T.: A technique of breast reduction: Transposition of the nipple on a cutaneous vascular pedicle. Acta Chir. Scand. 126:453, 1963.

Stark, R. B.: Breast reduction and asymmetry. In Stark, R. B.: *Aesthetic Plastic Surgery*. Boston, Little, Brown, 1981, p. 409.

Strömbeck, J. O.: Mammaplasty: Report of a new technique based on the two pedicle procedure. Br. J. Plast. Surg. 13:79, 1960.

Strömbeck, J. O.: Reduction mammaplasty. Surg. Clin. North Am. 51:453, 1971.

Tanski, E. V.: A new method for prophylactic mastectomy, reduction mammaplasty, and mastopexy. Plast. Reconstr. Surg. 65:314, 1980.

Weiner, D., Aiache, A., Silver, L., et al.: A single dermal pedicle for nipple transposition in subcutaneous mastectomy, reduction mammaplasty or mastopexy. Plast. Reconstr. Surg. 51:115, 1973.

Weiner, D. L., Dolich, B. H., Michat, M. I.: Reduction mammaplasty utilizing the superior pedicle technique: A six-year retrospective. Aesthetic Plast. Surg. 6:7, 1982.

Wise, R. J.: A preliminary report of a method of planning the mammaplasty. Plast. Reconstr. Surg. 17:367, 1956.

21

Liacyr Ribeiro

Mammaplasties: The Triangle Technique

From Verchère, in 1898, through Morestin (1907), Lexer (1912), Kraske (1923), Passot (1923), Dufourmentel and Mouly (1961), Arufe (1977), and others, to our time, with Peixoto (1980), plastic surgeons have been concerned with breast shape and scars. Whenever they achieved excellent shape, they failed in the size of scars, and vice versa.

Breasts with small scars always left much to be desired: usually they were flat, frequently flaccid, and empty of content, in anticipation of skin retraction, according to Peixoto's concept. The immediate results in these cases were generally not pleasing to the eye or to the touch. Still within the scope of this concept, vertical scars were too long, resulting in a rather ungraceful look.

Our idea is based on Peixoto's concept of tissue retraction, combined with our pedicle, described for the first time in 1969 and published in 1973 (Ribeiro), when a better shape of breast was achieved, since the emptying of content was compensated for by the introduction of the inferiorly based pedicle originating from the inferior pole. We conceived a geometric figure marking (the isosceles triangle shape), which varied in accordance with each different case.

Because the marking, though triangle-shaped, becomes so much like a gothic arch, the technique is also known as the Gothic technique. Such variation in outline is applied mainly when vertical scars become lengthened.

According to our experience, indications are still restricted to ptoses, small hypertrophies, medium hypertrophies, and large hypertrophies; the latter situation is generally found among patients with juvenile hypertrophy. The technique is totally contraindicated for giant hypertrophies and for cases in which resections are larger than 750 gm on each side.

HISTORICAL BACKGROUND

We often think that we have described something new or created a new technique. However, very frequently, if not most of the time, we are simply rediscovering old ideas. This is easily explained, because the search for solutions to old problems leads us to the past. A brief search through the bibliographic references will prove

that many facts that appear to be new and sensational, were described over 50 years ago. The objective of this historical background is precisely to focus on this.

In 1898, Verchère excised a small triangle from the inferior pole of the breast for the purpose of reducing ptosis, obviously leaving scars and shapes short of the ideal. Thirty years later, by means of daring methods, Dartigues (1928) would obtain the same results.

In 1905, Morestin's technique demonstrated that by excising a segment of skin, gland, and fat or simple skin, an elevation of the breast was achieved and the outcome was a single but long scar in the fold.

Like Passot (1923), who attained a single final scar only on the inframammary fold, we published (Ribeiro and Backer, 1973, Ribeiro, 1975) a technique that resulted in a horizontal scar on the fold and another one around the nipple.

Whereas Passot used to immobilize the skin, we utilized the vascular supply of the nipple-areola complex through the inferior pole of the breast. Some time later, Robbins (1977), Courtiss and Goldwyn (1977), Reich (1979), Georgiade (1979), and other authors would corroborate our idea.

Passot obtained the same kind of scarring and the same problems we incurred. Actually, unsightly scarring always occurred in the horizontal incision line that extended above the sternum (internally) and toward the axillary line (externally), in which areas poor cicatrization is unquestionable.

With Lexer's (1912) technique the lengthening of the scars occurred in the caudocephalad manner, directly the inverse of that of Peixoto's (1980) method and similar to Arié's (1957) technique. To compensate for the fold overpassing, Lexer conceived a horizontal scar and was considered the father of the inverted T method. Eleven years later, by improving Lexer's idea, Kraske (1923) would enlarge the incisions and scars, obtaining the same inverted T as the end result (Fig. 21–1A to C).

In 1922, Thorek (1942) reported the first nipple-areola free graft technique, a procedure used by many surgeons to this day.

Lotsch (1955) published a report of his technique in 1928 following Lexer's method, although Lotsch indicated the undermining of the skin for the areola elevation.

The result—a single vertical scar and, naturally, the

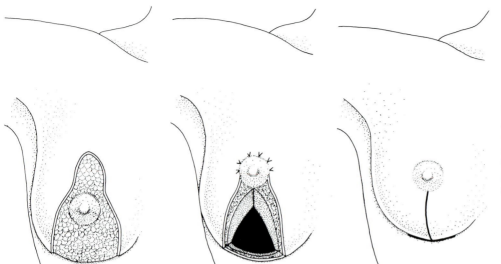

FIGURE 21–1
A, Lexer-Kraske triangular outline. *B*, Tissues are resected, and the areola is fixed in its new position. *C*, End result: inverted-T–shaped scar.

areolar scar—was also achieved some time later by Arié, Peixoto, and others.

In 1925, Dartigues (1928) proved that a small elliptical incision between the areola and the fold, for the purpose of elevating the breast, would be an accurate indication for cases of minimal ptosis. Today we believe that prosthesis implanting is the most advisable procedure for such cases.

In 1928, Biesenberger published his technique, popular for many years. In many cases, though, wide undermining, followed by daring rotations, caused tissue necrosis.

In this historical review, stimulated by our interest in techniques used to obtain reduced scars, we could not fail to mention Holländer (1924), father of the L-shaped scar, and Dufourmentel and Mouly (1961), who adhered to the technique.

Other similar techniques followed, especially with regard to the handling of dermal lipoglandular flaps, whose results would always be the same L.

In 1930, Schwarzmann increased the previous contributions with his method of nipple maneuver, in which he diffused the dermal or subdermal vascularization of the nipple-areola complex.

More recently an analysis of our contemporary colleagues' procedures reveals the following.

In 1957, Arié presented his method, though the technique failed with regard to the final scar, which extended beyond the submammary fold. In 1957, Pitanguy (1957) achieved optimal results by using Arié's technique through a lateral approach. This procedure originated his well-known technique: wider markings and a consequent lengthening of the scars.

By analyzing Peixoto's technique, we can see that, even though it may be similar to those of Lexer, Dartigues, Arié, Lotsch, and others, it presents a different

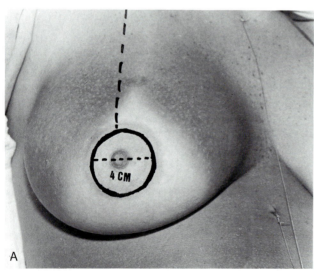
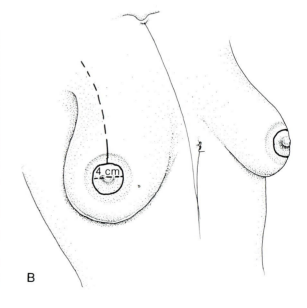

FIGURE 21–2
A and *B*, The new areola outline with a 4-cm diameter.

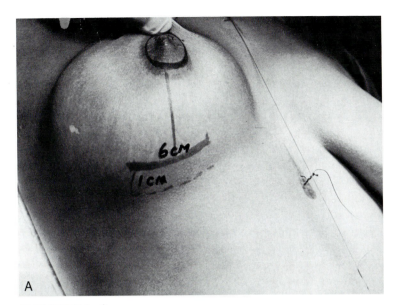

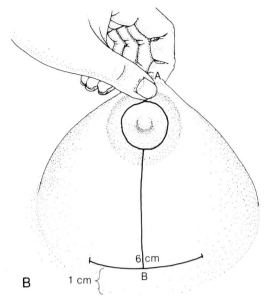

FIGURE 21–3
A and *B*, The new fold line is drawn 1 cm above the original fold. This line should be 6 cm long.

approach, for it is based on the progressive retraction of the dermoepidermal complex.

The results obtained by Peixoto, published in 1980 and 1984 (variation), were accomplished differently from those of the previous techniques used and are indicated for any kind of hypertrophy. However, our experiences with large hypertrophies and with breasts with little stretching quality brought about poor immediate results, because of the flattening and the flaccid consistency those breasts acquired. The solution found to correct such deficiencies was the introduction of an inferiorly based pedicle (pedicle 1) in the triangle technique outline. Such a technique, combined with Peixoto's concepts, brings forth a satisfactory outcome in breast shape and length of scars as well as firmness and consistency.

OPERATIVE TECHNIQUE

The preoperative markings are made with the patient in a half-seated position on the surgical table under general anesthesia.

The outline of the new areola size is determined, which, in keeping with the limitations of the technique, should have a diameter of 4 cm (Fig. 21–2).

A line is drawn from the middle portion of the clavicle down to the areola and is extended down to the mammary fold. Above this line, a new fold trace is marked, based on the fact that the retraction of the breast will move the fold down. The new fold line should be 6 cm long and equidistant to the middle line originating from the border of the areola (Fig. 21–3).

FIGURE 21–4
A and *B*, Point A is designated.

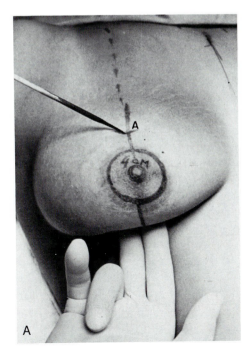

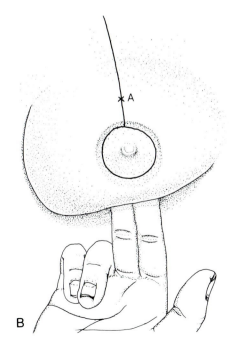

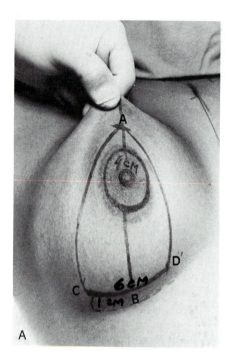

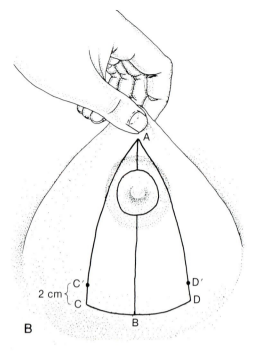

FIGURE 21–5
A and *B*, Points A, B, C, and D are joined to shape the triangle. Points C′ and D′ are located 2 cm above points C and D.

Point A is designated by means of the classic maneuver of projection of the fold on the upper pole of the breast (Fig. 21–4). The edge of the semiclavicular line is joined to the new fold line for determining point B.

Once points A and B are determined, they are linked to points C and D to shape the triangle (Fig. 21–5). Points C′ and D′ are placed 2 cm above C and D. Such points are variable according to the length (shorter or longer) of the final vertical scar.

Point B, as well as the midsternal line, serves as the base for good symmetry and to facilitate the transposi-

tion of the pattern to the second breast. The distance should be approximately 10 cm (Fig. 21–6).

The marked area, or triangular area, is de-epithelialized (Fig. 21–7), an incision is made 1 to 2 cm below the areola, and a lateral and medial incision is made into the de-epithelialized area to the muscular wall to establish the inferiorly based pedicle.

After establishing the pedicle, variable in thickness and length, the excess tissue is excised from the superior pole of the breast. The fat and/or glandular tissue can be resected either in segments or in a unique block (Figs. 21–8 to 21–10).

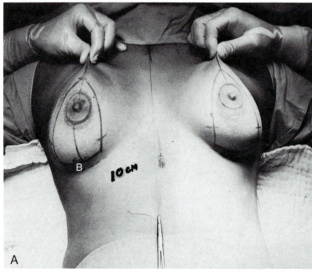

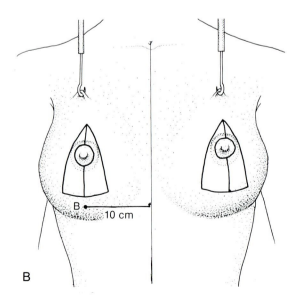

FIGURE 21–6
A and *B*, Point B is about 10 cm from the midsternal line.

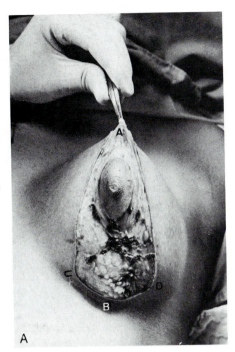
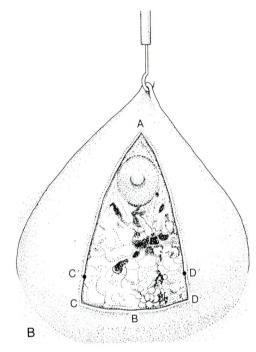

FIGURE 21–7
A and *B*, The outlined area is de-epithelialized.

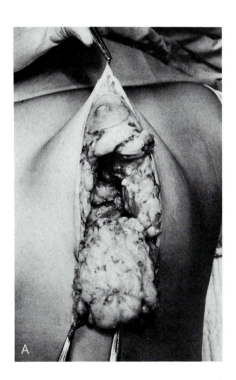
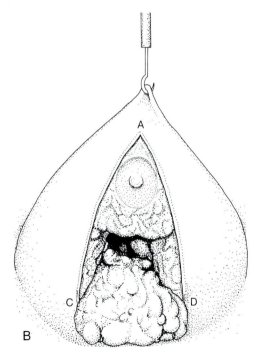

FIGURE 21–8
A and *B*, The making of the pedicle is initiated.

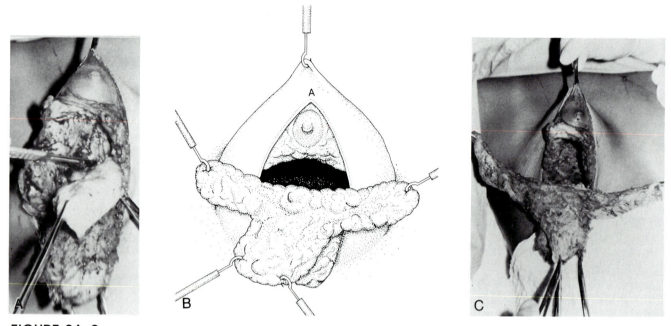

FIGURE 21–9

A to *C*, Excess *en bloc* tissue excision. Note the lateral and medial extensions of the resection.

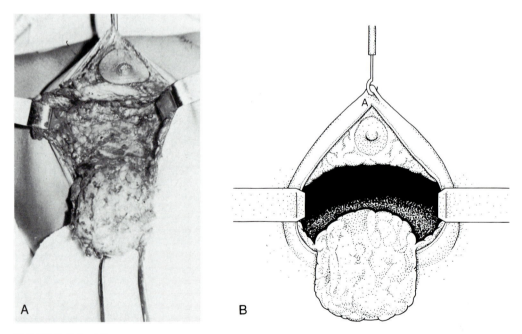

FIGURE 21–10

A and *B*, The pedicle is finished and the resection completed.

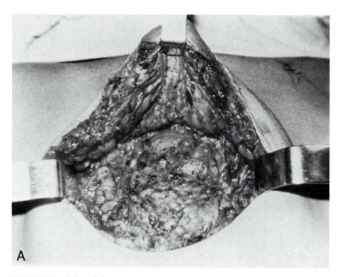
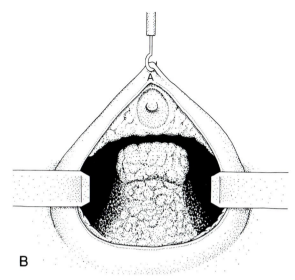

FIGURE 21-11
A and *B*, Fixation of the pedicle, with its tip bent over itself, on the muscular wall.

The pedicle is fixed on the aponeurosis of the pectoralis major muscle, with interrupted nonabsorbable sutures, with the tip of the pedicle bent, or not, over itself (Fig. 21–11).

The closure is accomplished by joining points C′ and D′ to B, which will originate the formation of two dog-ears, because points C′ and D′ measure 2 cm and come together at the center of the horizontal line, which is 6 cm long (Fig. 21–12). As a result of that, the new fold line will be shortened from 6 to 4 cm. Nevertheless, the resection of the dog-ears will bring the fold line to 6 cm again (Figs. 21–13 and 21–14).

REMARKS

The marking of the new areola site is based on a distance of approximately 4 cm, starting from point B, or the convergence of points C′ and D′ at B, up to the inferior border of the new areola.

The suture is realized in two ways (dermal and epidermal), with nonabsorbable sutures (5-0 nylon) in the vertical and horizontal lines.

The same kind of suture is used for the areola, following the "Greek bar" or the "U stitches" pattern (Fig. 21–14).

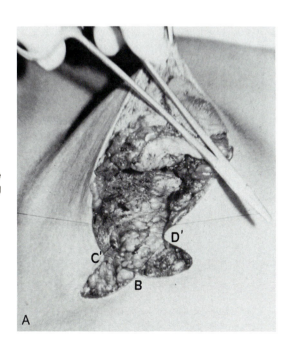
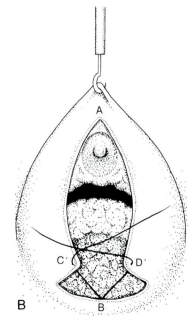

FIGURE 21-12
A and *B*, Points C′ and D′ are joined at B to allow the framing of the breast.

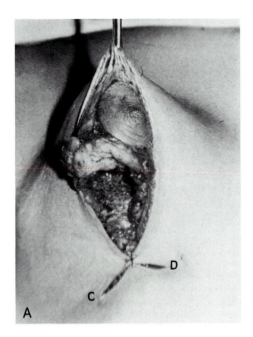

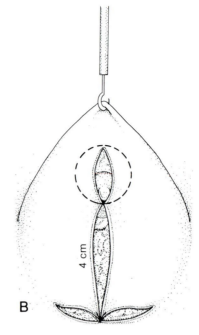

FIGURE 21–13
A and *B*, The lower border of the areola is 4 cm from the submammary fold.

INDICATIONS

The technique is applicable to small, medium, or large mammary hypertrophies. In the small hypertrophies (Fig. 21–15) generally associated with ptosis, there is no need for glandular tissue resection in most cases. Util-

izing a pedicle and changing the position of the tissues are enough to obtain excellent results.

In medium hypertrophies, with or without ptosis, some tissue (fat and/or glandular), which, in general, does not exceed 300 gm on each side, is resected (Fig. 21–16).

Text continued on page 277

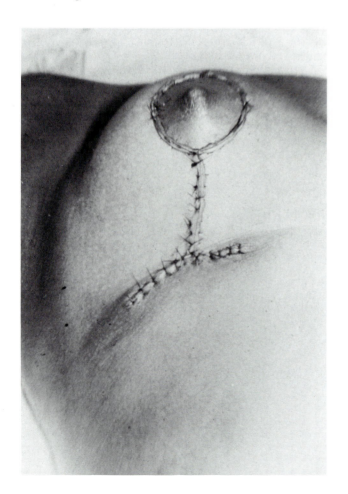

FIGURE 21–14
End result: a 6-cm scar on the new submammary fold.

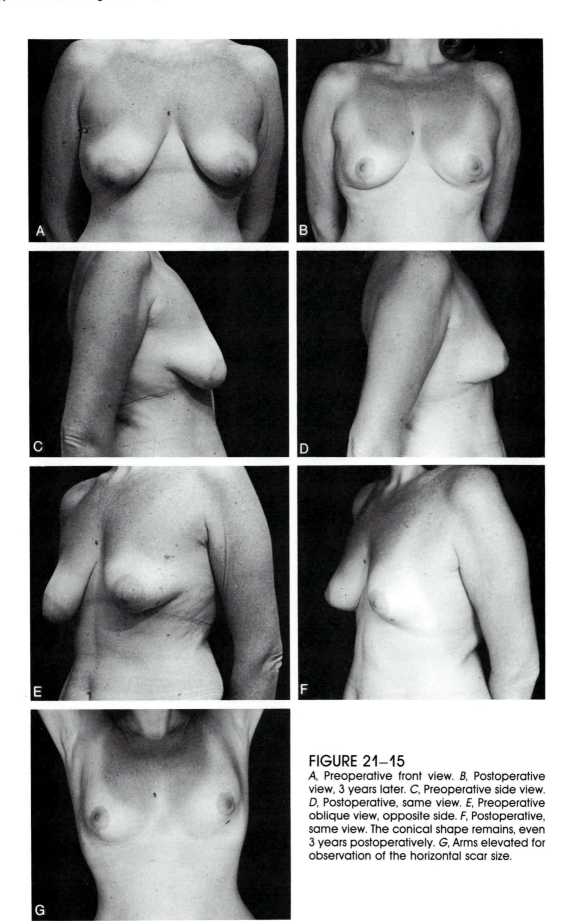

FIGURE 21–15
A, Preoperative front view. *B*, Postoperative view, 3 years later. *C*, Preoperative side view. *D*, Postoperative, same view. *E*, Preoperative oblique view, opposite side. *F*, Postoperative, same view. The conical shape remains, even 3 years postoperatively. *G*, Arms elevated for observation of the horizontal scar size.

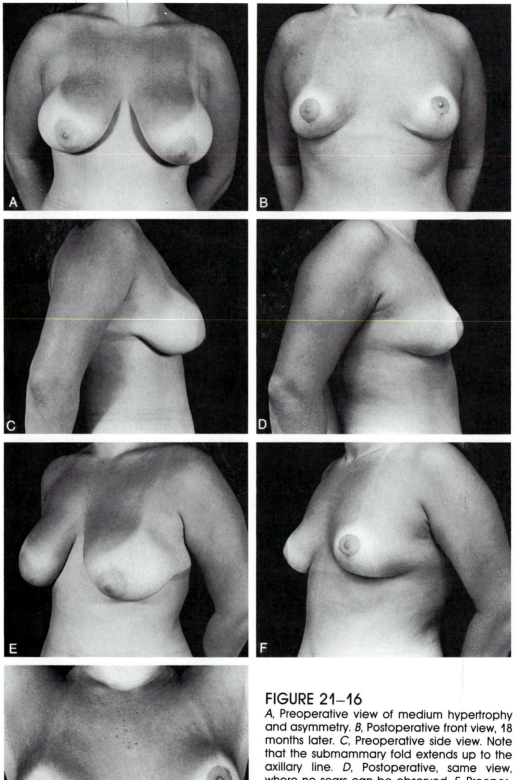

FIGURE 21–16

A, Preoperative view of medium hypertrophy and asymmetry. *B*, Postoperative front view, 18 months later. *C*, Preoperative side view. Note that the submammary fold extends up to the axillary line. *D*, Postoperative, same view, where no scars can be observed. *E*, Preoperative oblique view for evaluation of the degree of ptosis and hypertrophy. *F*, Postoperative view with areolar elevation. The lateral and medial scar edges cannot be seen. *G*, Arms elevated for observation of the horizontal scar, measuring approximately 6 cm.

For large hypertrophies the technique is limited to juvenile hypertrophy. In young patients the skin is more resilient and retracts better after the resection (base of the technique procedure). Between 400 and 750 gm of breast tissue is resected from each breast (Fig. 21–17).

The technique is not indicated for patients with skin with little elasticity or for older patients with large hypertrophy, but it is perfectly suitable for those with simple ptosis, who do not require a prosthetic implant and in whom resection of the triangle is sufficient.

It is obvious that in the cases of simple ptosis, with manipulation of the tissue and the pedicle, there will not be significant augmentation of the breast. However, the breasts will be more conical, with aesthetic shapes more consistent and in the correct position (Fig. 21–18).

In giant hypertrophies, where the resections exceed the average of 1 kg on each side, the technique is not indicated. The largest resection possible in this technique is 750 gm on each side, even in young patients.

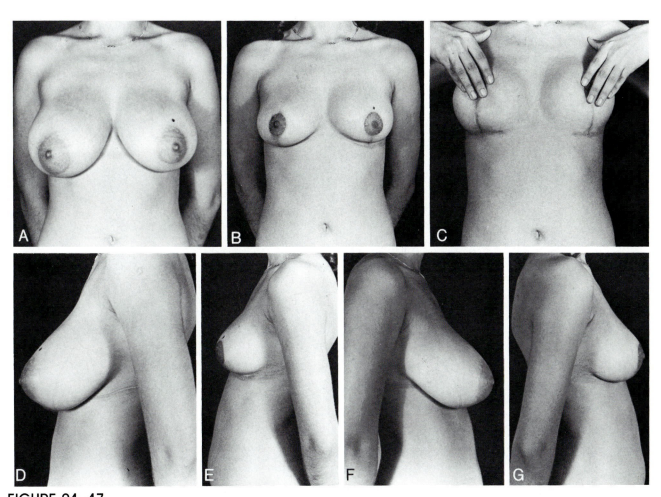

FIGURE 21–17

A, Preoperative front view of a young patient with severe hypertrophy. *B*, Postoperative, 1 year later. A resection of 700 gm on each side was required. *C*, The horizontal scar of approximately 6 cm can now be judged. *D*, Preoperative left side view. *E*, Postoperative side view, in which it can be seen that the retraction occurred in the anteroposterior direction. *F*, Preoperative opposite side view. Asymmetry can be noted between the breast and the torso. *G*, Postoperatively, same view. Note the good symmetry and the pleasing shape achieved.

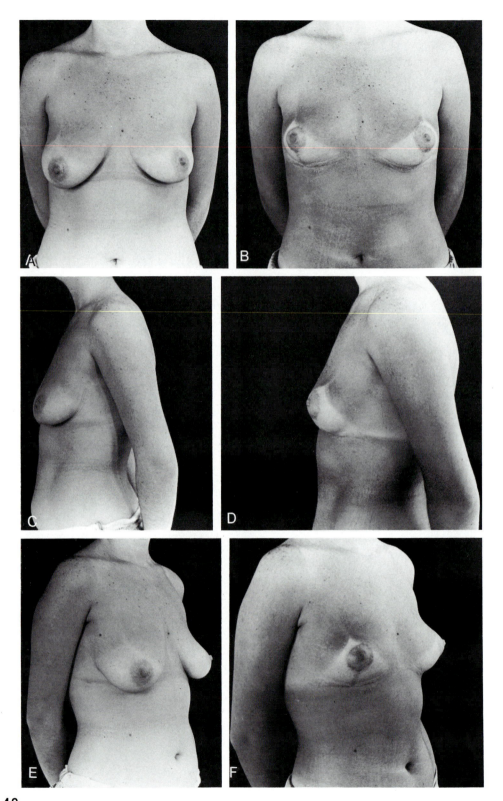

FIGURE 21–18

A, Preoperative ptosis and mild asymmetry. *B*, Postoperative front view, 9 months later. *C*, Preoperative side view of the flat breast. *D*, Postoperatively, same view. An aesthetic shape has been achieved. *E*, Preoperative oblique view of flattening of the upper pole. *F*, Postoperatively. Ptosis has been corrected, and the upper pole is filled.

COMPLICATIONS

Over the past 6 years, the most frequent complications, either immediate or delayed, have derived from (1) hypertrophic scarring (12%), (2) asymmetry (10%), (3) dehiscence of the suture at the convergence level of points C' and D' and B (2%), (4) hematomas (1%), (5) infection of one of the breasts (0.1%), (6) infection of both breasts (0%), and (7) necrosis of the areola (partial or total) (0%).

CONCLUSIONS

We consider valid any attempt to reduce scars while achieving better shapes. From our standpoint, conical-shaped breasts are the most aesthetic; however, we believe that this procedure cannot be indicated for every case. We wish to emphasize here that our experience proves that this technique is restricted to ptosis, small hypertrophy, medium hypertrophy, and large hypertrophy (juvenile only). Patients with large and giant hypertrophy whose resections are estimated to be over 750 gm on each side should not undergo this type of procedure.

References

Arié, G.: Una nueva técnica de mastoplastia. Rev. Latinoam. Cir. Plást. 3:22, 1957.

Arufe, H.: Mammaplasty with a single vertical superior pedicle to support the nipple-areola. Plast. Reconstr. Surg. 60:221, 1977.

Backer, E., Ribeiro, L.: Technical considerations. In: Georgiade, N. G. (ed.): *Reconstructive Breast Surgery*. St. Louis, C. V. Mosby, 1976, p. 195.

Biesenberger, H.: Eine neue Methode der Mammaplastik. Zentrl. Chir. 55:2382, 1928.

Bozola, A. R.: Mamoplastia: Técnica de Arié invertida (no ta prévia). Anais da la Jornada Sul Bras. Cir. Plást. 157:160, 1984.

Bozola, A. R.: Sistematizacao tática da mamoplastia em "L." Anais da la Jornada Sul Bras. Cir. Plást. 365:374, 1984.

Courtiss, E. H., Goldwyn, R. M.: Reduction mammaplasty by the inferior pedicle technique. Plast. Reconstr. Surg. 59:500, 1977.

Dartigues, L.: État actuel de la cirurgie esthétique mammaire. Monde Med. 38:75, 1928.

Dufourmentel, C., Mouly, R.: Plastique mammaire par la méthode oblique. Ann. Chir. Plast. 6:45, 1961.

Georgiade, N. G., Serafin, D., Riefkohl, R., Georgiade, G.: Reduction mammaplasty utilizing an inferior pedicle nipple-areolar flap. Ann. Plast. Surg. 3:211, 1979a.

Georgiade, N. G., Serafin, D., Riefkohl, R., Georgiade, G.: Is there a reduction mammaplasty for "all seasons"? Plast. Reconstr. Surg. 63:765, 1979b.

Holländer, J.: Die Operationen der Mammahypertrophie und der Hängebrust. Dtsche. Med. Wochenschr. 50:1400, 1924.

Joseph, J.: Zur Operationen der Hipertrophischen Hängebrust Dtsche. Med. Wochenchr. 51:1103, 1925.

Kraske, H.: Die Operationen der Atrophischen und Hipertrophischen Hängebrust. München Med. Wochenschr. 70:672, 1923.

Lexer, E. Hypertrophie Bei Der Mammae. München Med. Wochenschr. 52:2702, 1912.

Lexer, E.: *Die Freien Transplantation*. Stuttgart, Ferdinand Enke, 1919.

Lexer, E.: Die Gemste Wiederherstellangs. *Chirurgie*, Vol. 2. Leipzig, 1931.

Lotsch, G. M.: Operationen und der weiblichen Brust. In: Bier, Braun, Kummel (eds.): Chirurgische Operationslehre. Leipzig, A. Barth Verlag, 1955.

Morestin, H.: Hypertrophie mammaire traitée par la resection discoide. Bull. Soc. Chir. Paris 33:649, 1907.

Passot, R.: La cirurgie esthétique pure. Hôpital Paris 11:184, 1923.

Peixoto, G.: Reduction mammaplasty: A personal technique. Plast. Reconstr. Surg. 65:217, 1980.

Peixoto, G.: Reduction mammaplasty: Conceptual evolution. In: *Transactions of the VIII International Congress of Plastic and Reconstructive Surgery, Montreal, 1983*, p. 543.

Peixoto, G.: Reduction mammaplasty. Aesthetic Plast. Surg. 8:231, 1984.

Pitanguy, I.: Breast hypertrophy. In: *Transactions of the 2nd International Congress of Plastic Surgery*. Edinburgh, Livingstone, 1960, p. 509.

Prudente, A.: Sep. Arg. Cir. Clin. Exp. Vol. 6, No. 2, 3rd Abril-Junho, 1942.

Prudente, A.: *Contribuicrão ao estudo da plástica mamária: Cirurgia Estetica dos Seios*. Sao Paulo, Ed. Publicatas, 1936.

Reich, J.: The advantages of a lower central breast segment in reduction mammaplasty. Aesthetic Plast. Surg. 3:47, 1979.

Ribeiro, L.: Mastoplastia: Modificación personal de técnica. Prensa Med. Arg. 60:944, 1973.

Ribeiro, L.: A new technique for reduction mammaplasty. Plast. Reconstr. Surg. 55:330, 1975.

Ribeiro, L.: Late follow-up in reduction mammaplasty: Importance of the inferior pedicle. In Williams, B. (ed.): *Transactions of the VIII International Congress of Plastic and Reconstructive Surgery, Montreal, 1983*, p. 547.

Ribeiro, L., Backer, E.: Mastoplastia con pediculo de seguridad. Rev. Esp. Cir. Plást. 16:223, 1973.

Ribeiro, L., Backer, E.: Based pedicles in mammaplasty. In: Georgiade, N. G. (ed.): *Aesthetic Breast Surgery*. Baltimore, Williams & Wilkins, 1983, p. 260.

Ribeiro, L.: In: *Transactions of the VIII International Congress of Plastic Surgery, Montreal, 1983*.

Ribeiro, L.: Mastoplastia, una nova conduta: Forma com pequenas cicatrizes. Anais do XXI Cong. Bras. de Cirur. Plást. Rio de Janeiro, 1984, p. 43.

Robbins, T. H.: A reduction mammaplasty with the areola-nipple based on an inferior dermal pedicle. Plast. Reconstr. Surg. 59:64, 1977.

Schwarzmann, E.: Die Tecnik der Mammaplastik. Chirurg 2:932, 1930.

Sepulveda, R. A.: Tratamento das assimetrias mamárias. Rev. Bras. Cir. 71:11, 1981.

Thorek, M.: *Plastic Surgery of the Breast and Abdominal Wall*. Springfield, Ill., Charles C Thomas, 1942.

Verchère, F.: Mastopexie laterale contre la mastoptose hypertrophique. Méd. Mod. 9:540, 1898.

22

Ronaldo Pontes

Reduction Mammaplasty: The Lateral Technique

Among surgeons who perform reduction mammaplasty, there is a general trend toward techniques resulting in minimal scars. Attempts to attain this goal are commendable, and many papers have been published, some of them presenting excellent ideas (Peixoto, 1980).

Although I join this trend, I think that breast shape should not be jeopardized in favor of a small scar. The lateral technique is directed toward obtaining small scars and breasts of good shape.

RATIONALE

The basis of this technique is essentially a lateral incision shaped like a curve with internal concavity. This leads to short horizontal and vertical scars and allows an outward displacement of the inferomedial quadrant of the breast. The medial extremities of the horizontal scars are thus pulled apart.

INDICATIONS

The lateral technique is indicated for breasts with a slight or medium degree of hypertrophy on which skin resection must also be performed.

ANESTHESIA

General anesthesia is used in all cases. Estriol succinate, flurazepam, metoplamide, metoclopramide, and cimetidine are given the night before the operation.

Alprazolam, metoclopramide, and cimetidine are administrated 60 to 90 minutes before the operation. Anesthetic induction starts with thiopetal, diallilbisnortoxiferin, and fentanyl. Oxygen is given for 3 to 5 minutes, and the patient is intubated. The patient is slowly raised to the sitting position while cardiac function and blood pressure are checked, and anesthesia is maintained with halothane and fentanyl or halothane, nitrous oxide, and fentanyl. No blood transfusion is given. Ringer's lactate is used for fluid replacement.

After surgery is completed, oxygen is given for 10 to 15 minutes under assisted respiration. Atropine and neostigmine are administered. The endotracheal tube is removed as soon as the patient is breathing normally.

TECHNIQUE

Reduction mammaplasty by the lateral technique is based both on new skin markings (see Figs. 22–21 C and 22–29B) and on a type of glandular surgery that I have performed for some years (Pontes, 1973, 1981).

Two variations are used. In variation I a plane resection is done perpendicular to the thoracic wall. Variation II starts as does variation I, but another incision is made in a plane parallel to the thoracic wall. The amount of reduction is increased as the level of that plane is raised.

The photographic sequence (Figs. 22–1 to 22–37) describes the technique in detail.

COMPLICATIONS

The technique does not seem to lead to any particular complication. If the skin is too tense, the medial segment of the horizontal scar can become slanted downward.

Otherwise, complications do not differ from those encountered in other techniques, such as hematoma, hypertrophic scars, and residual dog-ears.

POSTOPERATIVE CARE

Stitches are removed by the ninth day. A brassiere must be worn during the 6 weeks following surgery. Then the patient may resume her normal life.

Text continued on page 308

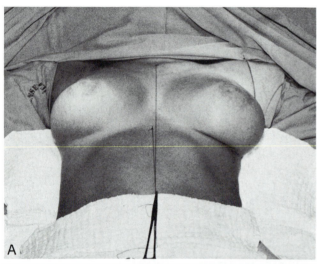

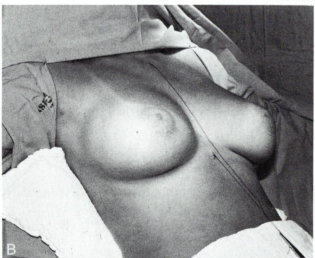

FIGURE 22–1

A and *B*, Patient ready for surgery, in a half-sitting position, with abducted arms. Front and side views.

FIGURE 22–2
Marking for incisions of the lateral technique. Note the curved lines AF and AB. Distance AB to AC measures 5 to 7 cm. Note the short submammary markings.

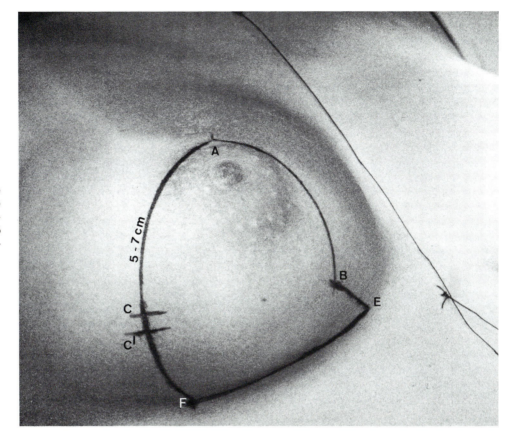

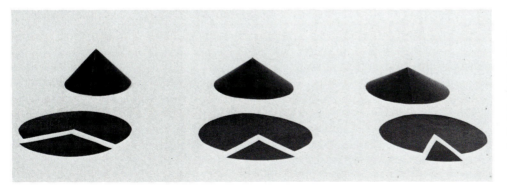

FIGURE 22–3
Aperture of angle ABC determines the base and shape of the cone. The same principles apply to the mammary cone. A wider angle will result in a narrower and higher breast cone with a smaller basis.

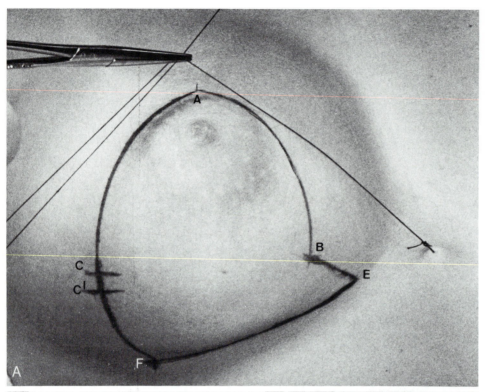

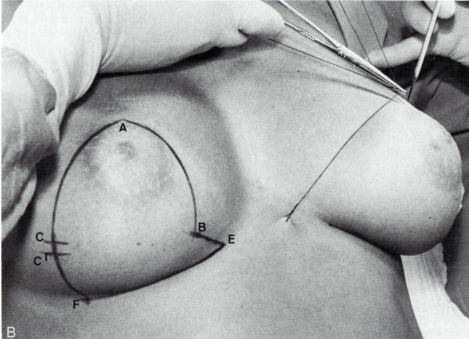

FIGURE 22–4
A and *B*, Markings are transferred to the opposite side by means of threads anchored at the xyphoid and sternal furcula.

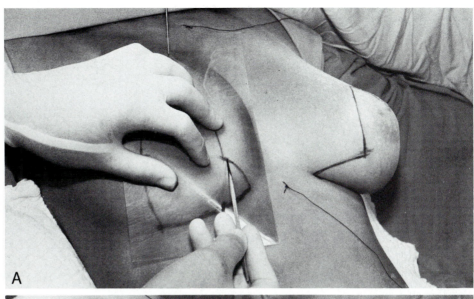

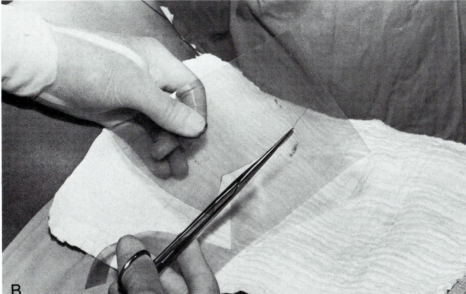

FIGURE 22–5
A to *C*, A template made of a piece of x-ray film is precise enough to check markings from one side to the opposite.

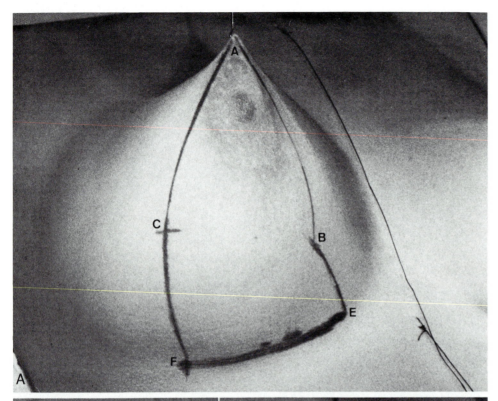

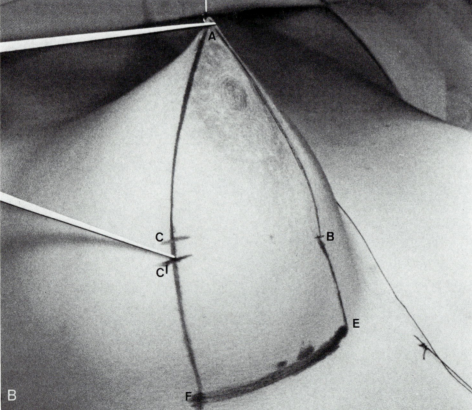

FIGURE 22–6
A and *B*, When the breast is raised by point A, distance AB becomes longer than AC. A new marking is then placed at C′ about 1.5 to 2 cm below C.

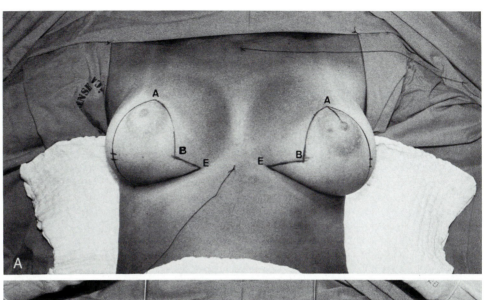

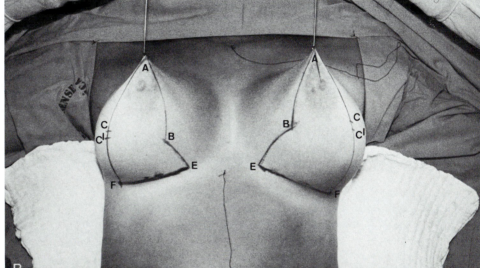

FIGURE 22–7
A to *C*, Completed markings. The breast is at rest and raised by point A. Note distance EE. EB is greater at the left because of breast asymmetry.

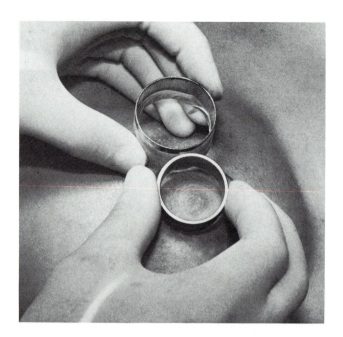

FIGURE 22–8
Areolar marking devices: a 3.5-cm diameter for initial incision around the areola and a 4-cm diameter for the incision through which the areola will emerge.

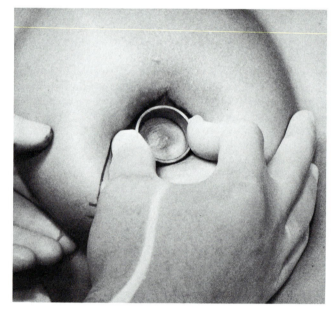

FIGURE 22–9
Areolar marking.

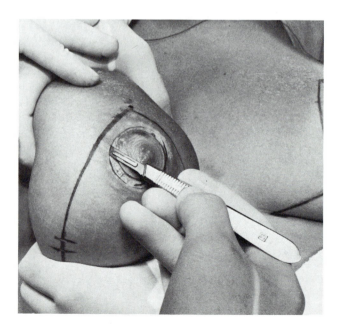

FIGURE 22–10
Assistant holding the breast at its base and squeezing it for an easier Schwarzmann's maneuver.

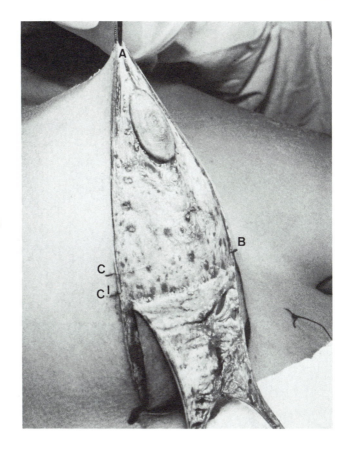

FIGURE 22–11
The skin triangle ABC' is preserved.

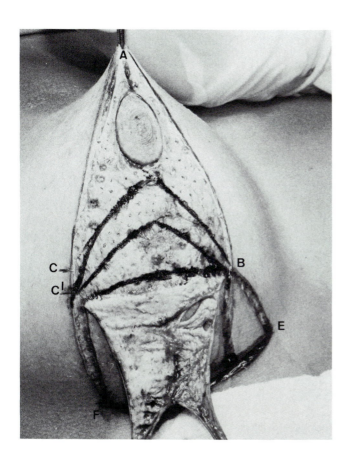

FIGURE 22–12
Different incision planes according to breast shape and reduction intended by the surgeon.

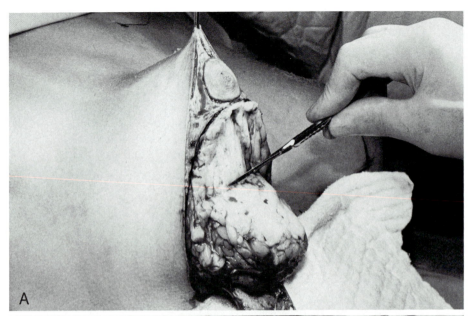

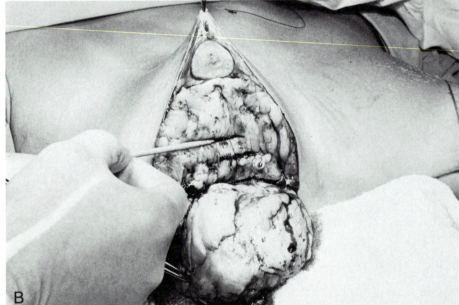

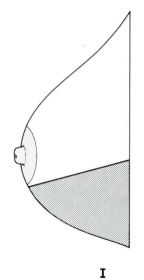

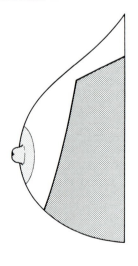

I

II

C

FIGURE 22–13
A, Plane resection. Variation I. *B,* Marking the different levels of incision for different amounts of reduction. Variation II. *C,* Vertical section showing glandular resection according to variations I and II.

FIGURE 22–14

A and *B*, Measuring the distance for the desired amount of glandular resection. It will be then transferred to the opposite side.

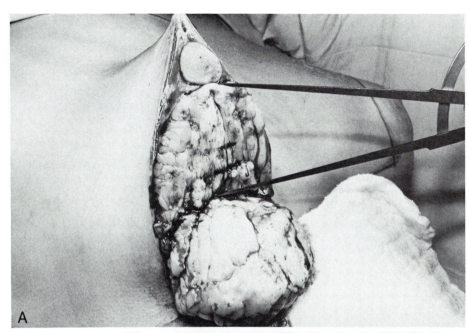

A

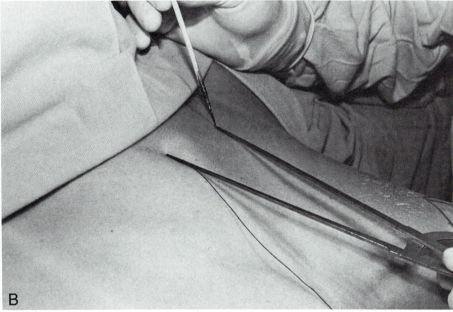

B

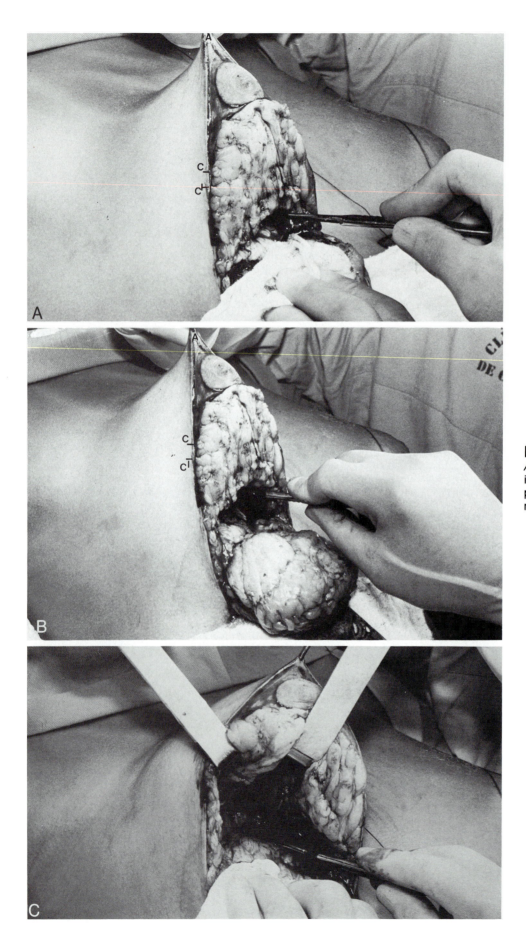

FIGURE 22–15
A to *C*, Stages of glandular incision in the horizontal plane. The surgeon determines the level of resection.

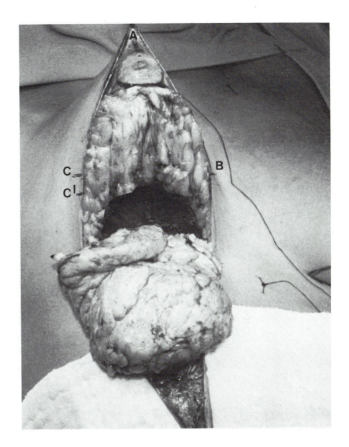

FIGURE 22–16
Breast raised to show the amount of tissue that can be resected by this technique.

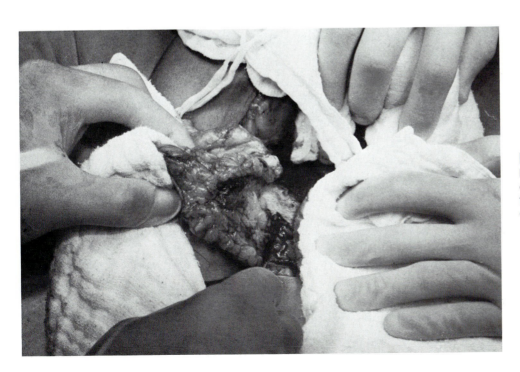

FIGURE 22–17
Resection is completed laterally. The assistant applies the compress in order to reduce bleeding.

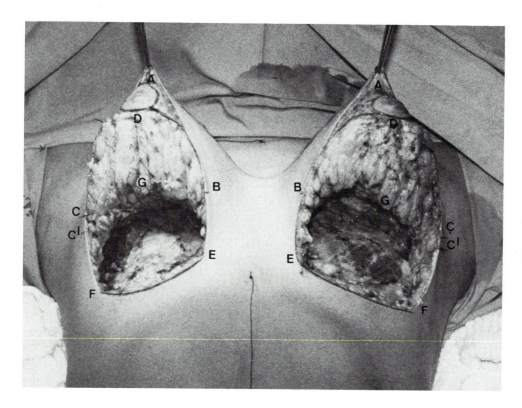

FIGURE 22–18
After hemostasis is completed, the mammary stumps are compared, and further resection is performed if necessary. In this case, resection was 230 gm on the right and 380 gm on the left because of asymmetry.

FIGURE 22–19
Skin slightly undermined at lines AB and AC'.

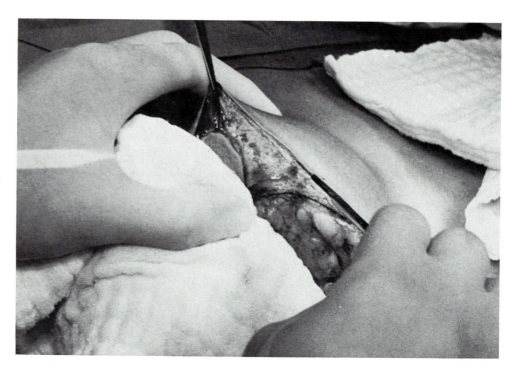

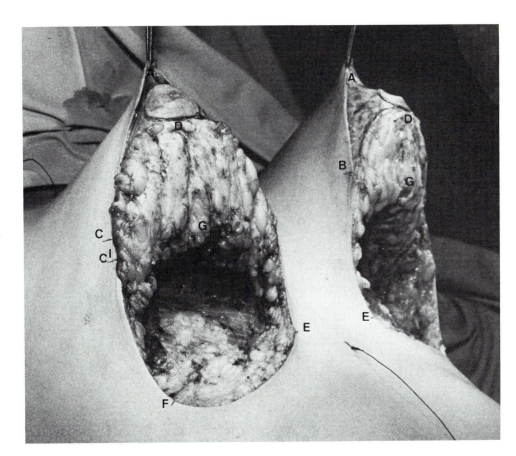

FIGURE 22-20
The two mammary stumps, oblique view. Note point G.

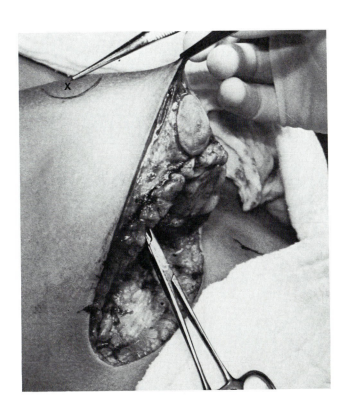

FIGURE 22-21
Rotation of point G inward and upward to fill the superior pole of the breast at point X, determined by the surgeon.

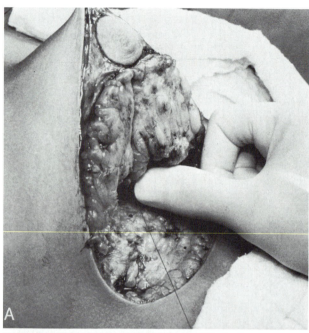

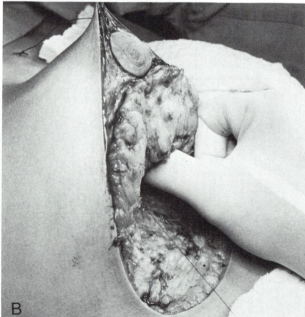

FIGURE 22–22
A and *B*, Fixation of point G with one or two stitches of Mersilene 3-0.

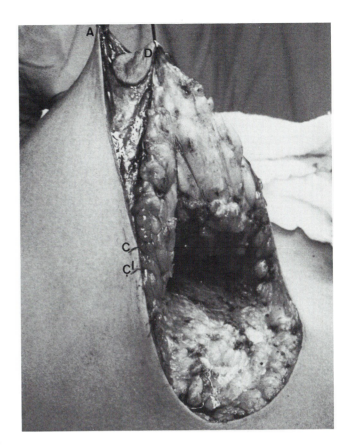

FIGURE 22–23
Breast raised by point A. A hook at D forms pillars.

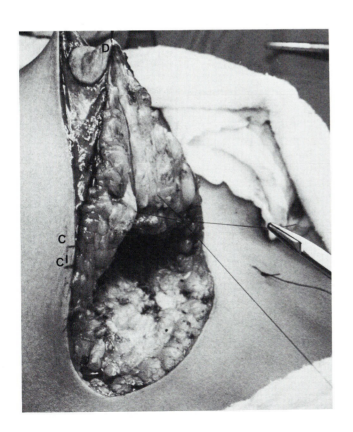

FIGURE 22–24
The pillars are sutured together with one or two stitches of nylon 4-0 for shaping the new breast cone and decreasing its base area.

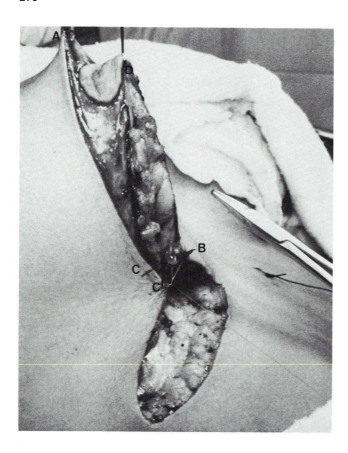

FIGURE 22–25
Dermal suture of the points BC′ and lines DC′ and DB with colorless nylon 5-0.

FIGURE 22–26
Initial stitches for skin suture with nylon 4-0.

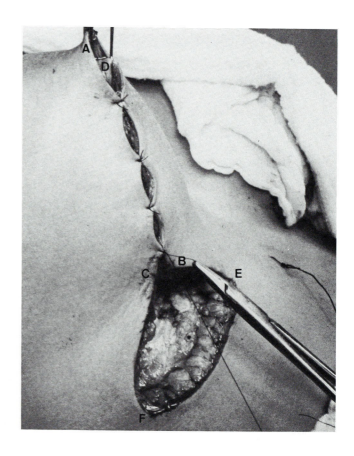

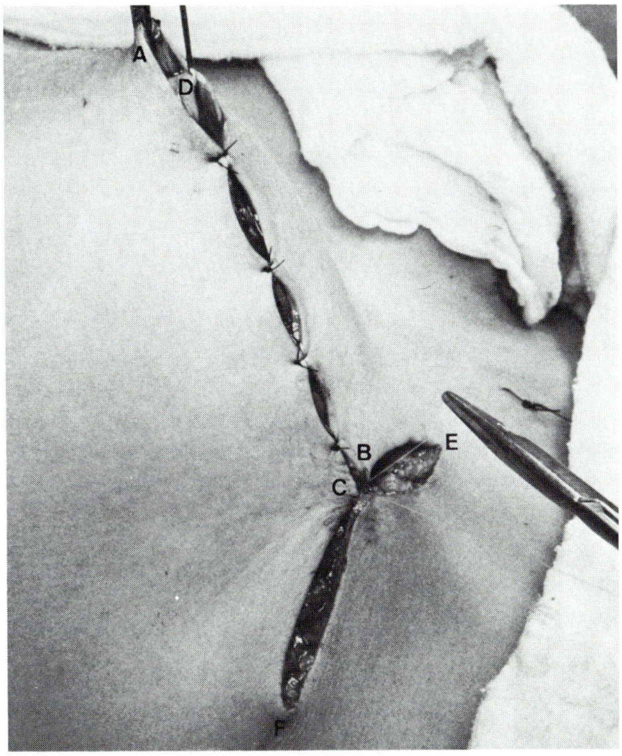

FIGURE 22–27
Breast remains raised by points A and D until the inverted T has been formed.

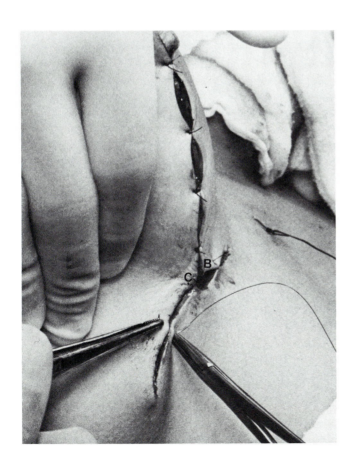

FIGURE 22–28
The assistant pulls the breast inward to reduce the lateral dog-ear.

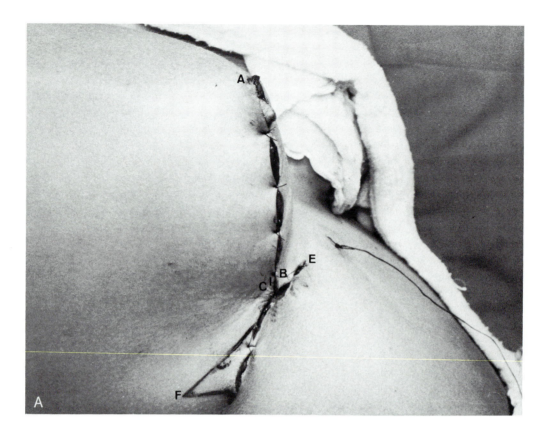

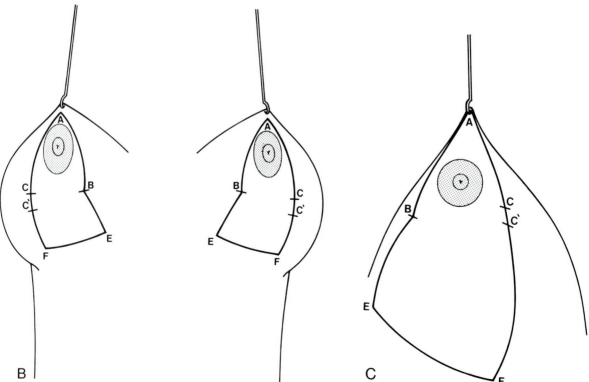

FIGURE 22–29

A, In order to avoid postural distortions, the surgeon should remove the lateral dog-ear only after the surgical table has been reset in the horizontal. B, Illustration showing details. Note small horizontal line EF in comparison with lines BE and C'F. C, Oblique view. Note the curved, continuous line from A to F.

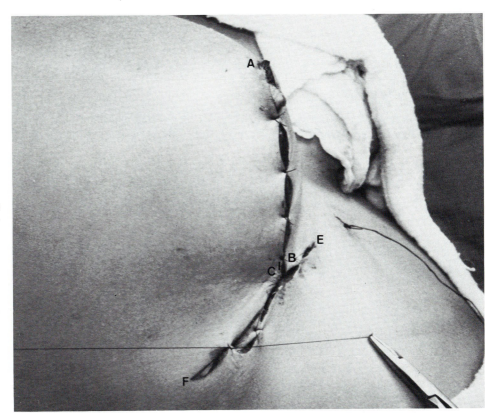

FIGURE 22–30
Provisional stitch for marking the definitive correction of the residual dog-ear.

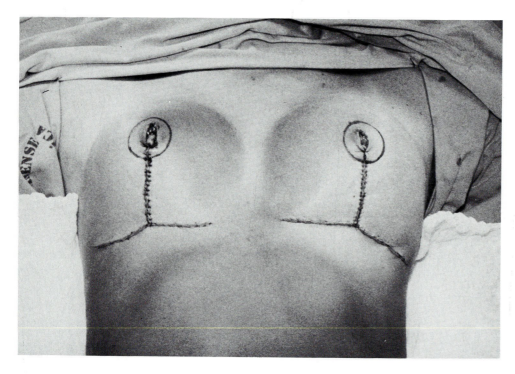

FIGURE 22–31
Completed skin suture. Nylon 5-0 single stitches are used for the vertical suture; and nylon 6-0 running stitches, for the horizontal one. Note the circular marking (done with a 4-cm ring) for position of the areola. Before placing the running stitches, the horizontal wound is anchored with 5-0 colorless nylon single stitches in order to ensure that the scar is of good quality.

FIGURE 22–32
Oblique view showing the apex of the superior pole formed by rotation of the gland. The areolae are spontaneously protruding through their future site. Note the short line of the future submammary scar.

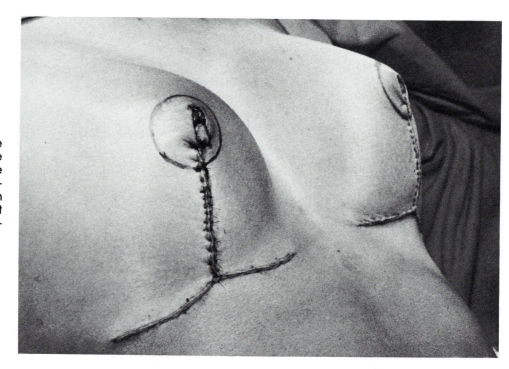

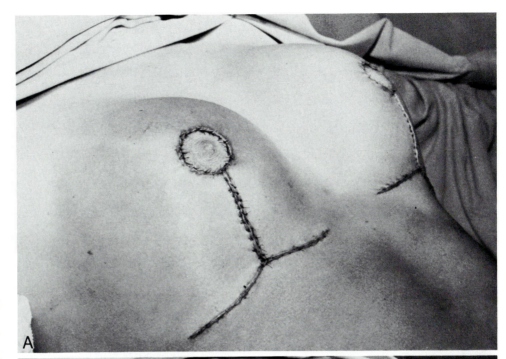

FIGURE 22–33
A and *B*, Completed operation immediately after closed suture and Micropore covering. No blood transfusion, drainage, or prophylactic antibiotic treatment is used. A slight temperature reaction is common during the first postoperative days and is treated with symptomatic medication.

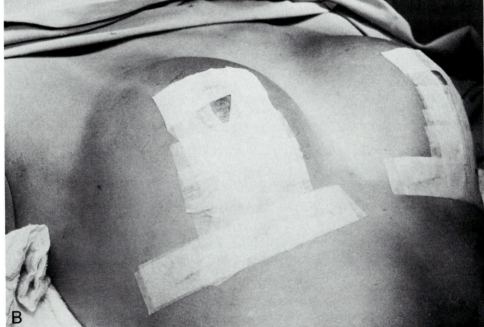

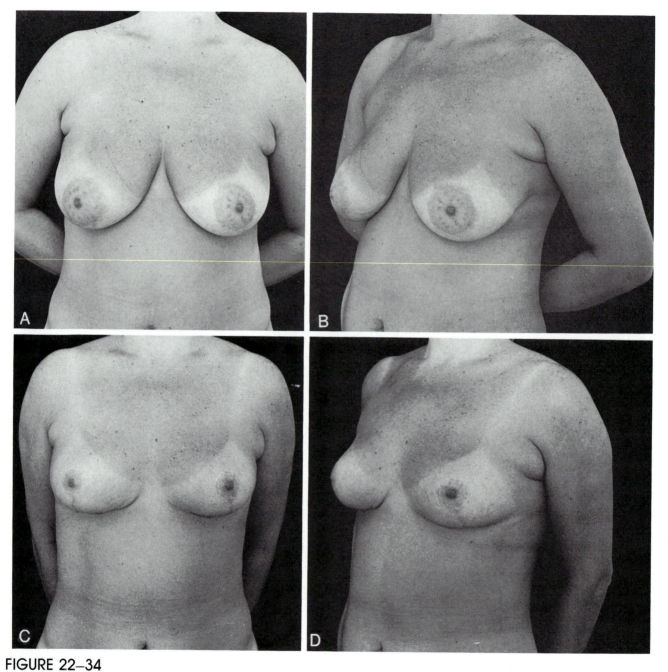

FIGURE 22–34

A and *B*, Hypertrophy of medium degree. Observe that the breasts are quite near one another. *C* and *D*, A satisfactory postoperative position and reduction were obtained by lateral technique variation II and glandular resection (250 gm on the right and 270 gm on the left).

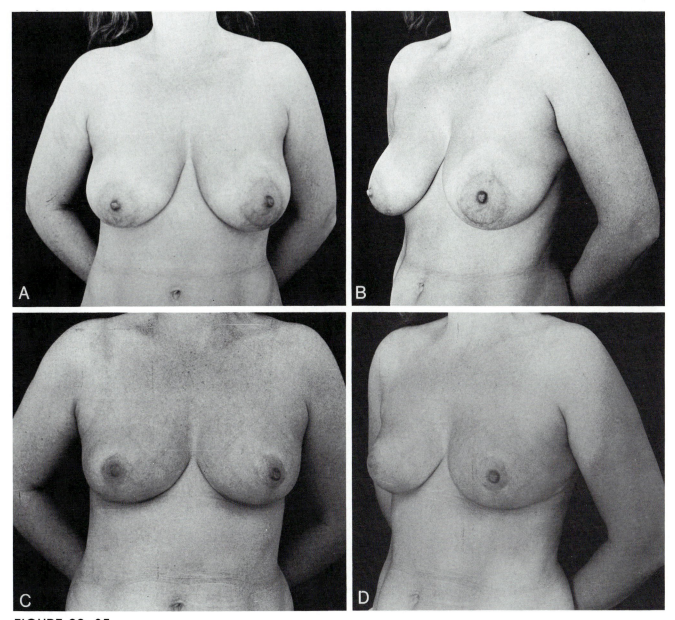

FIGURE 22–35

A and *B*, Same technique: glandular resection, variation II. The right breast contained a pathologic papilla. A free graft of the areola was thus performed. The graft took perfectly; a slight reduction of nipple projection occurred. *C* and *D*, Three-month postoperative views of same patient.

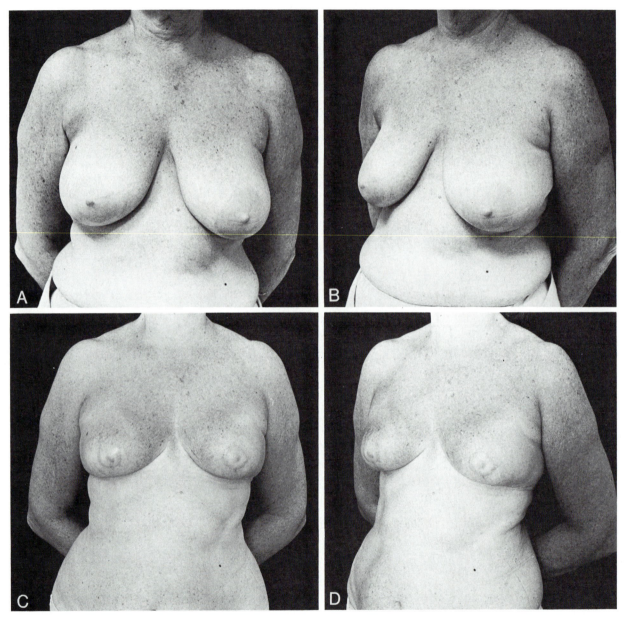

FIGURE 22-36
A and *B*, A case of hypertrophy with asymmetry. Operation by the lateral technique. Resection of 345 gm on the right and 215 gm on the left. *C* and *D*, Six-month postoperative views of the same patient.

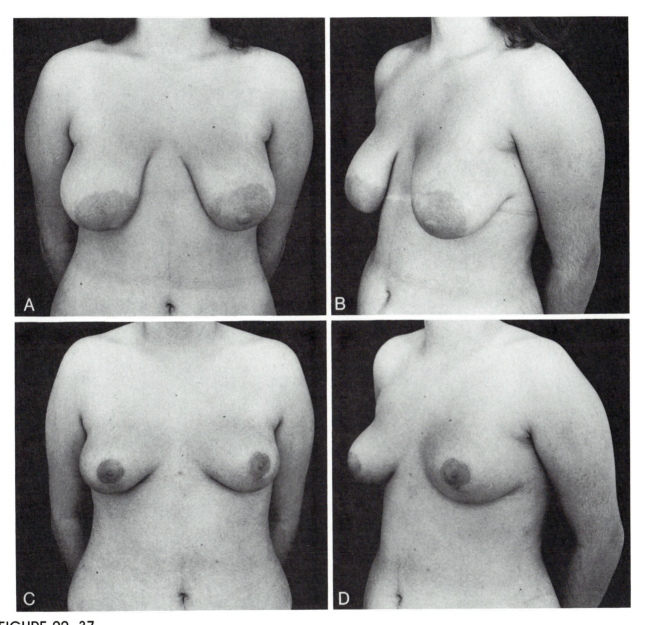

FIGURE 22–37

A and *B*, Ptotic flaccid breasts with giant areolae. There is a small scar left by the lateral incision. Variation I, glandular resection. Submammary scars remain completely hidden. *C* and *D*, Three-month postoperative views of same patient.

References

Arié G.: Una nuéva tecnica de mastoplastia. Rev. Latinoam. Cir. Plast. 3:23, 1957.

Cardosa de Castro, C.: Mammaplasty with Curved Incisions. Plast. Rec. Surg. 57:619, 1976.

Dufourmentel, C., Mouly, R.: Plastie mammaire par la méthode oblique. Ann. Chir. Plast. 6:45, 1961.

Dufourmentel, C., Mouly, R.: Développements récents de la plastie mammaire par la méthode oblique laterale. Ann. Chir. Plast. 10:227, 1965.

Franco, T., Rebello, C.: *Cirurgia Estetica*. Rio de Janeiro, Ed. Livraria Atheneu, 1977.

Georgiade, N. G., Serafin D., Riefkohl R., Georgiade G. S.: Is there a reduction mammaplasty for "all seasons"? Plast. Reconstr. Surg. 63:765, 1979.

Goldwyn, R. M.: *Plastic and Reconstructive Surgery of the Breast*. Boston, Little, Brown, 1976.

Holländer, E.: Treatment of hypertrophic breast: Replay to Lexer. Dtsch. Med. Wochenschr. 51:26, 1925.

Marino, H.: Plasticas mamarias. Buenos Aires, Editorial Cientifica Argentina, 1958.

Peixoto, G.: Reduction mammaplasty: A personal technique. Plast. Reconstr. Surg. 65:217, 1980.

Pitanguy, I.: Surgical treatment of breast hypertrophy. Br. J. Plast. Surg. 20:78, 1967.

Pontes, R.: A technique of reduction mammaplasty. Br. J. Plast. Surg. 26:365, 1973.

Pontes, R: Reduction mammaplasty: Variations I and II. Ann. Plast. Surg. 6:437, 1981.

Ribeiro, L.: A new technique for reduction mammaplasty. Plast. Reconstr. Surg. 55:330, 1975.

Strömbeck, J. O.: Mammaplasty: Report of a new technique based on the two pedicle procedure. Br. J. Plast. Surg. 13:79, 1960.

Schwarzmann, E.: Die Technik der Mammaplastik. Chirurg 2:932, 1930.

Hans Holmström
Clas Lossing

23

Reduction Mammaplasty Utilizing the Sliding Nipple Technique

The sliding nipple technique in reduction mammaplasties has been used regularly by us for more than 10 years. Like most new methods of breast reduction, the sliding nipple technique may be regarded as a refinement of existing different methods. Basically, it is a development of the bipedicle Strömbeck technique (1960), with its use of preoperatively designed skin-glandular flaps and the help of a pattern. To reduce its cosmetic drawbacks, such as a retracted nipple-areola complex and flatness of the breast, and to simplify the operative procedure, the sliding nipple technique was developed. Its important contributions are *exclusion of upper resection* and *mobilization of the nipple-areola complex* by a bilateral dermal relaxing incision, which result in a conical shape of the breast and projection of the nipple-areola complex. These principles have standardized and simplified reduction mammaplasty and resulted in a short operation time and a minimum of complications.

RATIONALE

We believe that exact preoperative determination of the new site of the nipple-areola complex is of central value because it creates an optimal position and shape for the reduced breast. A special pattern has been developed for the design of the skin-glandular flaps (Fig. 23–1). The resection of the inferior quadrants and of the deep portion of the gland is adapted to the need to fill the mold of the new breast, as determined by the skin excision.

The de-epithelialized dermis and subcutis are incised on both sides of the nipple-areola complex within the keyhole area. In this way the nipple-areola complex is released 6 to 8 cm on each side, which makes it easy to move to its new site. This technique relies on the concept described by Lalardrie (1988) that the most important contribution of blood flow to the nipple-areola complex comes from anastomoses within the upper 2 cm of glandular tissue and not exclusively from the subdermal network, as in the superior pedicle technique (Weiner et al., 1973). The subdermal network closest to the nipple-areola complex is, however, preserved and participates in the circulation through anastomoses to the underlying glandular tissue.

By the sliding nipple technique, tension on the nipple-areola complex, which is the greatest problem in its circulation, is avoided. In most cases the nipple-areola complex will float freely at its new site, which will result in a good nipple projection.

ANESTHESIA

Patients are operated on under general anesthesia. Prior to incision, 50 ml lidocaine (2.5 mg/ml) and epinephrine (2.5 µg/ml) is injected following the incision lines on each breast. The administration of local anesthesia has reduced the total blood loss to no more than 500 ml in large resections, and in the author's experience, there has never been a need for blood transfusion.

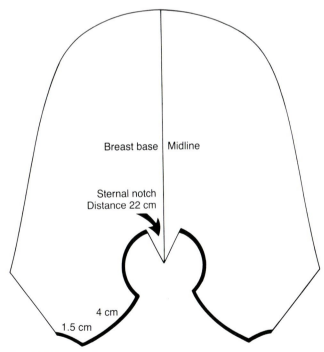

FIGURE 23–1
Pattern for reduction mammaplasty. Incision follows thick lines. Note the triangle in the upper part of the keyhole and slightly convex curved vertical incision lines ending in cut 1.5-cm corners. The triangle will ensure exact nipple positioning; and the curved vertical incisions, a convex lower profile of the breast.

PREOPERATIVE PLANNING

Preoperative drawing (Table 23–1) is performed with the patient in a sitting position with her arms hanging relaxed. The midclavicle line has been abandoned. Instead, the first step in planning the incision lines is to define the center of the base of the breast on a horizontal line measured from the midsternum to the anterior axillary fold. A line along the axis of the breast from the midpoint of the base determines the new nipple site. The midpoint is generally localized 8 to 9 cm from the midsternum and should be the same on both sides (Fig. 23–2A and B). Patients with asymmetric positions of the nipples or with extreme convergence or divergence of the nipples will, in this way, have the nipple horizontally corrected after operation. The vertical positioning of the nipple is mostly planned 21 or 22 cm from the sternal notch, but that it corresponds to the submammary fold must be checked. To ensure an exact symmetric vertical positioning of the nipples, the tip of the

TABLE 23–1
Scheme for Preoperative Planning

1. The patient is in the sitting position with the back straight and shoulders and arms relaxed.
2. The base of the breast is measured from the sternal midline to the anterior axillary fold. From the center of the base a line is drawn downward along the axis of the breast. This line does not meet the nipple when the nipple is located eccentrically.
3. The sternal notch is marked.
4. The new position of the nipple is marked on the midline, usually 22 cm from the sternal notch, and checked to be at the level of the submammary fold.
5. The breast pattern is applied with the triangle inside the keyhole on the new position of the nipple and the central line of the pattern along the midline of the breast.
6. The keyhole is drawn on the breasts.
7. With the patient still in a sitting position, medial and lateral points are marked at the ends of the submammary fold to the corner marking of the keyhole pattern.
8. With the patient lying down, the submammary fold is marked. On this a 1.5-cm triangular flap is placed corresponding to the intersection of the skin flaps. The distance from this triangle to the medial end point is checked carefully on both sides.

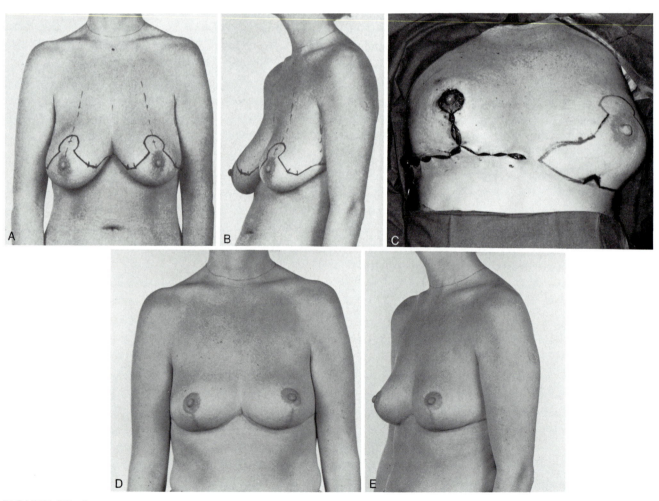

FIGURE 23–2
A and B, Moderate breast hyperplasia with preoperative marking using the breast midline and a special pattern. C, Intraoperative view. Note the submammary triangle. D and E, Six months after a 275-gm resection of each breast. Adequate nipple projection is noted.

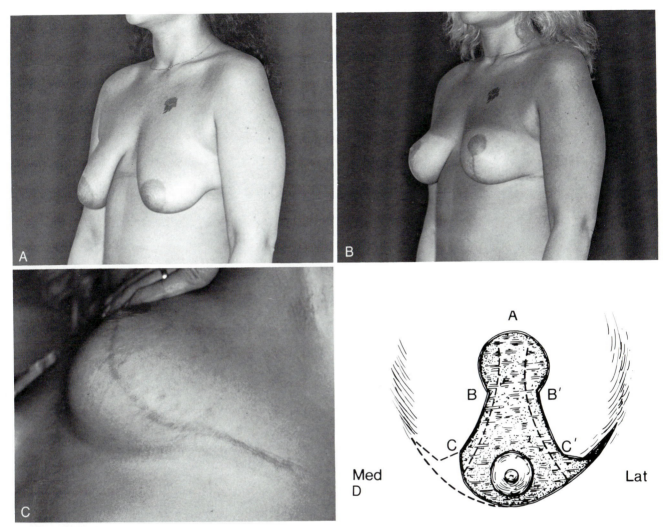

FIGURE 23–3
A and *B*, Ptotic breasts needing minor reduction. *C*, The medial inverted T (dotted) can be omitted, leaving only an L-shaped scarline. *D*, The sliding technique is used with transection of dermis and subcutis bilaterally of the nipple-areola complex. (Lat, lateral; Med, medial.)

triangle in the keyhole of the transparent pattern is placed exactly on the new nipple site.

The lower horizontal line is placed in the submammary crease, as in a traditional inverted-T reduction mammaplasty. However, an additional 1.5-cm skin triangle is designed to correspond to the cut lower corners of the lateral and medial breast flaps (Fig. 23–2C). This will reduce the risk of edge necrosis of the skin flaps. The position of the skin triangle coming up from the submammary crease is determined by the length of the medial breast flap (Fig. 23–2D and E). The length of the medial part of the inverted T can be shortened or even omitted in minor hypertrophy and ptotic cases (Fig. 23–3).

SURGERY

The patient is placed on the operating table with her arms along the sides of her body. A stabilizing tourniquet is applied around the base of the breast. A 4.5-cm

standard "cookie-cutter" is used for marking the areola incision. De-epithelialization is performed around the areola and at the predetermined new areola site, which is almost free of bleeding after the intradermal injection of lidocaine and epinephrine (Fig. 23–4A). After de-epithelialization, the tourniquet is removed. The detachment of the breast is started from the submammary incision line. The dissection follows the prefascial space laterally to the anterior border of the latissimus dorsi muscle, cranially to the level just above the new areola site, and medially to the sternum (see Fig. 23–4A). Caution is taken not to dissect too far in the axillary direction, so as not to interfere with the main lateral intercostal nerve branches. After detachment, the assistant is instructed to press down the upper lateral part of the breast tissue, which simplifies the resection. It is performed in the lower and central part of the breast in a discoid manner, leaving a glandular flap at least 2 cm in thickness, which will provide adequate blood supply to preserve the possibility of lactation (Lossing, 1985) and in most cases an intact innervation of the areola

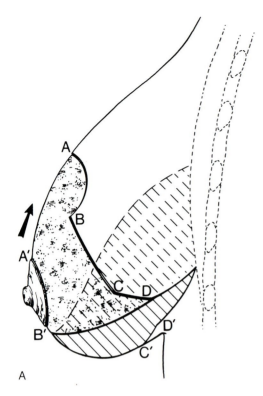

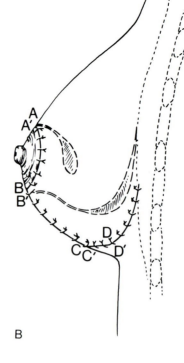

FIGURE 23–4

A and *B*, Resection is performed in the lower and deeper central portions of the breast (shaded area). By the sliding maneuver the de-epithelialized area above the nipple-areola complex will be displaced under the nipple-areola complex and improve its projection.

A

B

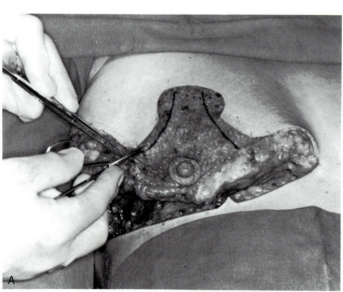

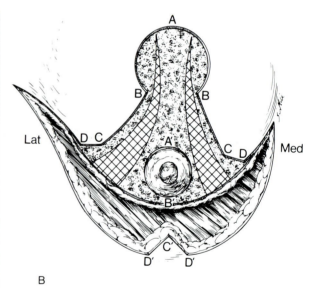

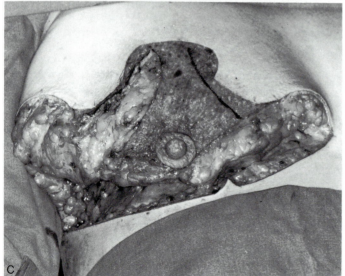

B

FIGURE 23–5

A and *B*, The dermis and subcutis are cut bilaterally, which releases the nipple-areola complex 6 to 8 cm on each side (here shown only on the first side). Lat, lateral; Med, medial.) *C*, The transposition of the nipple-areola complex is simplified by this sliding nipple technique without endangering the blood supply to the nipple-areola complex.

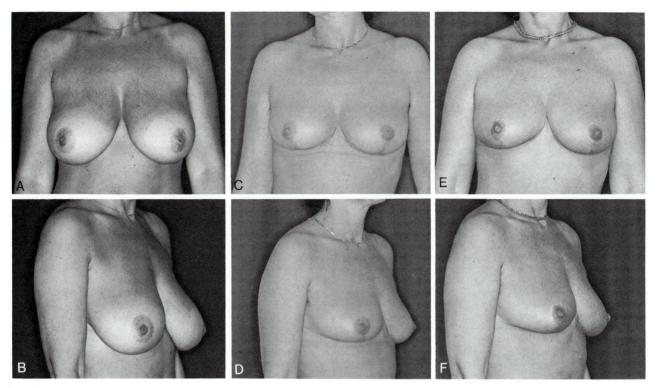

FIGURE 23–6

A and *B*, Preoperative views of medium mammary hyperplasia. *C* and *D*, Postoperative views 3 months after resection of 350 gm on each side. *E* and *F*, Stable conditions 6 years after reduction mammaplasty.

and nipple. The nipple-areola complex is mobilized through vertical dermal and subcutaneous incisions on both sides of the areola in the de-epithelialized region. If necessary, the incisions are carried into the superficial glandular tissue. By this maneuver the distance from the areola to the intact breast skin is increased 6 to 8 cm on both sides, which makes it possible to slide the areola nipple to its new superior position without tension (Figs. 23–4B and 23–5). When performing the sliding maneuver, the subareolar tissue is concentrated, giving the breast good central projection (Fig. 23–6).

Stitching is performed with resorbable sutures in the superficial fascia as well as intradermally in the horizontal submammary scarline, and nonresorbable skin sutures in vertical and periareolar scar lines. The triangle in the submammary incision line will fit adequately and relax the skin tension in the lower corners of the lateral and medial skin flaps. Suction drains are seldom used, and then only for 1 day after operation.

COMPLICATIONS

The traditional disadvantages of the Strömbeck method, such as a flat, square-shaped breast and a retracted or dimpled nipple, are avoided by the sliding maneuver. In some cases, particularly in breasts with a stiff fibrotic or sclerotic parenchyma and with a long sliding distance, tension can be applied to the nipple. This situation is managed by transection through the

glandular tissue on either the medial side or the lateral side of the areola. This will relax the tension and allow a combined sliding and rotating maneuver (Orlando and Guthrie, 1975).

Broad-chested women have a tendency toward a flat breast shape. Making a more aggressive resection of the breast laterally and stitching the remaining lateral gland portion to the superficial fascia of the lower horizontal line medially will provide a more conical and projecting shape of the breast.

Necrosis of the nipple has never occurred with the sliding nipple technique, but theoretically it is certainly possible. If the blood supply of the nipple-areola complex at the end of the operation were compromised in such a way that nipple necrosis might be anticipated, it would always be possible to transform this method into a free nipple grafting procedure, because the dermal surface of the new nipple-areola site has been saved.

POSTOPERATIVE CARE

The suture lines are taped, but the breasts need not be firmly dressed. The patients stay overnight at the hospital and are sent home with a brassiere. The breasts are checked after a week, and during the second week the stitches are removed. Taping of the scars for another month is advised. Severe physical activities should be avoided for a month, but the patient may return to work after 2 (sedentary work) or 3 weeks (physical labor).

References

Bolger, W., Seyfer, A., Jackson, S.: Reduction mammaplasty using the inferior glandular "pyramid" pedicle: Experiences with 300 patients. Plast. Reconstr. Surg. 80:75, 1987.

Lalardrie, J. P.: Reduction mammaplasty: Basic procedures. In: Gonzales-Ulloa, M., Meyer, R., Smith, J., Zaoli, G. (eds.): *Aesthetic Plastic Surgery*. Vol. 4. Padova, Piccin, 1988, p. 1.

Lossing, C., Holmström, H.: Reduction mammaplasty with preserved ability to suckle. [In Swedish.] Läkartidningen 82:2878, 1985.

Meyer, R., Kesselring, U. K.: Reduction mammaplasty with an L-shaped suture line: Development of different techniques. Plast. Reconstr. Surg. 55:139, 1975.

Müller, F.: Late results of Strömbeck's mammaplasty. Plast. Reconstr. Surg. 54:664, 1974.

Orlando, J. C., Guthrie, R. H.: The superomedial pedicle for nipple transposition. Br. J. Plast. Surg. 28:42, 1975.

Strömbeck, J. O.: Mammaplasty: Report of a new technique based on the two pedicle procedure. Br. J. Plast. Surg. 13:79, 1960.

Weiner, P. L., Aiache, A. E., Silver, L., Tittiranonda, T.: A single dermal pedical for nipple transposition in subcutaneous mastectomy, reduction mammaplasty or mastopexy. Plast. Reconstr. Surg. 51:115, 1973.

24

G. Stephenson Drew
E. Ronald Finger
Kenna S. Given

Superior Medial Pedicle Technique of Reduction Mammaplasty

The primary objective of the reduction mammaplasty procedure is to reduce the size of the hypertrophic breast with appropriate redraping of the skin envelope while maintaining a viable nipple-areola complex. The secondary objectives are to provide lasting conical projection, to preserve nipple-areola sensation, and to minimize scars. Finally, the procedure should be quick, relatively bloodless, and reproducible with regard to different types and sizes of enlarged breasts.

The superior pedicle technique of breast reduction has generally met these objectives and is thought by many to be technically easier while producing a longer-lasting aesthetic effect. Classically, however, it has been limited to smaller resections. By incorporating the medial quadrant in the superior pedicle, more aggressive reductions can be safely undertaken with the same excellent results. In fact, resections as large as 4100 gm per breast with nipple-areola transpositions up to 30 cm have been performed with reliable nipple-areola survival. Details of the procedure, as well as avoidance of complications, are discussed.

HISTORY

Breast reduction has been attempted by means of several approaches, from amputation with nipple-areola grafting to a host of nipple-areola transpositions. The trend during the last 25 years has been toward a variety of dermoglandular pedicles for nipple-areola transposition. Bipedicle procedures have been proposed horizontally and vertically, and single pedicles have been based laterally, inferiorally, superiorly, and superomedially.

Weiner et al. (1973) showed that a single superiorly based dermal pedicle could sustain nipple-areola viability solely with its cutaneous vascular supply. Others (Georgiade et al., 1979; Bostwick, 1983), however, have reported problems with tension on the pedicle if it is too long, with a resultant decrease in viability and nipple-areola sensation.

Orlando and Guthrie (1975) reported a series of 12 patients who underwent surgery using a superior medial pedicle and who retained complete nipple-areola viability and sensation. They attributed the increased sensation over the superior pedicle to its added medial component, which carries fibers from the anterior cuta-

neous branches of the fourth and fifth intercostal nerves. Ten years later Hauben (1984) published a report of a series of 78 patients operated on by the same technique. Nipple-areola transpositions of up to 15 cm were performed without vascular compromise or significant sensory deficit. Over the last several years my colleagues and I have experienced the same success with this technique.

SURGICAL TECHNIQUE

Preoperatively the patient is kept in a sitting position while the new nipple position is marked according to the inframammary line, which has been transposed to the anterior aspect of the breast. The new nipple location lies on the breast meridian (a line drawn between the midclavicular point and the nipple) usually between 19 and 22 cm. A modified Wise (1956) pattern is then employed with the vertical limbs measuring approximately 5 to 5.5 cm in length. The inframammary line is marked, and straight lines are drawn from the medial and lateral limbs of the Wise pattern to the respective ends of the inframammary incision. The lateral extent of the incision is usually the anterior axillary line, although removal of the breast tissue may extend even further laterally. The design of the superior medial pedicle is demonstrated in Figure 24–1. Notice that with longer pedicle lengths the base is slightly widened to ensure adequate vascularization (see Fig. 24–1C). The proposed areola site will be designed with a 38- to 42-mm diameter, and the areola itself will be reduced to about 42 to 45 mm. This discrepancy in size allows for the primary contraction of the areola as well as the retraction of the skin edges at the new areolar site.

Following induction of general anesthesia, infiltration with 0.5% lidocaine with 1:200,000 epinephrine is done in the prepectoral and incisional areas except for the region of the pedicle.

The actual procedure is technically simple. The details are illustrated in Figure 24–2. De-epithelialization is performed. The nipple-areola complex is held with double hooks under tension while being undermined at a 2-cm thickness and is made progressively thicker at the base. Only 60% to 70% of the de-epithelialized flaps need to be elevated for ample rotational capacity. The

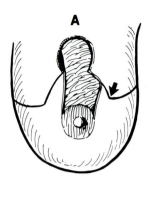
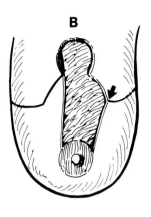
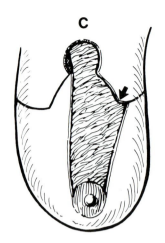

FIGURE 24–1
Variations in design of the superior medial pedicle.

nipple-areola complex is then rotated laterally and sutured into its new position with a temporary suture so that the remaining breast tissue can be easily excised. The breast tissue is excised, leaving a small layer of tissue overlying the pectoral fascia. To maximize the blood supply, no undermining of the breast flap is performed. When excising the breast tissue it is important to slightly bevel the flaps inferiorly along the inframammary line at *c* and *d* but not along the medial and lateral vertical edges marked *a* and *b*. This provides for better contour at the inframammary line while retaining enough tissue to ensure adequate projection. Much of the central projection is provided by breast tissue at the base of the pedicle. In fact, the proximal portion of the superior medial pedicle is often nearly full thickness to the chest wall. Additional sculpturing of the medial and lateral flaps can be done as necessary. Often no reduction of breast tissue is performed medially, most being removed from the lateral segment. The

incisions are temporarily closed with staples, and the breasts are checked for symmetry. Final closure is then performed in layers with 3-0 and 4-0 absorbable sutures. Steri-Strips are used to approximate the skin edges. Drains are used if needed (Fig. 24–3).

With increasing pedicle lengths, the base is widened to ensure adequate vascularization (see Fig. 24–1C). Notice, however, that the lateral aspect is not changed and begins approximately at the 10 o'clock position (right breast). This allows for a full-thickness wedge of lateral tissue to be excised to facilitate rotation. As in other methods of breast reduction, care must be taken to prevent tension on the pedicle during insetting of the nipple-areola complex. The rotation required by this procedure actually creates less torsion and tension on the pedicle with increased pedicle lengths. With shorter pedicles, rotation is enhanced by making a small (1 to 2 cm) relaxing incision medially (see arrow, Fig. 24–1A).

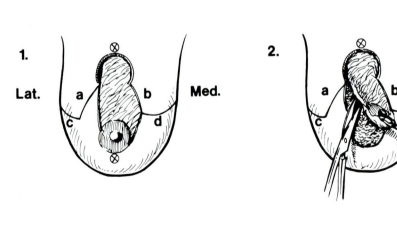
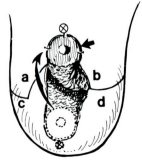

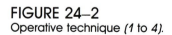

FIGURE 24–2
Operative technique *(1 to 4)*.

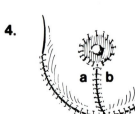

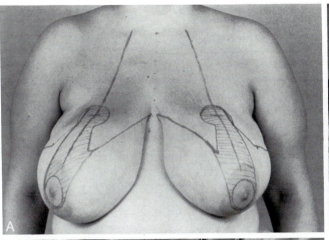

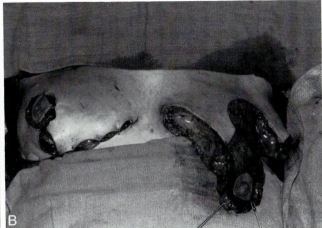

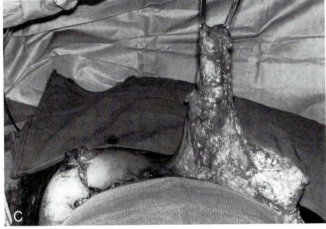

FIGURE 24–3

A, Preoperative markings and design of flap. *B,* The left breast has been reduced. Superior medial pedicle prior to rotation. The right breast, following reduction, has been temporarily closed with staples. *C,* Elevation of the superior medial pedicle.

POSTOPERATIVE CARE

The patient's breasts are placed either in a bulky dressing or in a brassiere postoperatively. The operative sites are examined at regular intervals over the next 24 to 48 hours for evidence of hematoma or impaired vascularity to the nipple-areola complex. Drains, if used, are usually removed on the first or second postoperative day. The patient is discharged on the second postoperative day. Any permanent sutures are removed by the tenth postoperative day, at which time the patient has generally returned to normal activity. Over the past 10 years over 300 reductions using the superior medial pedicle technique have been performed. Reductions up to 4100 gm per breast (mean, 692 gm) and nipple-areola transpositions up to 30 cm (mean, 11.6 cm) were performed. Representative examples are shown in Figures 24–4 to 24–7.

COMPLICATIONS

The complications were grouped as either early or late (Table 24–1). The early complications totalled 5.6%, which compares favorably with those reported in other series (Strömbeck, 1960; McKissock, 1972; Hugo and McClellan, 1979). Most complications involved small areas of necrosis or dehiscence, usually at the T portion of the incision. There were two cases of partial nipple-areola loss involving less than 25% of the areola. Both healed satisfactorily by secondary intention without need of revision.

Late complications consisted mostly of nipple-areola sensory loss, found in approximately 15% of the reduced breasts. This also compares favorably with previous reports utilizing the superior medial pedicle as well as

TABLE 24–1

Complications of the Superior Medial Pedicle Technique

COMPLICATIONS	% BREASTS
Early	
Skin necrosis	2.0
Fat necrosis	1.2
Nipple-areola necrosis	0.8
Dehiscence	1.2
Cellulitis	0.4
Late	
Sensory changes	14.8
Not enough reduced	1.6
Too much reduced	0.8
Recurrent ptosis	1.2
Scar hypertrophy	1.2
Nipple retraction	0.8
Dog-ears	0.8

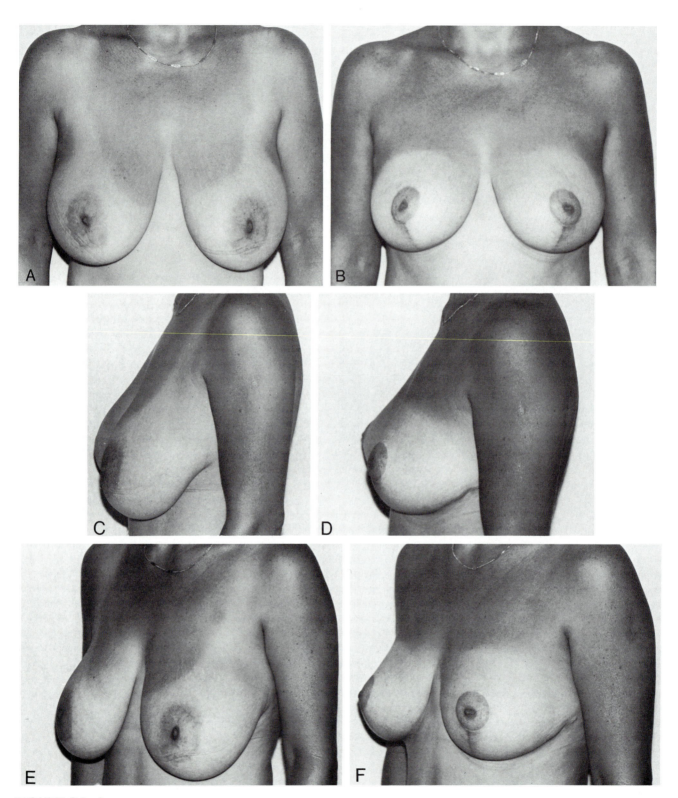

FIGURE 24–4
A 30-year-old patient with moderate hypertrophy and ptosis. From each breast, 425 gm of tissue was removed. Nipples were transposed 5.5 cm bilaterally. *A, C,* and *E,* Preoperative views. *B, D,* and *F,* Postoperative views at 8 months.

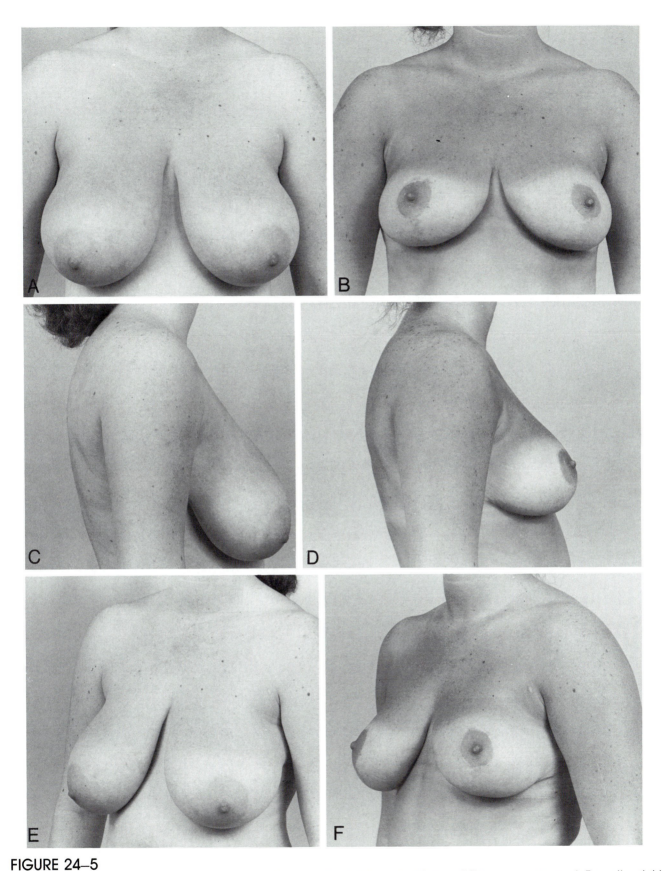

FIGURE 24–5
A 22-year-old woman with moderate hypertrophy. From the left breast, 680 gm of tissue was removed. From the right breast, 700 gm was removed. Nipple transposition of 11 cm was performed bilaterally. *A, C,* and *E,* Preoperative views. *B, D,* and *F,* Postoperative views at 1 year.

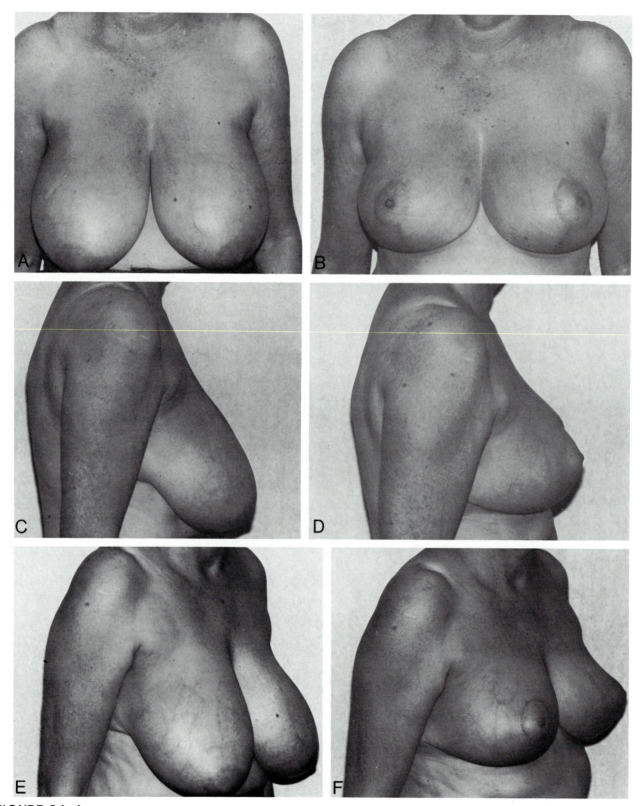

FIGURE 24–6

A 58-year-old patient with marked hypertrophy and ptosis. Bilateral 650-gm reduction and 12-cm bilateral nipple transposition. *A, C,* and *E,* Preoperative views. *B, D,* and *F,* Postoperative views at 18 months.

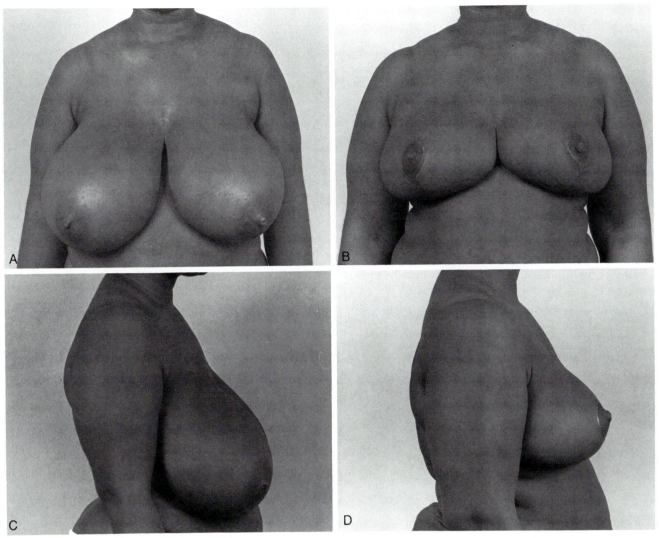

FIGURE 24–7
A 26-year-old woman with severe hypertrophy who underwent a 2560-gm reduction on the right and a 2260-gm reduction on the left. Nipple transposition of 16 cm was performed bilaterally. *A* and *C*, Preoperative views. *B* and *D*, Postoperative views at 11 months.

other techniques including the bipedicle (McKissock, 1972), inferior pedicle, and superior pedicle (Orlando and Guthrie, 1975; Hauben, 1984; Courtiss and Goldwyn, 1976).

AVOIDANCE OF COMPLICATIONS

Intraoperative Blood Loss

Although not a complication, blood loss can be greatly reduced by infiltration of lidocaine with epinephrine. The blood loss in many cases has been below 250 ml.

Necrosis of the Nipple-Areola Complex

It should be emphasized that the impairment of vascularity to the nipple-areola complex results not as much

from the length or thickness of the pedicle as from the tension placed on the pedicle by rotation. On several occasions the excellent vascularity to the nipple-areola complex was temporarily impaired by rotating the pedicle under too much tension. After reducing the tension by small adjustments in the pedicle thickness or by a slight back cut at the pedicle base, rotation was possible with maintenance of vascularity.

Skin Necrosis of the Vertical Incision

Skin necrosis of the vertical incision can be minimized by reducing the angle of the Wise pattern and thus reducing the tension of the vertical limb closure.

Nipple-Areola Inversion

Nipple-areola inversion can have several causes. It may occur when too much breast tissue has been excised from the lateral aspect of the areola recipient site. Also, when there is excessive tension on the pedicle, the areola may tend to retract at the lateral inferior aspect of the new areola site. Both of these problems result from technical errors and should be prevented. Fortunately, inversion seems to correct itself over the first few days after surgery.

SUMMARY

The superior medial pedicle technique was designed to avoid the late loss of projection and "bottoming out" of breast tissue while allowing easy transposition of the nipple-areola complex. The procedure was found to be simple and quick to perform. It combines the simplicity of the amputation technique and the advantage of maintaining the nipple-areola complex on a dermoglandular pedicle. In fact, this procedure has obviated the need to use amputation with the free nipple grafting technique. The procedure has proven useful on all types of reductions, from the firm globular hypertrophy of youth to gigantomastia, and even extreme ptosis of age and major weight loss. Furthermore, the results are reproducible and aesthetically pleasing.

References

Bostwick, J., III: *Aesthetic and Reconstructive Breast Surgery*. St. Louis, C. V. Mosby, 1983.

Courtiss, E. H., Goldwyn, R. M.: Breast sensation before and after plastic surgery. Plast. Reconstr. Surg. 58:1, 1976.

Finger, R. E., Vasquez, B., Drew, G. S., Given K. S.: Superomedial pedicle technique of reduction mammaplasty. Plast. Reconstr. Surg. 83:471, 1989.

Georgiade, N. G., Serafin, D., Riefkohl, R., Georgiade, G. S.: Is there a reduction mammaplasty for "all seasons"? Plast. Reconstr. Surg. 63:765, 1979.

Hauben, D. J.: Experience and refinements with the supero-medial dermal pedicle for nipple-areola transposition in reduction mammaplasty. Aesthetic. Plast. Surg. 8:189, 1984.

Hugo, N. E., McClellan, R. M.: Reduction mammaplasty with a single superiorly-based pedicle. Plast. Reconstr. Surg. 3:230, 1979.

McKissock, P. K.: Reduction mammaplasty with a vertical dermal flap. Plast. Reconstr. Surg. 49:245, 1972.

Orlando, J. C., Guthrie, R. H.: The supero-medial pedicle for nipple transposition. Br. J. Plast. Surg. 28:42, 1975.

Serafin, D.: History of breast reconstruction. In: Georgiade, N. G. (ed.): *Reconstructive Breast Surgery*. St. Louis, C. V. Mosby, 1976, p. 1.

Strömbeck, J. O.: Mammaplasty: Report of a new technique based on the two-pedicle procedure. Br. J. Plast. Surg. 13:79, 1960.

Weiner, D. L., Aiache, A. E., Silver, L., Tittiranonda, T.: A single dermal pedicle for nipple transposition in subcutaneous mastectomy, reduction mammaplasty, or mastopexy. Plast. Reconstr. Surg. 51:115, 1973.

Wise, R. I.: A preliminary report on a method of planning the mammaplasty. Plast. Reconstr. Surg. 17:367, 1956.

25

Mario S. L. Galvao

Reduction Mammaplasty: The Galvao Method

The importance of preserving the subdermal vascular plexus surrounding the nipple-areola complex during mammaplasties was first demonstrated by Schwarzmann (1937, 1930, 1931). Several techniques were later described (Goldwyn, 1976; Lalardrie and Jouglard, 1974; Marc, 1952), and the use of dermal pedicles became widely accepted.

Obviously, the broader the dermal pedicle, the better the supply to the nipple; therefore, a method was evolved with preservation of the superior, medial, lateral, and inferior pedicles. The aim of this method (Galvao, 1978, 1979, 1980, 1981) is to isolate the nipple-areola complex from the gland prior to proceeding to the reduction itself so that once the nipple-areola complex is safely lifted, any amount of breast tissue can be removed without endangering its viability. Moreover, the nipple-areola complex is easily transposed to its new position. The procedure is carried out in a "cut as you go" manner, allowing the surgeon to visualize the new breast mold being fashioned throughout the operation.

The technique of breast reduction without a medial scar was described by Marc (1952) and Dufourmentel and Mouly (1961) but became widely accepted only in the last decade or so following publications by Regnault (1974), Elbaz and Verheecke (1972), Meyer (1978), and others (Georgiade, 1976; Goldwyn, 1976; Lalardrie and Jouglard, 1974).

The aim of an ideal mammaplasty is a shorter scar, a better shape, and a procedure more easily performed. Our method, described previously, is now being used only for severe breast hypertrophy, and in some selected moderate cases of hypertrophy.

Since 1981, we have been using a method to correct mild and moderate breast hypertrophy without a medial scar. Our contribution to this method was presented at the Ninth International Congress of Plastic and Reconstructive Surgery in New Delhi (1987).

TECHNIQUE FOR REDUCTION OF UP TO 600 GRAMS FROM EACH SIDE: MAMMAPLASTY WITHOUT A MEDIAL SCAR

Marking the Breast

It is mandatory to carefully plan and outline the procedure 1 day before surgery. Both breasts must be fully examined with the patient sitting up and in a supine properly aligned position. The patient's shoulders and posture must be properly aligned. Often the breasts are of different size, and the measurements are made accordingly.

With the patient sitting up, the sternal notch, the xyphoid process, and the midclavicular line are outlined (Fig. 25–1).

Both breasts are pinched simultaneously, and the new nipple-areola complex position is outlined at point A on the right breast. It roughly corresponds to the level of the inframammary fold, and its real position is outlined later slightly lower, as shown in Fig. 25–2. Points B and C are calculated with slight tension between them (Fig. 25–3).

With the patient still sitting up, points A, B, and C are rechecked as shown in Fig. 25–4, and the new breast size is visualized (AB = AC = 8 cm).

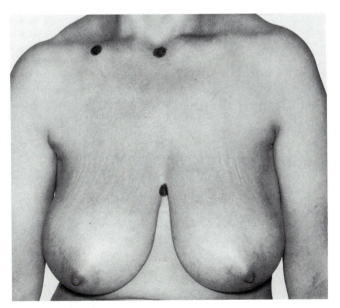

FIGURE 25–1
The three points necessary for marking the breast prior to a reduction mammaplasty are shown: the sternal notch, the xyphoid process, and the midclavicular point.

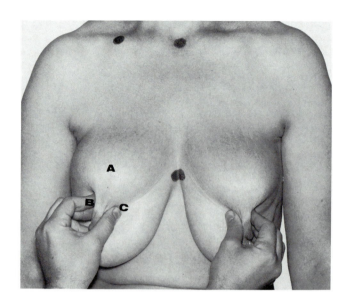

FIGURE 25–2
The new nipple-areola position is marked as shown at the approximate position of the inframammary fold.

FIGURE 25–3
Points B and C are established with slight tension as shown.

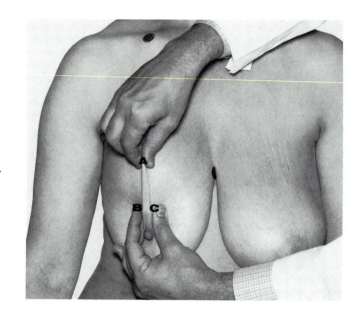

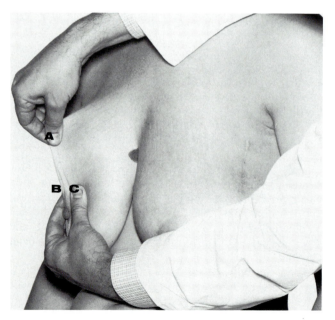

FIGURE 25–4
Patient in an upright position. Points A, B, and C are rechecked with slight tension.

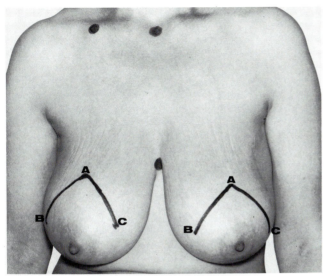

FIGURE 25-5
Points A, B, and C are marked with lines AC and AB equal to 8 cm in length. Point A is 16 to 22 cm from the sternal notch.

The same maneuvers are used to mark the left breast. Here the distances of the right breast (from point A to the jugular notch and from point A to the xyphoid process) are transposed to the left breast to ensure symmetry (Fig. 25-5).

From point A a new marking, A', is made 2 cm medially and inferiorly, following the line AC (AA' =

2 cm). This point A' corresponds to the site of the new nipple position when it is replaced at the end of the procedure (Fig. 25-6).

A curved line is now drawn from point A' to point B (Fig. 25-7).

With the patient in a supine position, two curved lines are marked from points B and C downward, and toward the middle of inframammary fold, where point D is outlined. Point D corresponds to a vertical line coming from the midclavicle and passing through the nipple-areola complex, finally reaching the inframammary fold (Fig. 25-8).

The lateral aspect of breast is outlined with the following maneuver: Point A is pinched and lifted by the fingertips while point B is pushed medially toward a point approximately 2 cm above point D. This maneuver will create a lateral dog-ear where point E is outlined on its outer aspect.

A line is, therefore, marked from point D to point E, which is placed most often about 1 cm above the original inframammary fold. After repeating the same procedure described above, a curved line is made from point E to point B with demarcation of a lateral dog-ear to be resected (Figs. 25-9, 25-10, and 25-11).

Discussion

It is sometimes difficult to decide whether to perform a T-shaped or an L-shaped mammaplasty. The L technique undoubtedly reduces postoperative scarring, although the lateral scar is occasionally slightly extended. However, if one makes the lines A'B and A'C curved, the amount of dog-ear to be resected is much smaller,

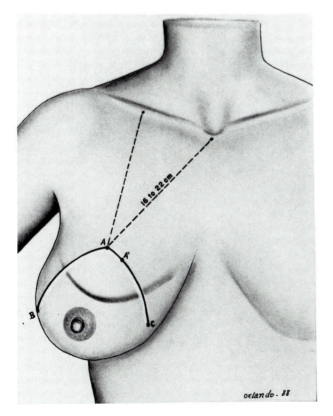

FIGURE 25-6
Note the position of A' placed 2 cm medially and inferiorly. This will correspond to the new nipple-areola site at the termination of the procedure.

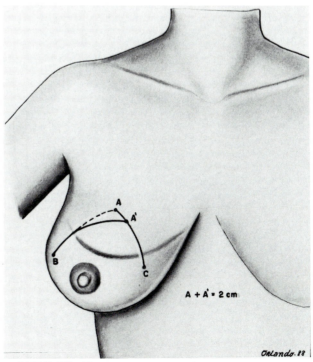

FIGURE 25-7
A new curved line is drawn from point B to A'.

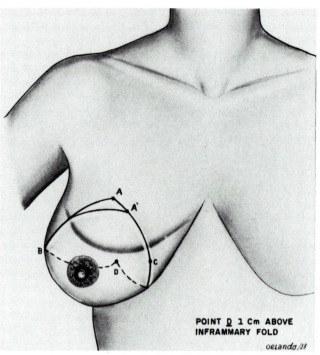

FIGURE 25–8
Point D in the inframammary fold is marked and corresponds to a neutral line from the midclavicular point. Two curved lines are then drawn from D to connect with B and C.

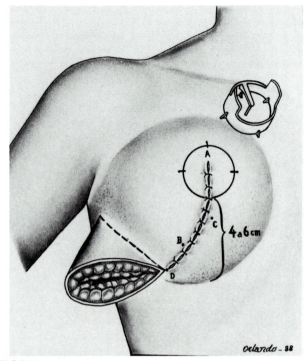

FIGURE 25–10
Excess breast tissue is resected as a pyramid, leaving a lateral dog-ear. Note the new sites of points B and C.

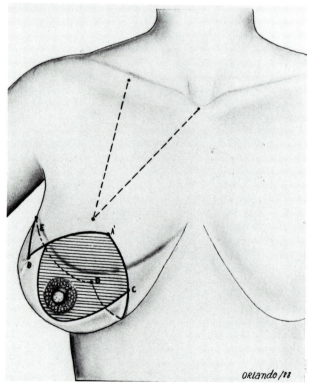

FIGURE 25–9
Point E is marked by elevating point A in the fingertips and pushing D medially, which creates a dog-ear laterally, with point E at its lateral aspect.

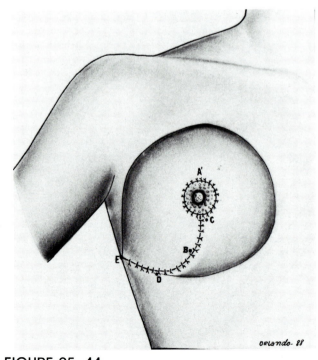

FIGURE 25–11
Appearance of the breast after closure following excision of excess tissue.

minimizing the extension of incision necessary to remove the dog-ear. On the other hand, if the lines A'B and A'C are drawn too curved, more tissue excess will show at point A', making the reposition of the nipple-areola complex more laborious. As a result, a distorted nipple-areola complex is produced because of unequal tension surrounding it.

In our experience minor and moderate breast hypertrophy up to 600 gm in a single breast can be safely reduced with the L procedure. For a large breast the technique preserving the superior, medial, lateral, and inferior pedicles is the safest choice.

TECHNIQUE FOR REDUCTION OF OVER 600 GRAMS FROM EACH SIDE, INCLUDING GIGANTOMASTIA: MAMMAPLASTY USING SUPERIOR, MEDIAL, LATERAL, AND INFERIOR PEDICLES

Marking the Breast

Points A, B, and C are marked as previously described for mammaplasty without a medial scar. Then the pa-

tient is asked to lie in a supine position, and the markings are rechecked by repeating the maneuvers previously described.

With the patient still in a supine position, a line is drawn from point A to the inframammary fold, passing through the nipple. Often this line is slightly oblique outward. A small triangle is then drawn at the inframammary fold where points B and C will meet (Fig. 25–12A).

The inframammary line is, thereafter, outlined determining points D and E (DE = 10 to 12 cm) (Fig. 25–12B). Dotted lines are placed from point B to D and from C to E that correspond to the full-thickness incision lines (Fig. 25–13).

With the patient sitting up, the angle at point A varies between 90 and 140 degrees. For this reason, we do not recommend the use of patterns to mark the breast. The distance from point A to the jugular notch measures between 16 and 22 cm, according to the size and the shape of the patient's chest (Fig. 25–14). The preoperative markings are as follows: AB = AC = 8 cm; DE = 10 to 12 cm. The new areola size, which measures 4 cm in diameter, is outlined by means of our nipple-areola template* (Fig. 25–15).

---

*The Galvao nipple marker is manufactured by Chas. F. Thackray Ltd., P.O. Box 171, Park Street, Leeds LSI IRQ, England.

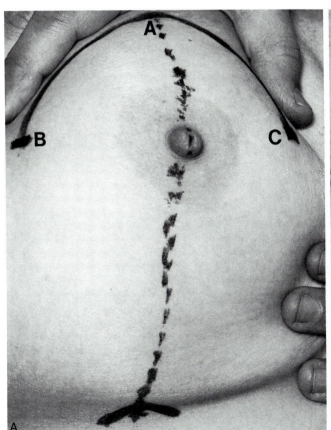 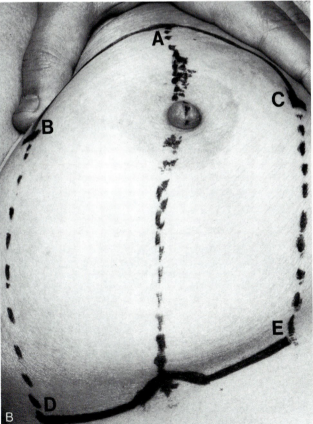

FIGURE 25–12

A, Note the position of the line from point A through the nipple to the inframammary fold. A small triangle is marked in the inframammary fold and represents the point where B and C will meet. *B,* The inframammary line is then outlined, determining points D and E (DE is 10 to 12 cm). Dotted lines are placed from points B to D and C to E, which correspond to the full-thickness incision lines.

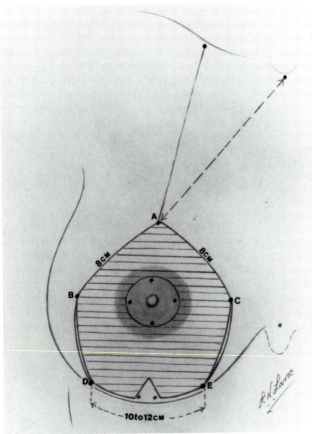

FIGURE 25–13

The distance from point D to point E is marked at 10 to 12 cm. Points B to D and C to E represent the areas of full-thickness incision lines.

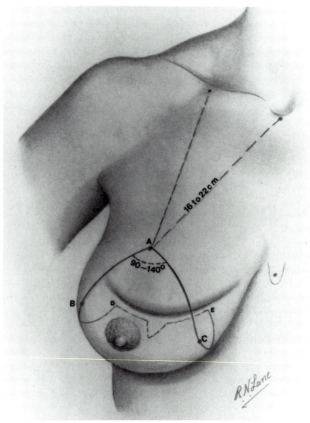

FIGURE 25–14

Note that AC and AB are each 8 cm in length. D to E equals 10 to 12 cm in length. The angle at point A varies from 90 to 140 degrees, depending on the size of the breast.

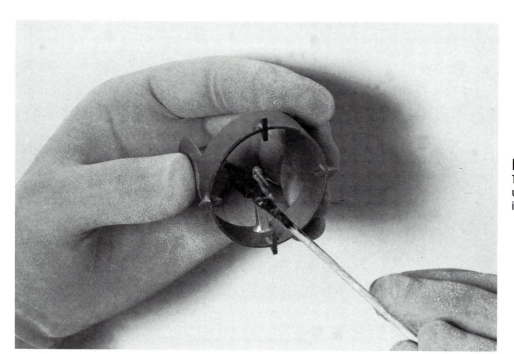

FIGURE 25–15

The nipple-areola template used in marking the areola is shown.

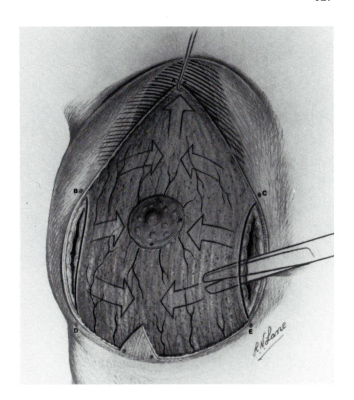

FIGURE 25–16

The area of de-epithelialization is shown. The area of dissection of the dermofat pedicles is shown through the incision from BD and CE. The nipple-areola complex and this large pedicle are detached from the gland. A small area is undermined at point A superiorly to allow easy folding of the upper pedicle. (From Galvao, M. S. L.: Reduction mammaplasty using dermofat pedicles. Br. J. Plast. Surg. 32:285, 1979.)

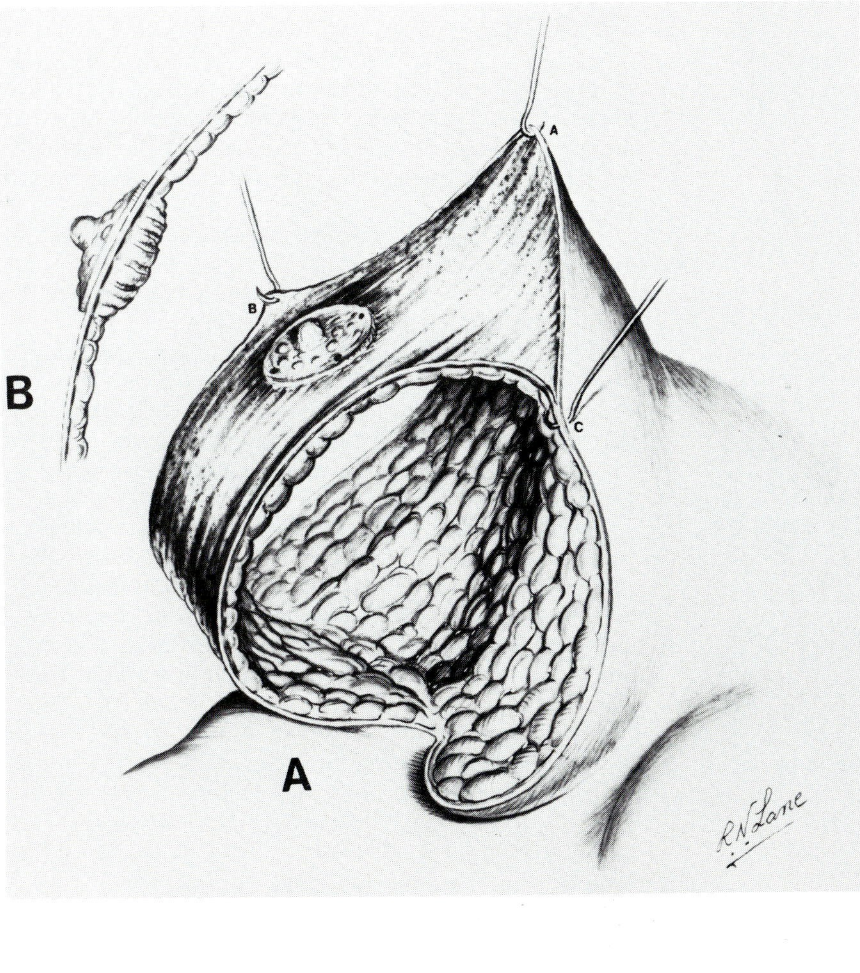

FIGURE 25–17

A, The appearance of the breast is shown following a pyramidal resection of breast tissue. A thickness of at least 1 cm is maintained at the pedicle. *B,* Note the increased thickness of breast tissue at the base of the nipple-areola complex. (From Galvao, M. S. L.: Reduction mammaplasty using dermofat pedicles. Br. J. Plast. Surg. 32:285, 1979.)

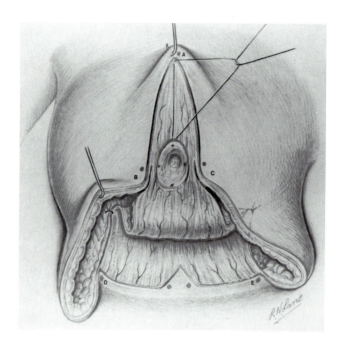

FIGURE 25–18

A suture is placed between point A and the areola prior to closure of the vertical suture line. A hook is placed at point A and held upward by the assistant, thus elevating the breast. Points B and C are approximated by the surgeon's fingers of the left and right hands, which allows one to visualize the new breast shape to be fashioned. Then the nipple-areola complex is pushed upward in the direction of point A, with the assistant still holding the breast upward. This maneuver is very important in determining whether the nipple-areola complex will reach its new position without excessive tension. Back cuts from points B and C upward for repositioning the nipple-areola complex can be carried out if necessary.

Operative Technique

The procedure is carried out with the patient under general anesthesia and in a semi-sitting position. Controlled hypotensive anesthesia is preferred but is not essential. Local infiltration of epinephrine reduces bleeding considerably.

Points A, B, C, D, and E, the small inframammary fold triangle, and cardinal points of the new areola are tattooed using Boney's blue ink. A partial-thickness incision is made around the outlined areola and also from point B to D, from C to E, and from D to E. The area demarcated is then de-epithelialized with a No. 22 blade.

A hook is now placed at point A, holding the breast upward for most of the operation. Full-thickness incisions are made from B to D and C to E, and the pedicles are dissected with the knife and the scissors. The nipple-areola complex is thereafter detached from the gland (Fig. 25–16).

Resection of the breast tissue is then performed as a pyramid shape with the gland incisions starting at point A downward (Fig. 25–17). The inferior pedicle is now fixed to the chest wall with 2-0 nylon sutures. It is important to suture the superior edge of the areola to point A before starting closure of the vertical suture line. Such a maneuver is helpful in checking whether the nipple-areola complex reaches its new position without excessive tension. It also facilitates its exteriorization (Fig. 25–18).

The vertical suture line is closed, and one is able to visualize the new breast to be fashioned. Excessive tension at the vertical suture line can be corrected by further excision of pedicles (Fig. 25–19).

After closure of the vertical suture line, two large dog-ears are produced. They are excised with removal of some breast tissue at an angle of 45 degrees for the desired contour. The lateral dog-ear contains some of the remaining axillary tail, which is usually excised (Fig. 25–20).

The new nipple-areola complex position is marked with our marker (Galvao, 1978), but it is cut slightly smaller, within the circle. The area is de-epithelialized, and the nipple is then hooked out. Cardinal tattoo dots inside and outside the areola are identified and approximated with fine nylon sutures. The inframammary fold suture line is always closed with subcuticular 4-0 nylon sutures, but interrupted stitches are preferred to close the tight vertical suture line (Fig. 25–21).

It is mandatory to place the nipple-areola complex pointing slightly downward. Gravitational forces will cause stretching of the suture lines, and the nipple-areola complex will later move upward (Fig. 25–22).

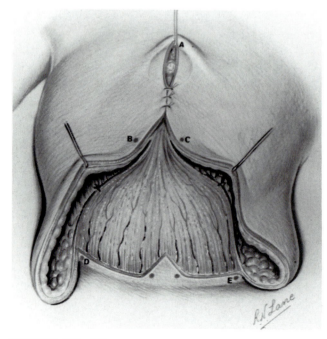

FIGURE 25–19

Closure of the vertical suture line.

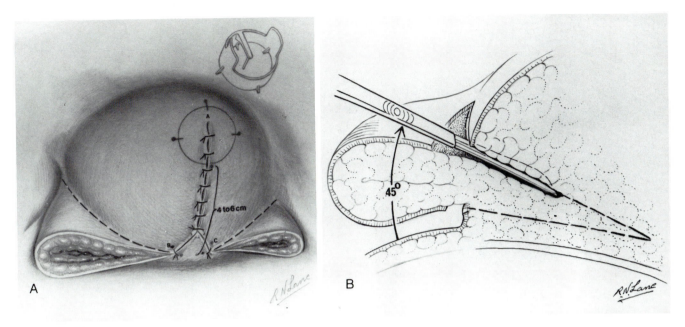

FIGURE 25–20

A and *B,* The resulting dog-ears must be sculptured at an angle of 45 degrees. The new nipple-areola complex position is outlined 4 to 6 cm from the inferior areola edge to the inframammary fold. (From Galvao, M. S. L.: Reduction mammaplasty using dermofat pedicles. Br. J. Plast. Surg. 32:285, 1979.)

FIGURE 25–21

The nipple-areola complex is repositioned following de-epi-thelialization of the outlined area, and the cardinal dots are approximated. (From Galvao, M. S. L.: Reduction mamma-plasty using dermofat pedicles. Br. J. Plast. Surg. 32:285, 1979.)

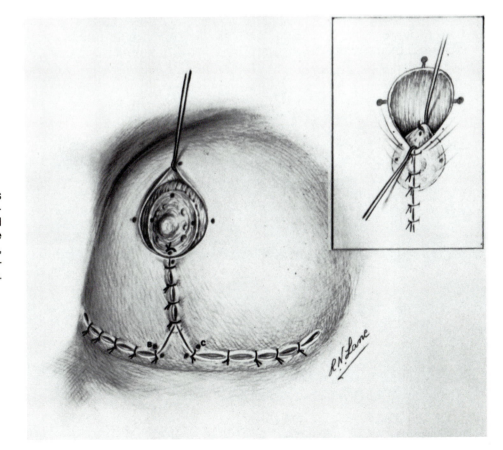

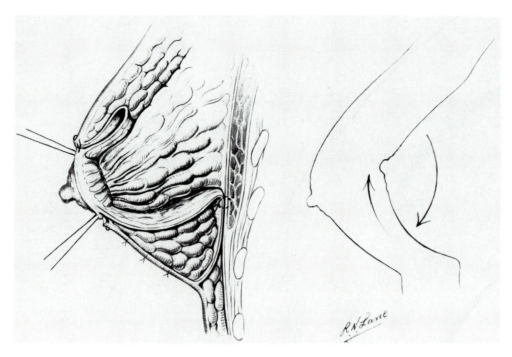

FIGURE 25–22
Buried dermofat pedicles. The breast is closed slightly tightly, the nipple-areola complex pointing downward. A normal breast contour is obtained some weeks later. (From Galvao, M. S. L.: Reduction mammaplasty using dermofat pedicles. Br. J. Plast. Surg. 32:285, 1979.)

Postoperative Care

Suction drains are inserted and left *in situ* for about 48 hours, and the breasts are immobilized with Steri-Strips and Elastoplast dressing. A fitted bra is worn from the second day continuously for 2 or 3 months after surgery. Steri-Strips are replaced weekly and used for about 6 weeks.

Prophylactic antibiotics are not given.

Results (Figs. 25–23 to 25–26)

Over 300 patients have been operated upon in the last 15 years with satisfactory results and negligible complications. Distortion of the nipple-areola complex has occurred in about 8 patients, which required minor trimming. This complication is not unusual for a mammaplasty without a medial scar, because the attempt to leave a small and short inframammary scar will undoubt-

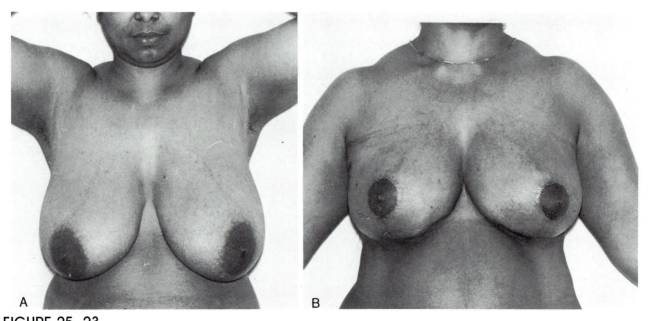

FIGURE 25–23
A, Young patient with gigantomastia. *B,* Same patient 6 months after reduction mammaplasty using the superior medial, lateral, and inferior pedicle technique.

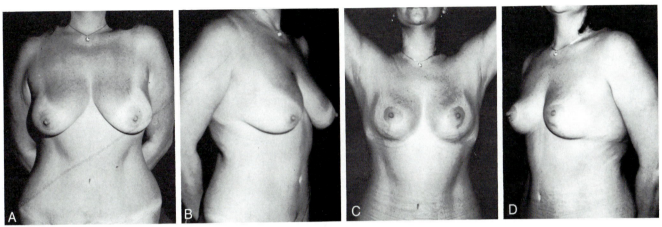

FIGURE 25–24

A and *B*, Young patient with a moderate degree of breast hypertrophy. *C* and *D*, Same patient 3 years after reduction mammaplasty using the technique described.

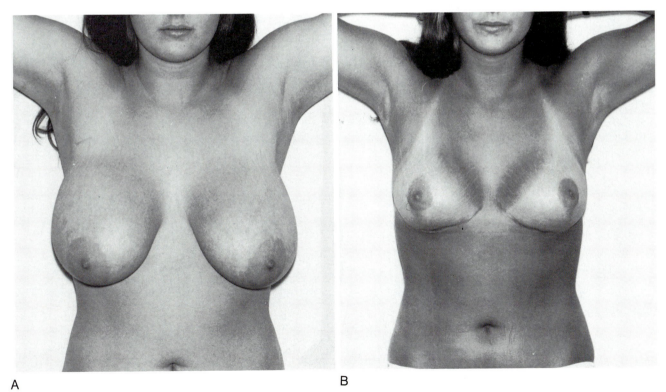

A   B

FIGURE 25–25

A, Young patient preoperatively with marginal hypertrophy. *B*, Same patient 8 months postoperatively after resection of approximately 750 gm from each breast.

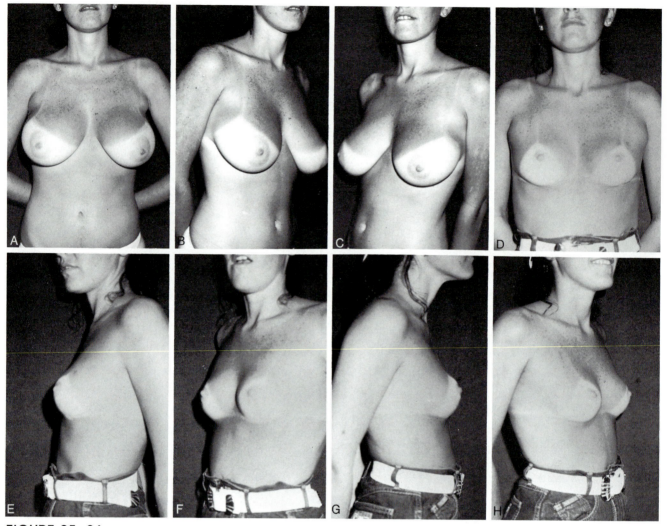

FIGURE 25–26
A to *C,* Patient 20 years old with a moderate degree of breast hypertrophy. *D* to *H,* Three years postoperative front, side, and oblique views of the same patient after a 600-gm resection of each breast.

edly leave skin excess at the vertical suture line, thus distorting the nipple-areola complex.

All the breasts are drained with suction drains. No hematomas have been observed. Prophylactic antibiotics have not been given and have been used only for patients whose breasts became infected.

References

Dufourmentel, C., Mouly, R.: Plastie mammaire par la méthod oblique. Ann. Chir. Plast. 6:45, 1961.

Elbaz, S. S., Verheecke, G.: La cicatrice en *L* dans les plasties mammaires. Ann. Chir. Plast. 17:283, 1972.

Galvao, M. S. L.: An instrument and technique for marking the nipple-areola complex during reduction mammaplasty. Br. J. Plast. Surg. 31:22, 1978.

Galvao, M. S. L.: Reduction mammaplasty using superior medial, lateral and inferior pedicles: A preliminary report. XXI World Congress of the International College of Surgeons. Abstracts. Jerusalem, Israel, 1978, p. 91.

Galvao, M. S. L.: Reduction mammaplasty using dermofat pedicles. Br. J. Plast. Surg. 32:285, 1979.

Galvao, M. S. L.: A method of reduction mammaplasty. In: Ely, J.

F. (ed.): *Transactions of the Seventh International Congress of Plastic and Reconstructive Surgery.* Sao Paulo, Cartgraf, 1980, p. 534.

Galvao, M. S. L.: *Year Book of Plastic and Reconstructive Surgery.* Chicago, Year Book Medical Publishers, 1981, p. 272.

Galvao, M. S. L.: A method of marking mammaplasty without medial scar. IX International Congress of Plastic and Reconstructive Surgery, New Delhi, India, 1987. Abstracts.

Georgiade, N. G.: *Reconstructive Surgery of the Breast.* St. Louis, C. V. Mosby, 1976.

Goldwyn, R. M.: *Plastic and Reconstructive Surgery of the Breast.* Boston, Little, Brown, 1976.

Lalardrie, J. P., Jouglard, J. P.: *Chirurgie Plastique du Sein.* Paris, Masson, 1974.

Marc, H.: Las plastie mammaire par la méthode oblique. Paris, G. Doin et Cie., Paris, 1952.

Meyer, R.: Personal communication, 1978.

Regnault, P.: Reduction mammaplasty by the "B" technique. Plast. Reconstr. Surg. 53:19, 1974.

Schwarzmann, E.: Die Technik der Mammaplastik. Chirurg 2:932, 1930.

Schwarzmann, E.: La técnica de la plástica mammaria. Dia. Med. 3:830, 1931.

Schwarzmann, E.: Beitrag zur Vermeldung von Mamillen-Nekrose bei einzeitiger Mammaplastik schwerer Fälle. Rev. Chir. Struct. 7:206, 1937.

26

Heinz H. Bohmert

Use of the Vertical Dermal Flap in Reduction Mammaplasty

The goals of an ideal reduction mammaplasty are to attain an aesthetically pleasant contour with proper nipple projection and with minimal scar deformity. The characteristics of attractive breasts have to be considered and include a pleasant fullness to the bosom; a slightly concave slope of the upper part to the point of maximum breast projection at the nipple; a shorter full curve to the submammary fold; and the natural obliquity of the nipple-areola complex, forward and outward, with a slight turn of the nipple upward. It is obvious that a perfectly aesthetically pleasing breast will never be achieved by any one surgical technique in all kinds of hypertrophied and ptotic breasts.

Techniques that avoid scars as much as possible have obvious appeal. However, a satisfactory contour and optimal symmetry without long scars are difficult to attain in large breasts. The safe transposition of the nipple-areola complex is the most important factor.

The operative procedure with which we have had the greatest success during the last years is the popular McKissock reduction mammaplasty using the vertical dermal pedicle.

OPERATIVE TECHNIQUE

McKissock (1972) described a technique for reducing moderate to severe mammary hypertrophy. With this method, the nipple and areola are transposed upward on a vertical dermal pedicle, based both superiorly and inferiorly. In this way distortion of the nipple and areola is avoided. Bolstering of the dermal pedicle under the nipple simultaneously increases the projection of the nipple.

The intended position of the nipple is marked before the operation. At operation, a caudocephalad dermal pedicle from the submammary fold to the new position of the nipple is de-epithelialized, apart from the areola (Fig. 26–1A and B). Depending on the degree of the hypertrophy, variously large tissue blocks can be removed both medial and lateral to the de-epithelialized skin zone (Fig. 26–1C).

Subsequently, tissue is also removed from under the de-epithelialized dermal pedicle so that the nipple and areola can be transported on the bridge flap (see Fig. 26–1C). The resection can be accomplished with excel-lent exposure because the incisions are long. The nipple and areola are transposed cranially, and the lateral skin flaps are opposed centrally over the caudal part of the dermal pedicle (Fig. 26–1D to F).

RESULTS

A comprehensive evaluation of results must include all important factors concerning the technique, extending from immediate postoperative complications to the final attitude of the patient. In our hospital, 367 women were treated by the McKissock method of reduction mammaplasty between 1978 and 1988. This operation was bilateral in 232 patients and unilateral in 135, of which 43 were being operated upon for asymmetry and 92 for making the contralateral breast symmetric with the other breast, reconstructed after mastectomy.

COMPLICATIONS

The frequency of complications was very low with this method. Partial necrosis of the nipple was noted in 2%, but in no case was the nipple lost. Reoperation to stop hemorrhage was required in 1% of patients and in 2% infection also required a second operation.

LONG-TERM RESULTS

We shall have a good idea of our results if we follow our cases at least 3 years after breast reduction. A recent survey was conducted of a group of 186 patients who had undergone the procedure more than 3 years before in order to evaluate long-term results. The survey was focused upon appraisals of contour, scar formation, nipple sensation, and the patient's attitude.

In order to judge whether deformation was produced by or after this operation, the distances between the sternal notch and the nipple and between the nipple and the submammary fold were measured before, during, and after the operation. It was found that the average intraoperative distance of 21 cm between the sternal notch and the nipple increased only very slightly to 22 cm after 3½ years. This average distance was 29 cm

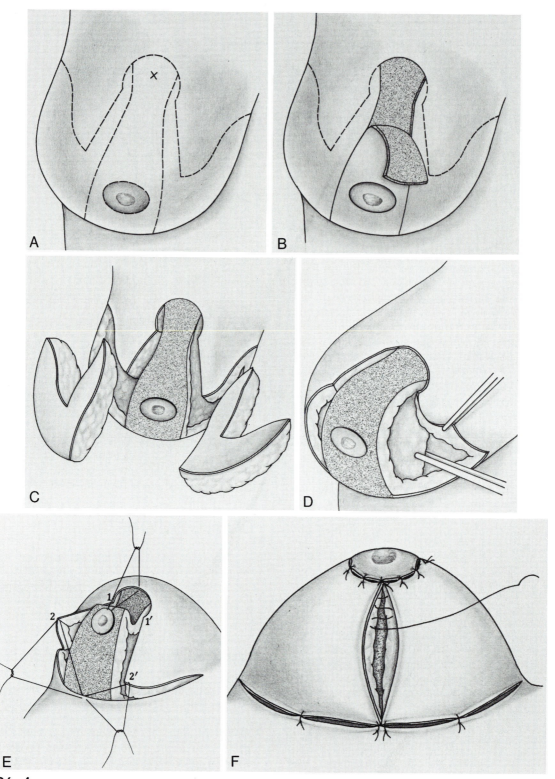

FIGURE 26-1

The McKissock technique. *A*, The vertical dermal pedicle is outlined. *B*, The dermal pedicle is de-epithelialized around the areola before blocks of tissue are removed bilaterally. *C*, Medial and lateral wedges of breast tissue are resected. *D*, Tissue resection behind the skin bridge and the cranial part of the breast. *E*, The nipple and areola are transposed on the vertical dermal pedicle to their new position, and the side wings of the mammary skin are joined over the caudal part of the vertical dermal flap. *F*, The medial and lateral skin flaps are sutured. Any discrepancy in the vertical line and inframammary fold can be adjusted as the flaps are sutured.

preoperatively. Similarly, the distance between the nipple and the submammary fold, which was on average 13 cm before operation, was 7 cm during the operation and on average 8 cm 3½ years later. This showed that there was no significant change in the shape of the breast after operation (Figs. 26–2 to 26–6).

With regard to the sensitivity of the nipple, 40% of the patients reported that it was unchanged and 60%

that it was decreased. In order to examine this objectively, the nipple was tested for erectility, and a positive response was almost always obtained.

The aesthetic results were reported at follow-up as good in 57%, fairly good in 31%, satisfactory in 6%, and poor in 6%. The unsatisfactory results were due to obvious scars.

Text continued on page 342

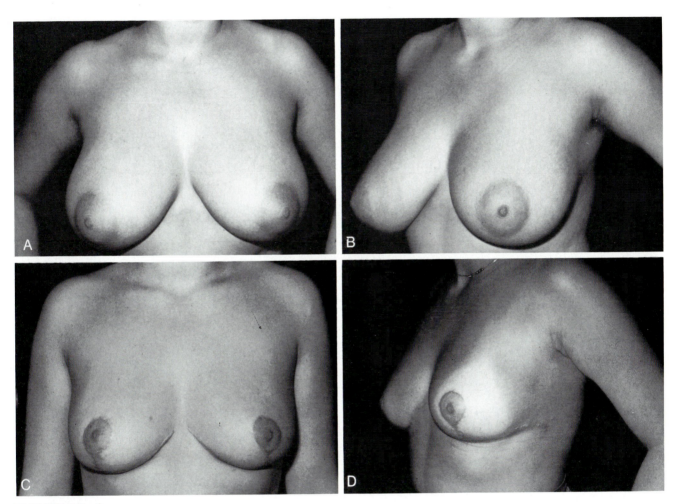

FIGURE 26–2
A and *B,* A 16-year-old female with juvenile hypertrophy of the breasts. *C* and *D,* The same patient 1 year after reduction mammaplasty by the McKissock technique, with removal of 650 gm from the right breast and 550 gm from the left breast.

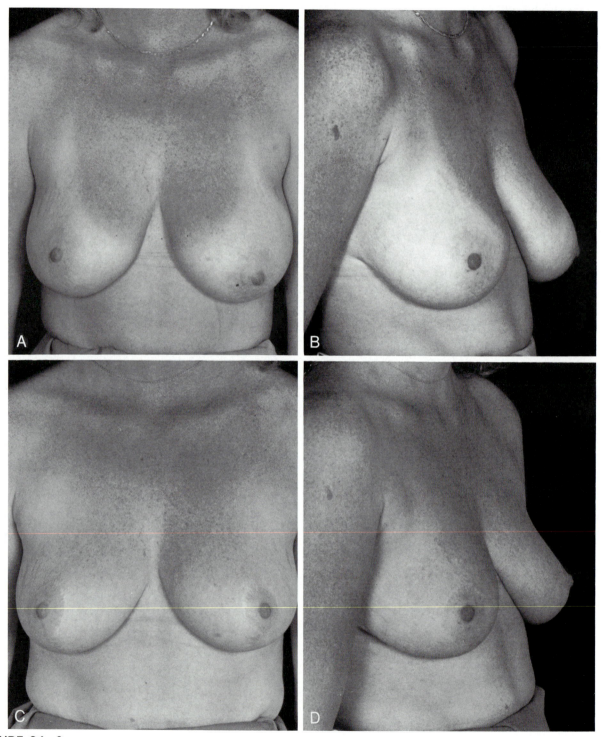

FIGURE 26–3

A and *B,* A 32-year-old patient with mammary hyperplasia with tense, firm, heavy breast tissue. *C* and *D,* The same patient 3 years after reduction mammaplasty, with removal of 210 gm from the right breast and 285 gm from the left breast.

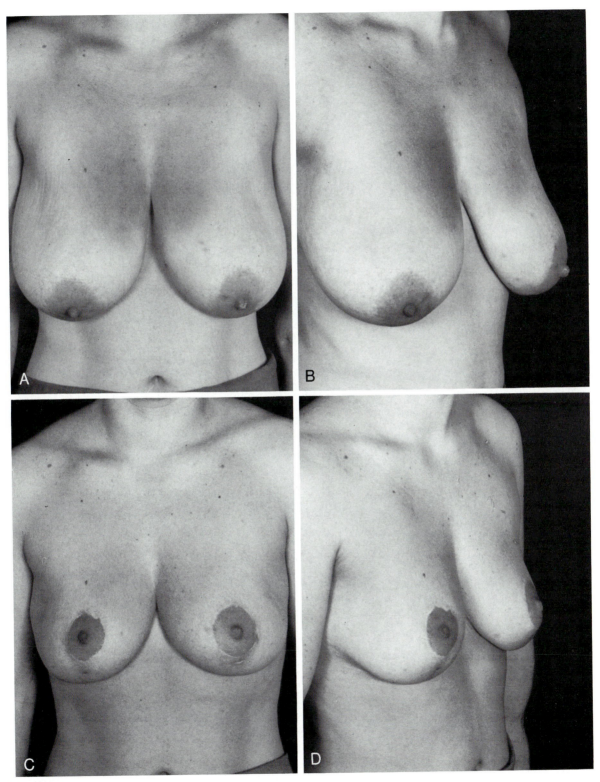

FIGURE 26–4

A and *B*, A 27-year-old patient with large, pendulous breasts. *C* and *D*, The same patient 2 years after reduction mammaplasty, with removal of 510 gm from the right breast and 490 gm from the left breast and elevation of the nipple position of approximately 12 cm.

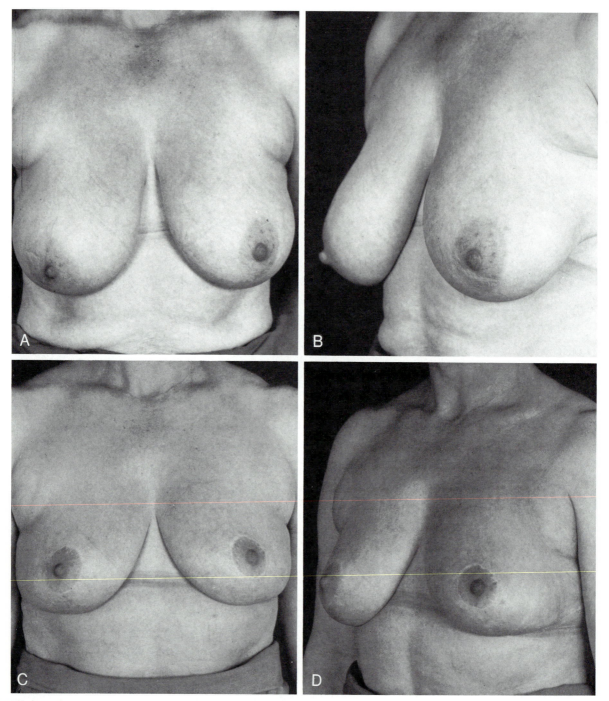

FIGURE 26–5

A and *B,* A 47-year-old patient with large, ptotic breasts and asymmetry. *C* and *D,* The same patient 3 years after reduction mammaplasty, with removal of 410 gm from the right breast and 370 gm from the left breast.

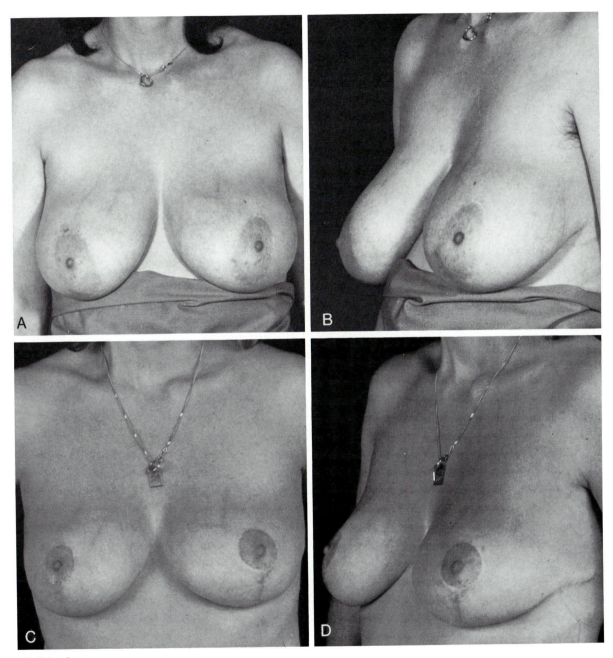

FIGURE 26–6
A and *B*, A 43-year-old patient with severe hypertrophy and ptosis of the breasts, reduced by the McKissock technique, with removal of 510 gm from the right breast and 570 gm from the left breast. *C* and *D*, The same patient 2 years after reduction mammaplasty.

DISCUSSION

As in the reduction mammaplasty described by Ström-beck (1960), major disadvantages of this method are the marked and often hypertrophic scars. Comparing the results with those of the methods from Marchac and de Olarte (1982) and Peixoto (1980), we found the most difficulties in these procedures in achieving optimal nipple projection and symmetry, and considerable experience is necessary.

In the McKissock operation, the vascularization of the nipple and areola is ensured by the presence of the bridge flap. This not only supplies blood but also increases the projection of the nipple, lying as it does under the areola.

Subsequent drooping of the breast is reported as one of the disadvantages of the McKissock reduction mam-maplasty, but the measurements on our patients did not show significant drooping.

McKissock's reduction mammaplasty is a well-standardized, reliable method that allows good operative exposure and is easy for the plastic surgeon in training to learn.

References

McKissock, P. K.: Reduction mammaplasty with a vertical dermal flap. Plast. Reconstr. Surg. 49:245, 1972.

Marchac, D. E., de Olarte, D.: Reduction mammaplasty and correlation of ptosis with a short inframammary scar. Plast. Reconstr. Surg. 69:45, 1982.

Peixoto, G.: Reduction mammaplasty: A personal technique. Plast. Reconstr. Surg. 65:217, 1980.

Strömbeck, J. O.: Mammaplasty: Report of a new procedure based on the two-pedicle procedure. Br. J. Plast. Surg. 13:79, 1960.

A. R. Moscona
Bernard Hirshowitz
Yaron Har-Shai

27

The Modified Bipedicle Vertical Dermal Flap Technique for Reduction Mammaplasty

The use of a dermal bridge for nipple transposition for reduction mammaplasty was popularized by Strömbeck in 1960 (Strömbeck, 1960).

In 1972 McKissock (McKissock, 1972, 1976) introduced his concept of a bipedicle vertical dermal flap technique and presumably was influenced a good deal by Strömbeck. According to McKissock, the bipedicle vertical dermal flap has definite advantages over the transverse dermal bridge.

With the bipedicle vertical dermal flap design, the anatomic siting of both the blood and nerve supply to the breast tissue is respected in that the inferior pedicle appears to incorporate many of these structures.

In addition, the superior pedicle, by virtue of its continuity with the nipple-areola complex, acts as a conduit for the subdermal plexus of vessels and nerves to the nipple-areola complex. Thus, this structure obtains a double blood and nerve supply through both pedicles, ensuring maximal vascularity and innervation.

In the course of our routine use of the McKissock technique some drawbacks to this method were encountered; and in an effort to improve on the results, we introduced various modifications (Hirshowitz and Moscona, 1982, 1983).

POINTS OF DIVERGENCE

The main points of divergence from the original description are as follows:

1. Limited raising of the new areolar site, together with a short and broad superior pedicle (Fig. 27-1).
2. Restricted length of the submammary incision (Fig. 27-2).
3. A narrow-based inferior vertical pedicle (Fig. 27-2).
4. Coring out in depth over much of the breast parenchyma (Fig. 27-3).

Limited Raising of the New Areolar Site

The areolar site can be raised only 2 to 6 cm. This is in contrast to the original McKissock design, in which the superior pedicle appears to be rather elongated. There is an intimate correlation between this limited raising of the nipple-areola complex and the extensive coring in depth of the breast parenchyma. The loss of breast mass results in contraction of the remaining superficial breast tissue (Cloutier, 1979) and skin around the central axis provided by the nipple-areola complex. The shrinkage of skin may be further explained by the previous stretching of the skin due to excessive bulk and weight of the underlying breast tissue. When these latter are reduced, the natural elasticity of the skin foreshortens the overall dimensions of the breast skin. Thus, the superior pedicle can be kept short by virtue of the natural tendency of tissues to contract (see Fig. 27-1).

Restricted Length of the Submammary Incision

The length of the submammary incision is restricted to approximately 15 cm. This enables the extremities of this incision to lie within the confines of the newly modeled breast. This line does not encroach medially on the sternal area nor into the axilla laterally. In the erect position this incision is largely hidden under the breast itself.

Notwithstanding the limitations imposed by the restricted length of this incision, there is no difficulty in mobilizing the medial and lateral breast flaps. These in turn can be readily brought together along the infra-areolar suture line (see Fig. 27-2).

Narrow-Based Inferior Vertical Pedicle of Adequate Bulk

The inferior pedicle markings start on either side of the newly outlined areola and descend by two parallel lines, which widen only slightly as the submammary fold is approached. Accordingly, the base of the inferior pedicle measures not more than 4.5 to 5.5 cm and only in markedly ptotic breasts 6 cm. In constructing the inferior pedicle in depth, both its medial and lateral faces are beveled outward somewhat as the pectoral

343

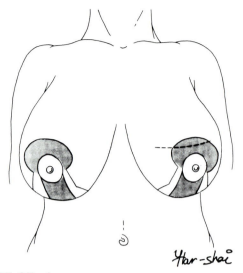

FIGURE 27–1
The preoperative design for reduction mammaplasty illustrates our modifications of the original McKissock concept, which include limited raising of the new areolar site, together with a short and broad superior pedicle. The dotted line represents on the front of a ptotic breast the submammary fold, underneath it.

fascia is approached. This, together with the coring under the areola, gives the inferior pedicle a somewhat truncated pyramidal shape.

Bulkwise, the inferior pedicle is adequate for providing the filling necessary to obtain a good contour of the lower half of the breast and good nipple projection. Should the base of the inferior pedicle be made any wider, there would be a corresponding reduction in the amount of dermoglandular tissue to be excised on either side of the inferior pedicle, because the length of the submammary incision is restricted in advance (see Fig. 27–2).

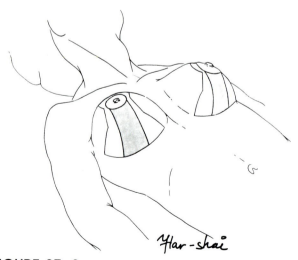

FIGURE 27–2
Restricted length of the submammary incision is dependent on the construction of a narrow-based inferior pedicle.

Deep Coring of the Breast Parenchyma

It is here that the main modification of the original McKissock concept is effected. Breast tissue is cored out in depth not only beneath the areola but also upward, under the superior half of the breast, and sideward, under the medial and lateral breast flaps, leaving a 2- to 3-cm-thick layer of breast tissue in all directions (see Fig. 27–3). Special attention is paid to coring out the lateral breast flap as far out as the axilla, because there is greater extension of the breast parenchyma laterally than medially. This step enables the breast to be made narrow in the transverse dimension and helps to avoid a broad shape in the re-formed breast.

A true "bucket handle" of the inferior pedicle, according to the original McKissock design, is not obtained because the coring out of the inferior pedicle is confined only to where it abuts against the areola.

The thickness of the areola is left at about 1.5 to 2 cm. Therefore, many of the lactiferous ducts to the nipple are divided, and their tethering effect is overcome. This permits the nipple-areola complex to be raised with ease. However, some lactiferous ducts do remain intact, because a few patients have been able, after this operation, to breast-feed their babies. In this regard, it may be worthwhile to consider subareolar scoring under the superior part of the areola in order to preserve as many lactiferous ducts to the nipple as possible (see Fig. 27–3).

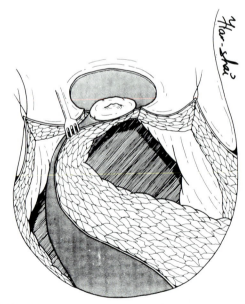

FIGURE 27–3
Coring out in depth over much of the breast parenchyma commences with subareolar coring. Special attention is paid to reaching as far out laterally as the axilla. It is here that we effect our main modification of the original McKissock operation. An effort is made not to expose the lateral pectoralis fascia for fear of damaging the lateral cutaneous branch of the fourth intercostal nerve (the special nerve to the nipple).

INDICATIONS FOR THIS PROCEDURE

We have found that the wide variety of shapes and sizes of pendulous and ptotic breasts can be adequately dealt with by means of the modified bipedicled vertical dermal flap technique. We believe that an affirmative answer can be given to the question raised by Georgiade and his associates (Georgiade et al., 1979): "Is there a reduction mammaplasty for 'all seasons'?"

The mammary gland extends in its vertical dimension from the second or third down to the eighth rib and transversely from the parasternal to the anterior axillary lines. Within these boundaries the shape and size of the breast can vary tremendously. The position of one structure that remains fairly constant within the gamut of different sizes and shapes of pendulous and ptotic breasts is the submammary fold. It is from this fold that the height of the nipple-areola complex is determined and the distance of it from the fold is fixed at about 5 to 6 cm.

These two almost constant features provide the basis for our preoperative markings. Both the outline of the oval superior pedicle, which is open inferiorly, and the lines of divergence from the extremities of this outline change, depending on the degree of breast size and breast ptosis. The range of height and width of the superior pedicle can vary between 2 to 6 cm and 6 to 10 cm, respectively.

In the small reduction mammaplasties, the extremities of the outline of the superior pedicle converge on the newly marked areola and may almost abut against it. As the need exists for excision of larger amounts of breast tissue and skin, the separation of the ends of this outline from the margins of the areola is made wider (Fig. 27–4).

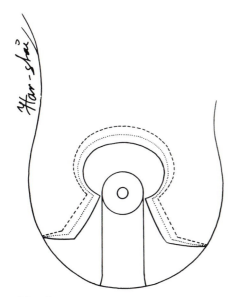

FIGURE 27–4
Schematic drawing showing increasing dimensions of the superior pedicle both in height and in width, with increasing degrees of pendulosity. By the same token, the spread of divergence of the descending limbs becomes correspondingly larger.

As previously stated, the submammary incision is kept as short as possible, to about 15 cm. However, in the very large pendulous and ptotic breasts, it is necessary to lengthen these measurements by some 1 to 2 cm. In these situations the descending limbs are correspondingly widely separated from the inferior pedicle. Their ends are joined to those of the submammary incision, and two dermoglandular areas scheduled for excision are outlined on either side of the inferior pedicle.

In the original McKissock operation, these two dermoglandular areas are made much larger than in our modified approach. However, with the addition of breast tissue obtained from deep coring, it is considered that a comparable amount of tissue is excised in both methods.

In the essentially ptotic breast in which the main element for excision is skin, deep coring would be done sparingly.

In the pendulous breast, the weight of the breast tissue contributes to the downward displacement of the nipple-areola complex. Both this and ptosis influence the distance between the midclavicular point (MCP) and the nipple. In the almost aesthetically perfect breast this distance is about 20 cm and is about 3.5 cm below the midhumeral point (Penn, 1954). Because one is dealing with the preceding two somewhat indeterminate factors, it is difficult to estimate preoperatively the planned postoperative distance of the nipple-areola complex from the midclavicular point. The implication of this is that when one is designing the superior pedicle, both breast weight and ptosis have to be considered.

In planning the shape of the superior pedicle, the following principle may act as a guideline: The greater the breast weight and degree of ptosis, the greater the height and width of the superior pedicle.

There is often a relationship between excess weight of the patient and pendulous breasts. In a subconscious effort to conceal the embarrassment caused by oversized breasts, the patient often tends to be overweight. After the operation, when breast size is normal, there is frequently an accompanying desire to lose body weight. This leads to further reduction in the size of the breasts. One estimation is that with every kilogram of body weight lost, there is a corresponding 10- to 12-gm loss of breast weight. This point also needs to be considered when one is planning the extent of the reduction mammaplasty to be performed.

TOTAL AMOUNT OF SKIN EXCISED

De-epithelialization of both the superior and inferior pedicles yields an amount of skin corresponding to the surface area of each pedicle. To this the excised skin of the two dermoglandular areas is added. When comparing this total amount with that excised in the McKissock method, one finds that in this latter method a larger area of skin is excised.

The obvious question that comes to mind is whether there is any skin redundancy in the modified method. The same rationale that applies to the limited raising of the nipple-areola complex, concomitant with deep coring of the breast parenchyma, also applies to the need for reduced skin excision.

Deep coring leaves a potential dead space within the breast wound, and the natural tendency of both breast tissue and skin to contract results in obliteration of this hollow. The skin brassiere readily adapts itself to the contents of the breast package.

THIRD-DIMENSIONAL CONCEPT OF THE POSITIONING OF THE NIPPLE-AREOLA COMPLEX

As the newly cut nipple-areola complex is being raised to its new position, the margins of the superior pedicle are wrapped around it. Provided that there is sufficient bulk to the inferior pedicle, this wrapping contributes to the overall elevation of the nipple-areola complex and tends to project the nipple forward. In this way a third dimension is added to the breast reduction (Fig. 27–5; see Fig. 27–7F).

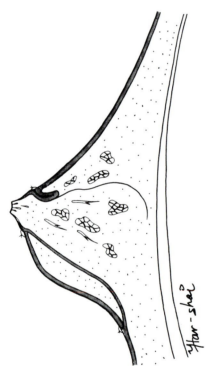

FIGURE 27–5
A third dimension of nipple projection is added to the breast reduction as the margins of the superior pedicle are wrapped around the nipple-areola complex. A sufficiently bulky inferior pedicle is necessary for obtaining this projection.

"DISHING OUT" POSTOPERATIVELY: IS IT PREVENTABLE?

One of the goals set for a satisfactory outcome following a reduction mammaplasty is the avoidance postoperatively of a downward projection of the inferior hem-

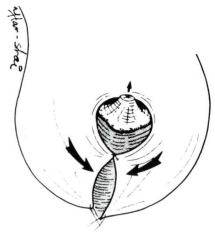

FIGURE 27–6
The continuous dermal sheet extending from the superior pedicle to the submammary fold has a reining effect on the nipple-areola complex, preventing "dishing out" post-operatively. The short and broad dimensions of our superior pedicle, in contrast to that of the original McKissock design, permit wide dermal contact with the infolding of the superior pedicle as the nipple-areola complex takes up its new position. This wide dermal contact probably contributes an element of strength to the infolding and may be an important factor in preventing postoperative dishing out.

isphere of the breast and an accompanying upward displacement of the nipple-areola complex (Dinner and Chait, 1977).

Following the routine use of our modified bipedicle vertical dermal flap technique, "dishing out" seems to be, in our experience, most uncommon. A possible explanation for the preservation of the breast shape by this method is the reining effect of a relatively short continuous sheet of dermis that extends from the superior pedicle to the submammary fold.

The short and broad dimensions of our superior pedicle, in contrast to that in the original McKissock design, permit wide dermal contact with the infolding of the superior pedicle as the nipple-areola complex takes up its new position (Fig. 27–6). This probably contributes an element of strength to the infolding and may be an important factor in preventing postoperative dishing out.

It is reasonable to assume that ordinarily the dermis is the main retaining element together with Cooper's ligaments in maintaining breast shape. In our bipedicle vertical dermal flap technique both these structures remain intact; and although the dermis strip is narrowed over the inferior pedicle and is buried somewhat in depth, it is sufficient to keep the nipple-areola complex permanently tethered in its immediate postoperative position.

PREOPERATIVE MARKINGS

Preoperative markings are made while the patient is in both a sitting position and a reclining position. The nipple-areola complex is encircled according to its planned new dimensions, which are generally about 4 cm in diameter. The submammary fold is drawn. More or less vertical lines connect the outer limits of the nipple-areola complex with the submammary fold, creating the inferior pedicle. The base of the inferior pedicle should be between 4.5 and 5.5 cm in width. In order to obtain this width, one may have to make these vertical lines diverge somewhat distally.

Only in the very ptotic breast would the base of the inferior pedicle be made 6 cm wide or more.

In ptotic breasts the submammary fold corresponds on the front of the breast to the projection of the fingers placed in the inframammary sulcus under the breast. In order to provide extra safeguards in the placement of the new nipple site, two additional lines are also drawn 19 to 22 cm in length, depending on the breast size, the body habitus, and the torso length. One is from the manubrium sterni to the nipple; the other, from the midclavicular point to the nipple. These two lines, together with the medial half of the clavicle, form a triangle, at the apex of which is the new nipple site. A measurement of 8 to 10 cm between the midline of the body and the medial limit of the superior pedicle acts as an added check on the positioning of the superior pedicle.

The markings will tend to produce a postoperative nipple site slightly lateral to the midclavicular line, with the nipple-areola complex pointing somewhat upward and outward.

Depending on the extent of the breast pendulosity and ptosis, the shape of the superior pedicle is delineated. As previously stated, the inferior limits of its outline can abut against the nipple-areola complex or can be separated from it on both its medial and lateral aspects by up to 2 cm.

From the points where the superior pedicle outline ceases, the descending limbs 5 to 6 cm in length begin. The spread of divergence of these limbs from the inferior pedicle will depend on the size of the superior pedicle (see Fig. 27–4). The smaller the superior pedicle, the narrower is this spread, because the terminating points of the descending limbs are joined to the ends of the submammary incision line, which has a fairly constant length of 15 cm. Only in cases of marked ptosis or pendulosity will the length of the submammary incision be elongated to 16 to 17 cm.

Thus, the size of the superior pedicle will have a direct bearing on the dimensions of the dermoglandular tissue to be excised on either side of the inferior pedicle. The larger the breast, the larger the superior pedicle and the larger the dermoglandular areas scheduled for excision.

OPERATIVE TECHNIQUE (Fig. 27–7)

The operation is performed with the patient under general anesthesia and in a semirecumbent position. A pillow is placed under the knees, and the soles of the feet are supported by a foot rest. Following skin preparation and draping, all the preoperative outlines are revised and are redrawn if necessary (Fig. 27–7A and B). They are incised through to the dermis.

Both the superior and inferior pedicles are de-epithelialized by means of sharp dissection (Fig. 27–7C). In this regard, it has been found helpful to de-epithelialize the skin on the outer margins of the pedicles first and then deal with the central bulging that remains. In this way one always has the plane of de-epithelialization under good vision, and this lessens the chances of button-holing of the skin. Care is taken not to expose the subcutaneous fat, since the integrity of the dermal sheet is considered important in preventing postoperative dishing out of the breast and preserving an intact subdermal vascular plexus. A strong hook is inserted into the dermis of the upper middle part of the superior pedicle (Fig. 27–7D). By applying traction to this hook, the breast is, as it were, suspended in space, enabling all the intramammary excisions to be conducted from the same point of reference. With either a diathermy cutting current or sharp dissection, both dermoglandular areas are excised. Starting with subareolar coring, which opening acts like a portal of entry, the whole extent of the breast is cored out except under the inferior pedicle, which is left intact (Fig. 27–7E). Subareolar coring leaves a somewhat thinner layer of tissue here than over the rest of the breast itself and is approximately 1.5 to 2.0 cm thick. Repeated assessments of the thickness of the breast flaps are made by means of apposing thumb to fingers; with both judgment and experience, the optimum thickness of between 2 and 3 cm is obtained (Fig. 27–7F). Deep coring needs to be performed superiorly, particularly in pendulous breasts, almost up to the level of the second rib.

Laterally, the coring in depth extends to the edge of the breast tissue in the axilla. The lateral breast flap is an important element in providing bulk to the inferior hemisphere of the breast. This and the inferior pedicle are the main factors in providing a pleasing contour to the breast, because the medial breast flap is rather limited in its amount of breast tissue.

It is necessary to incise the dermis of the superior pedicle, commencing at the apex of both dermoglandular areas on either side of the nipple-areola complex to a length of about 1.0 cm. This facilitates the raising of the nipple-areola complex to its new location and the suturing of the margins of the superior pedicle around it. These incisions do not in any way impair the blood supply of the superior pedicle.

Closure of the margins of the two descending vertical limbs along the infra-areolar suture line is performed with individual catgut or other biodegradable sutures. The skin edges are drawn together, and distally they meet at about the middle of the base of the inferior pedicle (Fig. 27–7G). But this point is not a precise one. Because of the predetermined length of the descending limbs of 5 to 5.5 cm, the infra-areolar suture line will be of an equal length (Fig. 27–7H). However, this can be somewhat adjusted by suturing the markings of the superior pedicle proximal to their terminating points.

This procedure will make for tighter closure around the nipple-areola complex and will elongate the infra-areolar line. The encircling skin margins around the nipple-areola complex can, if necessary, be enlarged by paring away their edges. A certain amount of leeway is

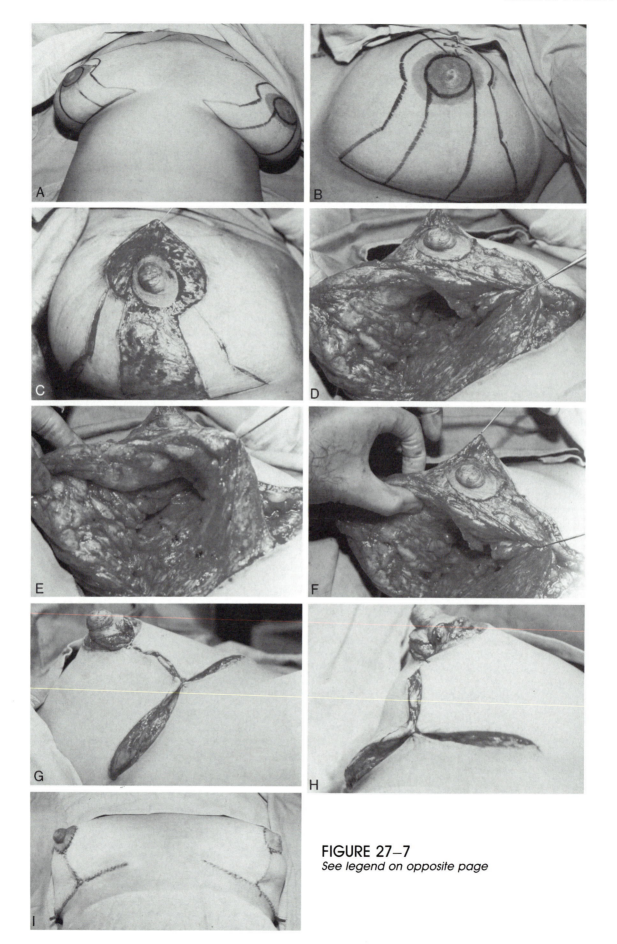

FIGURE 27–7
See legend on opposite page

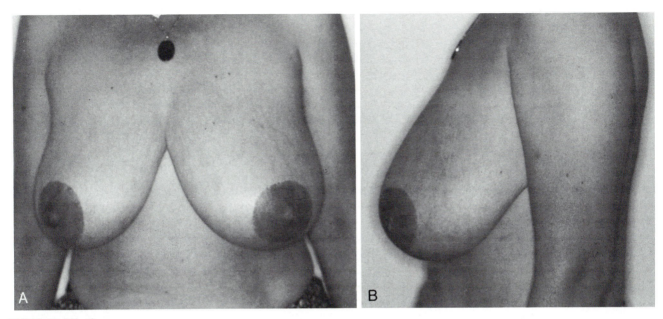

FIGURE 27–8
A and *B*, Front and side views of a woman who 20 years before had undergone partial amputation of the breasts with transplantation of the nipple as a free graft. When she was seen recently, her nipple sensation was virtually normal.

therefore provided in arriving at the final closure. There are rare instances when at the termination of the reduction mammaplasty a depression is noticed above the nipple-areola complex, which can be a cause for some concern. However, this rapidly disappears within a day or two as the breast tissue contracts and obliterates areas of dead space, which accounts for this depression.

An open-ended drain is inserted into the depths of the breast wound. It is usually removed after 24 hours.

Depending on one's preference, intracuticular or continuous running fine synthetic sutures are used for skin suture (Fig. 27–7I). In the latter case all sutures are removed by the tenth day.

COMPLICATIONS

Possible complications occurring with the operative procedure embodied in these modifications of the McKissock technique appear to be, in our hands, infrequent. They fall mainly into three categories: (1) vascularity, (2) delayed healing, and (3) loss of nipple sensation.

Vascularity

The integrity of the nipple-areola complex is inviolable, and the blood supply to the nipple-areola complex should be maximal. In view of the double blood supply to the nipple-areola complex through both pedicles,

adequate vascularity appears to be guaranteed. There is a rich blood supply through the subdermal plexus to the nipple-areola complex via the broad superior pedicle, which is contiguous with the nipple-areola complex. The well-constructed inferior pedicle carries with it a rich network of blood vessels, derived from the fifth, sixth, and seventh intercostal arteries, which give off numerous branches around the inferior border of the pectoralis major muscle prior to entering the gland. The nagging concerns of impaired nipple-areola complex vascularity that used to accompany the operation of reduction mammaplasty before the use of this present technique are for us largely a thing of the past.

Delayed Healing

The junction of the vertical infra-areolar suture line with the submammary incision is a potential source of weakness. We have encountered partial dehiscence of the skin margins here, causing delayed healing for 1 to 2 weeks and sometimes longer. It is important that all dead space beneath the skin margins at this point be eliminated by carefully approximating the subcutaneous tissue with absorbable sutures.

Loss of Nipple Sensation

In most of our patients, after this method of reduction mammaplasty, sensation of the nipple-areola complex

FIGURE 27–7
A and *B*, Preoperative skin markings. *C*, De-epithelialized superior and inferior pedicles. *D*, Skin hook inserted into the upper middle part of the superior pedicle. *E*, Coring out in depth over the whole of the breast parenchyma except under the inferior pedicle. *F*, Repeated assessments of the thickness of the breast flaps by apposing the thumb to the finger. *G* and *H*, The skin edges of the descending limbs are drawn together, and distally they meet at about the middle of the base of the inferior pedicle. *I*, Closure of all suture lines at the end of the procedure.

is, to a large extent, retained (Courtiss and Goldwyn, 1976). Our concern in adhering to two concepts may contribute to this retention of sensation. The nipple-areola complex was believed by Cooper (Cooper, 1840) to be innervated by nerve filaments lying superficial to the glandular tissue of the breast. Cathcart and associates (1948) and Craig and Sykes (1970), however, believe that this structure is supplied mainly from the depth of the breast tissue, with little extension of nerve fibers from the dermal areolar area.

We have reason to believe that the nipple-areola complex does derive innervation from the surrounding superficial nerves, as shown in one of our patients (Fig. 27–8A and B). If this is in fact the case, a broad superior

pedicle, because of its wide contiguity with the nipple-areola complex, would provide maximal innervation from this source. Second, an effort is made not to expose the fascia overlying the pectoralis major muscle, for fear of damaging the nerve to the nipple. This is the lateral cutaneous branch of the fourth intercostal nerve and, according to the anatomic cadaver dissections of both Hricko (Edwards, 1976) and Farina and co-workers (Farina et al., 1980), is a unique nerve to the nipple. The latter authors found that its anterior branch pierces the serratus anterior muscle in the midaxillary line where it turns anteriorly at a right angle, passing just lateral to the pectoralis major muscle, and enters the mammary gland on its posterior aspect, 1.5 to 2 cm from the edges

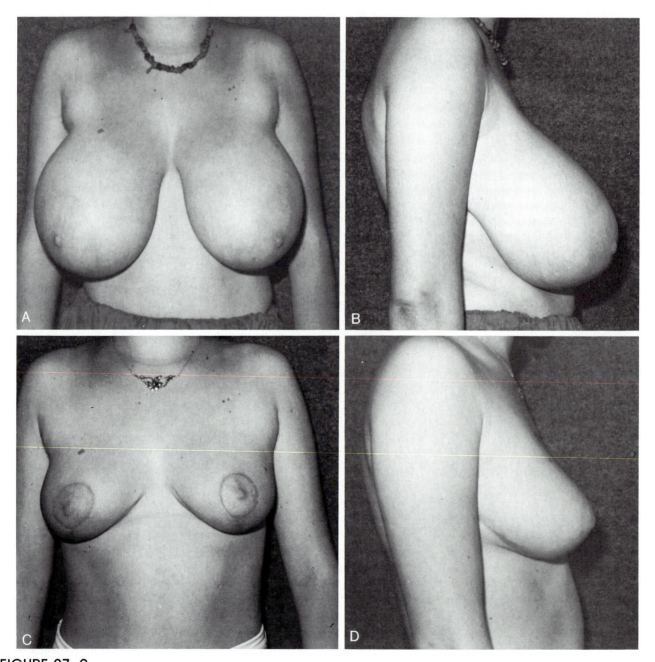

FIGURE 27–9

A and *B*, Preoperative front and side views of large, pendulous, ptotic breasts in a 17-year-old girl. *C* and *D*, The same patient 3 months after 860 gm of breast tissue was removed from the right breast and 900 gm from the left.

of the gland. This nerve consistently penetrates the left mammary gland at the 4 o'clock position and the right breast at the 8 o'clock position. It maintains the same depth in relation to the surface until midway to the nipple-areola complex, where it becomes more superficial as it reaches the areola. Retaining an adequate width to the inferior pedicle, it is hoped, keeps this nerve intact.

CONCLUSION

These modifications of the original McKissock bipedicle vertical dermal flap technique for reduction mammaplasty offer both safety and reliability in securing a pleasing operative result. This method appears to be based on sound anatomic principles and also incorporates the natural tendency of tissues to contract.

Senior residents training in plastic surgery are generally capable of grasping the broad principles of this operation, which can be performed by them under minimal supervision.

This procedure sets rather definite guidelines with regard to limited submammary incision length. It also allows for considerable freedom in determining the size of the superior pedicle, which is the focal area for determining the extent of the excision of breast parenchyma and skin. These modifications in our hands permit breast reduction to be performed for almost all shapes and sizes, with the reasonably certain expectation of achieving a satisfactory aesthetic and functional result (Figs. 27–9 to 27–11).

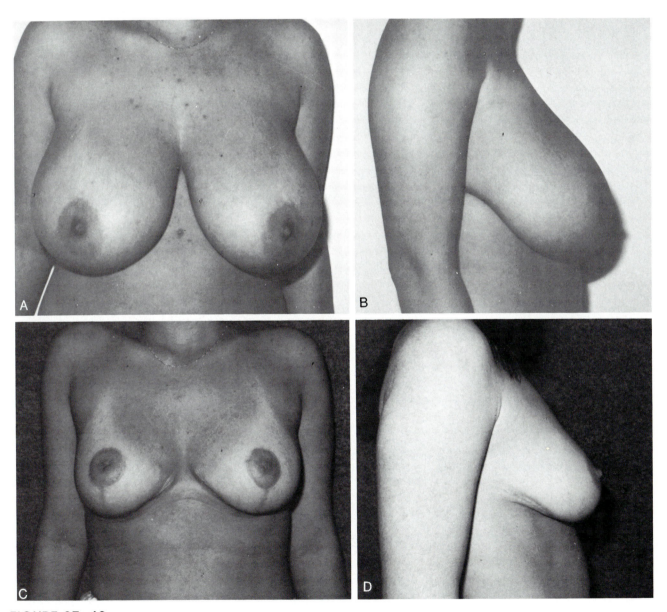

FIGURE 27–10
A and *B,* Preoperative front and side views of large and slightly ptotic breasts in an 18-year-old woman. *C* and *D,* Postoperative front and side views of the same patient after 550 gm of breast tissue was excised from each breast.

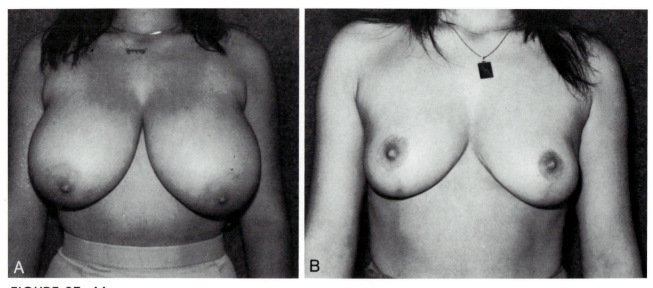

FIGURE 27-11
A, Enlarged and ptotic breasts. *B*, The same patient 4 months postoperatively.

References

Cathcart, E. P., Gairnes, F. W., Garxwen, H. S. D.: Innervation of the human quiescent nipple, with notes on pigmentation, erection and hyperneury. Trans. R. Soc. Edinb. 61:699, 1848.

Cloutier, A. M.: Volume reduction mammoplasty. Ann. Plast. Surg. 2:475, 1979.

Cooper, A.: *The Anatomy of the Breast.* London, Longmans, 1840.

Courtiss, E. H., Goldwyn, R. M.: Breast sensation, before and after plastic surgery. Plast. Reconstr. Surg. 58:1, 1976.

Craig, R. D. P., Sykes, P. A.: Nipple sensitivity following reduction mammoplasty. Br. J. Plast. Surg. 23:165, 1970.

Dinner, M. I., Chait, L. A.: Preventing the high riding nipple after McKissock breast reduction. Plast. Reconstr. Surg. 59:330, 1977.

Edwards, E. A.: Surgical anatomy of the breast. In: Goldwyn, R. M. (ed.): *Plastic and Reconstructive Surgery of the Breast.* Boston, Little, Brown, 1976, p. 37.

Farina, M. A., Newby, B. G., Alan, H. M.: Innervation of the nipple-areola complex. Plast. Reconstr. Surg. 66:497, 1980.

Georgiade, N. G., Serafin, D., Riefkohl, R., Georgiade, G. S.: Is there a reduction mammaplasty for "all seasons"? Plast. Reconstr. Surg. 63:765, 1979.

Hirshowitz, B., Moscona, A. R.: Modifications of the bipedicled vertical dermal flap technique in reduction mammoplasty. Ann. Plast. Surg. 8:363, 1982.

Hirshowitz, B., Moscona, A. R.: Technical variations of the Mc-Kissock operation for reduction mammoplasty. Aesthetic Plast. Surg. 7:149, 1983.

McKissock, P. K.: Reduction mammaplasty with a vertical dermal flap. Plast. Reconstr. Surg. 49:245, 1972.

McKissock, P. K.: Correction of macromastia by bipedicle vertical dermal flap. In: Goldwyn, R. M. (ed.): *Plastic and Reconstructive Surgery of the Breast.* Boston, Little, Brown, 1976, p. 215.

Penn, J.: Breast reduction. Br. J. Plast. Surg. 7:357, 1954.

Strömbeck, J. O.: Mammaplasty: Report on a new technique based on the two pedicle procedure. Br. J. Plast. Surg. 13:79, 1960.

28

28

Gregory S. Georgiade
Ronald Riefkohl
Nicholas G. Georgiade

Reduction Mammaplasty Utilizing the Inferior Pyramidal Dermal Pedicle Flap

The evolution of the technique utilizing a large central core of breast tissue resembling a pyramid with a layer of dermis on the inferior aspect was initially instituted by us in stages, starting in 1973. This early procedure was designed after the work of Ribeiro and Backer (Ribeiro and Backer, 1973; Ribeiro, 1975; Backer and Ribeiro, 1976). They utilized a dermal fat pedicle for breast "filling and contour" with their breast reduction technique that involved the nipple and areola being on a superiorly based dermal pedicle as described by Arié (1957) and Pitanguy (1963). Their original concept did not, however, contain the nipple and areola complex on the dermal pedicle. Ribeiro (1975), Robbins (1977), and Courtiss and Goldwyn (1977) described their technique for reduction mammaplasty using an inferior dermal flap with the nipple and areola on this inferiorly based dermal flap with minimal breast tissue. Georgiade and associates (Georgiade et al., 1979a) and Reich (1979) described their individual modifications of the use of this inferior dermal flap.

The importance of maintaining sufficient breast attachments to the pectoral muscle, yielding greater assurance of viability of the tissue pedicle, was emphasized by Georgiade (1979, 1981, 1983, 1986, 1987) and Ariyan (1980). The composite technique for carrying out this particular procedure for reduction mammaplasty has been utilized in over 1000 reduction mammaplasties with unilateral as well as bilateral breast hypertrophy.

The technique to be described emphasizes the use of a large pyramidal breast flap with an inferior dermal pedicle upon which the nipple-areola complex is attached.

PREOPERATIVE MARKINGS AND PREDETERMINATION OF THE SIZE OF THE BREAST MOUND AND NIPPLE-AREOLA POSITION

The patient is usually routinely marked preoperatively in a standing and upright position, although with large breasts the dermal pedicle and inferior mammary margins may be more easily marked when the patient is in a supine position. The initial marking on the breast is made at the sternal notch with a gentian violet marking pen. The midsternal point is then determined, and a vertical line is drawn along this midline. The new position for the areola is determined by placing the index finger at the inframammary crease and palpating this position on the outer breast surface. The new position is then marked at a slightly superior position and at the midclavicular line in the smaller breast or slightly medial in the large, hypertrophied breast (where there is a shift to a more lateral position of the nipple-areola complex). The final position of the areola is usually 20 to 22 cm from the sternal notch, in the region of the midclavicular line and slightly lower than the midhumeral line. Care must be taken to be assured that each areola is equidistant from the midsternal line, usually 9 to 12 cm from the midline (Fig. 28–1).

In order to expedite and accurately mark each breast, a steel wire loop (Duke design) has been used by us since 1976 (Georgiade, 1976, 1986; Georgiade et al., 1979) (Fig. 28–2). This wire loop is available in two diameters, 4.0 and 4.5 cm. The larger diameter is used for the older patient. The arms of the wire loop are serrated at 1-cm intervals and allow the operator to mark also the desired length of the breast flaps. The width of the flaps is determined by estimating the eventual final size of the breasts. For a moderate reduction (350 to 500 gm) the distance between the arms is 8 to 10 cm. For a larger reduction (600 to 800 gm) the distance is 10 to 12 cm (see Fig. 28–2). With the larger reduction mammaplasty (over 1500 gm), there is a proportional increase in the distance between the arms of the wire; the distance is approximately 14 cm. The inframammary marking is made just superior to the inframammary crease with a slight upward projection in the midportion of what will be the dermal pedicle, so as to minimize the tension at the time of approximation of the medial and lateral flaps at the inframammary line. Care is taken to minimize the medial and lateral extension of the markings, and the markings are never extended to the midclavicular line. The size of the dermal pedicle is now outlined with the breast in a midchest position. A 7-cm dermal pedicle base width is marked if a small breast mound is desired (A cup). The width

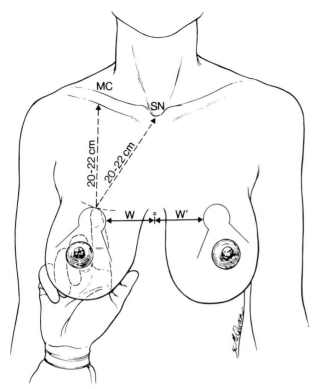

FIGURE 28–1
Note the markings established by palpating the inframammary crease and establishing the areola–sternal notch distance. The final markings must reflect the equal distance of each areola marking to the midline. MC, mid clavicle; SN, sternal notch.

flaps are identified by placing sutures in each position, at the most superior point of the areola, and also at the most superior point of the new position of the areola.

It is at this point in the procedure that a 1:300,000 solution of epinephrine is used to infiltrate the base of each breast. Approximately 40 ml of this solution is used for each breast (1 ml 1:1000 of epinephrine plus 300 ml solution).

The area of the predetermined dermal flap is now de-epithelialized (Fig. 28–3). At this time it is most important that the pyramidal flap of breast tissue be correctly sculptured. In order to accomplish this, the pyramid is developed by incising in a slanting manner away from the dermal pedicle in all directions and gradually widening the base of the newly created pyramid to the pectoral musculature. This is of particular importance in the lateral anterior axillary area, so that the innervation from the fourth and fifth intercostal nerves to the nipple-areola area is not disturbed.

The thickness of the breast parenchyma must be at least 5 cm at the apex of the pyramid in the subareola area and 10 cm at the base (Fig. 28–4). Incising of the breasts can be carried out in the small breast with sharp dissection; in larger breasts, cutting current or coagulation current (which is slower) can be used to minimize blood loss.

Resection of the redundant breast tissue is carried out by sharply incising along the previously determined

of this pedicle is increased up to 9 cm for the larger desired breast mound. It is important to maintain a dermal cuff of 1.5 cm along the periareolar area, and the markings should reflect this.

The larger, hypertrophied breasts are marked as to their new nipple-areola position with the breast supported so that the increased tension on the skin does not become a factor. If the tension is not corrected by adequate support, this will result in the new nipple position being placed 2 to 3 cm too high on the chest. There may be some discrepancy in the markings of the contemplated width of the reduction, because quite often there is asymmetry in the two breasts, which must be taken into consideration.

The markings, having now been determined, are then reinforced by the use of a brilliant green dye, in an alcohol base, which, when allowed to dry, will still be visible after skin preparation at the time of surgery.

TECHNICAL ASPECTS OF THE SURGICAL PROCEDURE FOR REDUCTION MAMMAPLASTY

The reduction of the breast is best carried out with the patient in a semi-sitting position. For proper orientation of the nipple-areola complex and the skin flaps at the time of closure, the corners of the predetermined

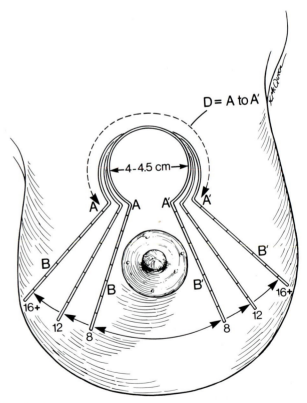

FIGURE 28–2
The use of the wire marker. The diameter of the circle is equal to the circumference of the wire loop, regardless of the distance between the arms of the wire, which will determine the distance between the medial and lateral breast flaps.

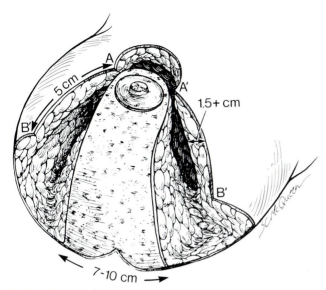

FIGURE 28–3
Breast pedicle shown after contouring and resection of the surrounding breast tissue.

outline of the new areola and flaps. One carries out the resection, maintaining an even thickness of the skin flaps of at least 1.5 cm. The tissue removed is weighed and compared with the amount of tissue removed from the opposite breast for proper balance and symmetry.

The coning of the breast is now initiated by approximating the medial and lateral flaps with 4-0 Vicryl or Dexon sutures. The areola is now positioned in relation to the preoperative suture markings.

The areola is positioned by placement of 5-0 sutures at the four points of the areolar circumference in the dermal layers. The inferior portion of the dermal pedicle is incised slightly at an angle beneath the skin in order to minimize the possibility of the buried sutures projecting above the skin postoperatively.

The inframammary crease line is created with the initial suture being placed so that the distance from the inferior areola point to the inframammary line is 5 cm. The redundant skin is then excised, care being taken to maintain the incision in the inframammary area. The medial and lateral flaps of redundant tissue are then excised and approximated with 4-0 Vicryl or Dexon sutures, care being taken to advance the tissue toward the midbreast pedicle so as to minimize the extension of the incisions medially and laterally (Fig. 28–5). The incisions are never extended to the midline (Fig. 28–6). In larger breast hypertrophy with associated severe ptosis and confluence of the two breasts at the midline, adjustments are made at the time of closure by excising the redundant subdermal fatty tissue in the medial and lateral inframammary area. Occasionally the inferior chest skin may be so redundant that a small oblique wedge of tissue is excised in the inferior lateral or medial breast shadow (see Fig. 28–2E).

A suction drain is then inserted laterally in each breast. Subcuticular pull-out sutures are inserted in order to approximate the skin edges. Sterile paper strips are then placed across the incision lines, further stabilizing the flaps.

FIGURE 28–4
Pyramidal breast tissue and dermal flap. Care must be taken to leave superior attachments of this breast pedicle to the upper pectoralis muscle.

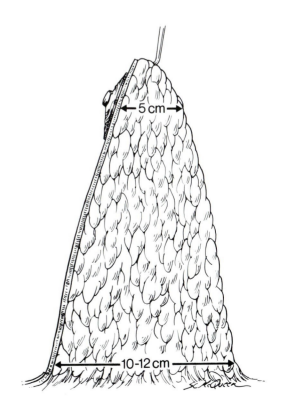

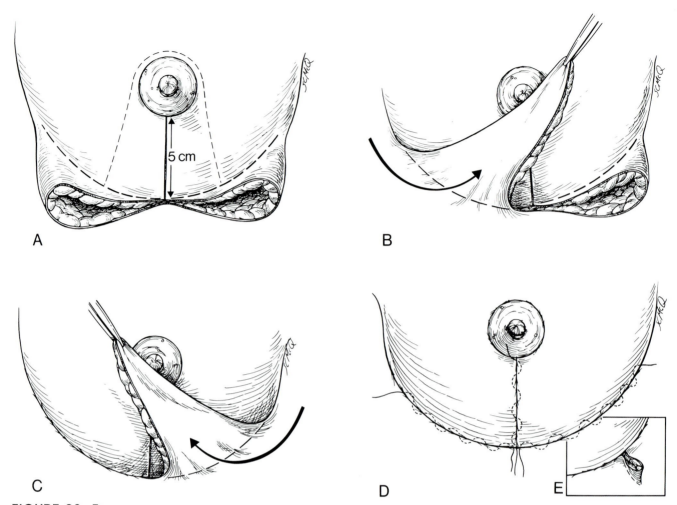

A   B

C   D   E

FIGURE 28–5

A, The initial point of closure with the length of flaps at 5 cm. The redundant tissue will be excised by following the contour of the new breast mound. *B* and *C,* The redundant tissue laterally and medially is advanced toward the midbreast, which minimizes the length of the eventual scar. *D* and *E,* The final closure, utilizing subcuticular sutures, supported by skin tape. Any excess redundancy of the inferior chest skin in the larger reductions can be excised with an inferior, oblique wedge of skin.

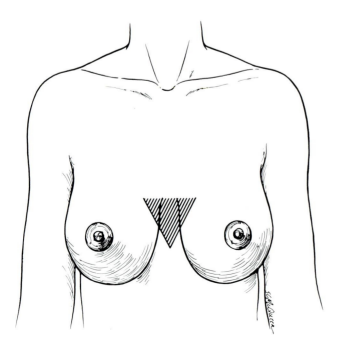

FIGURE 28–6

The final breast reduction incisions should never extend into this shaded triangular area.

POSTOPERATIVE MANAGEMENT

The newly created breasts are protected immediately postoperatively with a large, bulky mechanics waste dressing, which is applied in a "doughnut" fashion. The breasts are then re-dressed within 24 hours and inspected for hematomas, undue pressure, tension, or ischemia. The sutures are removed by the tenth postoperative day, and the paper strips are continuously applied across the suture lines for approximately 3 weeks. A suitable brassiere is worn most of the time for the next 2 weeks. The drains can usually be removed within 24 to 48 hours. The results of patients having had reduction mammaplasty are shown in Figures 28–7 to 28–11.

UNDESIRABLE RESULTS

The inferior pyramidal technique for reduction mammaplasty, like all other procedures for reduction mammaplasty, may result in some not completely satisfactory results.

The most common untoward result is the lack of sufficient resection of redundant breast tissue, particularly in the lateral component, but also occasionally in the medial aspect (Fig. 28–12). Correction of this necessitates a more critical evaluation of the breast mound configuration at the time of closure of the flaps. This is best attained with the patient placed in an upright sitting position. It is usually necessary to shave off additional
Text continued on page 362

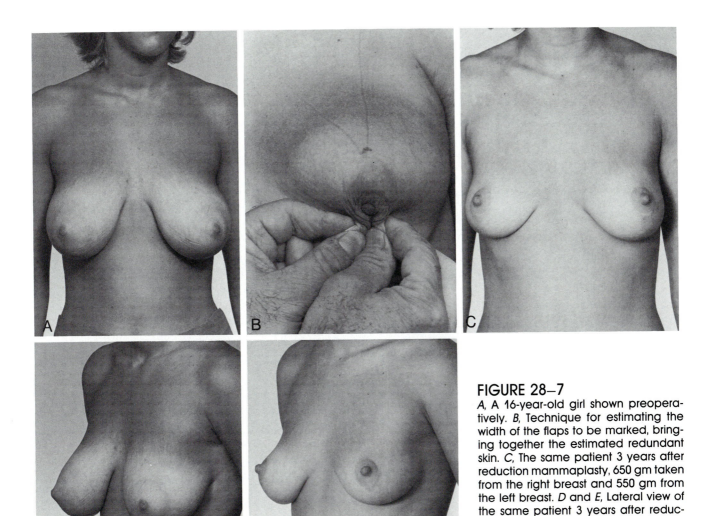

FIGURE 28–7
A, A 16-year-old girl shown preoperatively. *B*, Technique for estimating the width of the flaps to be marked, bringing together the estimated redundant skin. *C*, The same patient 3 years after reduction mammaplasty, 650 gm taken from the right breast and 550 gm from the left breast. *D* and *E*, Lateral view of the same patient 3 years after reduction mammaplasty.

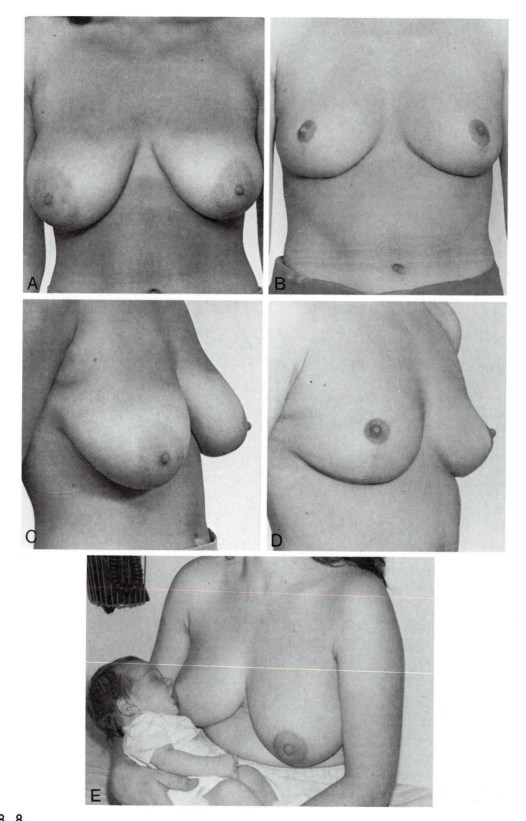

FIGURE 28–8

A and *B*, A 21-year-old woman preoperatively and 6 years after reduction of 650 gm from each breast. *C* and *D*, Lateral view of this same patient preoperatively and 6 years after reduction mammaplasty. *E*, The same patient breast-feeding 7 years after reduction mammaplasty.

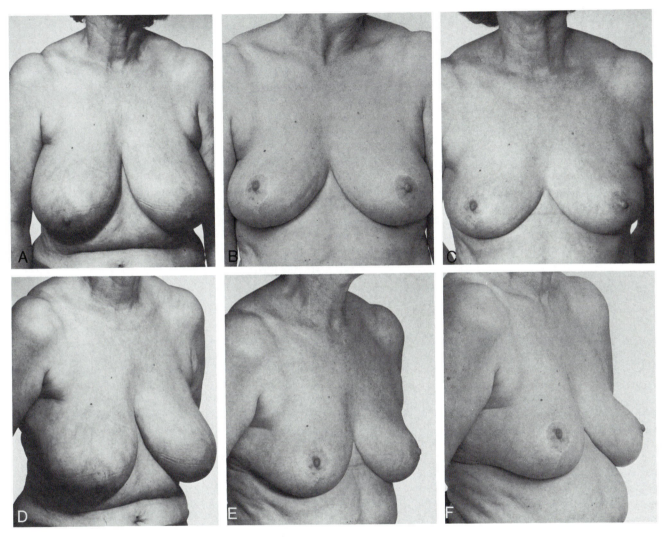

FIGURE 28–9

A to *C*, Front views of a 59-year-old patient preoperatively *(A)*, 1 year after reduction of 680 gm from each breast *(B)*, and 4 years after reduction mammaplasty *(C)*. *D* to *F*, Lateral views of the same patient preoperatively *(A)* and 1 *(B)* and 4 *(C)* years after reduction mammaplasty.

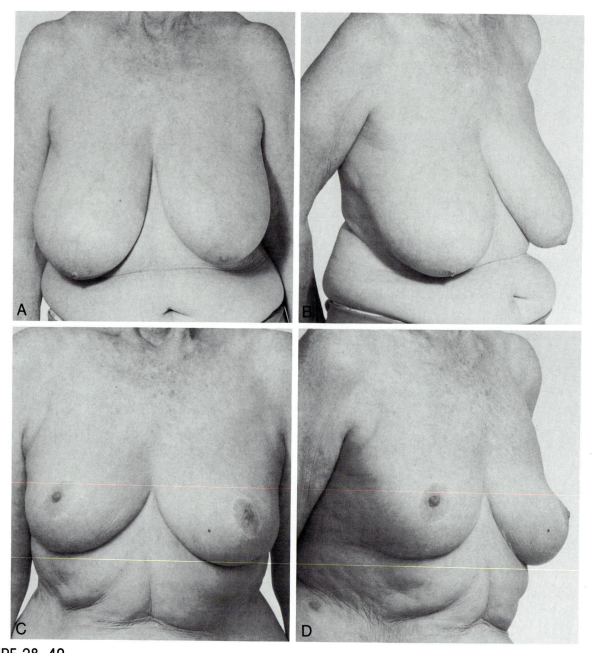

FIGURE 28–10

A and B, A 70-year-old patient with large, ptotic breasts. C and D, The same patient 2 years after removal of 1029 gm from the right breast and 850 gm from the left breast. Note the well-healed and concealed scars.

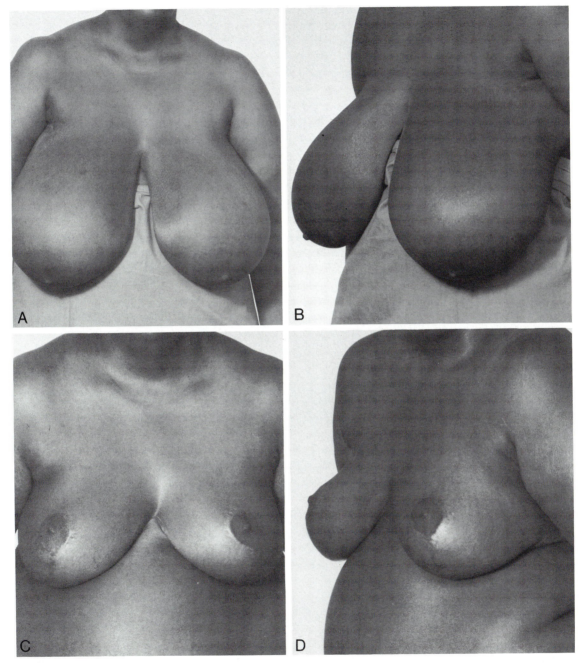

FIGURE 28–11

A and *B*, A 21-year-old patient with massive breast hypertrophy. *C* and *D*, The same patient 9 months after removal of 2800 gm from the right breast and 2800 gm from the left breast.

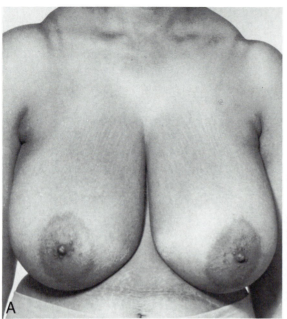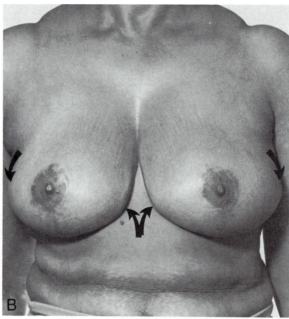

FIGURE 28–12

A, A 41-year-old patient with large, ptotic breasts. *B*, The same patient 2 years after removal of 1100 gm from each breast. Note the appearance of the breasts (arrows) when insufficient breast tissue is removed from the medial and lateral aspects at the time of contouring the pyramidal breast pedicle.

segments of the lateral portion of the breast pyramid and occasionally also segments of the medial aspect, with reduction of some of the bulk of the remaining skin flaps along the superior and lateral aspects of the resection.

Separation of the skin flaps occasionally occurs, particularly in the older patient at the most medial and inferior portion of the approximated flaps, where there is the greatest tension. This can be prevented by preoperatively marking the inframammary line with a projection of 1 to 2 cm at this point, where the medial and lateral flaps will be joined to the inframammary line. This most inferior projection will now replace the inferior areas of the medial and lateral flaps most likely to become ischemic and necrosed.

Inversion of the nipple can occasionally occur if sufficient thickness of the breast parenchyma has not been maintained for at least 5 cm of thickness at the base of the nipple-areola complex.

Partial thickness loss of the superior areola skin can occur if the superior base of the pyramid is not extended superiorly in relation to the areola at the time of sculpturing the pyramid.

ADVANTAGES OF THE INFERIOR PYRAMIDAL TECHNIQUE

The authors have found that this technique of maintaining a broad base of breast tissue attached to the chest wall maximizes the blood supply to the pyramidal flaps and allows the breast tissue to be easily coned. Lactation has been possible following the use of this technique, and nipple sensation has been maintained, with consistent nipple projection. The scars are minimal and maintained in the inframammary crease line, with the result that breast contour is not sacrificed for unnecessary short scars, because the scars produced by this technique are not visible.

References

Arié, B.: Una nueva técnica de mastoplastia. Rev. Latinoam. Cir. Plast. 3:23, 1957.

Ariyan, S.: Reduction mammoplasty with the nipple-areola carried on a single, narrow inferior pedicle. Ann. Plast. Surg. 5:167, 1980.

Backer, E., Ribeiro, L.: Reduction mammaplasty: Technical considerations. In: Georgiade, N. G. (ed.): *Reconstructive Breast Surgery*. St. Louis, C. V. Mosby, 1976, p. 195–201.

Courtiss, E. H., Goldwyn, R. M.: Reduction mammaplasty by the inferior pedicle technique. Plast. Reconstr. Surg. 50:500, 1977.

Georgiade, N. G.: *Reconstructive Breast Surgery*. St. Louis, C. V. Mosby, 1976, p. 115.

Georgiade, N. G.: *Breast Reconstruction Following Mastectomy*. St. Louis, C. V. Mosby, 1979.

Georgiade, N. G.: Reconstructive surgery of the breast. In: Sabiston, D. C., Jr. (ed.): *Davis Christopher Textbook of Surgery*. 12th ed. Philadelphia, W. B. Saunders, 1981, p. 665.

Georgiade, N. G.: Reconstructive breast surgery. In: Sabiston, D. C., Jr. (ed.): *Davis Christopher Textbook of Surgery*. 13th ed. Philadelphia, W. B. Saunders, 1986, p. 573.

Georgiade, N. G., Georgiade, G. S.: Reduction mammoplasty utilizing the inferior pyramidal dermal pedicle. In: Georgiade, N. G. (ed.): *Aesthetic Breast Surgery*. Baltimore, Williams & Wilkins, 1983, p. 291.

Georgiade, N. G., Georgiade, G. S.: Hypermastia and ptosis. In: *Essentials of Plastic, Maxillofacial and Reconstructive Surgery*. Georgiade, N. G., Georgiade, G. S., Riefkohl, R., Barwick, W. J. (eds.): Baltimore, Williams & Wilkins, 1987, p. 694.

Georgiade, N. G., Serafin, D., Morris, R., Georgiade, G. S.: Reduction mammaplasty utilizing an inferior pedicle nipple areola flap. Ann. Plast. Surg. 3:211, 1979a.

Georgiade, N. G., Serafin, D., Riefkohl, R., Georgiade, G.: Is there a reduction mammoplasty for "all seasons"? Plast. Reconstr. Surgery 63:765, 1979b.

Pitanguy, I.: Mammaplastias. Rev. Latinoam. Cir. Plast. 72:75, 1963.

Reich, J.: The advantages of a lower central breast segment in reduction mammaplasty. Aesthetic Plast. Surg. 3:47, 1979.

Ribeiro, L.: A new technique for reduction mammaplasty. Plast. Reconstr. Surg. 55:330, 1975.

Ribeiro, L., Backer, E.: Mastoplasia con pediculo de seguridad. Rev. Esp. Cir. Plast. 6:223, 1973.

Robbins, T. H.: A reduction mammaplasty with the areola-nipple based on an inferior dermal pedicle. Plast. Reconstr. Surg. 59:64, 1977.

29

Alan E. Seyfer

Reduction Mammaplasty Using the Inferior Glandular Pyramid Pedicle

The reduction mammaplasty operation ideally results in symmetric breasts having natural contour and volume, aesthetically situated scars, and sensate, properly situated nipple-areola complexes. In the past, the limiting factor for the procedure has been related to the preservation of normal blood flow to the nipple-areola complex and nipple sensation. This is especially true in the large breast that requires both a voluminous resection and a lengthy upward translocation of the nipple. In our experience, the procedure that best meets these exacting goals has been the "pyramid" pedicle technique (Bolger et al., 1987; Chow et al., 1984; Climo and Alexander, 1980; Georgiade et al., 1979; Mathes et al., 1980; Ribeiro, 1975). With this method, the circulation to the nipple-areola complex remains uninterrupted and is supplied by direct, perforating arterioles from the chest wall. These vessels, after supplying branches to the underlying pectoralis major muscle, enter the breast on its deep aspect. Because of the broad base of this "glandular pedicle," it also incorporates anterior branches of the intercostal nerves and results in preservation of normal sensation to the nipple-areola complex. Additional advantages have included excellent cosmesis and a good control of the final volume, which make it easier to correct asymmetry.

INDICATIONS

The most common indications for the procedure emphasize the reconstructive nature of the operation. In a longitudinal review of 300 patients, the most frequent preoperative symptom was upper back and shoulder pain. Other frequently voiced complaints, in addition to the perception of being "too large," were brassiere strap discomfort, shoulder notching, difficulty in sports activities, extreme heaviness, problems in performing job-related duties, and difficulties in finding properly fitting clothes (Bolger et al., 1987).

PREOPERATIVE MARKING

On the evening prior to the operation, the patient is seated erect with the hands resting on the thighs. Every effort is made to produce symmetric markings through measurements from established topographic landmarks

(Fig. 29–1). The suprasternal notch is marked, and another mark is made near each midclavicular line 7 to 8 cm from the suprasternal notch. The axis of each breast is traced, and this may be facilitated by draping the measuring tape around the neck and over the center of the nipples. The areola is marked at the 12 o'clock and 6 o'clock positions, and the line is continued down to the inframammary crease. The midline of the torso is marked over the sternum and epigastrium, and the proposed nipple position is chosen. This position may vary from 18 to 21 cm from the sternal notch to a point along the axis line of the breast according to the height and body habitus of the patient. This point is generally in the range of 18 to 20 cm for shorter patients and 19 to 22 cm for taller individuals. These new nipple positions should form the points of a roughly equilateral triangle with the suprasternal notch. Next, Wise's pattern (1956) is placed onto the breast with the new nipple position at the center. The pattern is outlined for assessment of the symmetry of the proposed flaps. It is important to keep the planned areola-to-inframammary fold distance in the range of 5 cm to avoid postoperative nipple positions that are too high. Medial and lateral flaps are marked so that their inferior borders are equal to or slightly longer than the length of the incision along the inframammary crease. After final adjustments, brilliant green dye is used to mark the final incisions.

OPERATIVE TECHNIQUE

As noted above, the technique, modified from that of Robbins (1977) and Georgiade et al. (1979), supports the nipple-areola complex with a three-dimensional pedicle of breast parenchyma having a wide base on the chest wall. The anterior base of the proposed pyramid measures 8 cm in width. Approximately 10 minutes prior to starting, 0.5% lidocaine solution with 1:200,000 epinephrine is injected into the subcutaneous tissues and beneath the marked incisions (AMA, 1983) (Fig. 29–2). With a breast tourniquet in place, the new areola is marked in the center of the existing areola complex so that it measures approximately 4 cm in diameter. The incisional markings are scored widely enough so that the electrocautery will not injure the skin that is to remain, and the excess skin and areola outside the new nipple-areola complex is de-epithelialized, leaving a 1-

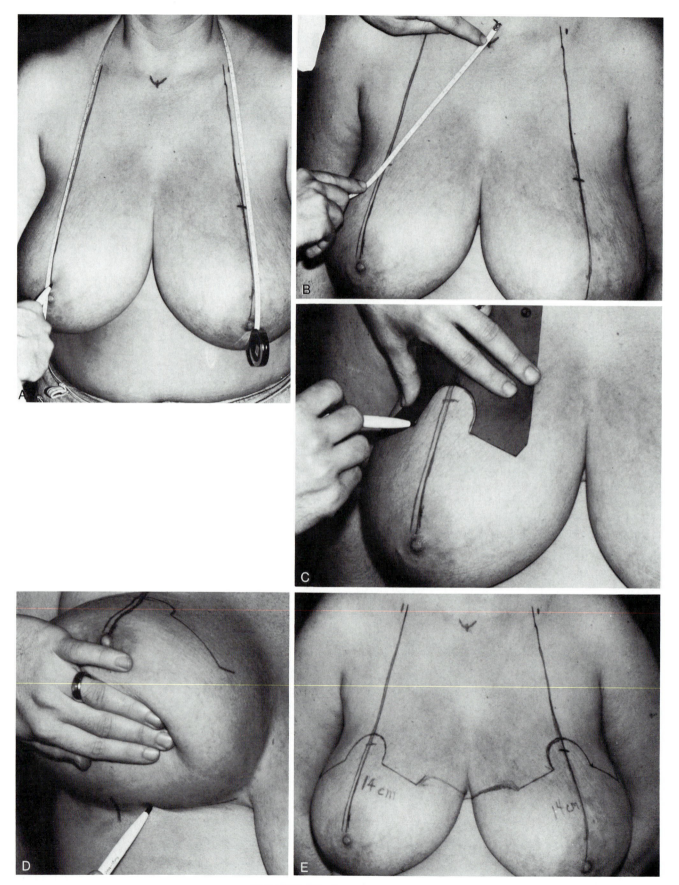

FIGURE 29–1
See legend on opposite page

to 2-cm border. The remaining skin is rapidly excised to the subdermal fat with the electrocautery. All incisions from this point forward are made with the cutting electrocautery. As the flaps are fashioned, the incision is beveled away from the axis of the breast so that the glandular pyramid is established with its wide base on the chest wall. The flaps are kept in the range of 1 inch in thickness, with the medial side slightly fuller for cleavage. The chest wall is approached medially and laterally down to the fascia (Fig. 29–2C). The flaps are widely elevated from the pectoral fascia to the level of the clavicle and away from the pyramid. This allows room for the pyramid to be inserted into this space at the time of upward translocation and closure. Next, the pyramid is stabilized with towel clips and generously trimmed with the electrocautery, leaving its broad three-dimensional base undisturbed and preserving 1 inch in parenchymal thickness posterior to the areola. The breast is bimanually palpated for assessment of the approximate size of the remaining tissue; and, when the size is deemed appropriate for the patient's body habitus, stay sutures are inserted for further assessment of the final volume and contour. Prior to inserting the stay sutures, the opposite breast is prepared by injecting the lidocaine-epinephrine solution. The same procedure is then followed on the opposite side. After any final adjustments on both sides, the contour, volume, and symmetry are assessed from the foot of the table.

The breast should have a pleasing contour, appropriate size, slight fullness medially, and good projection centrally. If necessary, the sutures are removed and further trimming done until these goals are met. The incisions are closed with absorbable sutures for the subcutaneous layer, subcuticular 3-0 Prolene for the inframammary crease, and 5-0 nylon for the periareolar sutures. Voluminous fluff dressings are applied, and a light circumthoracic expansile gauze is placed around the patient. The patient is then awakened and moved to the recovery room.

In our experience with over 500 individuals, there has been a significant decrease in blood loss since the introduction of the lidocaine-epinephrine solution (Bolger et al., 1987; Brantner and Peterson, 1985; Johnston et al., 1976; Katz et al., 1962; Mather and Cousins, 1979; Varejes, 1963). Previously, the patient was required to donate 2 units of autologous blood for the operation. Invariably, these units were returned to the patient because of operative blood loss. Although the average weight of tissue removed has remained relatively constant and in the range of 1300 gm, no transfusions have been necessary since this change in routine.

POSTOPERATIVE CARE

Intravenous maintenance fluid administration continues overnight, although the patient is allowed to drink clear liquids the evening of the day of the operation. Early ambulation and incentive spirometry are mandated, and the dressing is removed the morning after the operation. The patient is usually discharged on the second or third postoperative day.

COMPLICATIONS

The incidence of complications has been in the range of 13.6%, of which 11% were minor self-limited problems (Bolger et al., 1987). The most frequent has been the localized loss of skin over the inverted T, where the flaps join the inframammary crease; and a few (0.4%) of these patients have required skin grafting. Approximately 2% have experienced a partial loss of nipple-areola sensation. The incidence of hematoma, infection, and other complications has been extremely low (Bolger et al., 1987).

DISCUSSION

This simple technique can be employed with excellent reliability to reduce the size of any breast. The cosmesis is excellent, and the reduced breast undergoes a gradual, yet mild, degree of ptosis over the years that seems appropriate to its new size (Figs. 29–3 and 29–4). With this technique, unlike other techniques, the length of the pedicle required for translocation of the nipple-areola complex is not a limiting consideration, and there is minimal risk of nipple-areola loss (McKissock, 1972; Strömbeck, 1973). Sensation, in fact, remains normal in most patients. As is also not the case with other methods, there is no folding of tissue behind the nipple-areola complex, which sometimes results in an artificial or boxlike shape to the breast. Because the bulk of the pyramid and the thickness of the flaps can be easily controlled, there is also good control of the final volume, making it easier to correct asymmetry (Bolger et al., 1987; Dowden et al., 1984) (Fig. 29–5).

Text continued on page 370

FIGURE 29–1

A, The patient is marked in the sitting or standing position, and the suprasternal notch is marked in the midline. A point on the clavicle is marked 7 to 8 cm from the sternal notch, and the axis of each breast is marked from this point to the 12 o'clock and 6 o'clock positions of the areola. This line is continued to the inframammary crease and marked at that point. *B,* The position of the new nipple is marked along the previously drawn axis 18 to 22 cm from the suprasternal notch, depending on the body habitus of the patient. *C,* The Wise pattern is placed on the breast, and the limbs of the flaps are marked. The vertical limbs should measure no more than 5 cm in length. *D,* The horizontal lines along the inframammary crease and along the flaps are marked so that the flap length is 2 to 3 cm greater in length than the inframammary crease. This will allow for decreased tension where the vertical line meets the horizontal limb. The flap length can be lengthened as necessary by moving the vertical line closer to the midline. *E,* The final markings are shown in this patient, in whom the nipple will undergo a 14-cm upward translocation. This technique has been employed successfully with up to 22 cm of upward translocation. (Courtesy of Col. George E. Smith.)

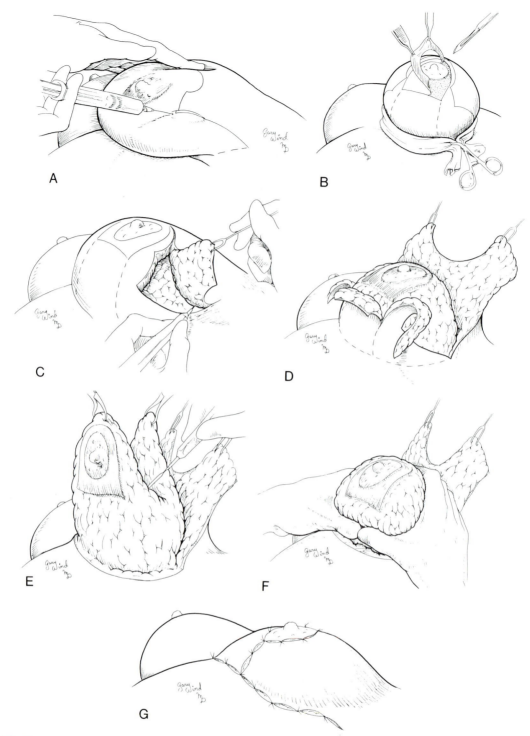

FIGURE 29–2

A, Prior to initiating the procedure, 0.5% lidocaine with 1:200,000 epinephrine solution is injected subcutaneously beneath the incisional markings as well as over the anticipated areas of resection. Approximately 35 ml of this solution (which totals approximately 175 mg lidocaine plus 0.175 mg epinephrine) is administered to the first breast and repeated for the second breast. *B,* With a long laparotomy sponge, a breast tourniquet is applied, and the new areola is marked. The area immediately about the areola is de-epithelialized. This allows for a convenient sewing ring during the final closure. *C,* After scoring the incisions, the flaps are developed medially and laterally down to the deep fascia of the chest wall, leaving the flaps at a uniform thickness of approximately 1 inch. For added hemostasis, all cutting is performed with the electrocautery. *D,* The flaps are mobilized at the fascial level to the border of the sternum medially, the clavicle superiorly, and the serratus muscle anterolaterally. The skin is removed from the central pyramid, which the surgeon bevels outward to ensure that the broad pyramidal base is undisturbed. *E,* The pyramid is suspended with a towel clip and trimmed, retaining its broad base. The excised segments are wider at the top of the pyramid and progressively thinner at the base so that the base remains undisturbed. *F,* Throughout the resection the breast is grasped intermittently and appropriately "sized" through bimanual palpation. This is accomplished with a view toward the final volume and is adjusted to the patient's body habitus. *G,* After the final volume is attained, stay sutures are inserted for assessing the size and contour of the breast. The reduction is then commenced on the contralateral side.

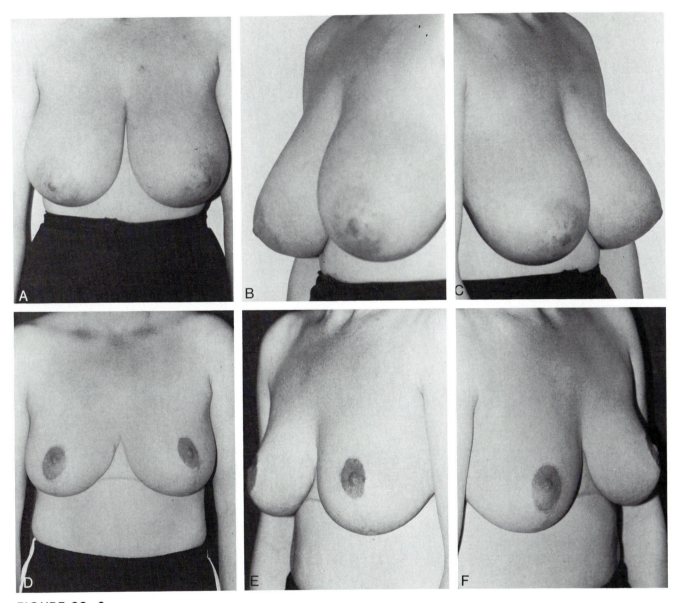

FIGURE 29–3

A to C, Preoperative front and lateral views of a 23-year-old woman who underwent a pyramid pedicle reduction mammaplasty with removal of 900 gm of breast tissue on the left and 840 gm on the right. *D to F,* Postoperative front and lateral views of the same patient 3 years after the reduction operation. There is a natural volume and contour to the breasts, along with an appropriate degree of ptosis.

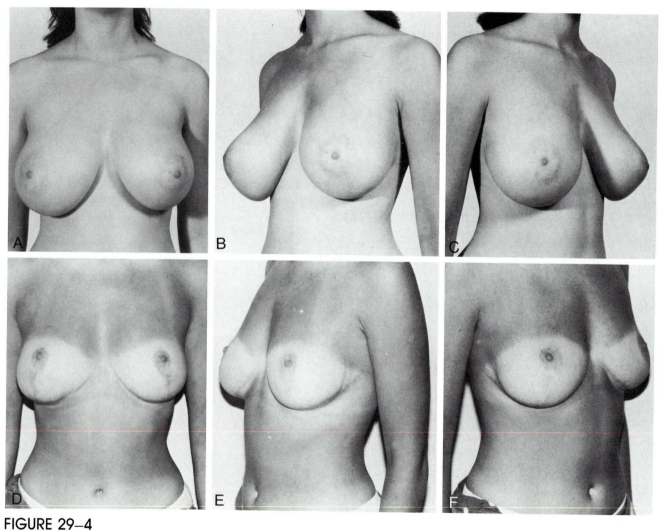

FIGURE 29–4

A to *C,* Front and lateral views of a 19-year-old woman who underwent a pyramid pedicle reduction with removal of 454 gm from the right breast and 422 gm from the left breast. *D* to *F,* Front and lateral views of the same patient 3 years after the reduction procedure. There is a natural degree of ptosis, reasonable contour, and appropriate volume.

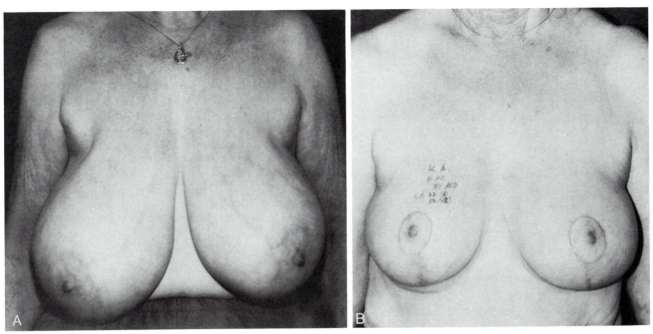

FIGURE 29–5

A, Front view of a 59-year-old woman who underwent a pyramid pedicle reduction mammaplasty for asymmetric bilateral hypertrophy. A reduction of 738 gm from the left breast and 1026 gm from the right breast was performed. *B*, The same patient 8 months postoperatively. Her breasts have reasonable symmetry and more natural volume and contour.

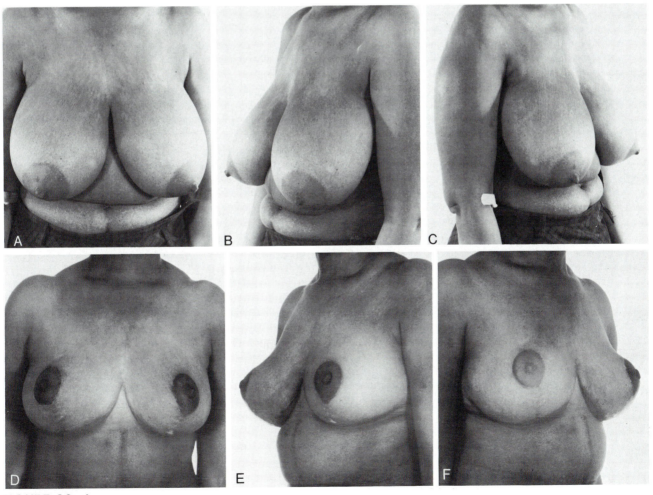

FIGURE 29–6

A to *C*, Front and lateral views of a 43-year-old woman prior to the removal of 1100 gm from the right breast and 1050 gm from the left breast by the pyramid reduction technique. *D* to *F*, Front and lateral views of the same patient 8 months postoperatively.

DISADVANTAGES

One disadvantage has been the length of time the operation requires. Although it is permissible to "double-team" the development of the pyramid, the mobilization of the flaps, and the suturing duties, it is best if one surgeon is responsible for resecting the tissue on both sides. This routine seems to avoid asymmetry in judging the final remaining volumes of the breasts. However, this is somewhat time-consuming, and the operation usually requires 2½ to 3 hours.

The scars are comparable to those of other techniques, and there is a gradual development of recurrent ptosis with time. However, this seems to be appropriate to the new volume and size of the breast (see Figs. 29–5 and 29–6). Likewise, this technique shares with other methods the problem of transient minor wound separation at the inverted-T area.

Several patients have attempted to nurse their offspring after having undergone this operation. Although they were successful in producing milk, the volume was not sufficient for adequate neonatal nutrition, and the patients were forced to cease this activity.

It is worth emphasizing that the subcutaneous administration of epinephrine has dramatically decreased the loss of blood during this operation. Prior to the routine use of lidocaine and epinephrine, the blood loss averaged 800 ml (n = 129 patients). Over the last few years, although the amount of tissue resected remains around 1300 gm, the average loss of blood has been 300 ml (n = 136 patients). This change in routine has eliminated the necessity for transfusions and the requirements for autologous blood (Bolger et al., 1987).

Acknowledgment

The author is grateful to the teaching staff and residents who participated in the care of the patients shown in this chapter.

References

AMA Drug Evaluations. 5th ed. Chicago, American Medical Association, 1983.

Bolger, W. E., Seyfer, A. E., Jackson, S. M.: Reduction mammaplasty using the inferior glandular "pyramid" pedicle: Experiences with 300 patients. Plast. Reconstr. Surg. 80:75, 1987.

Brantner, J. N., Peterson, H. D.: The role of vasoconstrictors in control of blood loss in reduction mammaplasty. Plast. Reconstr. Surg. 75:339, 1985.

Chow, J. A., Slade, C. L., Jackson, S. M., and Peterson, H. D.: Sensation of nipple-areola complex before and after reduction mammaplasty. Presented at the Annual Combined Meeting of the National Capital Society of Plastic Surgeons and the John Staige Davis Plastic Surgical Society, Baltimore, 1984.

Climo, M. S., Alexander, J. E.: Intercostothelial circulation: Nipple survival in reduction mammaplasty in absence of a dermal pedicle. Ann. Plast. Surg. 4:128, 1980.

Courtiss, E. H., Goldwyn, R. M.: Reduction mammaplasty by the inferior pedicle technique. Plast. Reconstr. Surg. 59:500, 1977.

Dowden, R. V., Dinner, M. I., Labandter, H. P.: Breast reduction for asymmetrical hypertrophy. Plast. Reconstr. Surg. 73:928, 1984.

Georgiade, N. G., Serafin, D., Morris, R., Georgiade, G.: Reduction mammaplasty utilizing an inferior pedicle areolar flap. Ann. Plast. Surg. 3:211, 1979.

Johnston, R. R., Eger, E. I., Wilson, C.: Comparative interaction of epinephrine with enflurane, isoflurane, and halothane in man. Anesth. Analg. 55:709, 1976.

Katz, R. L., Matteo, R. S., Papper, E. M.: The injection of epinephrine during general anesthesia with halogenated hydrocarbons and cyclopropane in man. Anesthesiology 23:597, 1962.

McKissock, P. K.: Reduction mammaplasty with a vertical dermal flap. Plast. Reconstr. Surg. 49:245, 1972.

Mather, L. E., Cousins, H. J.: Local anesthetics and their current clinical use. Drugs 18:185, 1979.

Mathes, S. J., Nahai, F., Hester, T. R.: Avoiding the flat breast in reduction mammaplasty. Plast. Reconstr. Surg. 66:63, 1980.

Ribeiro, L.: A new technique for reduction mammaplasty. Plast. Reconstr. Surg. 55:330, 1975.

Robbins, T. H.: A reduction mammaplasty with the areola-nipple based on an inferior dermal pedicle. Plast. Reconstr. Surg. 59:64, 1977.

Schultz, R. C., Markus, N. J.: Platform for nipple projection: Modification of the inferior pedicle techniques for breast reduction. Plast. Reconstr. Surg. 68:208, 1981.

Strömbeck, J. O.: Reduction mammaplasty. In: Grabb, W. C., Smith, J. W. (eds.): Plastic Surgery. 2nd ed. Boston, Little, Brown, 1973.

Varejes, L.: The use of solutions containing adrenaline during halothane anesthesia. Anesthesia 18:507, 1963.

Wise, R. J.: A preliminary report on a method of planning the mammaplasty. Plast. Reconstr. Surg. 17:367, 1956.

The Total Dermoglandular Pedicle Mammaplasty

Mammaplasty has to the extent improved over the decades to the extent that it is now one of the operations for which the greatest number of surgical techniques have been described. All the authors introduced certain modifications for surgical improvements leading to a gradual development of the techniques, somewhat reminiscent of the evolution of species. However, this evolution, which followed a certain chronologic pattern, introduced some "avant-garde" techniques that were eventually abandoned and condemned because, used without an associated safety procedure, they were unsafe and could lead to various complications.

HISTORY

Historically, the purpose of mammary reduction was, as its name implies, reduction of breast volume. With it came the aesthetic need to add a grafted nipple, in a *trompe l'oeil* fashion. That technique is still in use in some surgical centers but has fortunately been replaced in most of them by reduction with transposition of the nipple, with consequent conservation of the nipple as a flap based on a vascular pedicle. There is no doubt as to the superiority of the quality of a transposed nipple in comparison with a grafted one. A large pedicle was not required to maintain the nipple alive; often a thin strip of subcutaneous fat was sufficient—but, alas, not always. If the nipple survived the ischemia of the fragile transposition, it remained inert, congestive for a long while, and insensitive, retaining only its position in relation with the subjacent tissue.

Thereupon, innovators, trying with reason to increase the safety of the nipple by thickening its pedicle, recommended thicker and thicker fatty flaps. The survival of the nipple increased; but the torsion of the pedicle, necessary for the new positioning of the so very important complex, often produced surprises.

The advantage of the option for a nipple of superior quality by adding to the fatty pedicle a glandular bridge was beyond hesitation, and the surgeons were quick to make use of it by thickening the pedicle of the nipple and combining, in addition to the subcutaneous fat, a few centimeters of glandular tissue.

These pedicles were always of superior origin—at the noon, 10, or 2 o'clock positions—or of lateral origin—at the 3 or 9 o'clock positions—or bifid, but never of inferior origin. That is easily understood. The resections were done in the inferior quadrant of the breast, cutting automatically all bridges for a glandular pedicle of that quadrant. Because the transposition was always made toward the top, these glandular pedicles could not be very thick; otherwise, the displacement and the torsion would be more damaging.

In 1971, McKissock (1972) made an important leap to the pedicle of the nipple-areola complex by choosing two glandular bridges. Among them, the inferior is quite large, and connects the nipple to a glandular tissue quite deep to allow the vascularity of the nipple from the perforating vessels emanating from the pectoralis major. Contrary to the previous techniques, McKissock's technique bases the nipple on a mass of the breast gland that could represent 10% to 15% of the total mass of the remaining breast after reduction. Only Biesenberger's (1928) reduction based the nipple on a larger mass of the remaining breast; unfortunately, this method had too many problems inherent in the detachment of the breast from the pectoralis major and consequently caused interruption of the perforating vessels. Therefore, this type of reduction was disregarded (Fig. 30–1A).

In 1976, Robbins (1977) carrying on McKissock's work, based the nipple on a simple inferior pedicle, probably a little larger than McKissock's. The mammary mass in connection with the nipple had to represent 15% to 25% of the remaining mammary volume (Fig. 30–1B).

Since 1979, we (Moufarrège et al., 1982) have used 100% of the remaining gland as a vascular support for the nipple-areola complex. This pedicle initially was in a posterior and inferior position and finally occupied the entire height of the gland; care is always taken to include the 100% of the remaining breast. This is the *total dermoglandular pedicle* (Fig. 30–1C).

CHARACTERISTICS

The basic characteristic of the total pedicle rests in the fact that this technique takes place openly, on a breast completely stripped on its anterior aspect. The resection is done at the periphery, and all of the remaining gland is in direct contact with the nipple and acts as the pedicle. In other words, the pedicle of the

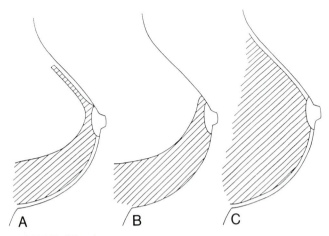

FIGURE 30–1
Amount of gland kept in the three techniques as a pedicle of the nipple-areola complex. A, The McKissock double vertical pedicle. B, The Robbins inferior pedicle. C, The Moufarrège total pedicle.

nipple-areola complex is composed of the whole remaining breast that extends from the lowest to the highest limit of the breast—hence the term "total pedicle."

This characteristic gives to the technique of the total pedicle all its other peculiarities and advantages, which will be enumerated.

TECHNIQUES

Sketches

Although the total pedicle is by no means limited to a drawing and can adapt to all sorts of incisions of pre-established drawings or not, we expose here a manner of drawing that we favor for reasons of simplicity, standardization, and, most importantly, conservation of reasonable scar length.

We divide the breast into three categories (Fig. 30–2A):

1. Category I. The hypertrophy is not or rarely accompanied by ptosis. The nipple stays more or less at the level of the inframammary fold.
2. Category II. The nipple is lower than the inframammary fold, but the breast at the level of this fold has a certain consistency and a real glandular projection.
3. Category III. The hypertrophy is accompanied by extreme ptosis, the nipple is very low, and the breast at the level of the fold is practically empty.

We start with the drawing of the keyhole described by Aufricht (1949), with certain modifications. The drawing is done on the patient in a sitting position; and the suprasternal notch and the axis of each breast passing through the nipple, which is not necessarily the midclavicular line, are marked.

We then choose the upper limit of the keyhole position at 19 cm from the suprasternal notch for women under 5 feet 3 inches tall (under 160 cm); 20 cm from the suprasternal hole for women between 5 feet 4 inches

and 5 feet 7 inches tall (160 to 170 cm); and 21 cm from the suprasternal notch for women over 5 feet 7 inches tall (over 170 cm).

These distances appear longer than those recommended in the past literature. The reason for this resides in the fact that the distance is measured out on skin already stretched down by the weight of the hypertrophy. Once the hypertrophy is treated, the new nipple site will spontaneously rise from 1 to 2 cm (Fig. 30–2B).

The upper curved part of the keyhole will not be a circle, but an oval drawing, with a longer horizontal axis, for two reasons: (1) Its closing (A joins C) has a tendency to give a circle; whereas if we started with a circle, its closing would give a vertical oval figure. (2) The natural tendency of the tissues, caused by the weight and the trimming, has a vertically elongating effect on the nipple-areola complex.

The opening of the keyhole arms (angle AB/CD) is from 90 to 100 degrees for category I, from 130 to 140 degrees for category II, and from 170 to 180 degrees for category III (see Fig. 30–2A).

We will see later why this technique allows such wide-angle openings of the keyhole (see Advantages [2]).

The keyhole arms are 5 cm long. We are aware that this length will be brought back to 4 cm because of the dermal stitches at 0.5 cm of each extremity closure.

The EF inframammary line, strictly in the submammary fold in its main central part, will be from 7 cm (slim candidate, 34-inch chest measurement) to 9 cm (more corpulent candidate, 38-inch chest measurement).

The BE and DF curved lines will have, on the first 2 to 3 cm, starting on B and D, a parallel direction to the tangent to the curved line of the keyhole at A and C. Then they curve in to join E and F, forming with the EF line angles of approximately 60 degrees in E (medial extremity) and 90 degrees in F (external extremity). The 90-degree angle at the external extremity will allow the subaxillary excess of skin to adhere more firmly to the lateral lining of the thorax, in such a way that the implementation base of the breast is really reduced without any cutaneous "drape" of skin excess in the subaxillary region (Fig. 30–2C).

The distance between E (left breast) and E' (right breast) accordingly will be from 9 to 15 cm (Fig. 30–2D).

Incisions

With the patient in the supine position, the circular periareolar incision is shaped for a 5 cm diameter that definitively will fit a space 4 cm in diameter, which will give the nipple-areola complex a certain interesting conical projection.

An inverted-U incision delimiting a dermal pedicle is performed. With a 6-cm width, it will extend from the superior part of the nipple-areola complex to the inframammary line. The area comprised in the interior of that inverted U is de-epithelialized.

The full-thickness incisions of the skin are then performed on the pre-established drawings. Only the junction between the de-epithelialized pedicle and the inferior incision is not cut full thickness (Fig. 30–3A).

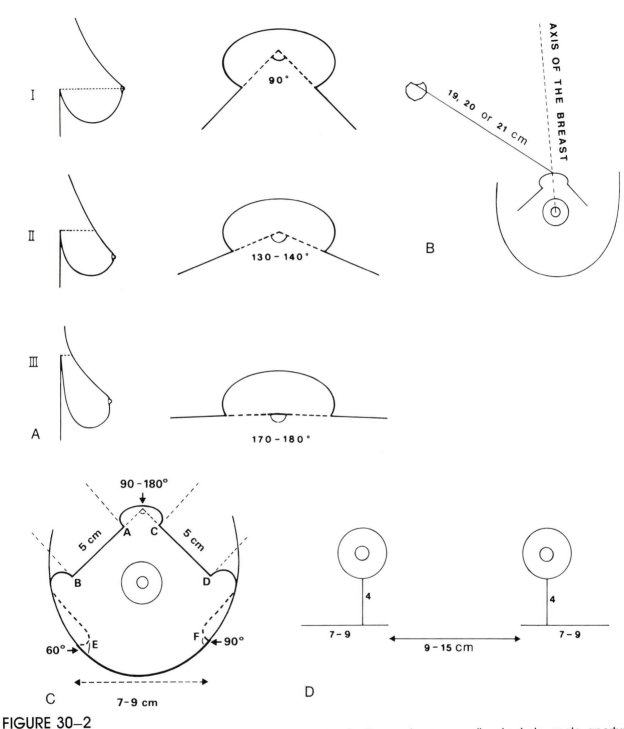

FIGURE 30-2

A, The three hypertrophy categories in the Moufarrège classification and corresponding keyhole angle apertures. *B,* Designing the axis of the breast and the distance from the areola to the suprasternal hole. *C,* Main drawing showing the oval design of the areola, the length and aperture of the keyhole arms, the pre-established inframammary incision (limited to 7 to 9 cm), and the curved lines joining the keyhole arm extremities to the extremities of the horizontal inferior incision. *D,* Final lines after the Moufarrège procedure with corresponding lengths.

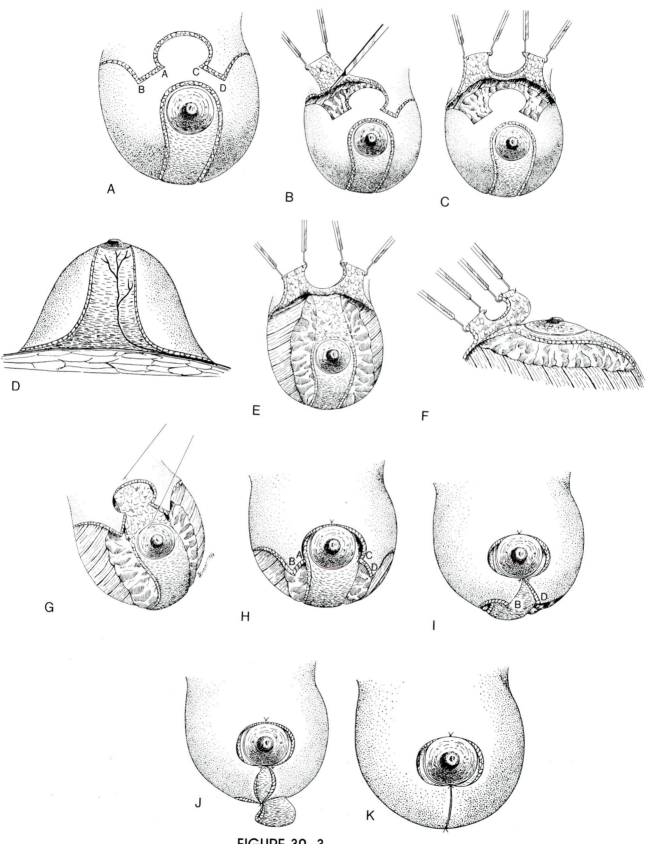

FIGURE 30–3
See legend on opposite page

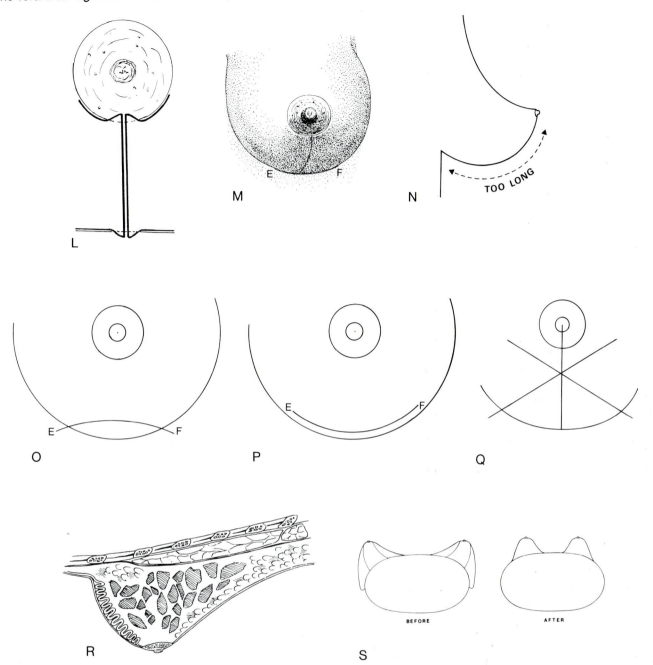

FIGURE 30-3

A, Incisions and de-epithelialization of the dermal pedicle. *B*, Consecutive undermining of the flaps, with one flap elevated.
C, Undermining of the flaps, with both flaps elevated. The breast will be sculptured while entirely exposed on its anterior
aspect for an open-sky resection. *D*, Transversal cut view of the breast in the Moufarrège procedure showing remaining
gland in the total pedicle (striped area), regions to be resected (dotted area), and the preservation of the intercostal
neural and vascular elements running along the pectoralis aponeurosis on the external side of the chest and through the
total pedicle toward the nipple. *E*, Resection focused on internal and mainly external quadrants. This figure shows the
remaining total pedicle after reduction. *F*, Profile view of the total pedicle after reduction. Notice that the pedicle extends
from the lowest to the highest limit of the breast without interruption. *G* and *H*, First stitch re-placing the upper limit of the
areola. *I*, First and second stitches completed the upper and lower limits of areola. *J*, Closure of the third cardinal point,
made easy by temporary extrusion of a part of the total pedicle. *K*, View after re-placing the luxate pedicle. *L*, Deer-foot
corner closure performed for prevention of small loss of skin at junctions. *M*, Final result, showing relative lengths of incisions.
N, Secondary ptosis and deformity in final trimming incisions (to be avoided). *O*, Possible deformity of the final lower
incision for the first weeks after surgery. *P*, The way to avoid deformity, by curving upward the extremities of the inferior EF
line in the initial drawing. *Q*, Classic "ship anchor" to be avoided. *R*, Adaptation of dermal pedicle on a shorter vertical
incision providing, through multiple consecutive folds, a strong inferior vault so that secondary ptosis can be avoided. *S*,
This drawing shows the rationale of implementation of base diminution through the resection of peripheral and particulary
the external quadrants.

Undermining the Flaps and Exposure of the Gland

The skin and subcutaneous fat flaps are detached from the breast gland up to the aponeurosis of the pectoralis major muscle. At the completion of that undermining, the breast is fully exposed on its frontal aspect while its posterior aspect remains entirely attached to the pectoralis major aponeurosis.

Technically, the undermining is done quite easily by holding separately the internal, then superior, and finally external flaps with skin hooks, successively placed in two positions at the same time in points A and B, A and C, and finally C and D. These points are raised by the assistant. It thus becomes easy for the surgeon, by putting some pressure with a sponge on the gland with one hand, to define, with the other one, with a No. 10 scalpel blade, the cleavage plane, established between the glandular tissue and the subcutaneous fatty tissue, which allows for a practically bloodless dissection (Fig. 30–3B and C).

Special attention is given to the detachment of the exterior flap in the subaxillary region. Cutting the areolar tissue at the extremity of the external quadrant of the breast is avoided so that the intercostal nerves are preserved, in particular the fifth, together with the tributary vessels of the external mammary system, which run along the aponeurosis of the pectoralis, through that areolar tissue, then medially toward the center of the breast and ascend through the mammary gland anteriorly to join the area of the nipple-areola complex (Fig. 30–3D).

Resection

One realizes immediately the advantage of working openly on a breast. The resection is done very easily in the areas most in need.

Classically, the large hypertrophies are characterized by a particular excess of the glandular tissue spreading quite far in the subaxillary region, for which the resection in the external quadrant is the most important. Here also, one saves that areolar tissue for the same reasons of safeguarding the intercostal nerves and the external mammary arteries, as explained previously. No resection will take place in the inferior or superior quadrants. These two quadrants are evidently the "protected zones" of the total dermoglandular pedicle. The resection in the internal quadrant is quite small (Fig. 30–3E and F).

Reconstitution

The nipple is set in its new position in the circle obtained by the closing of the curved line through the junction of the A and C corners. Technically, one begins by joining with a stitch the upper limit of the areola to the center of curved line AC (Fig. 30–G and H).

The second stitch brings in one stage the lower limit of the areola against points A and C (Fig. 30–3I).

The third cardinal stitch of the reconstitution brings the B and D corners against the line of the inframammary incision in a position chosen in terms of the respective lengths of the curved lines BE and DF.

The realization of this last stage is accomplished still more easily by leaving a part of the glandular pedicle outside the breast through the open space in the external part of the inframammary incision. Once the stitch is made, one re-enters the remaining glandular tissue, replacing it easily in position (Fig. 30–3J and K).

One should pay special attention at the closure of the two corners at the junction of the vertical line, with the circular one around the areola and the horizontal one in the inframammary fold. To avoid small loss of skin at these corners, it is advised to keep a small excess of skin in a deer-foot fashion, as seen in the drawing (Fig. 30–3L).

The rest of the suturing is completed in bringing lines BE and DF progressively against inframammary EF line. This is done by a certain puckering of lines BE and DF to adapt themselves to a shorter wound edge (EF). This puckering lessens within a few weeks and leaves practically no after-effects. This technique has the great advantage of keeping the lengths of the vertical scar (AB/CD) constant. The EF line is also kept constant, equal to the length already established at the beginning of the operation (7 to 9 cm) (Fig. 30–3M).

This contrasts in spectacular fashion with the final lines of mammaplasties performed with no pre-established drawing which bring the EF line to minimum length at the high cost of a longer and longer vertical line, which reaches as far as 10 to 12 cm in certain mammaplasties (Fig. 30–3N).

Because of the puckering of lines BE and DF, line EF may appear at the final stage of the operation as a curve with an inferior concavity. This spontaneously corrects itself within a few weeks, its center having a tendency to go down progressively with the softening of tissues and the relative lowering of all the mammary mass (Fig. 30–3O).

This problem could, however, be prevented during the drawing stage by exaggerating the upper curvature of extremities E and F of the inframammary fold EF line in order to compensate for the tendency of that line to take the opposite deformity (Fig. 30–3P).

This technique will avoid, because of skin undermining and centralization of all the remaining glandular mass, the classic anchor scar, traditionally tied to most of the techniques using pre-established sketches (Fig. 30–3Q).

Tissue Disposition

The 6-cm-wide dermal pedicle, which, according to the case, is originally between 2 and 5 times the length of the AB/CD vertical line, will be driven to occupy a 4- to 5-cm length at the end of the operation and consequently be compelled to intensively pucker itself, thus creating a dermal inferior vault all the more resistant to the traction and elongation, so that it is thicker and doubled up by the dermis of cutaneous flaps that cover it. This gives the total pedicle a certain capacity to resist the stretching and consequently classic pseudoptosis by lengthening of the vertical line, slipping of the gland in a subnipple position, and upper orientation of the nipples (Fig. 30–3R).

ADVANTAGES

1. *Absolute nipple security.* As a result of the pediculation of the nipple-areola complex on all of the remaining gland, the viability of the nipple-areola complex is ensured.
2. *Relative security of the cutaneous flaps.* The undermining of the lateral cutaneous flaps, entirely free of glandular tissue, allows the use of the skin to its maximum of elasticity and allows, therefore, an important cutaneous trimming and very secure ratio of width over length (1:1) in comparison with the ratios of 1:2 and 1:3 of classic techniques. This gives, in addition to superior viability of cutaneous flaps, a breast reshaping and lifting much more efficient and more homogeneous.
3. *Mammary projection.* Because the remaining gland is entirely in a central position, an exceptional projection of the breast and nipple is achieved (Fig. 30–3S), which is constant from patient to patient.
4. *Unique superior profile.* Undermining of the superior skin flaps up to the aponeurosis with the complete preservation of the superior quadrant of the breast gives a very pleasing projection over the nipple area.
5. *Reduction of pseudoptosis.* Pseudoptosis by stretching of the inferior vertical line is reduced because of the strong dermal inferior vault explained previously.
6. *Breast-feeding possible.* Postreduction breast-feeding is entirely possible and normal because galactophorous channels are preserved. Consequently, the remaining mammary gland, capable of galactogenous activity, is in direct communication with the nipple.
7. *Preservation of nipple sensation.* The preservation of intercostal nerves responsible for nipple-areola sensibility ensures without doubt a conservation of the nipple sensation.
8. *"Open sky" approach.* Surgery is performed openly, and therefore visualization is easier. Resection is performed in one or two sections. One is not compelled to go back after an attempt to suture to resect here and there some glandular fragments in search of a certain form or symmetry.
9. *Teaching.* Standardization of the technique, its method, and its execution under direct vision make the procedure easy to teach to residents.
10. *Execution time.* The time of the execution is relatively short with this technique because supplementary resection is unnecessary.
11. *Realization of equal breasts.* Direct visualization of the glandular tissue completely exposed makes the realization of equal breasts very easy, because the

quantity of gland to resect in the second breast is not evaluated by the amount taken from the first, but rather by the tissue left after resection.

12. *Reduction of the breast width.* This technique is particularly applicable to very wide breasts where the gland extends behind the midaxillary line. The undermining of pure cutaneous and subcutaneous flaps, the important resection in the external quadrant, and the trimming, much more extensive than in the classic techniques, allow the external wall to adhere properly on the lateral wall of the chest and allow a diminution of the implementation base of the breast at will.
13. *Form and surface.* The absence of parcels of mammary gland sequestered here and there under the skin gives a texture much more homogeneous, a breast with a more regular and natural look and pure lines. The skin acts like a rubber sack in which a gel (the mammary tissue) is placed and which will automatically take the most regular and harmonious shape.
14. *Realization of an immediately attractive form.* The total pedicle gives, in the immediate postsurgical stage, an attractive shape because of the disposition of the central pedicle and the potential of reshaping by the cutaneous flaps, which have become elastic.

DISADVANTAGES

1. *Difficulty of the first sketches.* Surgeons carrying out pre-established markings for the first time often experience difficulty in making the sketch correctly. That difficulty disappears with repetition.
2. *Prejudice against cutaneous flaps.* There is a legendary apprehension among surgeons with regard to real cutaneous fatty flaps completely undermined as far as the aponeurosis because of the possible loss of the flap skin.

A 10-YEAR EXPERIENCE

From 1979 to the first quarter of 1988, we performed 1500 bilateral reduction mammaplasties by the total dermoglandular pedicle. The age of the patients ranged from 14 to 72 years, with an average age of 30 years. The resection ranged from 100 to 1600 gm per breast; the transposition, from 4 to 32 cm. We experienced no loss of the nipple in the 1500 patients (Figs. 30–4 to 30–11).

In 2% of the cases, we have encountered skin healing problems, chiefly at the junction of horizontal and vertical incisions, mainly in the first 7 years. The wounds, which resulted in a certain amount of skin loss, healed eventually spontaneously without any skin grafting. In the last 3 years, this problem has diminished because we began to use the deer-foot closing technique at the junction of these incisions.

Of the 1500 patients, only 20 revealed a diminution of nipple sensation, a condition that nevertheless improved progressively with time. Curiously, a great number of our patients seemed to be agreeably surprised to

Text continued on page 386

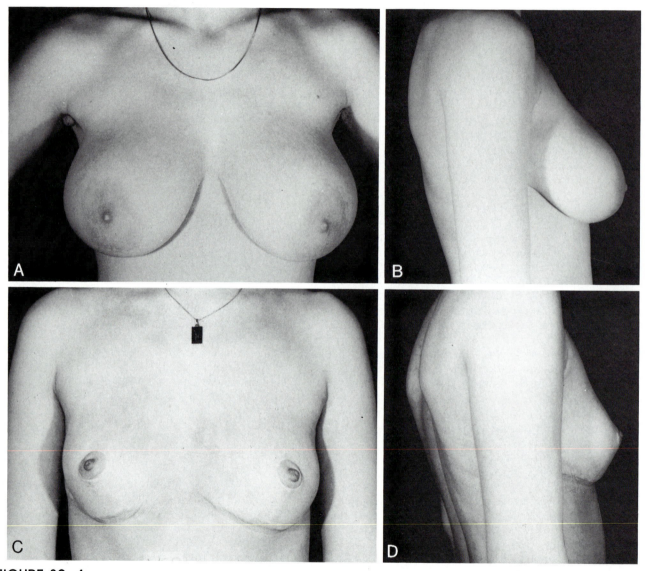

FIGURE 30–4

A and *B*, Preoperative views of a 24-year-old patient with hypertrophic breasts. *C* and *D*, Postoperative views 6 months after the patient underwent the Moufarrège procedure with removal of 515 gm from each breast.

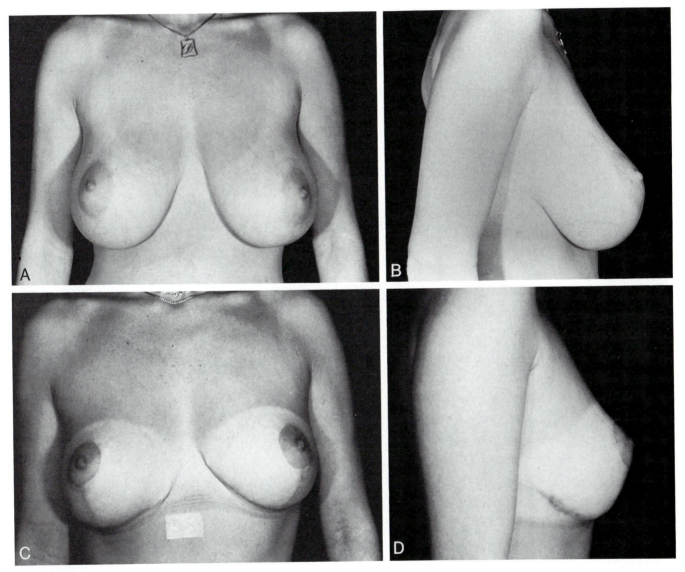

FIGURE 30–5

A and *B*, Preoperative views of a 27-year-old patient. *C* and *D*, One year after the patient underwent the Moufarrège procedure with removal of 450 gm from each breast.

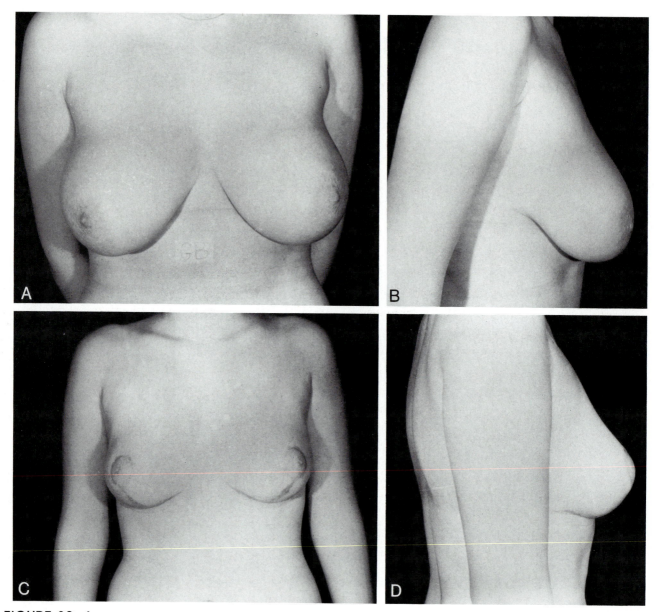

FIGURE 30–6

A and B, Preoperative views of a 20-year-old patient. C and D, Six months after the patient underwent the Moufarrège procedure with removal of 350 gm from each breast.

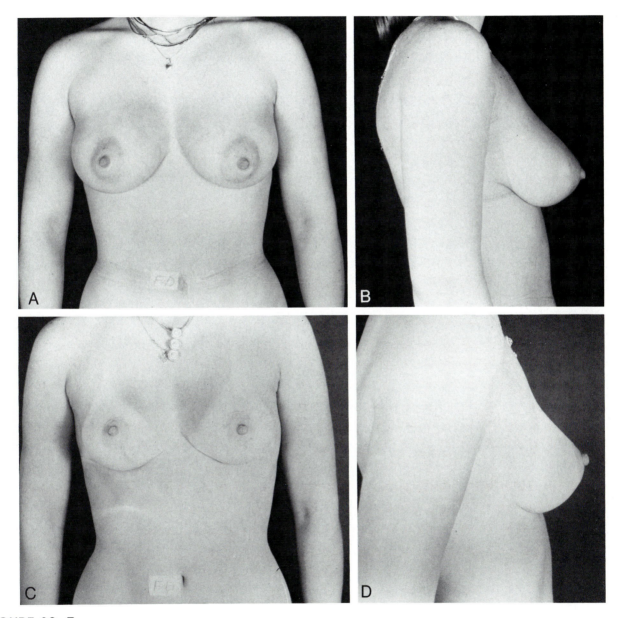

FIGURE 30–7

A and B, Preoperative views of a 25-year-old patient. C and D, Two years after the patient underwent the Moufarrège procedure with removal of 280 gm from each breast.

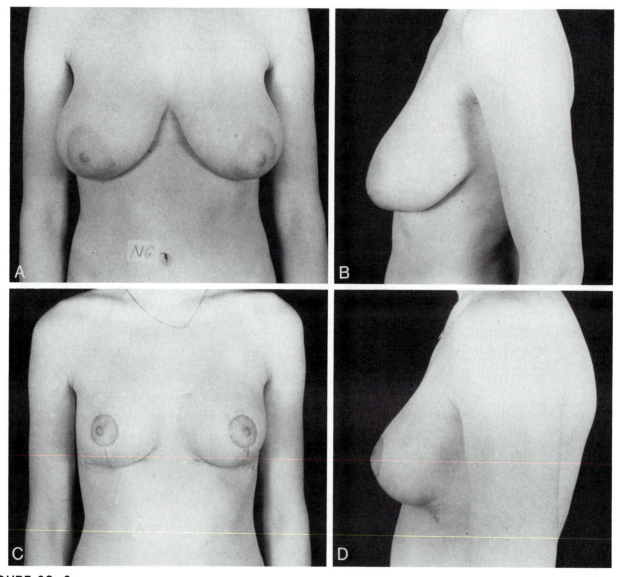

FIGURE 30–8
A and *B*, Preoperative views of a 23-year-old patient. *C* and *D*, Six months after the patient underwent the Moufarrège procedure with removal of 360 gm from each breast.

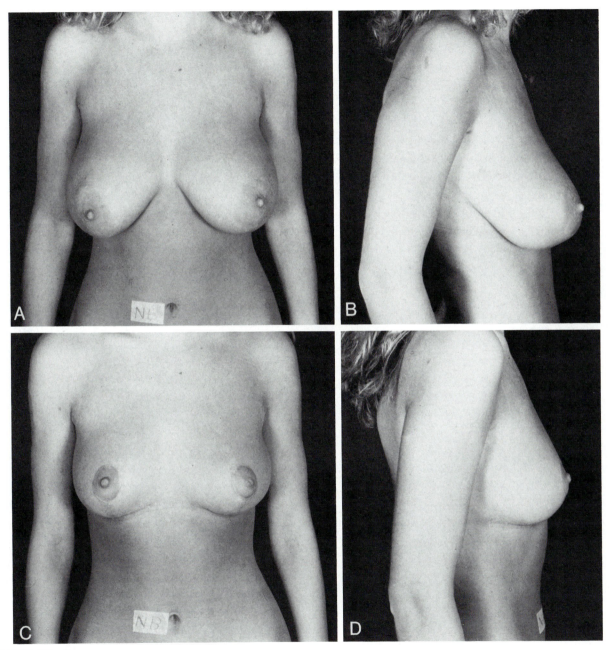

FIGURE 30–9

A and *B*, Preoperative views of a 20-year-old patient. *C* and *D*, Two years after the patient underwent the Moufarrège procedure with removal of 375 gm from each breast.

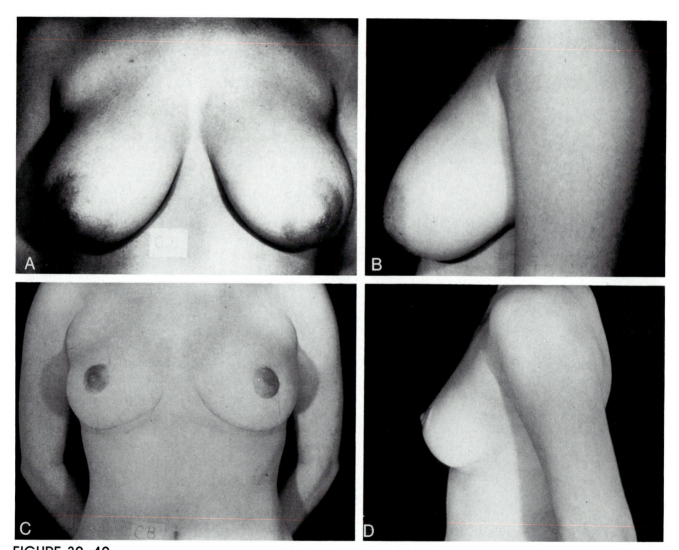

FIGURE 30–10

A and *B*, Preoperative views of a 21-year-old patient. *C* and *D*, Three years after the patient underwent the Moufarrège procedure with removal of 385 gm from each breast.

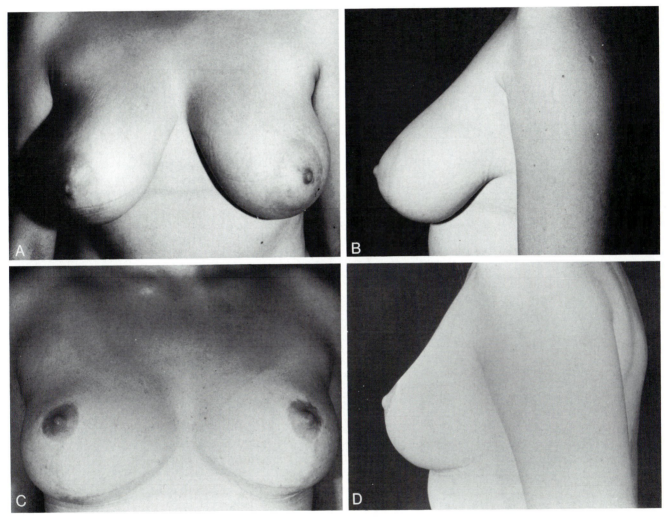

FIGURE 30–11
A and B, Preoperative views of a 35-year-old patient. C and D, Four years after the patient underwent the Moufarrège procedure with removal of 360 gm from each breast.

have an ameliorated nipple sensation either because of the diminution of the traction on the nerves or possibly because of psychologic factors.

Fifty-four of our patients became pregnant after this mammaplasty. They all carried through their pregnancy normally with normal lactation.

The psychologic impact on our patients is estimated to be good in 99% of cases.

References

Aufricht, G.: Mammoplasty for pendulous breasts: Empiric and geometric planning. Plast. Reconstr. Surg. 4:13, 1949.

Balch, C. R.: Central mound technique for reduction mammoplasty. Plast. Reconstr. Surg. 67:305, 1981.

Biesenberger H.: Eine neue Methode der Mammoplastik. Zentralbl. Chir. 55:2382, 1928.

Drzewiecki, A.: Breast reduction by central pedicle technique. Plast. Reconstr. Surg. 78:830, 1986.

Dufourmentel, C., Mouly, R..: Plastie mammaire par la méthode oblique. Ann. Chir. Plast. 6:45, 1961.

Georgiade, N. G., Serafin, D., Riefkohl, R., Georgiade, G. S.: Is there a reduction mammaplasty for "all seasons"? Plast. Reconstr. Surg. 63:765, 1979.

Georgiade, N. G., Serafin, D., Morris, R., Georgiade, G.: Reduction mammaplasty utilizing an inferior pedicle nipple-areolar flap. Ann. Plast. Surg. 3:211, 1979.

Isaacs, G., Rozner, L., Tudball, C.: Breast lumps after reduction mammaplasty. Ann. Plast. Surg. 15:394, 1985.

Lalardrie, J. P., Mitz, V.: Reduction mammoplasty using the technic of dermal vault. J. Chir. (Paris) 108:57, 1974.

Lalardrie, J. P., Jouglard, P.: Chirurgie Plastique du Sein. Paris, Masson, 1974.

McKissock, P. K.: Reduction mammaplasty with a vertical dermal flap. Plast. Reconstr. Surg. 49:245, 1972.

McKissock, P. K.: Reduction mammaplasty by the vertical bipedicle flap technique: Rationale and results. Clin. Plast. Surg. 3:309, 1976.

Mitz, V., Lassus, J. P.: Vascularisation du sein: Étude des rapports entre les vascularisations artérielles glandulaires et cutanée du sein. Arch. Anat. Pathol. 21:365, 1973.

Moufarrège, R., Muller, H., Beauregard, G., et al.: Plastie mammaire à pédicule dermoglandulaire Inférieur. Ann. Chir. Plast. 27:249, 1982.

Moufarrège, R., Beauregard, G., Bosse, J. P., et al.: Reduction mammoplasty by the total dermoglandular pedicle. Aesthetic Plast. Surg. 9:227, 1985.

Peixoto, G.: Reduction mammaplasty: A personal technique. Plast. Reconstr. Surg. 65:217, 1980.

Pitanguy, I.: Une nouvelle technique de plastie mammaire: Étude de 245 cas consécutifs et présentation d'une technique personnelle. Ann. Chir. Plast. 7:199, 1962.

Reich, J.: The advantage of a lower central breast segment in a reduction mammoplasty. Aesthetic Plast. Surg. 3:47, 1979.

Robbins, T. H.: A reduction mammaplasty with the areola-nipple based on an inferior dermal pedicle. Plast. Reconstr. Surg. 59:64, 1977.

Skoog, T.: A technique of breast reduction: Transposition of nipples on cutaneous vascular pedicle. Acta Chir. Scand. 126:453, 1963.

Strömbeck, J. O.: Mammoplasty: Report of a new technique based on the two-pedicle procedure. Br. J. Plast. Surg. 13:79, 1960.

Strömbeck, J. O.: Reduction mammaplasty. Surg. Clin. North Am. 51:453, 1971.

Thorek, M.: Plastic Surgery of the Breast and Abdominal Wall. Springfield, Ill, Charles C Thomas, 1942.

31

Jean-Marie Parenteau
Paule Regnault

Reduction Mammaplasty and Mastopexy Using the B Technique

Since the beginning of the practice of plastic and aesthetic surgery, surgeons have been searching for a technique of mastopexy and breast reduction that could be used for all sizes of breasts (with and without prostheses) and would be safe, with an average or less than average number of complications and with a minimal loss of blood.

Acceptable scars are a must, and avoidance of the medial aspect in the inverted-T incisions commonly used has been the object of many surgeons' experimentation. Also, the resultant breast should not be square or flat, but conical.

Initially patients and surgeons alike thought that reduction mammaplasty consisted only of a smaller and more comfortable breast. However, the aesthetic result has now taken precedence as the final goal.

The Strömbeck (Strömbeck, 1960) technique was commonly used in the l960s, often with an unsatisfying final result in breast shape and scars. Simultaneously, the Pitanguy technique (Pitanguy, 1967), with and without personal modifications, became very popular with many surgeons.

With experience, the aesthetic results were quite pleasing except for the medial aspect of the scar. There were also some limitations found in reducing breasts over 500 gm.

On the other hand, the B technique in breast reduction and mastopexy realizes these expectations with a minimal number of complications.

BREAST REDUCTION

Indications

The classic signs and symptoms of breast hypertrophy are back, shoulder, and neck pain; a feeling of discomfort and heaviness due to the size of the breast; hygienic problems, i.e., skin irritation at the inframammary line; and brassiere strap discomfort with notching at the shoulders.

Dr. Parenteau has used the B technique exclusively in over 1000 cases since 1975; and Dr. Regnault, in over 2500 cases since 1969. With this technique, up to 1500 gm per breast have been removed, and the greatest length between the sternal notch and the tip of the nipple was measured at 48 cm.

Technique

Measurements

The markings and measurements should be very precise. They are made with the patient in the sitting position as follows:

1. Point V is marked by measuring from the sternal notch to the upper limit of the areola (Fig. 31–1).
2. Then, with the patient in the supine position, point M is marked by measuring from the midsternal line to the median limit of the periareolar skin.
3. M′ is marked, symmetric with M in relation to the breast vertical axis.
4. The areola is reduced to about a 4 to 5 cm in diameter. It is very useful to draw the areolar axis, vertical and horizontal, to help suturing it with equal tension (Fig. 31–2).
5. The classic B marking as described by Regnault (Regnault, 1980) is as follows: From point M a slow curve is marked, continuing the median incision to the level of the new areola lower limit. Then, a second curve, forming an angle with the upper one, finishes the B appearance, going down to join the new submammary fold. The inframammary incision is marked 1 to 3 cm above the inframammary line. From point M′ a lazy-S curve joining the inframammary incision is made laterally (Fig. 31–3).

Anesthesia

General anesthesia with endotracheal tubing is utilized, but small reductions and mastopexies may be done under local anesthesia, with usual standard premedication.

Prior to starting the procedure, the incision and the full thickness of the skin at the periphery of the incisions and the mammary gland lying above the pectoral muscle to be dissected are infiltrated with lidocaine (Xylocaine), 1/4%, and epinephrine, 1:400,000. A total of 60 ml of this solution is used, on the average, on each side.

Surgical Technique

A periareolar *de-epithelialization* (Fig. 31–4) is started with an incision around the areola, down to its dermis.

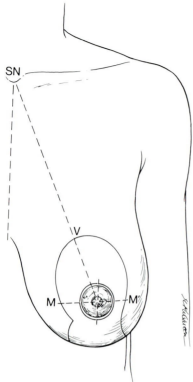

FIGURE 31–1
The patient is in the sitting position, with her arm alongside her chest. Point V (vertical height) is marked. The sternal notch (SN)–nipple axis is only for measurement of the upper areola limit. Points M and M′ are marked.

The periareolar skin is de-epithelialized with the knife up to point V superiorly, laterally to point M′, medially to point M, and inferiorly 1 cm below the new areola. This appears as an oval or circular area of de-epithelialization.

The *excision* of the breast tissue for breast reduction follows, with a deep incision below the de-epithelialized infra-areolar margin and from point M to the mid part

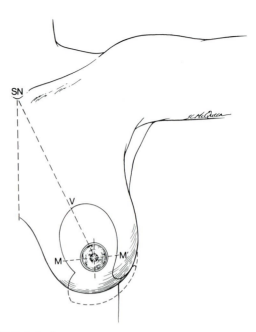

FIGURE 31–3
With the arm at a right angle, V is marked, as are points M and M′. The length of the subareolar incision is determined, and horizontal submammary and lazy-S incisions are made.

of the new inframammary line. The incision along the new inframammary line is made simultaneously. *Medially*, dissection with the cutting cautery is done down to the pectoral fascia, leaving some areolar tissue on the fascia and muscle, with beveling of the cautery at the desired angle so that the desired amount of glandular

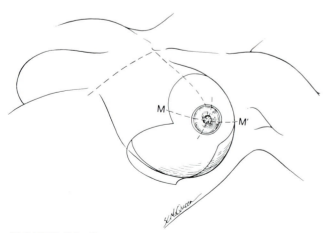

FIGURE 31–2
With the patient in the recumbent position, the periareolar, submammary, vertical length, and lazy-S incisions are made.

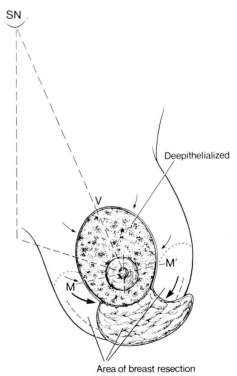

FIGURE 31–4
De-epithelialization and rotation of the flaps.

tissue is retained in the medial portion of the breast. *Inferiorly*, cutting with the cautery is done at a 45-degree angle down to the pectoral fascia and continuing the previous incision. No breast tissue should be left between the new and the previous inframammary lines. The breast tissue is lifted *en bloc* from the pectoral fascia up with the cautery to the second or third rib. In order to achieve a semispheric and even breast, it is advised that more tissue be removed medially than laterally because of the difference in tissue tension, the medial part of the breast being longer and looser than the lateral part, which is being pulled downward and medially.

Superiorly, a hook is placed at the de-epithelialized infra-areolar margin; and with the cautery from point M' to point M, the incision is deepened, with beveling at the desired angle for removal of more or less glandular tissue, eventually joining the dissection reached previously at the second or third rib. The flap underneath the nipple-areola complex is never thinner than 1 cm.

A *thick flap* is created, involving the full thickness of the glandular tissue, free at its superior, inferior, and medial aspects, but attached laterally. This lateral flap is pulled medially and downward into the maximal concavity of the initial lower curve of the B drawing. After estimating a correct and easy joining of these flaps, the lateral incision is finally determined, then executed with the knife and cautery.

This thick flap consists of the amount to be removed, and now the site of the lateral incision is definitely determined. By pulling medially on the flap, one can estimate the correct amount to be removed in order to obtain the desired volume and shape with moderate tension for clothing.

The *principle of a Z-plasty* is now used. The median flap is pulled laterally and the lateral flap is pulled medially and downward into the maximum concavity of the initial lower curve of the B drawing.

After verifying hemostasis, one applies a drain when necessary. For the closure, a few sutures of Prolene are put at key points through glandular tissue, holding the two flaps. Running sutures with Dexon 4-0 are made around the areola. At the four quadrants, four separate stitches secure the adequate tension, where a subareolar running suture is applied (Fig. 31–5). Steri-Strips are put on. Adaptic and soft gauze sponges are laid on the wounds. When used, drains are removed after 24 to 48 hours (Fig. 31–6).

Postoperative Care

An appointment at the office for subsequent care is made for the removal of Prolene stitches and Steri-Strips. The patient wears a soft brassiere continuously night and day for 3 weeks. Only minimal movement of the pectoral muscles is recommended. Patients are examined at 1 month, 3 months, 6 months, 1 year, and so forth.

The age range of patients for reduction mammaplasty is 15 to 72 years and for mastopexy, 19 to 50 years (Figs. 31–7 to 31–10).

Complications

The *early* complications are those of all reduction techniques: a hematoma occurs in 1% of all cases and skin flap necrosis in the upper part of the lateral flap in 1.5%. Nipple-areola necrosis may occur in 0.1% of cases, i.e., in those with poor vascularization and very large reductions. Infections are found in 1% of cases and are associated with hematoma and skin necrosis. Fat necrosis has not occurred in Dr. Parenteau's experience.

The *late* complications include scars and sensory changes. *True keloids* are exceptional and more often on the horizontal part of the incisions. The occurrence of hypertrophic scars is no greater than in other techniques, and medial scars are, of course, nonexistent. *Sensory changes* may occur, from complete loss of feeling in 0.5% to diminished sensitivity in 5% of cases. Recurrent hypertrophy of gland or fat is possible in young patients gaining weight and may be unilateral, and younger patients (under 20 years) are warned. Avoidance of complications is obtained by an avoidance of tension on the suture lines of the rotating flaps.

Text continued on page 394

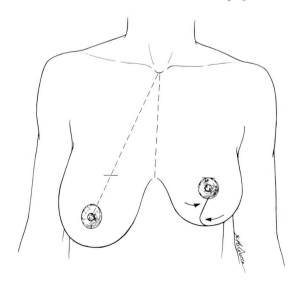

FIGURE 31–5
Preoperative and postoperative views of the breasts in the sitting position.

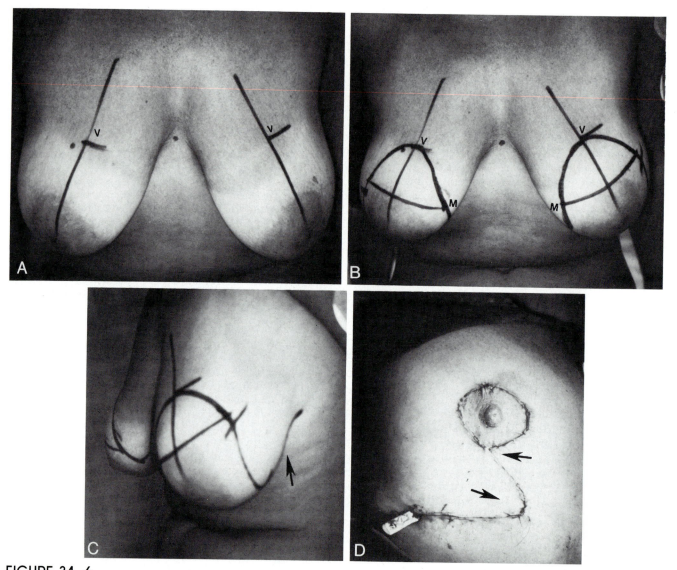

FIGURE 31–6

A, Preoperative markings with the patient in an upright position. The initial marking will be the point for the new margin of the areola. This is made 15 to 18 cm from the sternal notch (point V; see Fig. 31–1). *B,* Points V and M represent the medial margins of the areola. Points M and M′ are equidistant from the midsternal line. An arc is drawn to connect M and V, and the lateral margins are marked symmetrically with the medial coordinates. *C,* The submammary fold location is estimated, approximately 2 cm higher than the existing one. The new location is traced parallel to the present fold (Fig. 31–2). *D,* Immediate postoperative appearance. Notice how the lateral flap has been advanced medially and slightly downward. The medial flap is moved slightly laterally. Subcutaneous sutures are used to approximate the skin edge, and subcuticular running sutures are used to approximate the skin edge. A drain is inserted laterally for 24 to 48 hours.

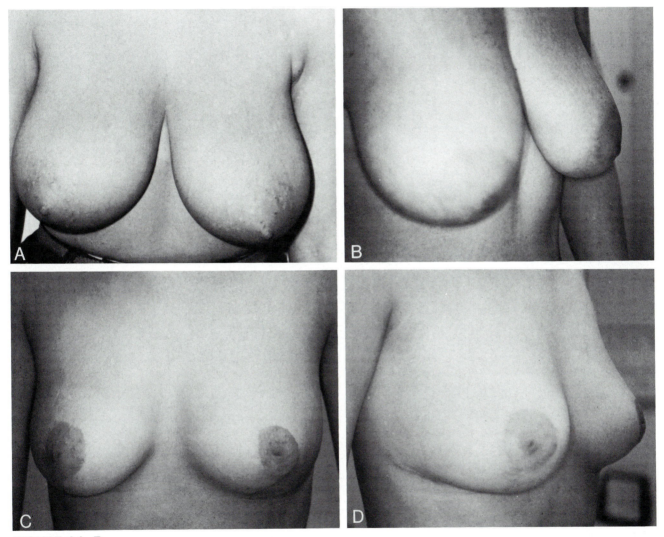

FIGURE 31–7
A and *B*, Preoperative front and lateral views of a patient with moderate hypertrophy. *C* and *D*, 6 months after surgery.

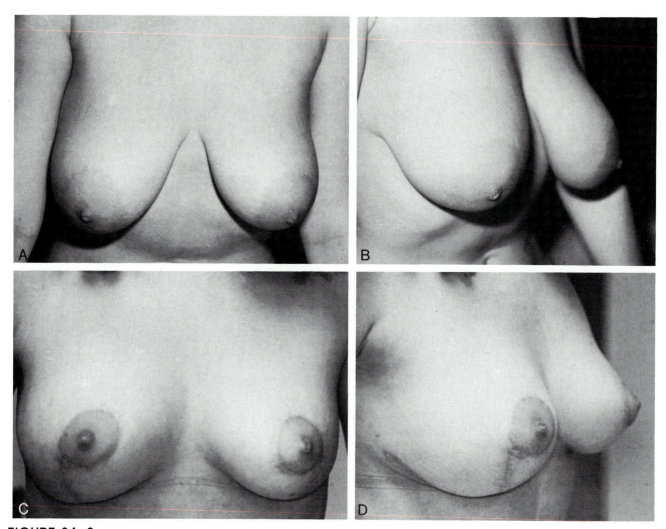

FIGURE 31–8

A and B, Preoperative front and lateral views of a 24-year-old patient with moderate hypertrophy. C and D, The same patient 6 months after removal of 550 gm from each breast.

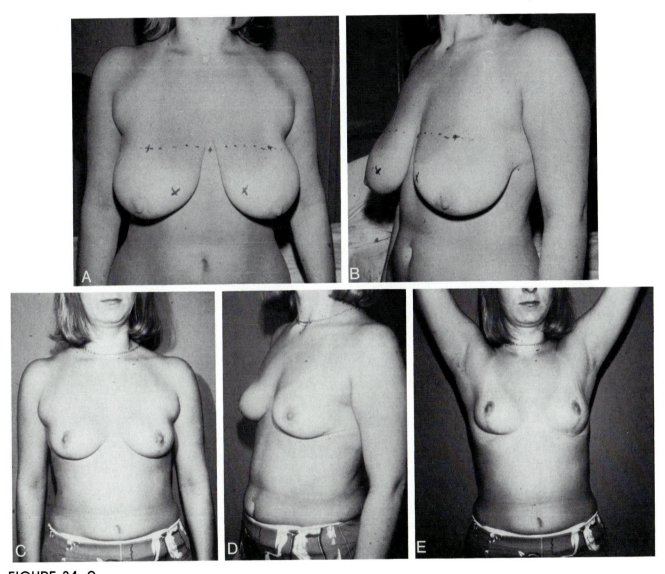

FIGURE 31–9

A and B, Preoperative view of a patient with breast hypertrophy and ptosis. Markings of the upper and medial limits of the peripheral skin of the new areola are shown. *C* and *D,* The same patient 2 years after B reduction of 550 gm of tissue from each side. *E,* The same patient with arms elevated, showing the typical scar of the B technique with complete elimination of the medial scar.

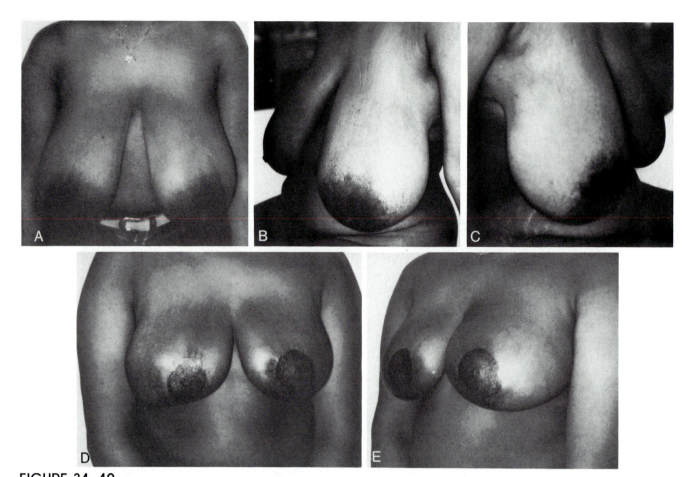

FIGURE 31–10

A to *C*, Preoperative views of a patient with hypertrophy and ptosis. *D* and *E*, Postoperative views at 3 months of the same patient after removal of 1300 gm of tissue from the right breast and 1150 gm of tissue from the left breast.

Pathology

Malignancy, though rare, is always possible; therefore, careful preoperative examination and possibly mammography are performed. Fibrocystic disease, fibroadenoma, and fatty hypertrophy, benign modifications, are common pathologic findings.

CONCLUSION

The advantages of the B technique are as follows:

1. Excision of excessive glandular tissue and skin is easily performed.
2. The result is aesthetically pleasing, with a symmetric shape and the nipple at its vertex.
3. The good results are lasting, and there is no tendency toward upward migration of the nipple-areola complex with aging.
4. There are minimal scars, and these are in the least visible locations. The operation is safe, simple, and short and can be used in breasts under 1500 gm in young patients and under 1200 gm in older ones.
5. Sensitivity is usually preserved.
6. There is usually minimal blood loss.

References

Ben Hur, N., Golan, J.: Some remarks on breast reduction by the B technique. Presented at the International Congress of Plastic and Reconstructive Surgery, Rio de Janeiro, May 23, 1979.

Pitanguy, I.: Breast hypertrophy. In: *Transactions of the International Society of Plastic Surgery,* Second Congress, London, 1959. Edinburgh, Livingstone, 1960.

Pitanguy, I.: Surgical treatment of breast hypertrophy. Br. J. Plast. Surg. 20:78, 1967.

Pitanguy, I.: Personal preferences for reduction mammaplasty. In: Goldwyn, R. M. (ed.): *Plastic and Reconstructive Surgery of the Breast.* Boston, Little, Brown, 1976, p. 167.

Regnault, P.: The hypoplastic and ptotic breast. A combined operation with prosthetic augmentation. Plast. Reconstr. Surg. 37:31, 1966.

Regnault, P.: Reduction mammaplasty by the B technique. Plast. Reconstr. Surg. 53:19, 1974.

Regnault, P.: Breast ptosis: Definition and treatment. Clin. Plast. Surg. 3:193, 1976.

Regnault, P.: Reduction mammaplasty by the "B" technique. In: Goldwyn, R. M. (ed.): *Plastic and Reconstructive Surgery of the Breast.* Boston, Little, Brown, 1976, p. 269.

Regnault, P.: Partially submuscular breast augmentation. Plast. Reconstr. Surg. 59:72, 1977.

Regnault, P.: Breast reduction. In: Owsley, J. Q., Peterson, R. A. (eds.): *Symposium on Aesthetic Surgery of the Breast.* St. Louis, C. V. Mosby, 1978, p. 58.

Regnault, P.: Breast reduction: B technique. Plast. Reconstr. Surg. 65:840, 1980.

Reich, J.: The advantages of a lower central breast segment in reduction mammaplasty. Aesthetic Plast. Surg. 3:47, 1979.

Strömbeck, J. O.: Mammplasty: Report of a new technique based on the two pedicle procedure. Br. J. Plast. Surg. 13:79, 1960.

Strömbeck, J. O.: Reduction mammaplasty. In: Gibson, T. (ed.): *Modern Trends in Plastic Surgery.* London, Butterworth, 1964, p. 237.

Strömbeck, J. O.: Reduction mammaplasty. In: Grabb, W. C., Smith, J. W. (eds.): *Plastic Surgery: A Concise Guide to Clinical Practice.* Boston, Little, Brown, 1968, p. 821.

Strömbeck, J. O.: Reduction mammaplasty. Surg. Clin. North Am. 51:453, 1971.

Strömbeck, J. O.: Late results after reduction mammaplasty. In: Goldwyn, R. M. (ed.): *Long Term Results in Plastic Surgery.* Boston, Little, Brown, 1980, p. 722.

Bernard Bodin
Roger Mouly

32

Reduction Mammaplasty: A Lateral Technique

Over the past 25 years, we have used a technique of mammaplasty characterized by a single lateral oblique external scar. This technique was first described in 1961 and presented during the following years by the same authors in several papers (Dufourmentel and Mouly, 1965, 1966, 1968, 1961; Mouly and Dufourmentel, 1971). The oblique scar in reduction mammaplasty was also recommended by other plastic surgeons: Marc (1952), Elbaz and Verheecke (1972), Fonseca-Ely (1978), and Schatten et al. (1971). The single vertical scar was proposed by Arié (1957).

The main principles of this technique are the absence of undermining between skin and glandular tissue and respect for cutaneous glandular continuity, which allow posterior stability of the breast; glandular resection extending as required on the posterior aspect of the gland; and, finally, a single lateral scar, which can improve the final result, avoiding the rather long horizontal scar, which is often hypertrophic, of the classic T pattern (Vandenbussche, 1979).

The method, with its possible variations and good and bad features, is discussed in this chapter.

OPERATIVE TECHNIQUE FOR MODERATE HYPERTROPHY

Preliminary Skin Markings

With the patient sitting, point A is marked, which represents the lower pole of the lateral cutaneous excision, located at the intersection of the submammary fold and the anterior axillary line.

Point B is the medial aspect 2 cm above and medial to the areola, which represents the upper pole of the excision (Fig. 32–1).

The upper lateral incision line joins the two dots in a straight or slightly curved line while the hand pushes the breast downward and inward.

The lower medial incision joins the same two dots while the breast is pushed upward and outward. These two lines define the area of skin that will be resected. The maximum width of this spindle-shaped area is usually 10 to 15 cm.

Next, the lines of the cutaneous resection are drawn, joining A to B, of equal length.

At the end of the operation, the nipple will be buried and exteriorized in symmetric positions on both sides.

As an alternative, one can mark at the onset of the operation, with a metal washer 4 cm in diameter, the new placement of the areola. The technique consists of placing the ring on the areola, with the nipple as a center, and marking the contour of the ring on the skin. The ring is opened and defines an arc of a circle the same length as the areola. One then marks three points (Fig. 32–2A): D, on a vertical line from the nipple to the submammary fold, 5.6 cm from the fold; C, on a horizontal line from the nipple to the midline, approximately 8.9 cm from the midline; and B, on a straight line from the suprasternal notch to the nipple, at a distance between 16 and 20 cm from the suprasternal notch. The arc must pass through these three points.

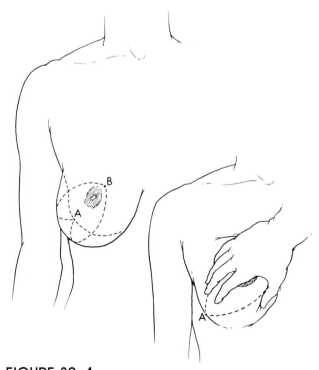

FIGURE 32–1
Preoperative markings outline incisions. Point B is located at the junction of the submammary fold with the anterior axillary line.

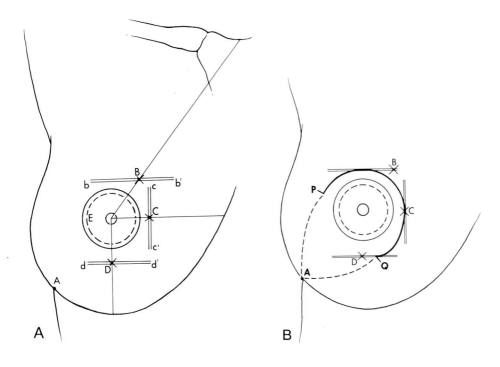

A

B

FIGURE 32–2
A and *B*, Preliminary skin markings with positioning of the nipple as described in the text at the onset of the operation.

The extremities P and Q of the arc are placed symmetrically to a line joining the submammary external point A to the new nipple. Segments AP and AQ are drawn and define cutaneous resection (Fig. 32–2B).

Incisions

The incisions are made along the drawn lines and around the areola. The skin around the areola is removed. Care is taken to preserve the deeper dermis and the veins (Fig. 32–3).

The lateral incisions are extended down to the plane of the gland. At the inferior external angle we open up the space between gland and fascia of the pectoralis major muscle. The posterior aspect of the whole breast is freed (Fig. 32–4).

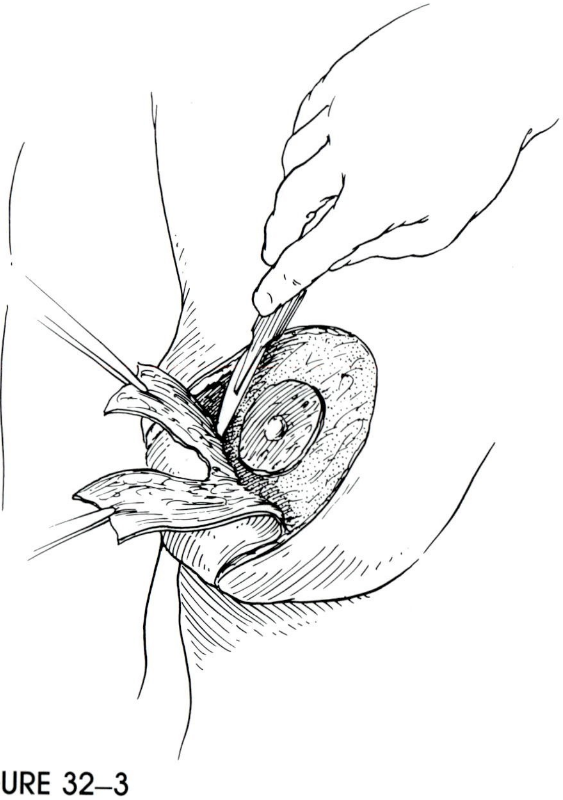

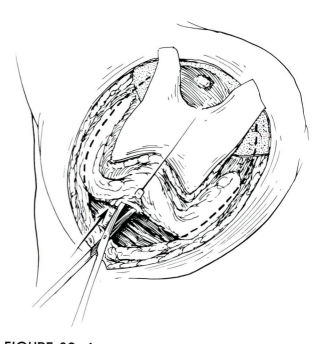

FIGURE 32–3
Periareolar dissection; intradermal dissection around the nipple.

FIGURE 32–4
Undermining at the deep aspect of the gland before resection.

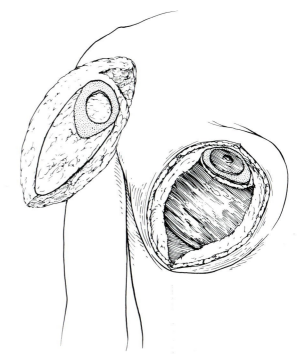

FIGURE 32–5
Resection of the gland. On the right is a gap left after glandular and skin resection; on the left is a piece of excised glandular cutaneous tissue.

The glandular incisions are made through the gland along the lateral borders of the wound and 2 cm around the lower lateral border of the areola; a layer of glandular tissue under the areola is retained.

A block of glandular tissue is resected in this way in continuity with the skin (Fig. 32–5). For large hypertrophic breasts, we perform an extra resection from the deep aspect of the breast.

The mammary cone is restored as the glandular cavity is closed by Vicryl sutures in two layers (Fig. 32–6).

Sutures and Dressings (Fig. 32–7)

The suture of the areola is not usually a problem, in spite of preservation of the periareolar dermal ring. If the apposition is difficult, we can easily undermine the cutaneous tissue 1 or 2 cm around the areola. We place a drain for 2 or 3 days in approximately one of four cases when there is some evidence of bleeding, following retromammary undermining. Strips are placed on the skin, followed by nonadherent mesh and elastic bandages. The dressing is changed on the second or third postoperative day.

Sutures for the areola and for the lateral scar are taken out on the seventh and twelfth day, respectively.

Figure 32–8 shows a patient with moderate breast hypertrophy operated on by the lateral method and the early result, with a close-up of the scars after removal of the stitches on the fourteenth day.

VARIATIONS

Ptosis

With ptosis, we use a similar approach, but in this case a dermoglandular flap is rotated under the upper part of the breast at its deep aspect.

We use what Gillies and Marins (1958) refer to as the periwinkle shell operation. However, we insert the flap deeply instead of superficially; the markings are the same as for the hypertrophic operation.

Two deep incisions are done, one along the upper lateral edge, the other around the lower lateral border of the areola, 2 cm away from this border (Fig. 32–9A).

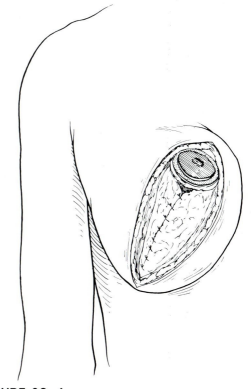

FIGURE 32–6
Sutures in the gland.

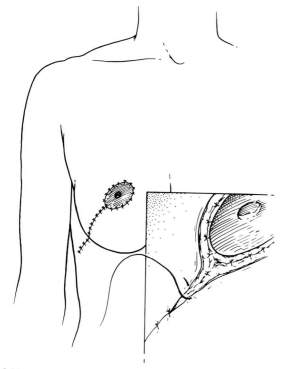

FIGURE 32–7
Suturing of the skin.

We preserve the deep dermis in the area of the resected skin for two purposes: protection of the blood supply of the underlying gland and strong support for the mastopexy. After the undermining of the breast, glandular resection is now performed.

The dermoglandular flap is triangular. The upper border corresponds to the skin incision and the internal border to the periareolar incision. It is rotated under the lateral aspect of the gland (Fig. 32–9B). The fixation

of the flap should not create any tension on the medial edge, which can make the cutaneous suturing difficult. We therefore orient the flap in a vertical direction and fix it under the upper pole of the breast slightly outward (Fig. 32–9C). With this technique (Fig. 32–10), we have achieved satisfactory projection of the areola, as shown in Figure 32–11.

Large Hypertrophy

In the case of large hypertrophy, with the previous markings, the scar passes over the new breast and goes on too far on the thoracic skin; so we have modified the markings as follows.

The purpose is to break the cicatricial line by a cutaneous resection.

The borders of the wedge resection are of different length; so we shorten the upper wedge and draw an isosceles triangle whose base represents the difference in length between the two lateral lines (Fig. 32–12A). The final scar will have the shape of an inverted L, with a radial part from the nipple to point A and an external mammary one going upward and backward (Fig. 32–12B).

Two goals are attained: the scar will remain under the brassiere, and the areola rotates externally.

Large Hypertrophy with Glandular Ptosis

In the case of large hypertrophy with glandular ptosis, the upper part of the breast is flattened. To restore the contour, we use the same dermoglandular flap as for a ptotic breast, but a glandular resection is done at the deep aspect of the breast and of the flap itself.

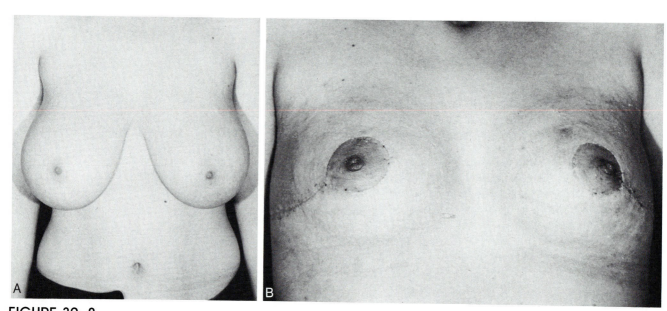

FIGURE 32–8
A and B, A 28-year-old patient with moderate breast hypertrophy before and after a 500-gm resection by the lateral method, with a close-up of the scars after removal of the stitches on the fourteenth day.

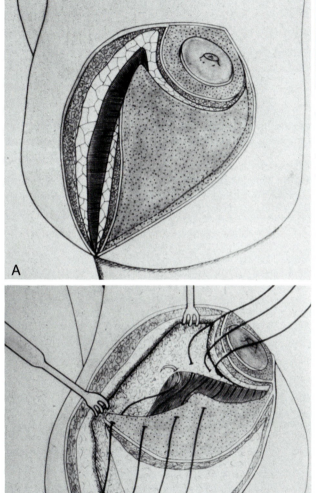

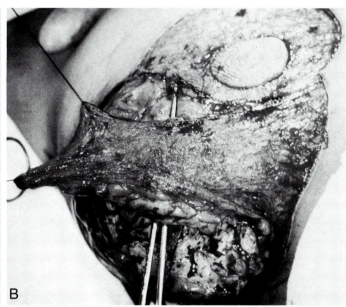

FIGURE 32–9

A, Lines of incision of the dermoglandular flap. *B,* Operative view. The flap is prepared and ready for rotation. *C,* The flap is rotated under the upper part of the breast and sutured with polyglactin 910.

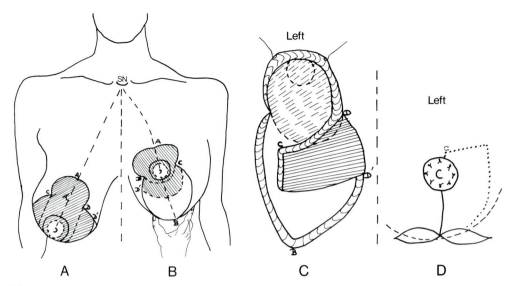

FIGURE 32–10

A, The preoperative design is shown on the right breast with the patient in an upright position. A line is drawn from the sternal notch to the nipple and then to the inframammary fold, as shown in B. Point A is marked on this line at a distance of 17 to 19 cm from the sternal notch. Point A′ is marked 5 cm inferior to point A. At right angles to A′, points C and D are marked each 4 to 5 cm and equidistant from A′. A curved elliptic line is then drawn connecting C, A, and D. Lines DB and CB are then drawn as shown in B. B, Operative design. The initial step involves the patient's being in an upright sitting position. The periareolar circle is completed (4 cm in diameter). The dermoglandular flap is outlined (DD′ = 6 cm). The shaded area is then de-epithelialized, and the skin is incised to the glandular plane from D′ to B and C to B. The gland is now separated from the prepectoral plane and the axillary extension from the skin. C, The glandular resection technique is shown of the left breast. The nipple coning flap is maintained at 1 to 2 cm thickness. The gland is resected, and a layer of constant thickness attached to the dermis and skin is left. The dermoglandular flap (A to A′, C) is freed, leaving a glandular layer that is easily adaptable and particularly useful in marked breast asymmetries. This flap as shown is rotated under the lateral aspect of the gland. The flap is oriented in a vertical direction and is fixed under the upper pole of the breast, slightly outward. This technique will achieve satisfactory projection of the areola, as shown in the postoperative results. D, Construction of the left side of the breast. The areola is closed with 8 U-type sutures. The flap is rotated superiorly and fixed by its two ends to the pectoralis muscle behind the level of the areola. Note the position of the flap (C). The closure of the inframammary incision is carried out with the resection of the dog-ear in the inframammary fold. Intradermal sutures are used to approximate the skin edges.

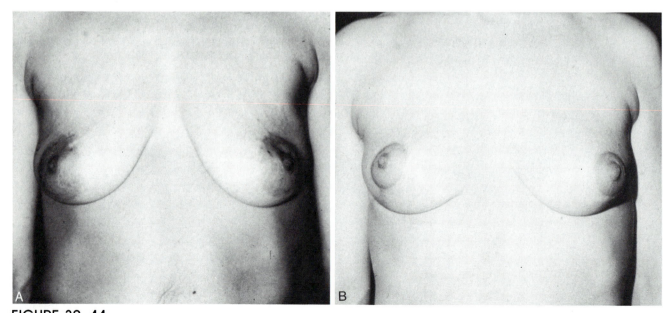

FIGURE 32–11

A, Moderate ptosis. Preoperative view. B, The same patient 1 year after operation. Note the good projection of the nipple.

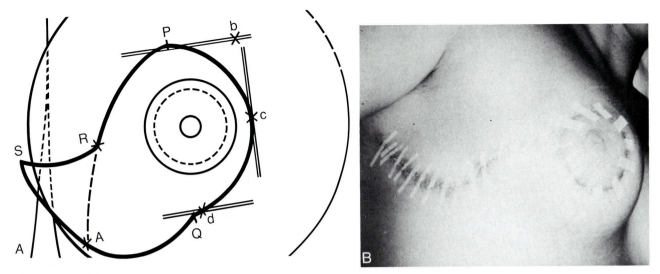

FIGURE 32–12

A, Marked hypertrophy. Preoperative markings and drawings of the isosceles triangle of additional skin resection. *B,* The scar after removal of the sutures on the fifth day.

DISCUSSION

After more than 25 years of experience with this technique, we believe that the lateral technique gives excellent results, particularly in moderate hypertrophy and ptosis; but we will be much more reserved when the indications call for another technique.

Moderate Hypertrophy

For mammary reduction of less than 300 gm with good adhesions between skin and gland, shaping of the breast with the lateral technique is easy and results in a short lateral scar. One of the main advantages of the lateral technique is also avoiding any circular incision around the areola in cases of small hypertrophy. In this situation, we propose that the tapered resection go as far as the top of the nipple with a V excision of the areola itself, which is often enlarged. Such a modification of the same technique can be used in cases of asymmetry. The smaller breast is reduced without a circular scar around the areola, even if the larger side has a periareolar incision and resultant scar (Fig. 32–10).

Moderate Ptosis

The lateral approach allows a very satisfactory correction of moderate ptosis. The wedge resection can easily reduce the skin brassiere. The dermoglandular flap inserted at the upper part of the breast restores a satisfactory contour (see Figs. 32–10 and 32–11; Figs. 32–12 to 32–14).

Two precautions must be pointed out for the beginner learning to utilize this technique. Too high and medial a position of the nipple is a sequela very difficult to correct. The residual volume presents sometimes an excess of glandular tissue in the medial portion.

Optional Indications

It is very satisfactory having the medial and lower aspect of the breast free of scars. We have, however, encountered many difficulties in patients with large hypertrophies and ptosis because there is a problem of shaping the breast with a tendency to external flattening when the cutaneous resection is too long. The external portion is then more conspicuous; and if it extends beyond the area of the brassiere, the advantage of the single lateral scar is lost.

At Saint Louis Hospital we routinely use a technique that we started in 1981. This is a modified version of lateral reduction mammaplasty, including two new concepts. The first concept concerns glandular resection according to Lalardrie's dermal vault method (1974), which is described in his book. The other concept comes from the ideas of J. Baruch (personal communication) on skin resection and regular use of a dermoglandular suspension flap. These two concepts are self-explanatory in the following diagrams illustrating the preoperative markings (Fig. 32–15).

The glandular resection is performed after keeping a residual portion of the gland, including its cutaneous dermis cover. This maneuver allows a glandular resection giving the desired "residual glandular volume" (Lalardrie).

The skin resection, according to Baruch, is more medial than in the initial lateral technique and has the shape of a spindle (Fig. 32–15A, B, C, E, and F). The main difference is the adaptation of the skin flaps at the lower portion to follow the inframammary fold (Fig. 32–15D). The dermoglandular flap appears similar to the one previously discussed for ptosis correction (see Fig. 32–9).

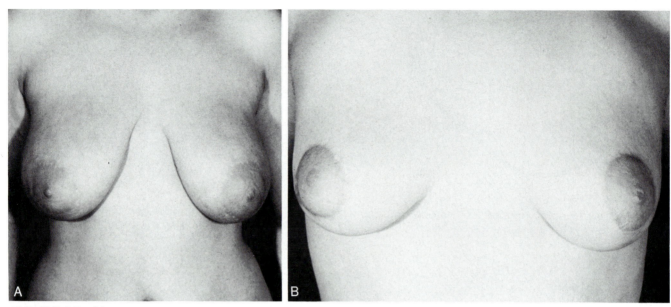

FIGURE 32–13
A, Moderate hypertrophy with good indication for the lateral method. *B,* The patient 1 year later.

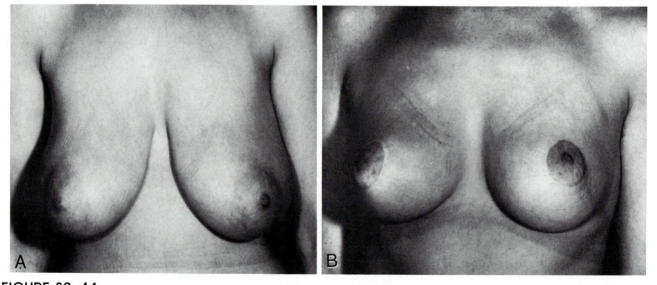

FIGURE 32–14
A, Hypertrophy and ptosis with optional indication for the lateral method. *B,* Postoperative view. Note the slight flattening of the external position of the breast, together with an excess of tissue in the medial part.

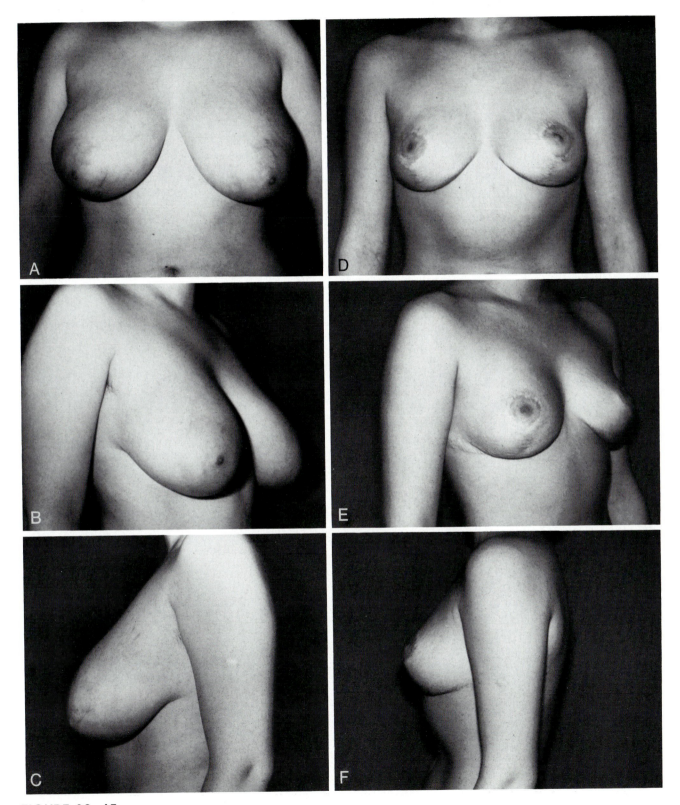

FIGURE 32–15

A to *F,* The Saint Louis technique is shown preoperatively and 18 years following resection of 60 gm. Front and side views.

This technique used in the plastic surgery unit of Saint Louis Hospital has, like any other technique, certain disadvantages and limitations.

Advantages

The advantages of the technique are as follows:

1. It provides good vascular safety (with no necrosis, even in inexperienced hands).
2. It has good training value.
3. It is well adapted to any kind of hypertrophy.
4. The result is pleasant shape and symmetry, which is often difficult to obtain in our practice because French women usually desire little residual volume.

Disadvantages

This technique is not as well adapted in cases of isolated ptosis and major ptosis where we have to modify the drawing and to leave space available around the periareolar incision.

Limitations

The relative inconvenience of the length of the inframammary scar may be a problem. This external scar is always more conspicuous; and if it is too long, it extends outside the lateral scar to the brassiere.

CONCLUSIONS

We have tried to point out the main advantages of the lateral technique, including its simplicity, safety, and single scar in cases of moderate hypertrophy and ptosis. In other cases we think that the disadvantages are too obvious to propose it to untrained surgeons. The Saint Louis procedure (Bricout et al., 1988) is a good alternative for large breast hypertrophies (see Fig. 32–15).

References

Arié, G.: Una nueva técnica de mastoplastia. Rev. Latinoam. Cir. Plast. 3:28, 1957.

Bricout, N., Groslières, D., Servant, J. M., Banzet, P.: Plastie mammaire—La technique utilisée à Saint Louis. Ann. Chir. Plast. Esthet. 33:7, 1988.

Courtiss, E. H., Goldwyn, R. M.: Reduction mammaplasty by the inferior pedicle technique. Plast. Reconstr. Surg. 59:500, 1977.

Dufourmentel, C., Mouly, R.: Plastie mammaire par la méthode oblique. Ann. Chir. Plast. 6:45, 1961.

Dufourmentel, C., Mouly, R.: Développements récents de la plastie mammaire par la méthode oblique latérale. Ann. Chir. Plast. 10:227, 1965.

Dufourmentel, C., Mouly, R.: Mammaplasty by the lateral method: Reconstructive surgery of thermal injuries and other subjects. Excerpta Medica International Congress, Series No. 141, 1966, p. 131.

Dufourmentel, C., Mouly, R.: Modifications of "periwinkle shell operation" for small ptotic breasts. Plast. Reconstr. Surg. 41:523, 1968.

Elbaz, J. S.: Traitement des hypertrophies mammaires avec ou sans ptose par la méthode dite "oblique externe." Thesis, Paris, 1963.

Elbaz, J. S., Verheecke, G.: La cicatrice en L dans les plasties mammaries. Ann. Chir. Plast. 17:282, 1972.

Fonseca-Ely, J.: Reduction mammaplasty—An eclectic approach. Aesth. Plast. Surg. 2:95, 1978.

Georgiade, N. G., Serafin, D., Riefkohl, R., Georgiade, G. S.: Is there a reduction mammaplasty for "all seasons"? Plast. Reconstr. Surg. 63:765, 1979.

Gillies, H., Marins, H.: L'Operation en colimacon ou rotation spirale dans les ptoses mammaires isolées. Ann. Chir. Plast. 3:87, 1958.

Lalardrie, J. P., Jouglard, J. P.: *Chirurgie Plastique du Sein.* Vol. 1. Paris, Masson, 1974, p. 156.

Lalardrie, J. P. Mouly, R.: History of mammaplasty. Aesthetic Plast. Surg. 2:167, 1978.

Marc, H.: *La Plastie Mammaire par la Méthode Oblique.* Vol. 1. Paris, G. Doin, 1952.

Mouly, R., Dufourmentel, C: Mammaplasty by the lateral method. *Transactions of the Fifth International Congress of Plastic and Reconstructive Surgery.* Melbourne, Butterworth, 1971.

Penn, J.: Breast reduction. Br. J. Plast Surg. 7:357, 1955.

Pitanguy, I.: Surgical correction of breast hypertrophy. Br. J. Plast. Surg. 20:78, 1967.

Ragnell, A.: Operative correction of hypertrophy and ptosis of the female breast. Acta Chir. Scand. 94:Suppl. 113, 1946.

Schatten, W. E., Hartley, J. H., Jr., Hamm, W. G., et al.: Reduction mammaplasty by the Dufourmentel-Mouly method. Plast. Reconstr. Surg. 48:306, 1971.

Skoog, T.: A technique of breast reduction: Transposition of the nipple on a cutaneous vascular pedicle. Acta Chir. Scand. 126:453, 1963.

Strömbeck, J. O.: Mammaplasty: Report of a new technique based on two pedicle procedure. Br. J. Plast. Surg. 13:79, 1960.

Vandenbussche, F., Vandervoord, J., Robbe, M., Decoopman, B.: Plasties mammaire de réduction. Aleas et malfaçons des techniques à cicatrice en T renversé. Ann. Chir. Plast. 24:319, 1979.

33

Trudy Vogt

Reduction Mammaplasty: The Vogt Technique

Today, when so many good techniques are available for this functionally and aesthetically important operation, it is easier to remember another new technique associated with the author's name, rather than struggling to recall the unipedicle technique, the bipedicle technique (Georgiade, 1976), and several permutations and combinations derived from them. This is a technique basically designed by a woman plastic surgeon for her female patients, incorporating her female preferences and aesthetic views. This technique is not a replacement of any procedure, but another addition to various wonderful procedures presently in existence that work well for many surgeons with experience and expertise.

GOALS

Our basic goals in performing this operation are (1) to relieve the physical and psychologic symptoms of hypertrophic breasts and (2) to recreate aesthetically pleasing, symptom-free, smaller, and newer breasts that are as close to normal as possible.

It is easy to achieve the first goal by simple amputation of the breast. The experience has also taught most of us how to estimate the amount of excision necessary to give proper relief from the symptoms of breast hypertrophy. It is the second goal that is difficult to achieve and the more important part of this operation, and it also dictates the modifications of simple amputation of the breast (Arié, 1957).

The following are specific criteria for aesthetically pleasing and normal-appearing breasts: (1) a rounded, conical shape; (2) nipple sensitivity and projection; (3) ptosis correction and nipple elevation; and if possible, (4) preservation of lactating function, especially in younger patients.

ANATOMIC BACKGROUND

It has been well demonstrated and proven beyond doubt that the breast derives its most important blood supply via the lateral pectoral artery and the perforating branches of the internal mammary artery medially (Hinderer, 1976; McKissock, 1972). The blood supply from the perforating branches of intercostal arteries through the pectoral muscle is insignificant and can be easily sacrificed without loss of breast tissue, as done in augmentation mammaplasty (Hinderer, 1976). The most important nerve supply is derived through the cutaneous branches of the second to fifth intercostal nerves, which also supply the skin surrounding the areola-nipple complex (McKissock, 1972; Schwarzmann, 1930). As long as the surrounding areolar skin is preserved in full thickness or as a dermal pedicle, the nipple sensation in the new location is not lost. The nipple-areola complex, after all, is an important part of the breast, from an aesthetic as well as functional point of view; above all, it is a secondary sex organ with psychologic and erotic value (Bames, 1948).

HISTORICAL BACKGROUND

Almost all of the procedures known today undertake the technique of breast reduction trying to preserve the blood supply from the medial and lateral aspect of the gland by converting the entire gland into a unipedicle or bipedicle mass (Cramer, 1976; McKissock, 1972; Pitanguy, 1960; Skoog, 1963; Strömbeck, 1960; Vinas, 1976; Weiner et al., 1973) and then moving the areola-nipple complex to its new location by transferring it either on a dermal pedicle or as a free nipple graft (Pitanguy, 1960). Finally, all of the techniques depend on the recreated skin brassiere to hold the reduced breast in its new form and shape forever. A fact is overlooked by many, that the skin covering a hypertrophic breast is already in an overstretched condition and has lost its normal elasticity under the constant stress of holding the excess weight of the hypertrophied gland. Cooper's ligaments, which are to some extent responsible for maintaining the shape of a normal breast in its aesthetically pleasing, rounded form, are overstretched, weakened, and sometimes totally destroyed in a hypertrophied breast under the constant stress of holding the excessive weight of hypertrophic breast tissue; these ligaments are further destroyed by surgical maneuvers and excision. One cannot, therefore, depend totally on the newly formed skin brassiere to hold and maintain the shape of the newly reconstructed breast for a long time. It is this underlying pathophysiology of the hypertrophic breast that led us to search for a different mechanism for maintaining the glandular shape permanently without depending too much on the skin brassiere. Thus the idea of a glandular prosthesis with a glandular-skin brassiere evolved. The remaining breast tissue, after resection and proper reduction, is split into two glandular flaps, one of which is fixed permanently to the chest wall, over which is draped the remaining skin-glandular flap as a covering brassiere. This technique has led to the permanency of results in our cases and has prevented widening of scars and recurrence of ptosis due to strong dermis-to-dermis and intraglandular scarring over a large interface. The permanently fixed glandular prosthesis gives a good, rounded, and conical shape to the newly formed breast because there is more fullness in the upper quadrants and better distribution of the breast tissue in all quadrants as compared with the emptiness seen at the upper pole and square contours observed in some other techniques (Goldwyn, 1976; Rees and Flagg, 1972).

TECHNIQUE

Preoperative Markings

These are very simple and easy to remember. A midmammary line is marked on either side as a line starting from a point 2 cm lateral to the suprasternal notch, through the nipple and extending to the inframammary fold (Fig. 33–1). Transposition of the nipple-areola complex will be done along this line. The new nipple site is located by placing the thumb on the inframammary fold and, while pushing it superiorly, palpating the new location with the index finger placed on the front of the breast along the midmammary line (Cramer and Chong, 1976). This point is marked O and represents the new nipple site on the midmammary line (Fig. 33–2). The nipple site on the opposite breast is located similarly, and both points ae matched as equidistant measurements from the suprasternal notch. An

individually modified Strömbeck pattern (Goldwyn, 1976) is used to mark the area of de-epithelialization, using O as the center of the keyhole (Fig. 33–3). The limbs of the keyhole pattern are then extended on either side beyond the inferior margin of the areola for the required estimated amount of excision. Care is taken to keep the limbs of equal length and symmetric in relation to the areola (Fig. 33–3). A curved line is then drawn joining the inferior ends of the limbs of the keyhole below the areola. A circle 4 cm in diameter is drawn around the nipple with the nipple as the center. This completes the markings, which are always done with the patient in an erect standing or sitting position (Fig. 33–4). It will be observed that the markings for the flaps are not predetermined, and there is ample leeway left for the final adjustment of these flaps toward the end of the operation so that they are of proper form and shape, without undue tension.

Surgical Technique

Actual surgery is begun by de-epithelializing the area within the keyhole. This is started from the 4-cm circle around the areola, which is left attached to the breast tissue. The rest of it is de-epithelialized with meticulous use of the blade of a knife (Schwarzmann, 1930; Strömbeck, 1960). This maneuver is facilitated by making the breast taut, either with a tourniquet or with the help of an assistant (Fig. 33–5). Good de-epithelialization is important from the point of view of maintaining good blood and nerve supply to the dermal pedicle, which in return preserves the same for the transposed nipple (Hinderer, 1976; Strömbeck, 1960). The first deep knife cut is made at the inferior border to the de-epithelialization, cutting all the way through the skin and the breast tissue up to the prepectoral fascia (Fig. 33–6A). Here, using blunt finger dissection as in augmentation, the entire upper breast tissue is undermined along the

Text continued on page 411

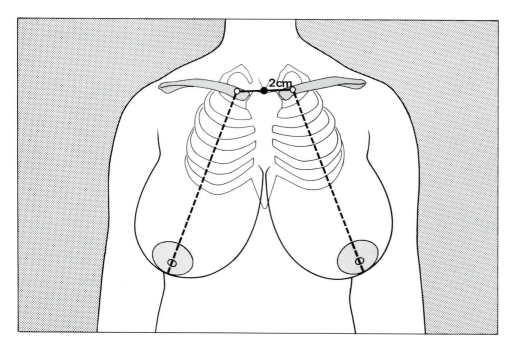

FIGURE 33–1
Midmammary line is drawn 2 cm from the suprasternal notch to the nipple and extended to the inframammary line.

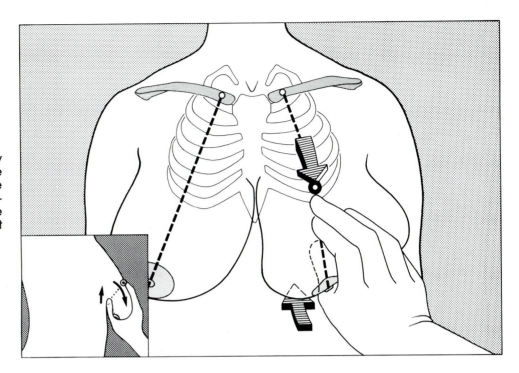

FIGURE 33–2
New nipple site located by placing the thumb on the inframammary line and the index finger on the midmammary line in front of the breast and palpating it through the breast tissue.

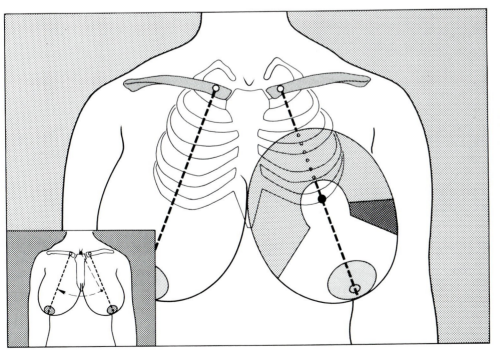

FIGURE 33–3
With the new nipple site located exactly in the center of the keyhole of the modified Strömbeck pattern, the area of de-epithelialization is marked out. Each limb of the keyhole is extended for at least 2 cm beyond the lower border of the areola.

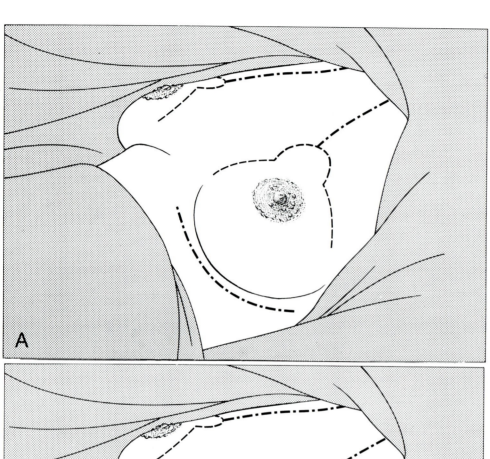

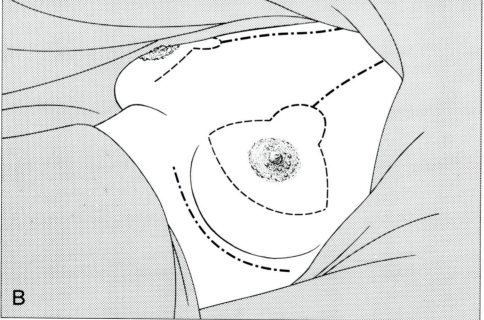

FIGURE 33–4
A and *B,* The markings are completed.

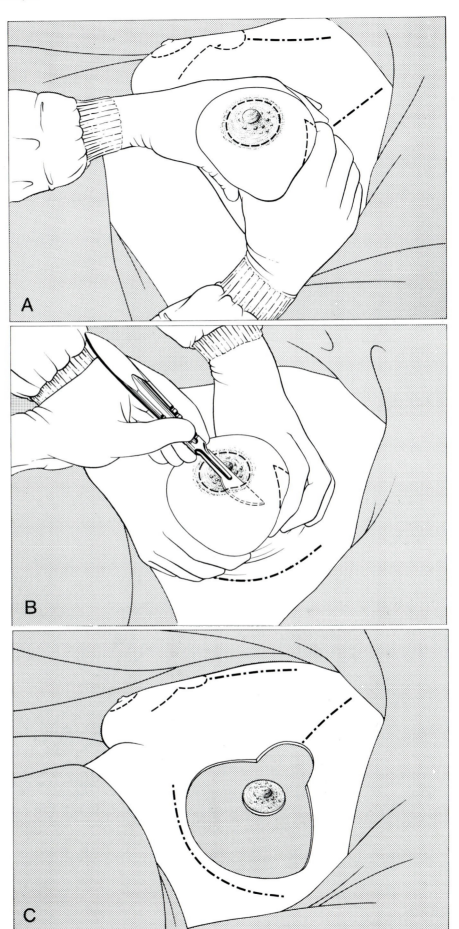

FIGURE 33–5

A, De-epithelialization technique. The assistant makes the breast taut. *B,* De-epithelialization is begun around the areola circle, 4 cm in diameter, which is left attached to the breast tissue. *C,* De-epithelialization is complete on the left side.

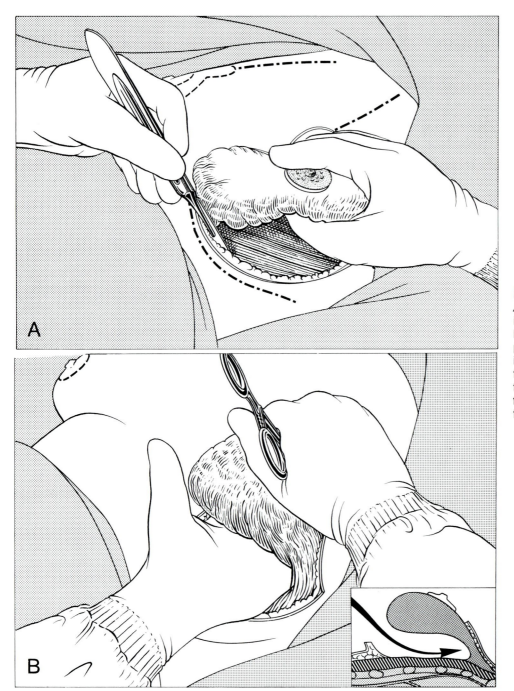

FIGURE 33–6
A, First deep cut made at the inferior margin of de-epithe-lialization all the way to the pectoral fascia. *B,* Undermin-ing of the breast tissue along the prepectoral fascia up to the second rib, done with the fingers. The level of dissec-tion is shown in the inset.

pectoral fascia all the way to the first intercostal space, care being taken not to disturb the medial and lateral blood supply (Fig. 33–6B). The breast at this point is divided into upper and lower portions, and the upper portion is undermined. When the amount to be resected is large, the lower portion is proportionately large. One then slices the upper breast tissue into two flaps with a coronal incision started at the lower end, cutting parallel to the nipple-areola complex, confining it to the width of the pattern, and extending the incision superiorly up to the superior areola border but not beyond it. The superficial flap with the nipple-areola complex is 2 to 3 cm thick (Fig. 33–7). Depending upon the amount to be further resected, the lower flap is sliced again into two slices. The lowermost flap is excised and discarded as a keel excision of Pitanguy (1960); this flap can be of variable thickness, depending upon the amount to be resected (Fig. 33–7).

This excision takes a keen eye and good judgment on the part of the surgeon in any type of procedure and can be expected only after a good amount of experience. It also requires a sense of sculpture on the part of the plastic surgeon.

The middle flap now becomes the lower flap, which is then rolled on itself and pushed upward into the submammary pocket. This forms the future glandular prosthesis over which a superficial flap of remaining breast tissue is draped, forming the skin-glandular brassiere. This maneuver gives one a rough idea as to whether more breast tissue needs to be resected from the lower flap. Adequate hemostasis is maintained throughout the procedure with electrocoagulation. At this juncture, the areola-nipple complex is transposed to its new location with three interrupted sutures of 4-0 Prolene (Fig. 33–8). One then passes a 3-0 Prolene suture through the middle of the inferior portion of the lower flap, taking a good "bite."

The flap is then rolled on itself in the submammary pocket; and the suture is fixed to the periosteum, the fascia, and the overlying muscles of the second rib. This is the future glandular breast prosthesis (Fig. 33–9). If necessary, two more sutures are placed, one on either side of the first one, to fix this breast flap firmly and securely to the chest wall in its desired position. This also prevents its future migration downward through the action of gravity.

The rest of the operation is quite simple. The areola circle is completed by placing the fourth suture below the areola. The lower border of this flap is then grasped in a clamp; with slight traction on it, a distance of 4.5 cm is measured along the vertical legs of the keyhole pattern. A 3-0 interrupted Prolene suture is placed at this point, marking the location of the inframammary line (Fig. 33–10). The upper and lower margins of the inframammary incision are then grasped in a towel clamp from the 4.5-cm mark on the upper border, which makes the medial and lateral dog-ears quite apparent. This is usually done in such a way that the medial dog-ear is shorter than the lateral one (Fig. 33–11A). Both of the dog-ears are next marked out and carefully excised with the remaining lower breast tissue (Fig. 33–11B). The wound edges are then carefully defatted for adequate coaptation, hemostasis is once again achieved with electrocoagulation, and a drain is placed inferiorly and brought out through the lateral end of the inframammary incision (Fig. 33–12). The areola is then sutured with 4-0 subcuticular suture. Both breasts are operated on and sculptured simultaneously so that a careful comparison for proper symmetry, size, and shape can be done from the lower end of the operating table before final closure at this time. The inframammary incision is closed with interrupted 4-0 Dexon sutures, and the skin is finally closed with subcuticular 3-0 Prolene sutures. Final closure is done quite meticulously

Text continued on page 417

FIGURE 33–7
Gland divided into two slices up to the inferior margin of the new areola site. The inferior flap may be further divided into two slices (inset), the inferior one being excised and discarded.

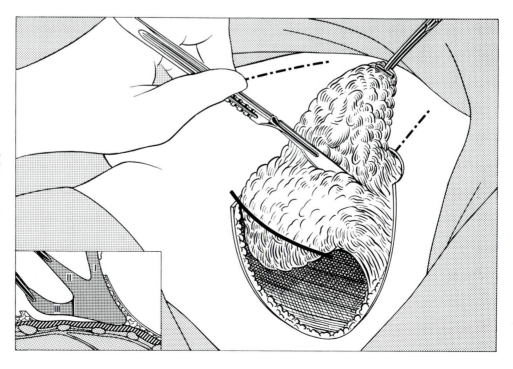

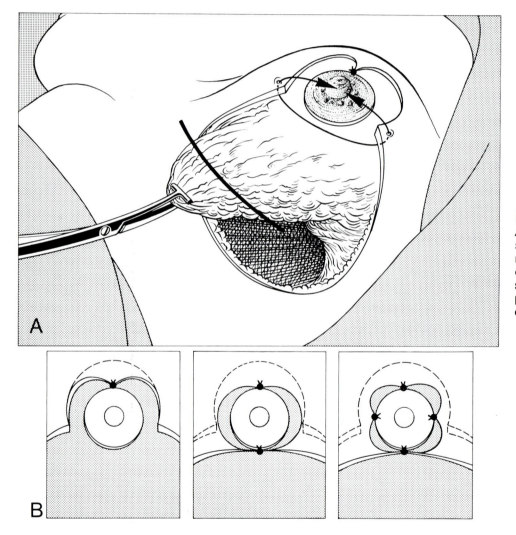

FIGURE 33–8
A and *B,* A 3-0 polypropylene suture is passed through the middle of the inferior border of the flaps, which is then sutured to the muscles and periosteum of the second and third ribs.

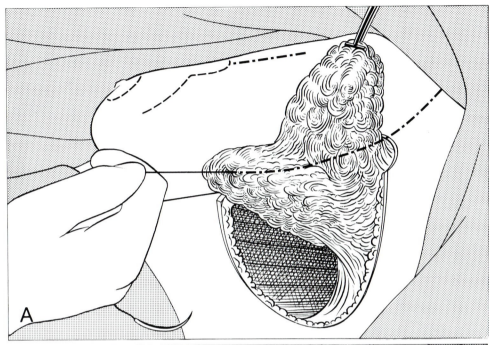

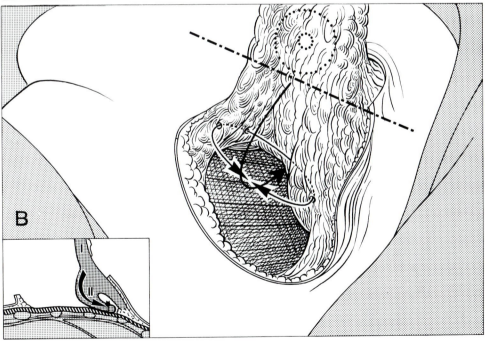

FIGURE 33–9
A and *B*, The areola is transposed in its new keyhole site with three interrupted sutures of 4-0 Prolene. *Inset*, Transposition of the flap to the new position.

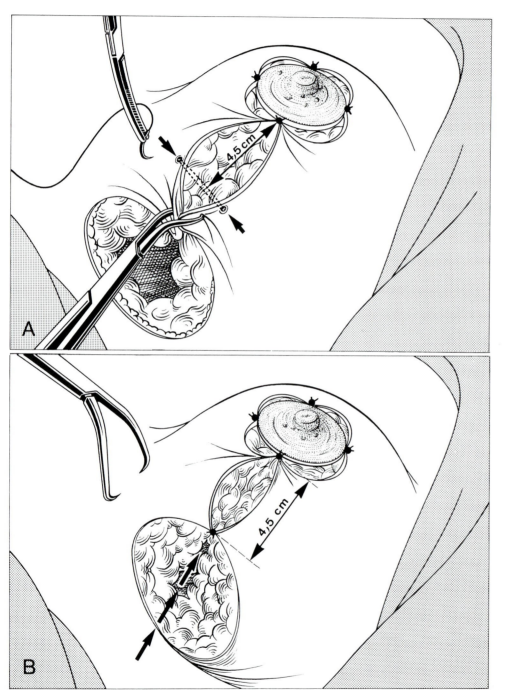

FIGURE 33–10
A, Taking the lower ends of the vertical legs of the keyhole and placing them on slight traction, a point 4.5 cm from the lower border of the areola is measured that marks the new inframammary line location. This may be done with a towel clip or a clamp. *B,* A 3-0 Prolene stitch is placed at this point.

FIGURE 33–11
A, Two sides of the inframammary incision are grasped in the towel clip at the new inframammary point, making the medial and lateral dogears, which are marked out, apparent. *B,* Excision of the dog-ears.

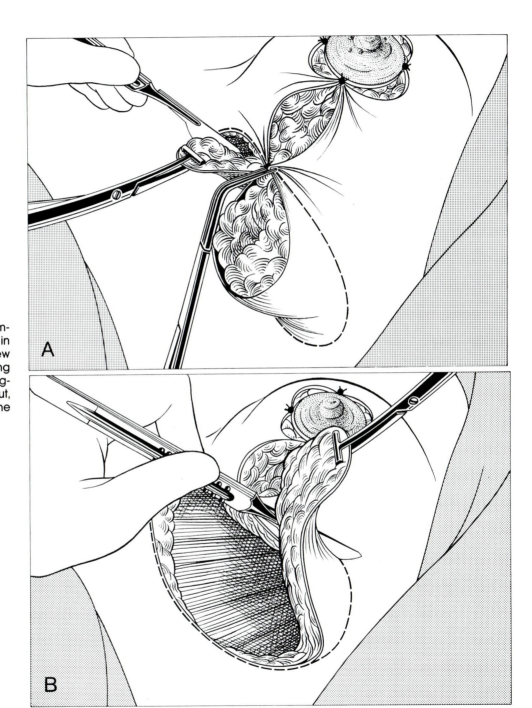

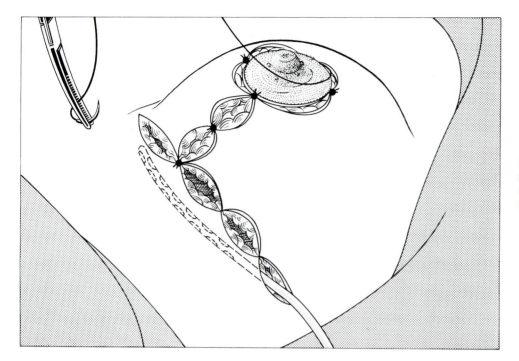

FIGURE 33–12
Suturing of the inframam-
mary incision with the drain
in place.

FIGURE 33–13
The final closure with intracuticular suturing is reinforced with Steri-Strips.

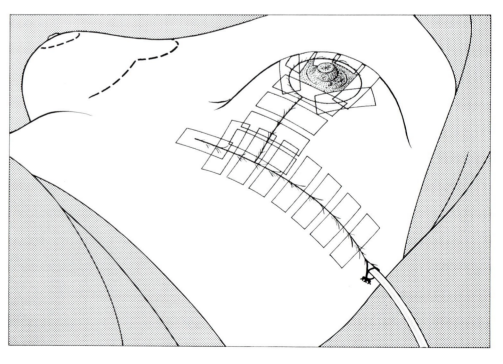

and further reinforced with 0.5-inch-wide Steri-Strips (Fig. 33–13).

Individual drains are connected to separate Hemovacs. A supportive dressing is then applied, creating a good brassiere with crossed strips of microfoam, leaving the nipple-areola complex exposed so that it can be observed in the postoperative period without disturbing the main dressing.

POSTOPERATIVE CARE

The drain is usually removed after 48 to 72 hours, depending upon the drainage, without disturbing the original dressing. The first dressing is changed on the fifth postoperative day and is replaced immediately with a similar dressing. This supportive dressing is continued up to 3 weeks. It is changed on every fifth day or sometimes twice a week, depending upon the circumstances. All sutures, including Steri-Strips, are removed at the end of 3 weeks, and the incision lines are reinforced with fresh Steri-Strips. At this point, the patient is placed in a tight, well-fitting bra, which she must wear day and night for the next 3 months or more. It is our belief that with this type of extensive surgery, good postoperative care with a strict regimen is mandatory in order to achieve a good and long-lasting result. During the follow-up period the incisions are always carefully checked at each dressing change. The patient is to avoid strenuous use of the arms involving pectoralis major activity and is restrained from participating in such sports as horseback riding, swimming, tennis, jogging, and so forth, for a period of 3 to 6 months following surgery. This restriction on activity is important in preventing hemorrhage and wound dehiscence and also contributes to good intraglandular and dermis-to-dermis scar formation around the breast tissue, holding it in its desired place and form for a long period of time. During the period of supportive wound dressing, the patient is not permitted to have a total body bath, thus maintaining the wound dressings dry. Most patients receive a transfusion of 1 or 2 units of blood intraoperatively, which, we believe, shortens convalescence and further improves healing in the postoperative period.

PITFALLS AND HOW TO AVOID THEM

As in any reduction mammaplasty technique, there exist certain pitfalls to which a young surgeon with limited experience can be a victim. This section is especially devoted to those who wish to try this technique for the first time. Following are the few important pitfalls of reduction mammaplasty, even with immediate good postoperative results, inherent to any technique:

1. Flattening in the upper quadrants due to the lack of breast tissue
2. Nipple pointing in upward direction
3. Square contour of the lower border of the breast
4. Unaesthetic, widespread postoperative scars

These complications are really the result of the basic pathologic condition of hypertrophied, heavy breasts, namely, the overstretched skin covering of the presurgical breast with loss of normal elastic tissue and supporting structures such as Cooper's ligaments and interlobular fibrous septa. Moreover, it has been our observation that most hypertrophied breasts also have an overabundance of adipose tissue, which interferes with proper surgical maneuvering of the breast tissue and with proper healing of the scars, both internal and external. With this etiologic background, when one starts firmly packing fat-laden postreduction breast tissue without any support, it continues to exert its weakening effect on the inferior breast skin, where most of the postoperative scars are placed and which also bears the brunt of the gravitational pull. It is therefore easy to understand why there is widening of well-stitched scar lines postoperatively. With lack of internal support, it is also impossible to prevent postoperative gravitation of the breast mass inferiorly behind the correctly located nipple-areola complex, which slowly begins to point upward. Already thinned-out inferior skin continues to stretch further, and soon this portion of the breast assumes a squared, instead of a rounded, appearance. These factors can lead to the previously mentioned pitfalls that are inherent to all techniques and are well counteracted by the Vogt technique in creating the "glandular prosthesis" flap, which is rotated upward and fixed to the chest wall and thus rolls the lower breast tissue toward the upper midline of the breast.

PITFALLS INHERENT TO OUR TECHNIQUE AND HOW TO AVOID THEM

Flaps That Cannot Be Easily Maneuvered for Rotation and Plication

If the flap that forms the glandular prosthesis is too thick, it cannot be easily rotated without undue tension on the flap, which, in turn, can interfere with its vascular supply. Fixation of this flap is also difficult if the fixation sutures should cut through it. Plication of the areola-bearing flap upward can also be problematic.

It has been observed that breast heavily laden with adipose tissue that one encounters in a hypertrophied breast is difficult to maneuver surgically, as in plication and upward rotation, and also that the fat interferes with proper scar formation and healing because of its poor vascularization. To avoid this, most patients in our clinic are first subjected to a weight reduction program prior to surgery, which helps in the reduction of breast adipose tissue along with fat in the rest of the body. These patients are thus rendered better surgical candidates for reduction mammaplasty. In order to facilitate the maneuverability of the glandular prosthetic flap, it must be made thin enough for its upward rotation but also thick enough to maintain its vascular supply. Then this flap must also be split along its side so that it can be exactly rolled up without tension.

Asymmetry in the Glandular Prosthetic Flap

On comparing the lateral and medial sides of the glandular prosthetic flap, one may find asymmetry between the two margins of the lower part of the flap. This asymmetry can be corrected by undertaking the keel resection from underneath the flap on the affected side only, as mentioned in the text previously. The lateral splitting should not be continued beyond the fifth costal cartilage, so that adequate blood supply to the nipple-areola complex is preserved.

Breast Flaps—Tension

Cutting-through of the fixation suture at the inferior margin of the lower flap is due to the excess of fatty tissue in the flap and a lack of elasticity. The problem has already been solved when the patient has been put on a weight reduction program preoperatively and most of this fat has withered away under the therapy. One can also place two or three such sutures with fairly large "bites" at the inferior margin of the lower flap in order to include some breast tissue along with fibroelastic tissue. More than one stitch ensures its permanence. The decision has to be made during the operation. Fixation sutures must be of the strong, nonabsorbable material, such as nylon, Mersilene, or Prolene. It has been our observation that it takes about 6 months for internal glandular and dermis-to-dermis fixation through scarring to become firm and strong and able to hold the breast tissue in its new shape and form permanently. If an absorbable suture like Vicryl, Dexon, or catgut is used, one may find that the gland no longer holds its immediate postoperative form and shape because of early, premature absorption of the fixation sutures. If this happens, one has simply to reopen and fix the glandular prosthesis flap to the second or third rib periosteum with strong, permanent, nonabsorbable sutures.

Widening of the Scars

The most common and serious objection to reduction mammaplasty is the obvious side scars following certain techniques.

Many techniques have evolved in reduction mammaplasty simply to avoid this complication, placing incisions in different locations and trying to conceal the scars, thus making them less obvious. It has been our observation that some patients are scar-formers, who cannot really be helped by any single technique or precaution. However, in most of our patients the following steps have been considerably useful in preventing formation of widespread scars.

Weight Reduction

It has already been mentioned that most of our patients undergo a weight reduction program before this

procedure that helps in reduction of fatty tissue from the breast. The presence of excess adipose tissue either in the glandular prosthesis flap or along the skin edges lining the incisions prevents formation of satisfactory and strong scars to hold the postoperative form of the breast tissue permanently; the loss of the excess fatty tissue provides good subcutaneous and cutaneous healing without dehiscence.

Defatting of the Skin Edges

The healing is much better and the scar is narrower if the skin edges along the inferior suture line are defatted before the final closure. This is the area that carries most of the weight of the breast tissue and also has the most tension, which is constantly aggravated by gravity. Interposed fatty tissue prevents good scar formation and, if excised prior to skin closure, will allow a good scar formation with reduced tendency toward scar-widening and dehiscence.

The following are also useful in strong and narrow scar formation:

1. Use of subcuticular skin closure using suture material, such as 3-0 Prolene, left in for 3 weeks
2. Deep and subcutaneous closure of the wound in layers, using absorbable material such as Dexon or Vicryl
3. Reinforcement of the wound edges with Steri-Strips immediately following surgery and up to 12 weeks postoperatively
4. Prophylactic prevention of severe physical activities, especially those involving strenuous use of pectoral muscles, such as tennis, swimming, golfing, and jogging

The Formation of "Peri-stitch Granuloma"

In some cases of reduction mammaplasty using the Vogt technique, a small granuloma formation around the permanent fixation stitch might be observed at the level of the second or third rib, along the midmammary line. One should make the patient aware of the presence of a permanent stitch and its location so that accidental opening of the breast tissue for biopsy purposes by other surgeons—not aware of the underlying pathologic condition—might easily be avoided.

In conclusion, a good surgical result can only be achieved with a well-planned and well-executed technique under a strict and uniform discipline. Experience on the part of the surgeon is important, but knowing and avoiding the possible pitfalls before embarking on an operation are most useful and beneficial adjuncts to this difficult task.

COMPLICATIONS

It will be no exaggeration to mention that there have been only two cases of major postoperative complications with a unilateral partial loss of areola-nipple complex and some fat necrosis underneath. This was in a series of 300 consecutive reduction mammaplasties performed in 600 breasts with this technique over a period of 11 years. The nipple projection and nipple sensation were uniformly good.

SUMMARY

The Vogt technique for reduction mammaplasty has been presented with details of the operative technique. In this procedure, the remaining gland after reduction is split coronally into two slices. The inferior flap is then

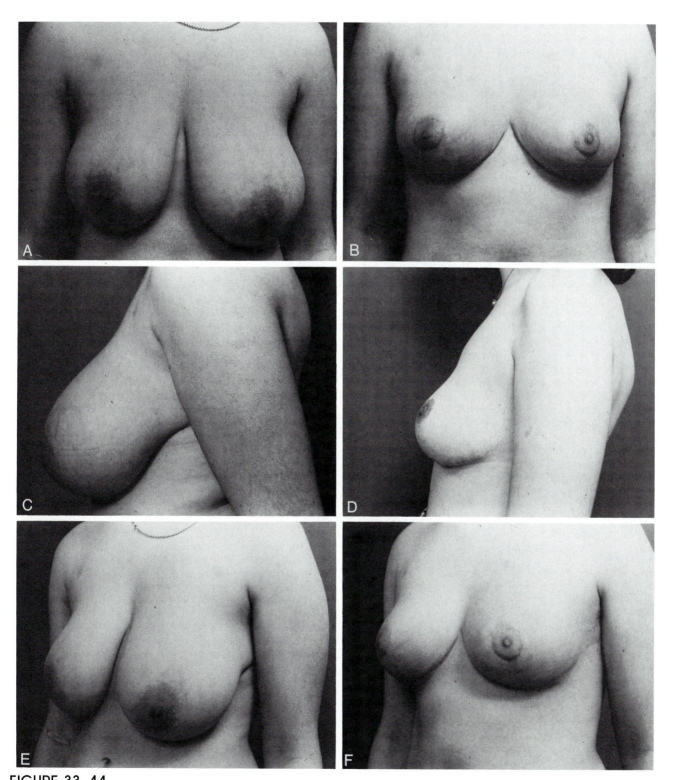

FIGURE 33–14

A, Front preoperative view. *B,* Front postoperative view, 2 years after surgery. *C,* Left lateral preoperative view. *D,* Left lateral postoperative view, 2 years after surgery. *E,* Left oblique preoperative view. *F,* Left oblique postoperative view, 2 years after surgery.

rolled and permanently fixed to the chest wall with nonabsorbable sutures as a glandular breast prosthesis. The superficial glandular flap, with skin, is then draped over the fixed glandular prosthesis, which gives the breast a natural-looking form and shape that lasts over a long period. The operation fulfills the basic criteria stipulated for this operation. A long follow-up has proven that there has been no recurrence of ptosis since we started fixation of the glandular breast prosthesis to the chest wall, and no reoperations were necessary to correct any recurrent deformities (Figs. 33–14 to 33–18).

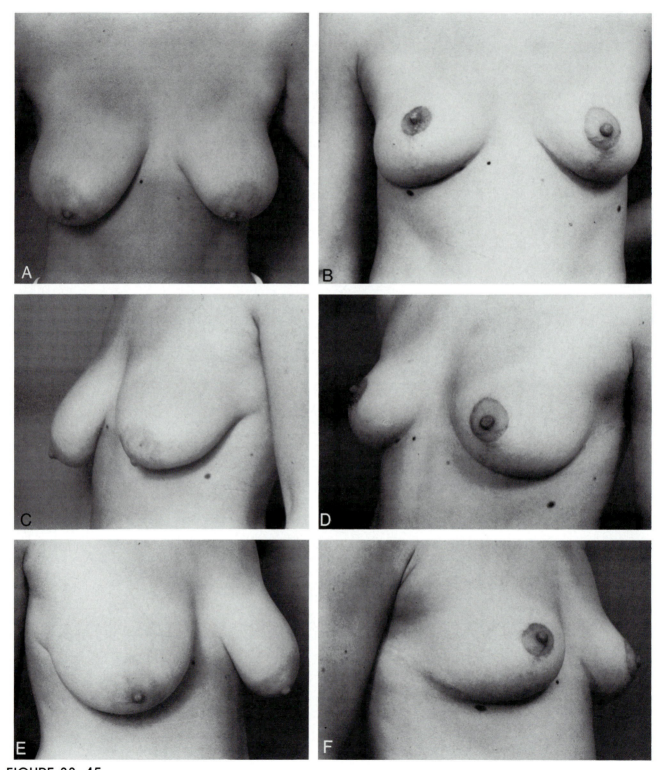

FIGURE 33–15

A, Front preoperative view. *B,* Front postoperative view, 2 years after surgery. *C,* Left oblique preoperative view. *D,* Left oblique postoperative view, 2 years after surgery. *E,* Right oblique preoperative view. *F,* Right oblique postoperative view, 2 years after surgery.

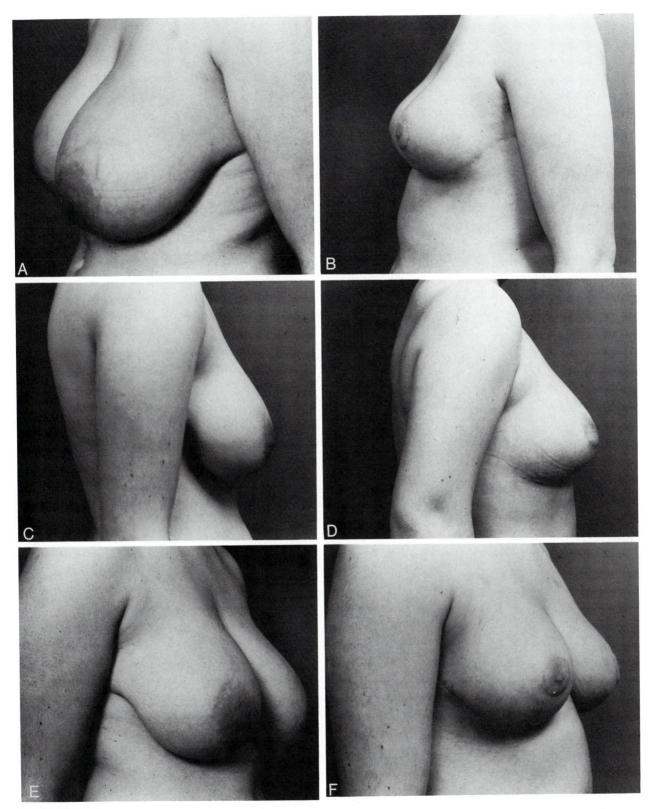

FIGURE 33–16

A, Left lateral preoperative view. *B,* Left lateral postoperative view, 2 years after surgery. *C,* Right lateral preoperative view. *D,* Right lateral postoperative view, 2 years after surgery. *E,* Right oblique preoperative view. *F,* Right oblique postoperative view, 2 years after surgery.

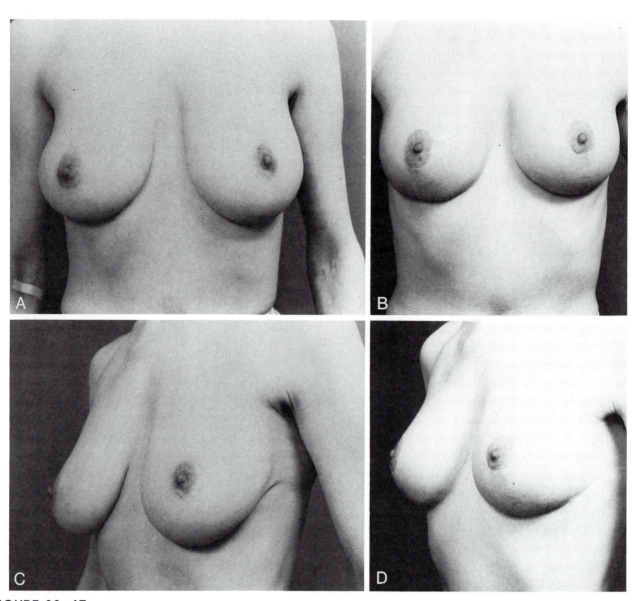

FIGURE 33–17
A, Front preoperative view. *B,* Front postoperative view, 5 years after surgery. *C,* Preoperative left oblique view. *D,* Left oblique postoperative view, 5 years after surgery.

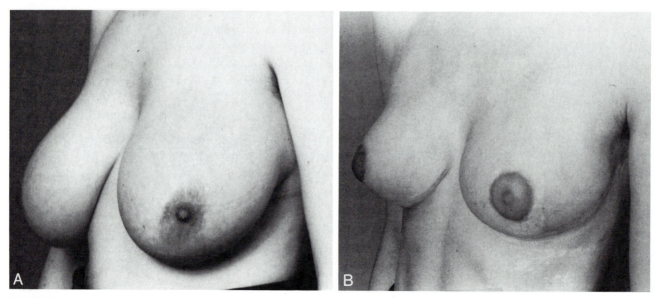

FIGURE 33–18
A, Left oblique preoperative view. *B,* Left oblique postoperative view, 3 years after surgery.

Acknowledgments

The author wishes to acknowledge the assistance of Sharadkumar Dicksheet, M.D., in the preparation of the manuscript, based on his observation of the technique in use. The author wishes to thank Mr. Bernard Struchen for preparation of the diagrams.

References

Arié, G.: Una nueva técnica de mastoplastia. Rev. Latinoam. Cir. Plast. 3:23, 1957.

Bames, H. O.: Reduction of massive breast hypertrophy. Plast. Reconstr. Surg. 3:560, 1948.

Conway, H., Smith, J.: Breast plastic surgery, mastopexy, augmentation mammaplasty and mammary reduction. Plast. Reconstr. Surg. 21:8, 1958.

Cramer, L. M., Chong, J. K.: Unipedicle cutaneous flap: Areola-nipple transposition on an end-bearing superiorly based flap. In: Georgiade, N. G.: *Reconstructive Breast Surgery*. St. Louis, C. V. Mosby, 1976, p. 143.

Georgiade, N. G.: Correction of the pendulous hypertrophied breast. In: Georgiade, N. G.: *Reconstructive Breast Surgery*. St. Louis, C. V. Mosby, 1976, p. 120.

Gillies, H., Marino, H.: The "periwinkle shell" principle in the treatment of the small ptotic breast. Plast. Reconstr. Surg. 21:1, 1958.

Goldwyn, R. M.: Remarks on reduction mammaplasty. In: Goldwyn, R. M. (ed.): *Plastic and Reconstructive Surgery of the Breast*. Boston, Little, Brown, 1976, p. 147.

Herman, S., Hoffman, S., Kahn, S.: Revisional surgery after reduction mammaplasty. Plast. Reconstr. Surg. 55:422, 1975.

Hinderer, U. T.: The dermal brassiere mammaplasty. Clin. Plast. Surg. 3:227, 1976.

Longacre, J. J.: Surgical correction of the flat discoid breast. Plast. Reconstr. Surg. 17:358, 1956.

McKissock, P. K.: Reduction mammaplasty with a vertical dermal flap. Plast. Reconstr. Surg. 49:245, 1972.

Pitanguy, I.: Breast hypertrophy. *Transactions of the International Society of Plastic Surgeons,* Second Congress, London, 1959. Edinburgh, Livingstone, 1960, p. 509.

Rees, T. D., Flagg, S. V.: *Reduction Mammaplasty in Unfavorable Results in Plastic Surgery*. Boston, Little, Brown, 1972, p. 317.

Ribeiro, L.: A new technique for reduction mammaplasty. Plast. Reconstr. Surg. 55:330, 1975.

Schwarzmann, E.: Die Technik der Mammaplastik. Chirurg 2:932, 1930.

Skoog, T.: A technique of breast reduction transposition of the nipple on a cutaneous vascular pedicle. Acta Chir. Scand. 126:453, 1963.

Strömbeck, J. O.: Mammaplasty: Report on a new technique based on two-pedicle procedure. Br. J. Plast. Surg. 13:79, 1960.

Vinas, J. C.: The double breasted. Clin. Plast. Surg. 3:227, 1976.

Weiner, D. L., Aiche, A. E., Silver, L., et al.: A single dermal pedicle for nipple transposition in subcutaneous mastectomy, reduction mammaplasty or mastopexy. Plast. Reconstr. Surg. 51:115, 1973.

Wise, R. J.: Treatment of breast hypertrophy. Clin. Plast. Surg. 3:289, 1976.

34
Rodolphe Meyer
Ulrich K. Kesselring

Reduction Mammaplasty with the L Technique

HISTORY AND PHILOSOPHY

The essential goal in a reduction mammaplasty is to achieve a good shape of the breast and to produce as short as possible postoperative scars. The first objective can actually be obtained by many procedures, the easiest being inverted-T methods, especially those in which the suture lines are already outlined at the beginning of the operation by a pattern (Fig. 34–1A). So with the technically easy methods of Wise (1956), Strömbeck (1960), Pitanguy (1961), Lalardrie (1972), McKissock (1972), Weiner et al. (1973), Ribeiro (1975), Reich (1979), Georgiade et al. (1979), Planas and Mosely (1980), and others, an experienced surgeon is able to model a breast in a beautiful shape, but to the detriment of the length of the suture line. At this point the surgeon's ambition in the search for improvement of his technique should be a maximal shortening of the scars in order to achieve an optimal result without spoiling the thorax skin. In our mind the incision lines should not be dependent on a pattern, but rather individualized and adapted to each preoperative size and shape of the hypertrophic and ptotic breast (Fig. 34–1B). The method for reduction mammaplasty with an L-shaped suture line that we have been using for more than 20 years is one of the methods that can be adapted to different aspects of breast deformity. Since we advocated our method (in 1971), many other plastic surgeons have applied it in the original or in a modified form.

The lateralization of scars in a horizontal or oblique manner had already been advocated by Holländer (1924), Gläsmer and Amersbach (1928), Marc (1952), and Dufourmentel and Mouly (1951). We published our procedure for the first time in 1971 (Meyer and Martinoni, 1971). At that time, we converted the methods of Lotsch and Gohrbandt (1955) and Arié (1957), with only vertical suture lines, changing the inframammary crease into an L procedure. We limited the length of the subareolar vertical suture line at the level of the newly created fold.

After our publication of 1971, Elbaz and Verheecke (1972) described a similar line obtained in modifying the Dufourmentel oblique method.

In 1973 we presented the L technique at the Congress of the International Society of Aesthetic Plastic Surgery in Jerusalem. At the same meeting, P. Regnault presented her B method, and a year later she published it.

Our procedure was then again described in its definitive form in 1975 (Meyer and Kesselring, 1975) and later in 1979, with the presentation of three different types of access incisions for resection and vascular pedicles, all with the same de-epithelialized zone and all with the same lateralizing L suture line (Meyer and Kesselring, 1979).

In that publication we showed that lateralization with an L-shaped suture line can also be applied with superior resection and inferior vascular protection of the nipple-areola complex by means of the inferior pedicle of Ribeiro (1975), Courtiss and Goldwyn (1977), Robbins (1977), Georgiade et al. (1979), and Reich (1979). This is actually, in our hands, indicated only in exceptional cases presenting a relatively short distance between the inferior areolar border and the submammary sulcus, cases in which the nipple is pointing downward. We also showed that even the vertical pedicle of McKissock (1972) may be used in our L procedure. In the original method of McKissock and in the modification of Galvao (1988), a reduction of the suture line seems not to be required.

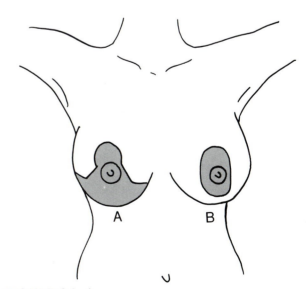

FIGURE 34–1

A, Technically easier method with the incisions reaching the sternal area. *B,* Outline of the incision for the L method.

425

A modification of our method was presented by our former resident Maillard (1986), who converted the L into a Z, beginning the descending line more laterally at the lower circumference of the areola (on the right side at the 8 o'clock position). In a similar way, Goland and Ben Hur (1982) converted the B of Regnault (1974) into a Z. In 1986 De Longhis added a dermal suspension to our L procedure by fixation of the lower end of the de-epithelialized superiorly based flap to the pectoral fascia. This anchoring flap acts as a brassiere-like suspension dermopexy in a similar way as advocated by Hinderer (1976). If it is well covered by the superficially rotated adipocutaneous flap, the result of the contour should be excellent.

Strömbeck also modified Regnault's technique for young patients (1983). Nicolle (1986) introduced another lateralization of the suture line, resulting in a very lateral inverted T. Some plastic surgeons, such as Cramer and Chong (1976), Fonseca Ely (1978), Lassus (1987), and Tafalla Pena (1988), have shown, with modifications of Arié's (1957) method, that all their procedures with only vertical suture lines are limited to cases of moderate ptosis, if one does not want to prolong the vertical line further than the inframammary sulcus, as Biesenberger (1931) and Lotsch and Gohrbandt (1955) did. Palacin et al. (1988) are also limiting the Peixoto (1980) technique to young, firm-breasted women with good skin and without ptosis, excising tissue varying from 150 to 380 gm. Thus, all these publications have shown that it is impossible to reduce severe hypertrophy with only a vertical scar in one stage if the shape has to be acceptable. In the hands of Piotti (1981) the vertical technique is limited to reductions of 500 gm per breast. He states that if the submammary groove will be higher by the mastopexy, the vertical suture line will be located 2 to 3 cm below it. In a few weeks' time the gland settles, and the suture enters almost completely the submammary groove. For this to happen, however, the breast must already have slight ptosis at the end of the operation. In our opinion, such a philosophy does not correspond to the actual goal of a sophisticated reduction with mammopexy.

One should not exaggerate in condensing the suture length. If one did so, the result of the procedure would become inevitably formless.

If one encounters too much skin left at the end of a mammopexy without tissue resection, the redundant skin has to be excised in one way or another. One has then to choose whether the excision is to be done in a prolonged vertical line or in a reversed T, staying in the horizontal crease, or by lateralization of the suture line. Cramer and Chong begin the reduction of severe hypertrophic breasts in the Arié way, but evidently a long anchor suture line results.

BASIC PRINCIPLES

Basically the original technique and all modifications have the five principles we and other authors have advocated, including the following:

1. Decreasing the circumference of the base of the breast cone (Meyer and Martinoni, 1971), in contradiction to the procedure of Garcia Padron (1976) (Figs. 34–2 and 34–3)
2. Elevation of the submammary crease (Meyer and Martinoni, 1971), (Fig. 34–3)
3. Resection of the basal layer of the breast cone tangential to the pectoral muscle, corresponding to the ground floor of a building (Meyer and Kesselring, 1975; Peixoto, 1980; Marchac and de Olarte, 1982; Maillard, 1986) (see Figs. 34–3 and 34–9)
4. Reduction of the length of the scars with the L technique (Meyer and Martinoni, 1971; Elbaz and Verheecke, 1972), in the B technique (Regnault, 1974), and in small inverted-T techniques (Peixoto, 1980; Marchac and de Olarte, 1982)
5. Keeping the distance between the areolar border and the submammary crease under 6 cm

To achieve a vertical scar with the shortest possible horizontal scar, we advance the vertical incision toward the areola and excise the redundant skin.

With great satisfaction we have observed in some publications, particularly in those of Peixoto (1980) and Marchac and de Olarte (1982), that their methods are based on the same principles: removal of the basal tissue of the breast cone, reduction of the basal circumference, elevation of the submammary fold, and scar minimization.

OPERATIVE TECHNIQUE

In the standing patient, the new nipple site is determined and marked. The point is usually on the horizontal projection of the submammary crease or 1 to 2 cm higher (Fig. 34–4; see Figs. 34–25, 34–26, and 34–34).

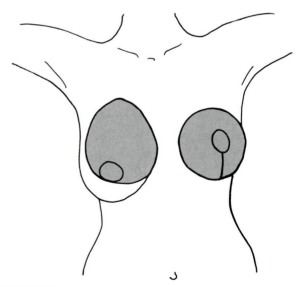

FIGURE 34–2
Decreasing the circumference of the breast cone.

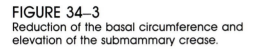
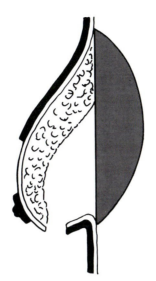
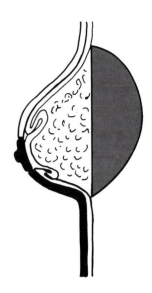

FIGURE 34-3
Reduction of the basal circumference and elevation of the submammary crease.

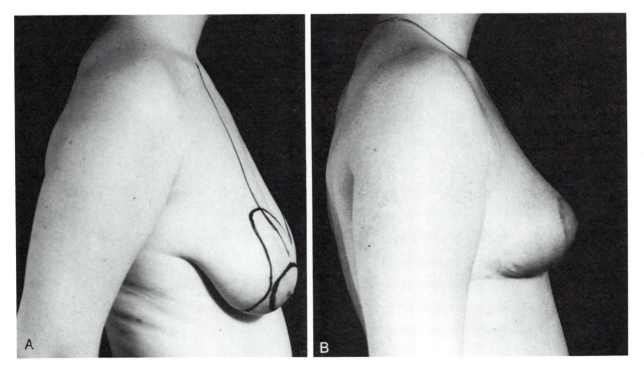

FIGURE 34-4
A and *B*, Juvenile hypertrophy before and after reduction. The operative sequences performed on this patient follow in the next figures.

The experience and the sense of proportion of the surgeon will allow him to position correctly the site of the new nipple-areola complex in each individual case.

The borders of the area to be de-epithelialized are determined by the future upper and lateral borders of the areola. The first two points are fixed measurements: 14 to 17 cm from the upper clavicular border and 8 to 10 cm from the midsternal line (see Fig. 34–4). The lateral point is dictated by the volume of the breast and reflects the reduction that has to be performed. The three points define the outline area of de-epithelialization and the new areola position (see Figs. 34–4 to 34–7, 34–18, 34–25, 34–26, and 34–34). The lower half is again determined by the skin redundancy, breast volume, and the intended reduction to be performed.

Once past the areola, the de-epithelialized zone follows a medially curved line, which then curves infero-laterally to pass 2 to 3 cm above the inframammary crease and to meet the lateral border outline, which is a cranially convex zone of de-epithelialization with an intact nipple-areola island. In most cases we leave a strip of skin in the outlined area, stopping the de-epithelialization 2 to 3 cm higher (see Fig. 34–5).

After de-epithelialization (see Fig. 34–7), the entire adipoglandular mass is released from the pectoral fascia superiorly to the third rib with tissue resection starting at the inferior pole of the breast (Fig. 34–8; see Figs. 34–22 and 34–35) and continuing in a parallel plane to the thorax through the entire breast. In this way the base of the cone is removed without the skin. Often, supplementary wedge resections of the adipoglandular tissue must be performed in the upper lateral quadrant and in the upper medial quadrant.

In order to facilitate the plication of the flap and fixation of the areola, the dermal layer of the flap can be severed superficially on either side without causing embarrassment of the areolar blood supply, provided that at least a 5-cm width of the dermal pedicle is preserved cranially (Figs. 34–9 and 34–10).

At this point the fixation of the areola in the new site can be performed before the modeling of the breast cone as we usually do, using strong resorbable mattress sutures to the pectoral fascia. The shaping of the cone may be done before fixation, as Regnault (1974) does it. We actually place the nipple-areola complex in the

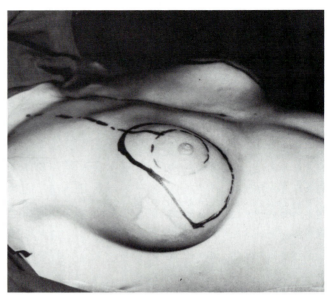

FIGURE 34–6
Same outline at the beginning of the operation.

correct position first (Fig. 34–11; see Fig. 34–23). The inferomedial quadrant is then defatted, which permits the skin to be easily rotated laterally to join the lateral skin border, thus reducing the ciircumference of the base of the mammary cone and raising the inframammary fold. Since the skin incision and excision do not reach the inframammary crease, the skin belonging to the inferior aspect of the breast can also be defatted, pulled against the thorax to the new level of the inframammary fold, and fixed there to the underlying muscle fascia (see Fig. 34–11; Fig. 34–12). Resorbable sutures are used to remodel the adipoglandular flap and to fix it to the pectoral fascia as needed. In order to obtain the L-shaped suture line, one must drape the skin in a rotating manner around the breast cone formed by the

Text continued on page 434

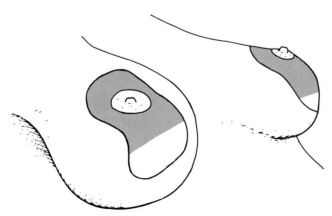

FIGURE 34–5
Outline of the area to be de-epithelialized.

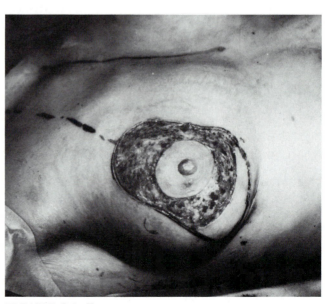

FIGURE 34–7
Breast after de-epithelialization. A lower strip of skin can be removed in full thickness.

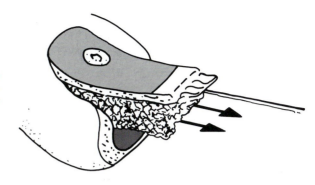

FIGURE 34–8
The adipoglandular tissue is dissected from the pectoral fascia up to the third rib. The basal tissue is about to be resected. The lower strip of skin has not yet been removed in the areola carrier flap, which is held horizontally taut.

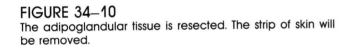

FIGURE 34–9
The adipoglandular tissue is resected in a plane parallel to the thorax wall. Bilateral wedge resection in the adipoglandular flap facilitates the remodeling of the breast cone. The remaining strip of skin in the flap is removed.

FIGURE 34–10
The adipoglandular tissue is resected. The strip of skin will be removed.

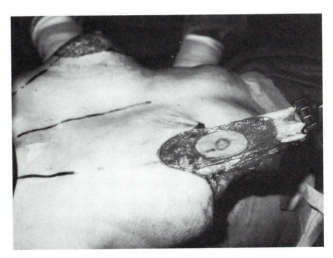

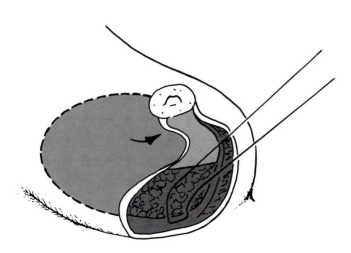

FIGURE 34–11
"Areola-pexy" and deep mattress suture for fixation of the adipoglandular flap facilitate the remodeling of the breast cone. The remaining strip of the skin in the flap is removed.

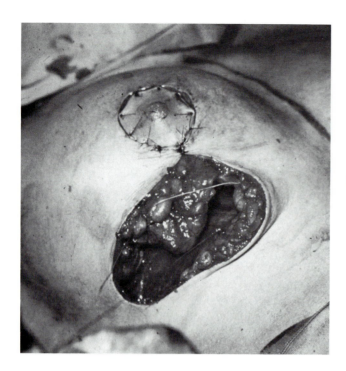

FIGURE 34–12
"Areola-pexy" and deep mattress suture.

FIGURE 34–13
Lateral dog-ear to be cut off.

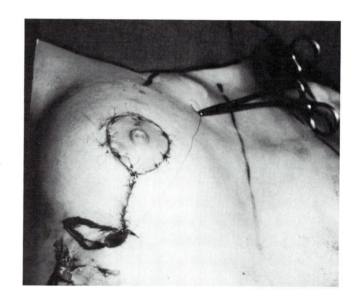

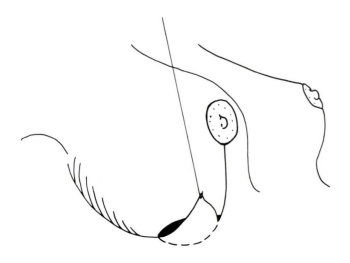

FIGURE 34–14
Small skin flap to be resected in a curved line to compensate the upper curve of the wound.

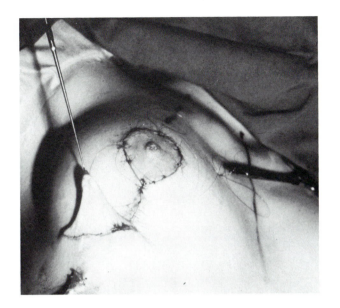

FIGURE 34–15
Skin flap of the dog-ear to be removed.

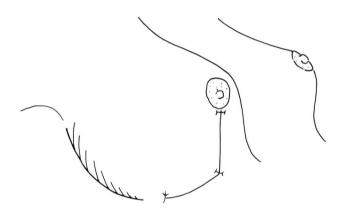

FIGURE 34–16
L-shaped suture. Around the areola we use semiburied sutures knotted on the inner side. For the L closure we use deep subcutaneous resorbable thread and intradermal running sutures of nonresorbable material.

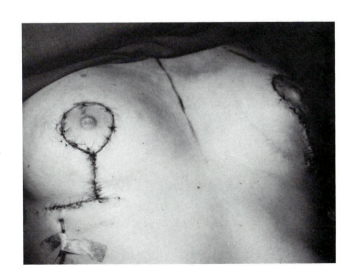

FIGURE 34–17
End of the operation.

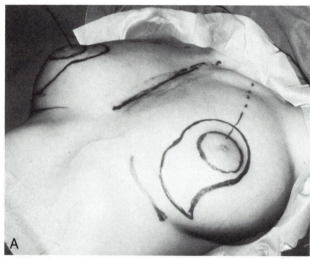

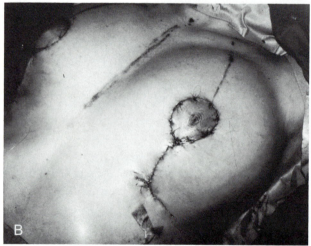

FIGURE 34–18
A and *B*, Moderate juvenile hypertrophy, allowing a very short horizontal suture line.

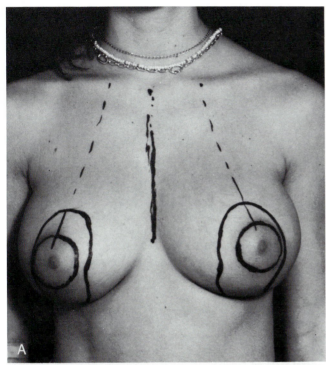

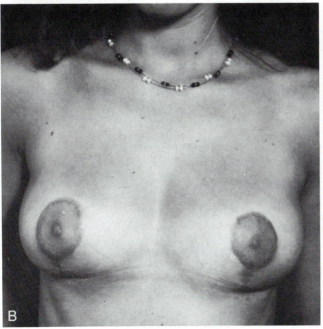

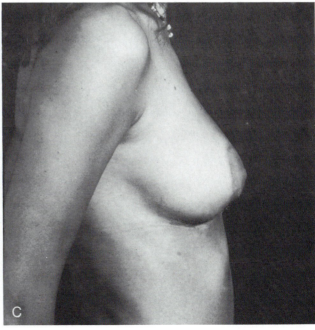

FIGURE 34–19
A to *C*, Patient shown in Figure 34–18 before and after surgery.

flaps. We make up for the additional length of the lower skin border wth a curved resection of the upper lateral skin border (Figs. 34–13 to 34–15).

It is important not to exceed 6 cm in distance from the lower areolar border to the new inframammary crease, because doing so tends to produce a late result of an upward-tilt nipple with a sagging inferior hemisphere (Figs. 34–16 to 34–25). With very large breasts it may not always be possible to end with a perfect L. In such cases we proceed to resect a medial dog-ear, thereby adding a short limb to the junction of the L, which results in an asymmetric T (Figs. 34–26 to 34–34). Still, the length of such an additional medial "heel" is considerably shorter than that achieved with the vertical bipedicle of McKissock (1972); the inferiorly based pedicle of Ribeiro (1975), Robbins (1977), Reich (1979), or Courtiss and Goldwyn (1977); or other methods with inverted-T sutures. With this the eventual medial scar is at least 7 cm away from the midsternal line. It is important to begin the operation by lateralizing the incisions and then rotating the skin of the inferomedial quadrant as much as possible laterally. We use the same technique following the same principles and an adequate assessment also for gigantomastia. Of course, in those cases an actual L suture line is not possible, but at least the procedure limits as much as possible the length of the horizontal inframammary scar and achieves a pleasant shape and minimal scarring (Fig. 34–35).

As already mentioned, we will under exceptional circumstances perform reduction mammaplasty by the same method, but utilizing an inferior pedicle of the nipple-bearing flap, in those rare cases with a downward-pointing nipple (Fig. 34–36). In those cases the distance from the nipple-areolar complex to the inframammary crease is short, and so the well-vascularized flap can be lifted and stretched upward once the adipoglandular mass is resected through an upper incision. The inferior pedicle has to be de-epithelialized down to the very base and lifted and covered with a medial skin flap that will be rotated laterally (Figs. 34–37 to 34–39). Then the upper areolar circumference is sutured to the previously outlined semicircle into the new position with Dexon sutures. The skin can now be draped around the properly positioned remaining breast cone (see Fig. 34–39). The dissection of the inferior skin border below the de-epithelialized area must be carried out very superficially so as not to interfere with the blood supply coming from below. We have abandoned the lateralization of McKissock's procedure (1972) with the vertical bipedicle flap.

For all aesthetic breast surgery we use 2-0 Vicryl for fixation of the adipoglandular mass to the new level, Dexon 2-0 for subcutaneous separate or running sutures 4-0 and 5-0 Prolene for subcuticular running sutures.

Text continued on page 446

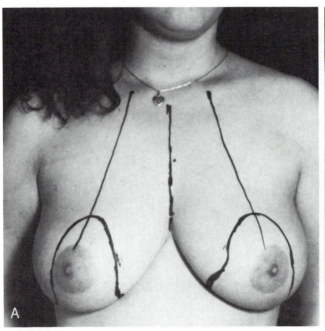 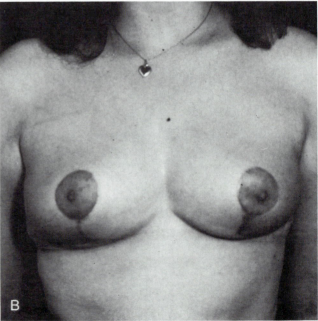

FIGURE 34–20
A and *B,* Juvenile hypertrophy before and after reduction.

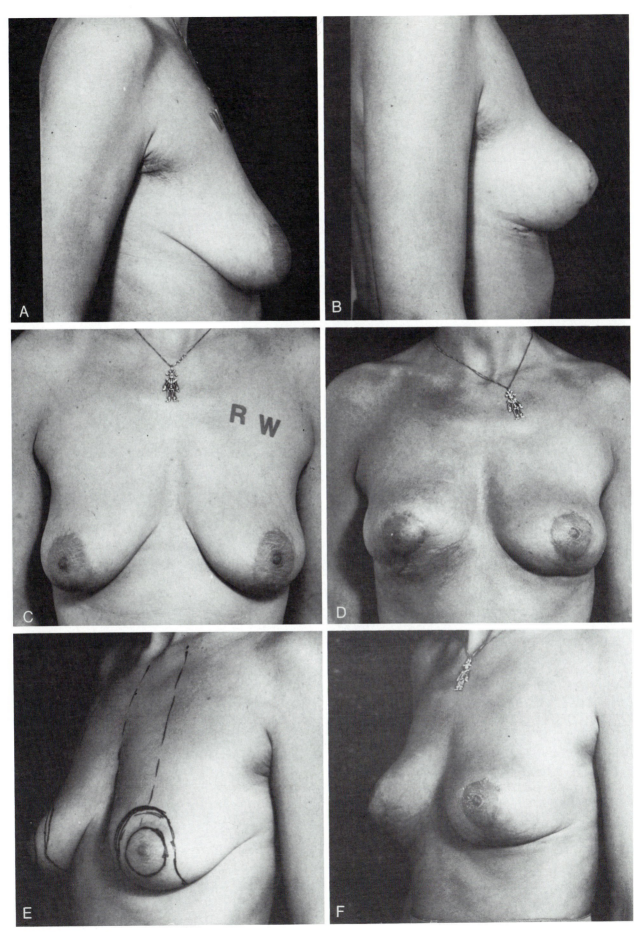

FIGURE 34–21
A to *F*, Middle-aged woman with marked ptosis, before and after intervention.

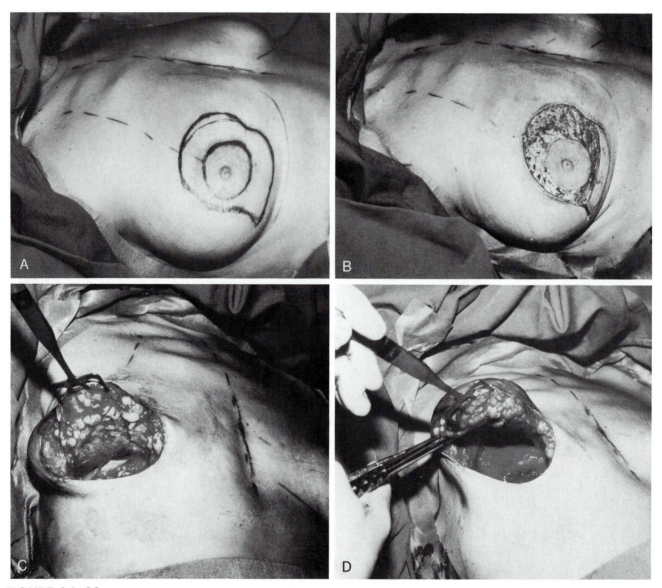

FIGURE 34–22

A, Patient shown in Figure 34–21 at the beginning of the operation. *B,* Same patient after de-epithelialization. *C* and *D,* Beginning and end of tissue dissection from the pectoral fascia.

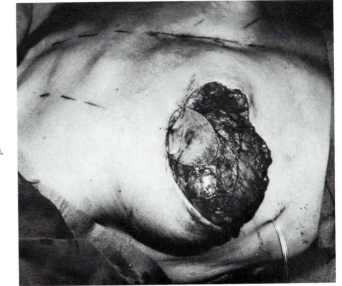

FIGURE 34–23
"Areola-pexy" beginning at the 12 o'clock position.

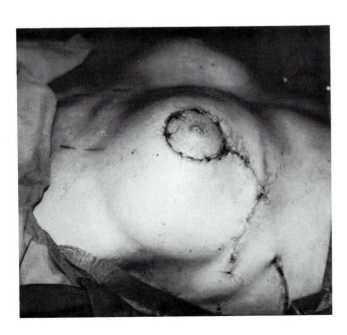

FIGURE 34–24
End of the L-shaped suture.

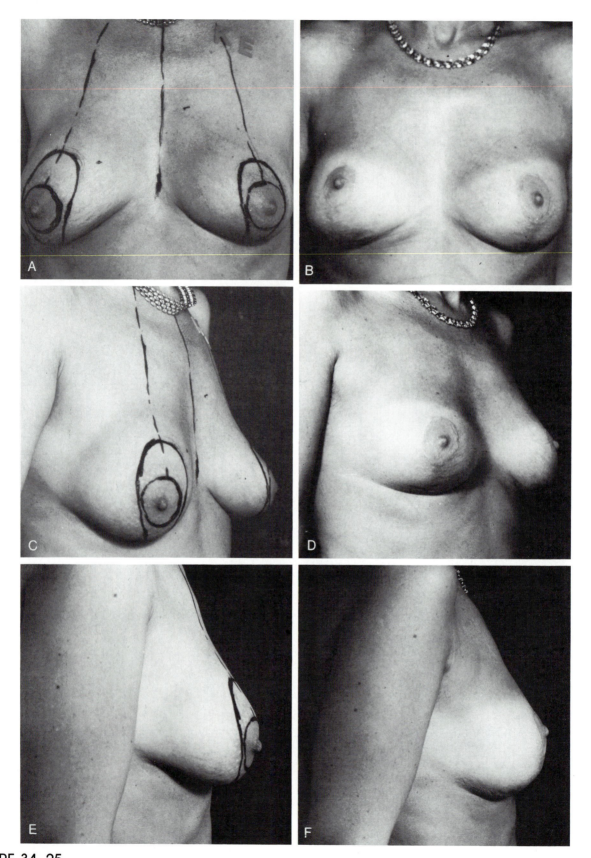

FIGURE 34–25

A to *F*, A 40-year-old patient with severe ptosis after augmentation mammaplasty with prostheses *in situ*, before and after mammopexy including new prostheses.

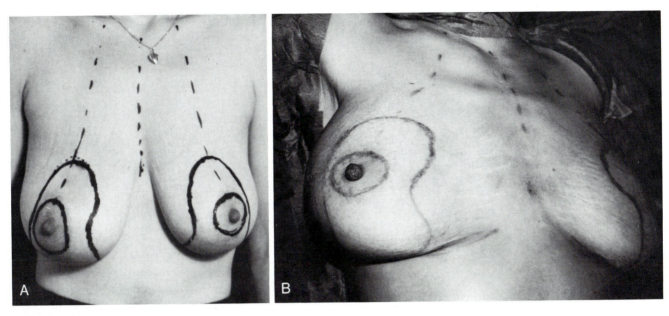

FIGURE 34–26
A and *B*, Marked hypertrophy with many striae. The incisions are outlined with the patient in the standing position and lying on the operating table.

FIGURE 34–27
De-epithelialization in the patient shown in Figure 34–26.

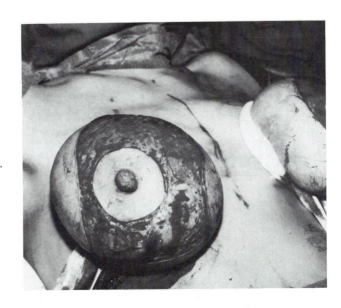

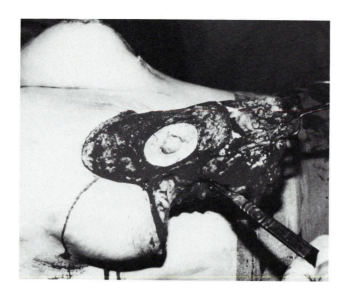

FIGURE 34–28
Removal of the adipoglandular mass.

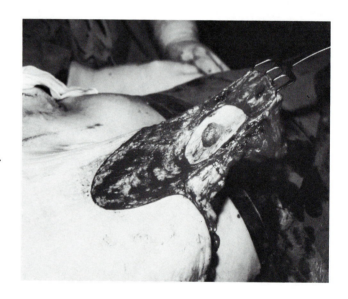

FIGURE 34–29
Areola-carrying flap after tissue resection.

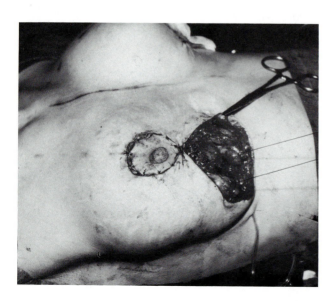

FIGURE 34–30
"Areola-pexy" and mattress suture attaching the flap to the pectoral fascia.

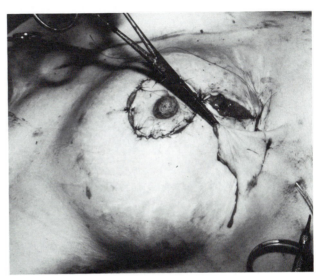

FIGURE 34–31
The skin is draped around the new cone. The lateral skin excess is about to be resected.

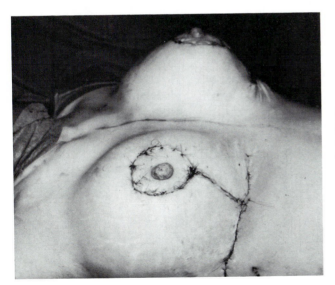

FIGURE 34–32
End of the operation. In this case of important hypertrophy and ptosis, a horizontal medial suture limb was necessary, giving to the whole suture an asymmetric, inverted-T aspect.

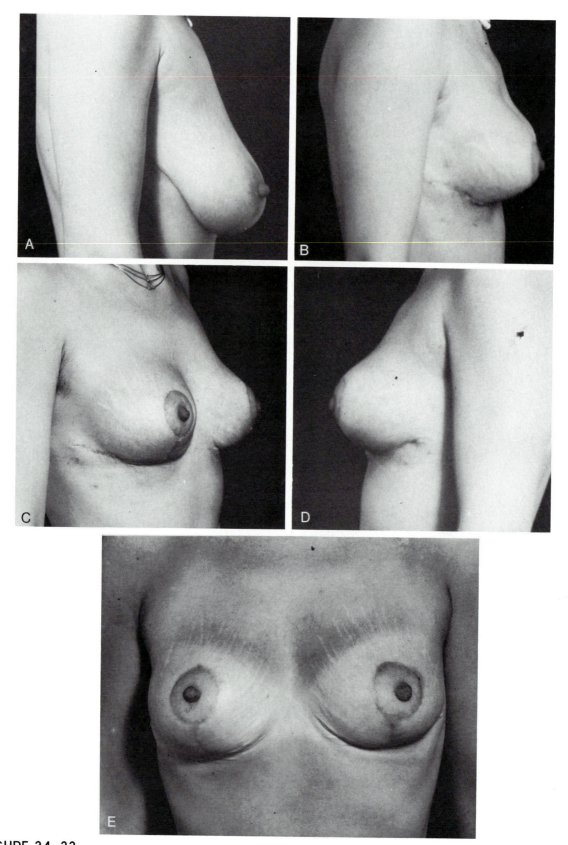

FIGURE 34–33
A to *E,* Other preoperative and postoperative views of the *same* patient shown in Figures 34–26 through 34–32.

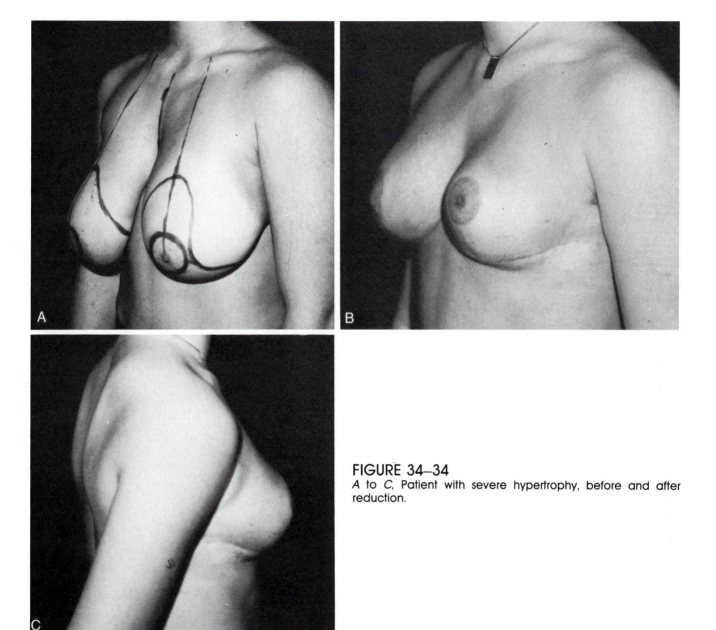

FIGURE 34–34
A to *C*, Patient with severe hypertrophy, before and after reduction.

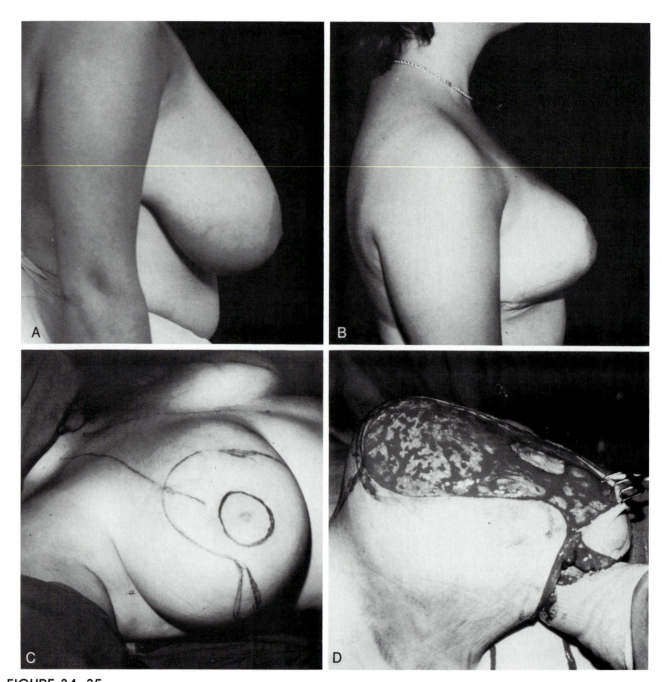

FIGURE 34–35
A to *D*, Patient with juvenile gigantomastia in preoperative and postoperative side views and on the table with incisions outlined and during the basal blunt dissection.

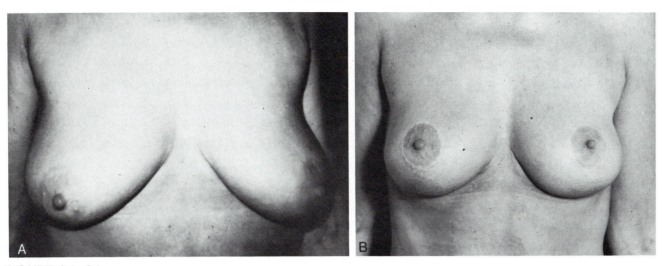

FIGURE 34–36
A and *B*, Middle-aged woman with a short distance between the areola and the inframammary crease, an indication for the use of the inferior flap. Preoperative and postoperative front views.

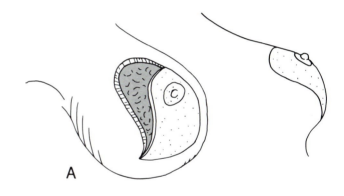

FIGURE 34–37
A, Lower nipple-areola vascular protection with the inferior flap and lateralized incisions and suture lines. *B*, Section showing access and amount of tissue resection.

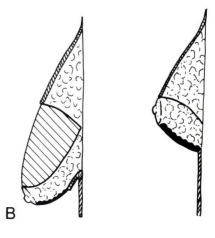

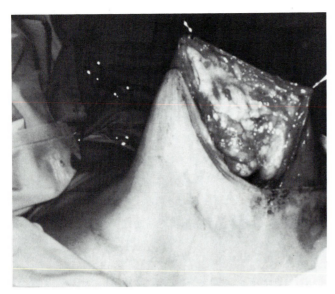

FIGURE 34–38
The adipoglandular tissue resection is performed from the incision above the nipple-areola complex.

SUBCUTANEOUS MASTECTOMY WITH THE L TECHNIQUE

In order to gain the benefit of a large dermal flap after a subcutaneous mastectomy we use superolateral access for tissue resection and an inferior dermal pedicle for covering the required prosthess. In this way, we achieve maximal protection of the prosthesis with good continuity of the blood supply to the skin and nipple-areola complex.

The approach is through a lateral incision at the border of the de-epithelialized zone, giving comfortable access to the gland and permitting an exact resection of the upper lateral quadrant, which often extends to the

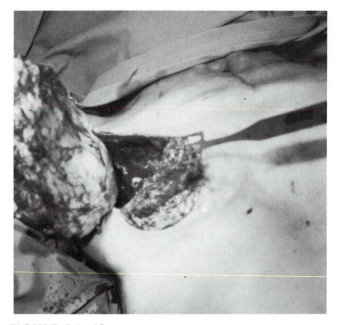

FIGURE 34–40
Subcutaneous mastectomy with the same inferior flap and superior access for tissue resection.

axilla (Fig. 34–40). Once the prosthesis is introduced, the dermal flap is draped around it as far as possible to provide, in effect, a second-layer covering (Figs. 34–41 and 34–42). The subpectoral placement of a prosthesis is also possible with this incision. The principles of skin resection and closure remain the same as described previously.

DISCUSSION

It seems obvious that the lateralization of the scar in an L shape can be achieved with many other types of resections in reduction mammaplasty. We believe that nowadays a scar line extending medially to the sternum

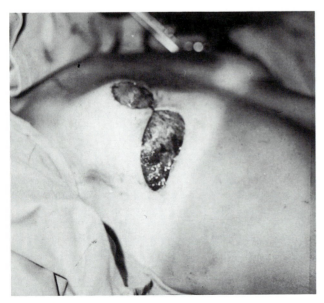

FIGURE 34–39
Lateralization of the suture line ending in an L.

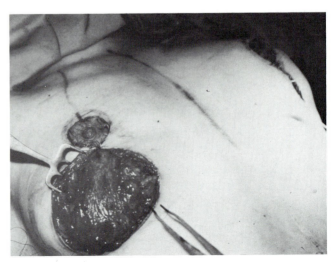

FIGURE 34–41
The prosthesis is covered with a de-epithelialized inferior dermal flap.

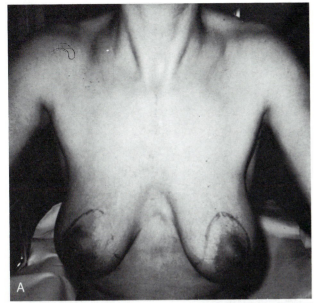

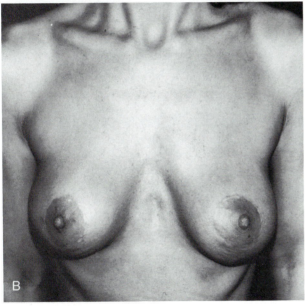

FIGURE 34–42
A and *B,* Patient with fibrocystic mastopathy before and after surgery, including the use of mammary prostheses.

obtain small inverted T scars on closure, and Maillard's closure results in a Z-shaped scar.

At the International Society of Aesthetic Plastic Surgery course in Montreal, Canada, in 1983, we had the opportunity to be involved in a televised demonstration of simultaneous breast reductions in a young woman. Dr. P. Regnault operated on the left breast, using her B method, and we operated on the right one, using our technique. The results of the procedures were practically the same, the two techniques being very similar. We both operate in the same manner, the only technical difference being that Regnault first shapes the breast cone using basal sutures before suturing the nipple-areola complex into its predetermined site, whereas we proceed in the reverse order.

In any event, we have found that both methods are effective, and that the result depends more on the amount of tissue to be resected and on the strength of the basal pexis than on the sequence of steps followed.

Many plastic surgeons, in different countries, are now using the L technique, and modifications of it, to avoid or reduce a long T scar line.

In conclusion, we can state that after 20 years' experience using the L technique, we have realized what we set out to achieve from the beginning: a significant glandular resection with maintenance of vascularity to the nipple-areola complex; proper form of the remodeled breast; and a significant reduction in the resulting scar line, especially medially, where it is most important. For this, good assessment and a meticulous execution are required.

The main *advantages* are the good vascular nipple protection and the short L suture lines, which result in a scar easily concealed, leaving unspoiled the inframammary medial area. Another advantage is that with minimal scar length in relatively young patients, even if the shape becomes with time unsatisfactory, there is always the possibility of performing a secondary correction while staying in the reduced scar length. If with other techniques the scar reaching the frequently exposed sternal area is once set, it will be visible all the patient's life.

The unique *disadvantage* of our method is that it is not a simple one. The novice, not possessing the necessary sense of sculpturing, had better start with a completely pre-assessed procedure.

It is indeed a method for exigent surgeons and exigent patients.

References

Arié, G.: Una nuéva tecnica de mastoplastia. Rev. Latinoam. Cir. Plast. 3:23, 1957.

Biesenberger, H. H.: *Deformitäten und kosmetischen Operationen der weiblichen Brust.* Wien, W. Maudrich, 1931.

Courtiss, E., Goldwyn, R. M.: Reduction mammaplasty by the inferior pedicle technique. Plast. Reconstr. Surg. 59:500, 1977.

Cramer, L. M., Chong, J. K.: Unipedicle cutaneous flap: Areola-nipple transposition on an end-bearing superiorly based flap. In: Georgiade, N. G. (ed.): *Reconstructive Breast Surgery.* St. Louis, C. V. Mosby, 1976, p. 143.

De Longhis, E.: Mammaplasty with an L-shaped scar and retropectoral dermopexy. Aesthetic Plast. Surg. 10:171, 1986.

Dufourmentel, C., Mouly, R.: Developpements récents de la plastie mammaire par la méthode oblique latérale. Ann. Chir. Plast. 10:227, 1965.

should not be allowed unless absolutely necessary. It is obvious that the advantage of this minimal scarring technique is important, especially in young patients, in whom spoiling of the middle of the thorax would really be a pity. The surgical improvement of the shape of the breast should not be compromised by unaesthetic scars extending toward the midline, which may be visible in décolleté dresses. Once a scar is placed, it is placed for life. Another important principle of our technique, advocated nearly 20 years ago, is that of keeping the incision line about 2 to 4 cm above the inframammary crease, thereby allowing the skin of the lower part of the breast to be converted into thoracic wall skin. Peixoto (1980) and Marchac (1982), as well as Maillard (1986), have also adopted this principle. The first two

Elbaz, J. S., Verheecke, G.: La cicatrice en L dans les plasties mammaires. Ann. Chir. Plast. 17:283, 1972.

Fonseca Ely, J.: Reduction mammaplasty: An ecletic approach. Aesthetic Plast. Surg. 2:95, 1978.

Galvao, M. S. L.: Reduction mammaplasty with preservation of the superior, medial, lateral and inferior pedicles. In: Georgiade, N. G. (ed.): *Aesthetic Breast Surgery*. Baltimore, Williams & Wilkins, 1983, p. 175.

Garcia Padron, J.: Mammareduktions plastik. Transacta der III Tagung der Vereinigung der Deutschen Plastichen Chirurgen, Koln, 1976, p. 82.

Georgiade, N. G., Serafin, D., Riefkohl, R., Georgiade, G.: Reduction mammaplasty utilizing an inferior pedicle nipple-areola flap. Ann. Plast. Surg. 3:211, 1979.

Gläsmer, E., Amersbach, R.: Zur feineren Technik der Hängebrustoperation. Münch. Med. Wochenschr. 75:1547, 1928.

Golan, J., Ben Hur, N.: Simplified design of the "B" technique mammaplasty. Aesthetic Plast. Surg. 6:2, 1982.

Hinderer, U. T.: The dermal brassiere mammaplasty. Clin. Plast. Surg. 3:227, 1976.

Holländer, J.: Die Operation der Mammahypertrophie und er Hängebrust. Dtsche Med. Wochenschr. 50:1400, 1924.

Lalardrie, J. P.: The "dermal vault" technique: Reduction mammaplasty for hypertrophy with ptosis. Transacta der III Tagung der Vereinigung der Deutschen Plastichen Chirurgen, Koln, 1972, p. 105.

Lassus, C.: Breast reduction: Evolution of a technique: A single vertical scar. Aesthetic Plast. Surg. 11:107, 1987.

Lotsch, G. M., Gohrbandt, E. E.: Operatichen und der weiblichen Brust. In: Bier, A. K. G., Braun, H., Kummel, H., (eds.): *Chirurgische Operationslehre*. Leipzig, A. Barth Verlag, 1955.

Maillard, G.: A Z-mammaplasty with an L-shaped scar and retropectoral dermopexie. Aesthetic Plast. Surg. 10:171, 1986.

Marc, H.: *La Plastie Mammaire par la Méthode "Oblique."* Paris, G. Doin, 1952.

Marchac, D., de Olarte, G.: Reduction mammaplasty and correction of ptosis with a short inframammary scar. Plast. Reconstr. Surg. 69:1, 45, 1982.

McKissock, P. K.: Reduction mammaplasty with a vertical dermal flap. Plast. Reconstr. Surg. 49:245, 1972.

Meyer, R., Kesselring, U. K.: Reduction mammaplasty with an L-shaped suture line. Plast. Reconstr. Surg. 55:139, 1975.

Meyer, R., Kesselring, U. K.: Reduction mammaplasty with an L-shaped suture line. In: Georgiade, N. G. (ed.): *Reconstructive Breast Surgery*. St. Louis, C. V. Mosby, 1976, p. 157.

Meyer, R., Kesselring, U. K.: Various dermal flaps with L-shaped suture line in reduction mammaplasty. Aesthetic Plast. Surg. 3:41, 1979.

Meyer, R., Kesselring, U. K.: Reduction mammaplasty with an L-shaped suture line: Development of different techniques. Plast. Reconstr. Surg. 65:217, 1980.

Meyer, R., Kesselring, U. K.: L-shaped suture lines in mammaplasty. In: Gonzalez-Ulloa, M., Meyer, R., Smith, J. W., Zaoli, G. (eds.): *Aesthetic Plastic Surgery*. Padova, Piccin Nuova Libraria. St. Louis, C. V. Mosby, 1988, p. 209.

Meyer, R., Martinoni, G.: Mastoplastica di riduzione in ATTI XXI Congresso Nazionale della Societa Italiana di Chirurgia Plastica Ricostruttiva, 1971.

Nedkoff, N.: Eine neue Schnittmethode der Brustkorrektur. Zentralbl. Chir. 65:1503, 1938.

Nicolle, F. V.: Some methods for improving results of reduction mammaplasty and mastopexy. In: Georgiade, N. G. (ed.): *Aesthetic Breast Surgery*. Baltimore, Williams & Wilkins, 1983, p. 300.

Palacin, J. M., Del Cacho, C., Johnson, D., Planas, J.: Reduction mammoplasty with the Peixoto technique. Eur. J. Plast. Surg. 11:132, 1988.

Peixoto, G.: Reduction mammaplasty: A personal technique. Plast. Reconstr. Surg. 65:217, 1980.

Piotti, F.: Experience with a vertical technique in mammaplasty. Aesthetic Plast. Surg. 5:349, 1981.

Pitanguy, I.: Mamaplastias. Rev. Bras. Cir. 42:201, 1961.

Planas, J., Mosely, L. W.: Improving breast shape and symmetry in reduction mammaplasty. Ann. Plast. Surg. 4:297, 1980.

Regnault, P.: Reduction mammaplasty by the B-technique. Plast. Reconstr. Surg. 53:19, 1974.

Reich, J.: The advantages of a lower central breast segment in reduction mammaplasty. Aesthetic Plast. Surg. 3:47, 1979.

Ribeiro, L.: A new technique for reduction mammaplasty. Plast. Reconstr. Surg. 55:330, 1975.

Robbins, T. H.: A reduction mammaplasty with the areola-nipple based on an inferior dermal pedicle. Plast. Reconstr. Surg. 59:64, 1977.

Skoog, T.: Technique of breast reduction: Transposition of the nipple on a cutaneous vascular pedicle. Acta Chir. Scand. 126:453, 1963.

Strömbeck, J. O.: Mammaplasty: Report of a new technique based on the two pedicle procedure. Br. J. Plast. Surg. 13:79, 1960.

Strömbeck, J. O.: Reduction mammaplasty. In: Georgiade, N. G. (ed.): *Aesthetic Breast Surgery*. Baltimore, Williams & Wilkins, 1983, p. 146.

Tafalla Pena, M., Lorda Barraguer, E., Rodes Perez, A.: Mastoplastia reductiva: Conceptos personales. Cir. Plast. Ibero-Latinoamericana 14:231, 1988.

Vogt, T., Dicksheet, S.: Reduction mammaplasty: Vogt's "glandular prosthesis" and "glandular brassiere" technique. In: Gonzalez-Ulloa, M., Meyer, R., Smith, J. W., Zaoli, G. (eds.): *Aesthetic Plastic Surgery*. Padova, Piccin Nuova Libraria. St. Louis, C. V. Mosby, 1988, p. 209.

Weiner, D. L., Aiache, A. E., Silver, L., Tittiranonda, T.: A single dermal pedicle for nipple transposition in a subcutaneous mastectomy, reduction mammaplasty, or mastopexy. Plast. Reconstr. Surg. 51:115, 1973.

Wise, R. J.: Preliminary report on method of planning the mammaplasty. Plast. Reconstr. Surg. 17:367, 1956.

35

Claude Lassus

A Single Vertical Scar for Breast Reduction

Large breasts have apparently always been a matter of concern to women. Durston, in 1731, proposed what is supposed to have been the first aesthetic breast surgery.

Today, heavy breasts are less accepted than ever before because of the change in the fashionable female silhouette, which is becoming longer, thinner, and in a certain way very often androgynous, as shown in the clothing of the day. This is certainly one reason women, young and old, object to large breasts. This condition is also bothersome with regard to physical and athletic activities in which women are becoming more and more involved.

The weight of the breasts and their large size can lead to uncomfortable fullness; neck and back pain; shoulder grooving; and difficulties with moisture, intertrigo, and other dermatoses beneath the breast in the inframammary area because of constant skin-to-skin contact. For these reasons women seek breast reduction. The request is acceptable from this point of view and reasonable also because large breasts are difficult to assess for lumps or masses.

Patients are now more and more demanding about this specific operation. They want perfect results: smaller breasts with a beautiful appearance persisting over years and minimal scarring. The breast reduction technique must fulfill these goals as much as possible and must provide

1. Reduction of the breast to a satisfactory size
2. Local and general safety without any necrosis of the gland, skin, or areola and without any impairment of sensibility
3. Minimal scarring, since no scarring is impossible
4. A pleasant and persisting result

In the mid-1960s I was performing a reduction technique based on (1) resection *en bloc* of skin, fat, and gland; and (2) transposition of the areola on a dermal flap, for safety, as recommended by Skoog (1963). This technique resulted in a single vertical scar even in large-breasted patients (Fig. 35–1).

However, there was a drawback in these cases; part of the scar appeared 2 or 3 cm below the brassiere line (Fig. 35–2). For this reason I modified the technique in 1977. The addition of a short horizontal scar succeeded

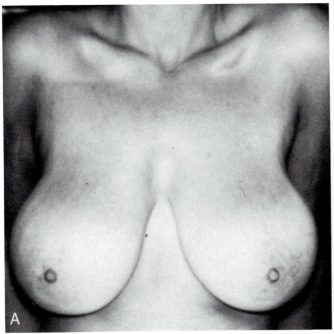 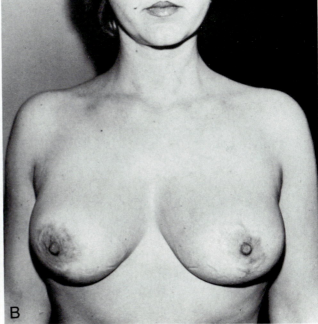

FIGURE 35–1
A, Before. *B,* After.

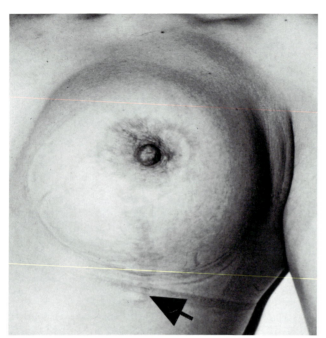

FIGURE 35–2
Part of the vertical scar appearing below the brassiere line.

in eliminating this drawback. Later, Peixoto (1980), Marchac, and de Olarte (1982), and others described similar techniques with a short horizontal scar.

One of the goals of reduction mammaplasty is minimal scarring. This challenge is, perhaps, the last one, because safe techniques have now been available for a number of years, as well as techniques providing a good final shape. In the last few years I have used all my efforts to diminish the scarring and to finish with a single vertical scar remaining above the new inframammary

fold, because the resection *en bloc* of skin, fat, and gland and the transposition of the areola on a dermo-glandular flap make reduction mammaplasty a very safe procedure.

PREOPERATIVE PLANNING

Determining the new nipple position (A) is the first step in planning the technique. This should be determined while the patient is upright, as should all the other markings (Fig. 35–3A).

The nipple position (A) will be on a point located where a vertical line coming from the nipple crosses a horizontal line coming from a point located 2 cm lower than the midhumeral distance (Fig. 35–3B).

The second important point is point B, located 2 or 4 cm above the crossing of the vertical line coming from the nipple with the inframammary crease (Fig. 35–4).

The amount of resection to perform to attain a satisfactory reduction of volume is determined by pinching the breast skin in the area located between A and B (Fig. 35–5A). The points where the fingers touch each other are marked, and A is joined to B with an internal and an external line connecting the points marked by the pinching (Fig. 35–5B). This area shows the glandular resection to be performed, but this resection will possibly be modified at the end of the operation if the result does not look right at that time (Fig. 35–5C).

The areolar flap is then drawn. It is generally a superiorly based one. The inferior border is located 5 cm beyond the nipple so that the vascularization and innervation are preserved (Figs. 35–6 and 35–7). When the nipple ascension is greater than 8 or 9 cm, the lateral pedicle as advocated by Skoog (1963) and others is preferable.

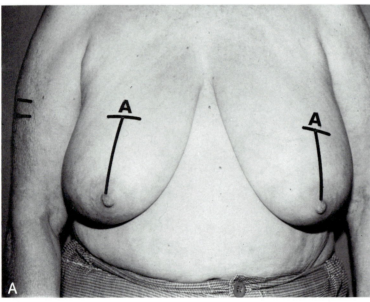

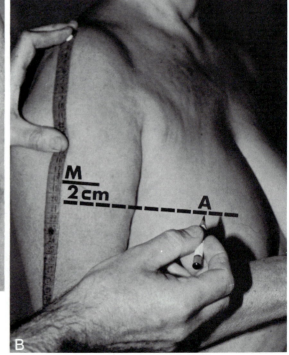

FIGURE 35–3
A and *B*, Marking point A.

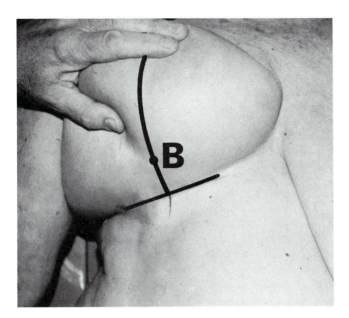

FIGURE 35–4
Marking point B.

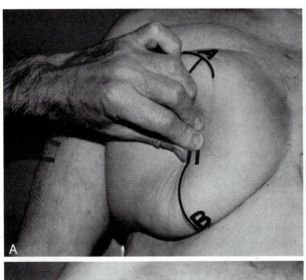

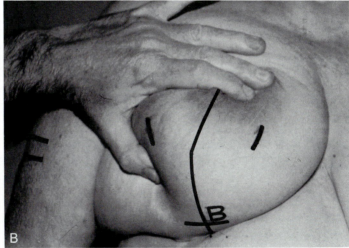

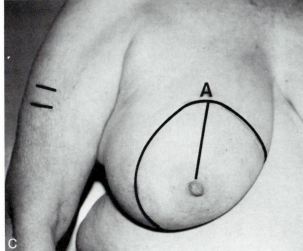

FIGURE 35–5
Drawing of the resection area. *A*, Determining the width. *B*, Marks of the limits. *C*, Joining A to B through these marks.

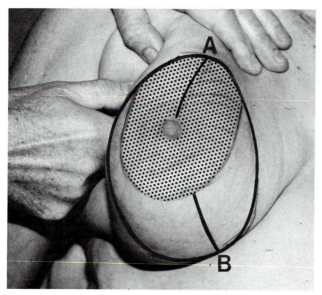

FIGURE 35–6
The areolar flap is drawn.

When the drawings are completed on both sides, the width of each area is measured very carefully so that good symmetry will be obtained, and the breasts are reshaped with the hands for determining whether the preoperative drawings of the resection area are correct (Fig. 35–8).

OPERATION

It is important that the patient be in a semi-sitting position during the operation. All the markings are

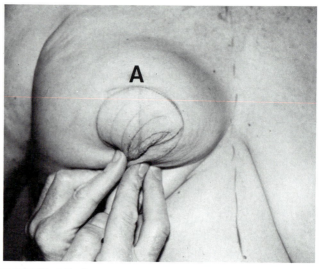

FIGURE 35–8
Checking whether the drawing of the resection area is correct.

superficially incised with a No. 15 blade so that they are not lost during the operation.

The nipple-areola complex is marked and incised, and a circle of 4 cm is generally retained (Fig. 35–9). Then a careful de-epithelialization of the areolar flap is performed with a No. 15 blade (Fig. 35–10A). When this has been done, one should check very carefully that not a single portion of epithelium has been left, in order to avoid the occurrence of a dermal cyst in the postoperative period (Fig. 35–10B).

Except in the area of the areolar flap, the outer and inner line outlining the resection is incised down to the pectoral fascia (Fig. 35–11). The breast is elevated from this fascia up to a position a little higher than the new

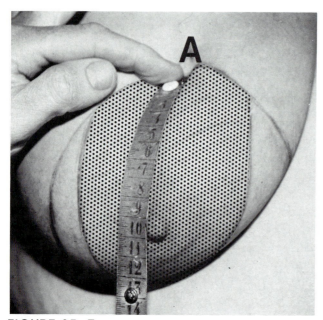

FIGURE 35–7
Measurement of the distance between the nipple and point A.

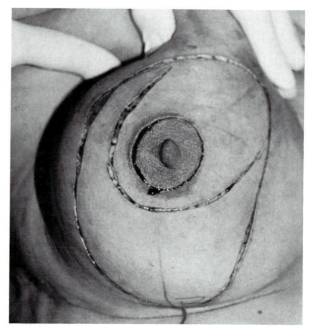

FIGURE 35–9
Superficial incision of the drawings.

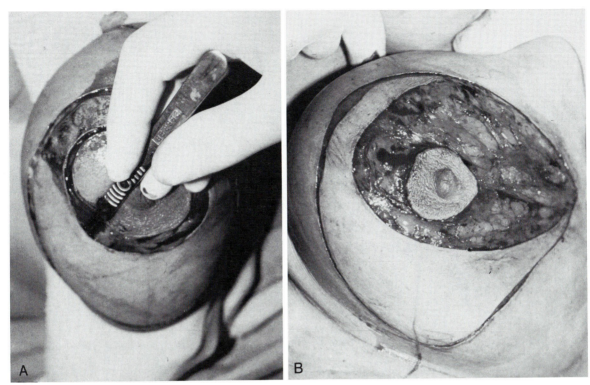

FIGURE 35–10
A and *B*, De-epithelialization of the areolar flap.

nipple level (Fig. 35–12). The inferior border of the areolar flap is cut down to a 5-cm depth (Fig. 35–13). From this level the glandular resection is performed beneath the areolar flap and leaves a glandular lining 0.5 cm thick (Fig. 35–14). This resection is carried out

as high as needed for achieving satisfactory volume (Fig. 35–15). Sometimes lateral tissue has to be resected to narrow a wide breast and to avoid bulging on the outer or inner side or on both sides of the breast.

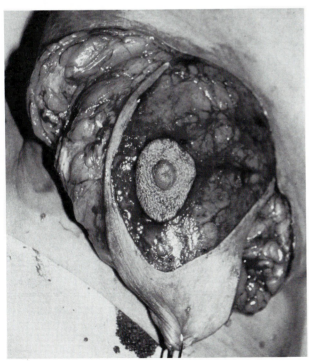

FIGURE 35–11
Incision of the lateral borders of the wedge resection down to the pectoral fascia.

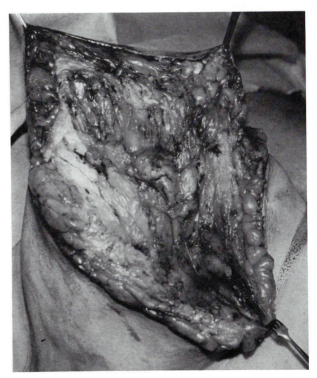

FIGURE 35–12
Elevation of a gland from the pectoral fascia from beneath to a position a little higher than the new nipple position.

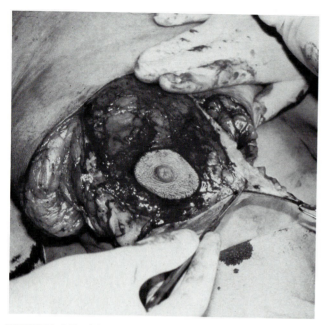

FIGURE 35–13
The inferior border of the areolar flap is cut down to a 5-cm depth.

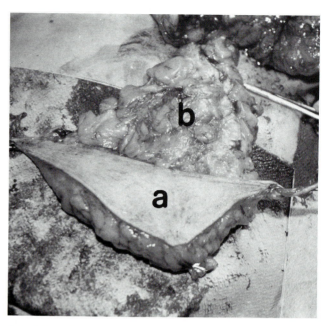

FIGURE 35–15
Piece of resection. *a*, Lower tissue resected *en bloc*. *b*, Upper tissue resected (fat and gland).

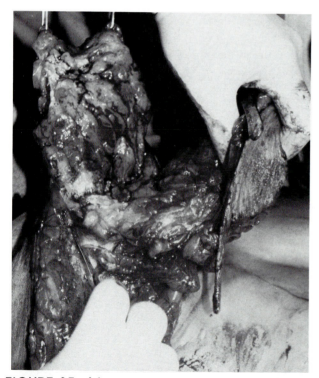

FIGURE 35–14
Glandular resection beneath the areolar flap.

Skin edges are now approximated by framing stitches going first downward and then upward (Fig. 35–16). This maneuver allows the checking of (1) the volume and (2) the shape. Sometimes they are both good, but more often it is necessary to check either the volume or the shape, or both, again.

When the resection has been insufficient, the suture lines are reopened and more is resected in the area where it is needed (Fig. 35–17). After resuturing, the shape is rechecked. If the shape is unsatisfactory (Fig. 35–18), the breast is reshaped with skin stitches (Fig. 35–19A). When good shape is obtained, this new suture line is marked with methylene blue (Fig. 35–19B). The stitches are cut, and the drawings on the skin mark the exact amount of the new resection to be done (Fig. 35–20).

Beforehand three or four lines are drawn on both sides; each line has a number, the same on the left as on the right (see Fig. 35–19B). This is very helpful. When the new resection has been completed, it is easy to reapproximate the skin edges, uniting 1 to 1, 2 to 2, 3 to 3, and 4 to 4. It saves time (Fig. 35–21A).

The operation is finished in the usual manner (Fig. 35–21B), with subcutaneous stitches to reapproximate the skin (I never reapproximate glandular edges) and an intradermal running suture to complete the suturing of the areola and of the skin. No drainage is used. It is unnecessary because there is no skin or glandular undermining (Fig. 35–22A and B).

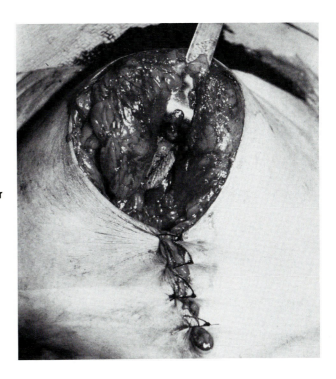

FIGURE 35–16
Approximation of the skin edges starting at the inferior position of the longitudinal incision.

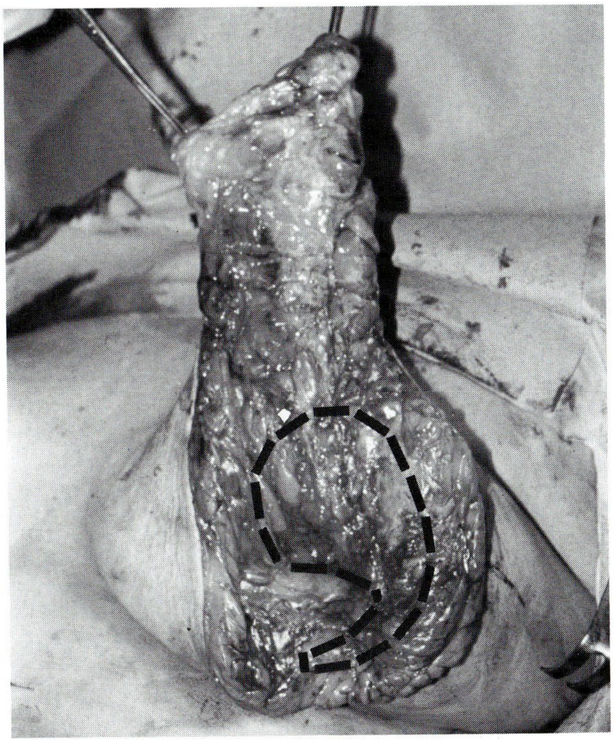

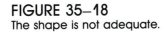

FIGURE 35–17
Outline of an additional resection to reduce the breast to the desired size and shape.

FIGURE 35–18
The shape is not adequate.

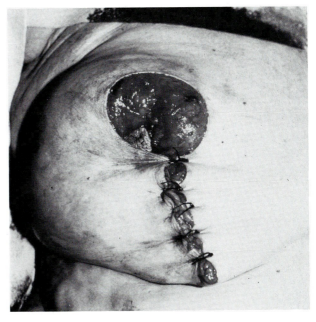

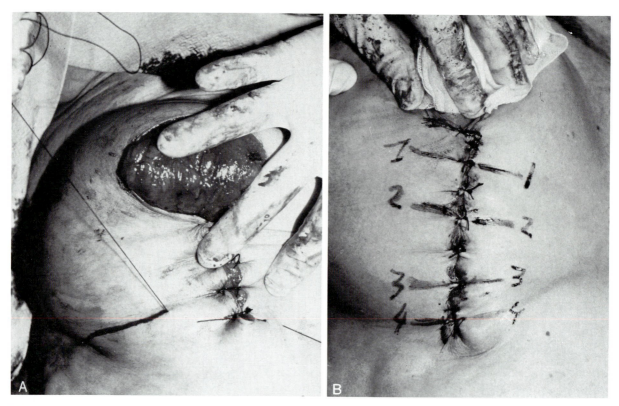

FIGURE 35–19

A and *B,* By this maneuver a good shape has been created. Methylene blue is applied along the new suture line, and horizontal lines are drawn, each having the same number on the left as on the right.

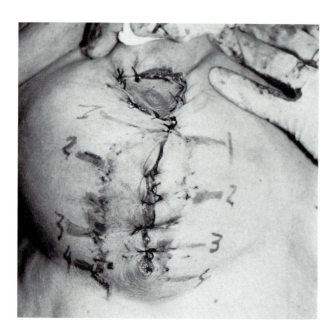

FIGURE 35–20

The new resection to be performed is marked.

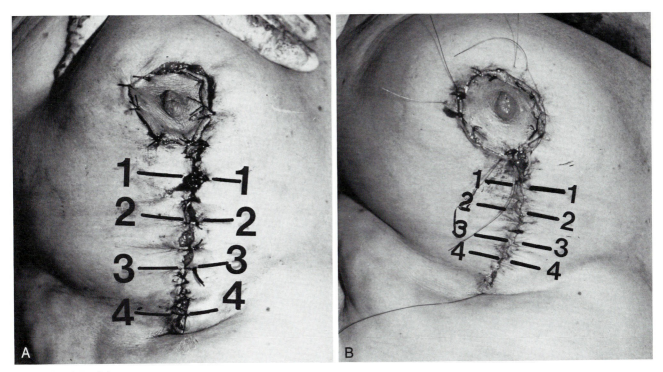

FIGURE 35–21

A, Easy approximation of skin edges uniting *1* to *1*, *2* to *2*, *3* to *3*, *4* to *4*. *B*, The operation is finished.

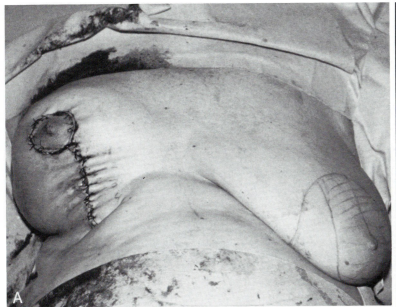

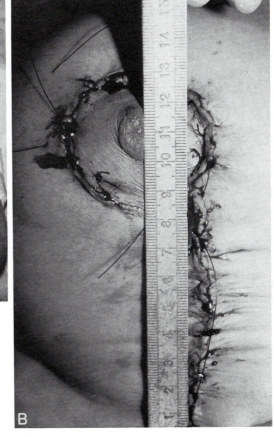

FIGURE 35–22

A, One side is completed. *B*, The length of the scar is 8.5 cm.

COMPLICATIONS

This procedure is very safe, for the following reasons:

1. The nipple-areola complex is transposed on a dermoglandular flap, which is very secure unless this complex has to move up more than 9 cm. At greater than this distance, it could be difficult and dangerous to use this superiorly based pedicle. A lateral pedicle is more adapted to this situation.
2. There is no skin undermining and no glandular undermining, which ensures that there is no hematoma and no infection postoperatively.

The possible complications are as follows:

1. Impending nipple necrosis.
   a. Some superficial incisions with a No. 15 blade in the blue areola are often sufficient to help the venous drainage and to obtain the recovery of adequate circulation in this area. Sometimes, however, this is not enough.
   b. Then all the stitches suturing the areola to the skin must be released, and the flap is left in a relaxed position for 2, 3, or 4 days to recover. It is possible to suture it again, with the patient under local anesthesia, 5, 6, or 7 days postoperatively (Fig. 35–23).
2. Hypertrophic scarring or keloid. This is generally foreseeable by observation of old scar sequelae. In young patients without any previous scars, hypertrophic scarring may occur after the operation. If it does, it is advantageous to have been able to reduce the breast by a single vertical scar. After 12 to 18 months a revision of the scar can be performed with the patient under local anesthesia. The revision may improve the scar at that time because there is less tension on the scar.
3. An inadequate volume. Some patients want a breast smaller than what was obtained by the operation. The volume can be reduced by performing a new wedge resection, removing skin, fat, and gland. During this step more can be removed from the lateral aspect of the breast. This is done without moving up the nipple, which is now in a normal position.
4. An inadequate shape. This can be corrected by the same technique I have described in the realization of the operation (see Fig. 35–19A). With some skin sutures the breast cone is reshaped. Methylene blue is applied along this new suture line. The stitches are cut. The exact amount to be resected is delineated, and an adequately shaped breast can be obtained (Fig. 35–24).
5. Too long a scar. When this occurs, it can be shortened by a triangular skin resection that ends in a short horizontal scar (Fig. 35–25).

POSTOPERATIVE CARE

The postoperative care is simple. The approximating stitches are removed around the fifth postoperative day, and the intradermal sutures are left for 2 weeks. After this period one can apply some Steri-Strip bandages to obtain a scar that is as inconspicuous as possible.

The initial shape of the breasts is rarely good. The patient must be informed before the operation that she may have to wait for 2 or 3 months before the breasts obtain a pleasant appearance. At first the nipples point downward. The upper part of the breast is bulging and the lower part of the breast is concave on the profile. But after 2 or 3 months, because of the weight of the breast, there is a transfer from the high to the low, and the form has improved. A brassiere or bandage is forbidden until the breast has achieved a satisfactory shape.

In summary, the patient must wait 2 or 3 months before the exact breast volume and shape are attained. Just after the operation the breast looks larger than it will be 3 months postoperatively. The patient should not be concerned if in the immediate postoperative period the shape is not ideal.

INDICATIONS

This procedure is mainly suitable for young patients with hypertrophy that will not need resection of more than 500 gm from each breast (Figs. 35–26 to 35–29).

In this case the result will be quite aesthetically pleasing because of the elasticity of the skin, which will contract nicely after the operation, and because of the predominant glandular texture of the breast.

The less there is to resect, the easier the procedure to be done. This is why I recommend when first performing this technique that one do so with mildly hypertrophic, ptotic breasts in young patients. When one becomes experienced in this approach, where no exact pattern can be followed until the end of the operation, it is possible to apply this procedure to large hypertrophic, ptotic breasts. In these cases it is somewhat more difficult to finish with a vertical scar above the new inframammary fold. The surgeon must want to achieve this goal as it is shown in the case used to demonstrate the technique (Fig. 35–30) and in another large breast (Fig. 35–31).

TYPE OF ANESTHESIA

It is important that the patient be operated on in a semi-sitting position. The procedure is carried out with the patient under general anesthesia after hydroxyzine (100 mg) has been injected intravenously 15 minutes before the operation. Then 1 to 2 mg of phenoperidine plus 5 to 10 mg of droperidol is injected intravenously. Two or 4 mg of flunitrazepan is injected intravenously within 30 seconds.

The patient is then intubated, and the anesthesia is conducted by inhalation of N_2O plus O_2 during the operation, which lasts generally 2 to 2½ hours.

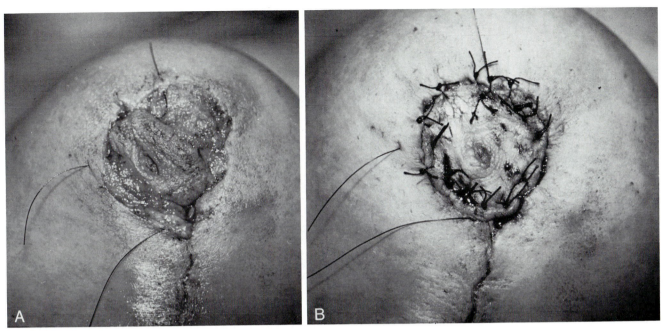

FIGURE 35–23
A, Stitches suturing the areola to the skin were released 5 days before. *B*, They are now sutured again under local anesthesia. The areola has fully recovered.

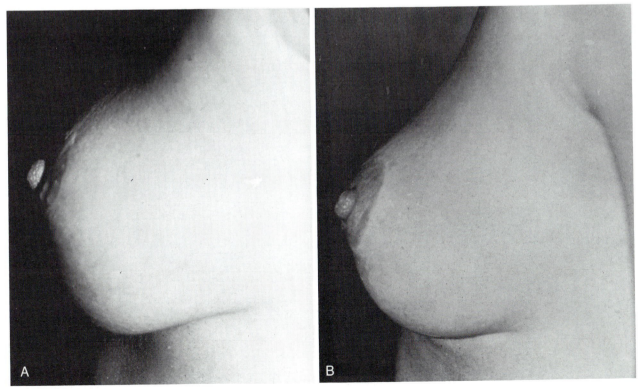

FIGURE 35–24
A, Poor shape after 3 months. *B*, Final result after correction according to the maneuver shown in Figure 35–19A.

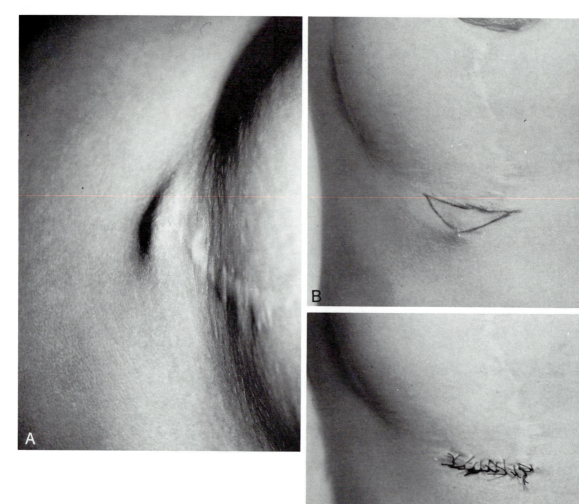

FIGURE 35–25
Correction of a too long scar. *A*, Long scar. *B*, Triangular skin resection. *C*, Final result.

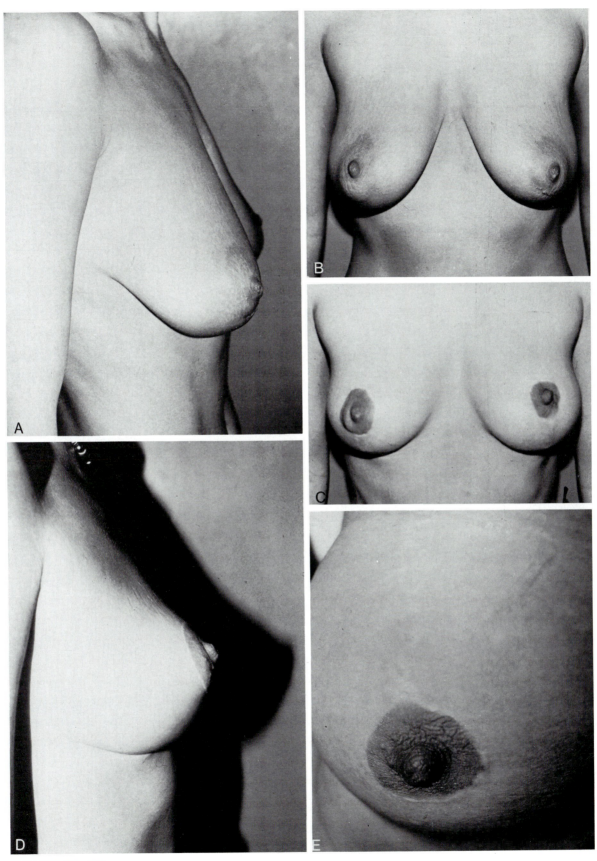

FIGURE 35–26
A and *B,* Before. *C* to *E,* After.

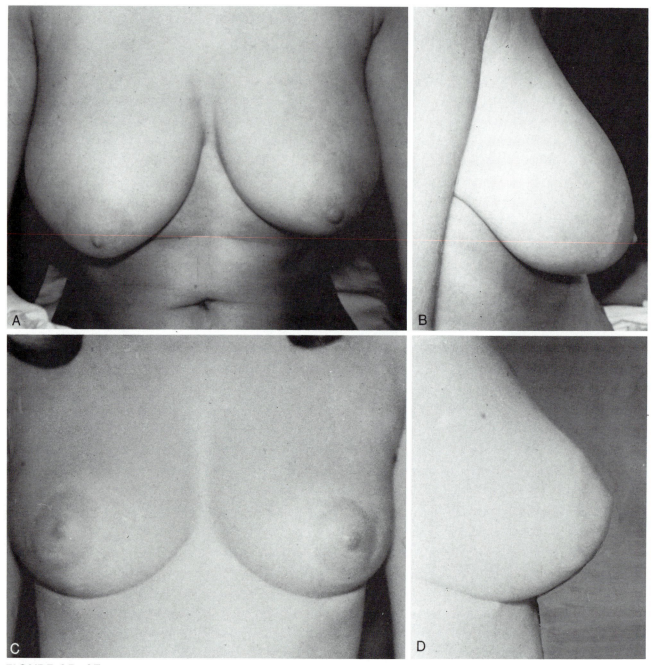

FIGURE 35–27
A and *B*, Before. *C* and *D*, After.

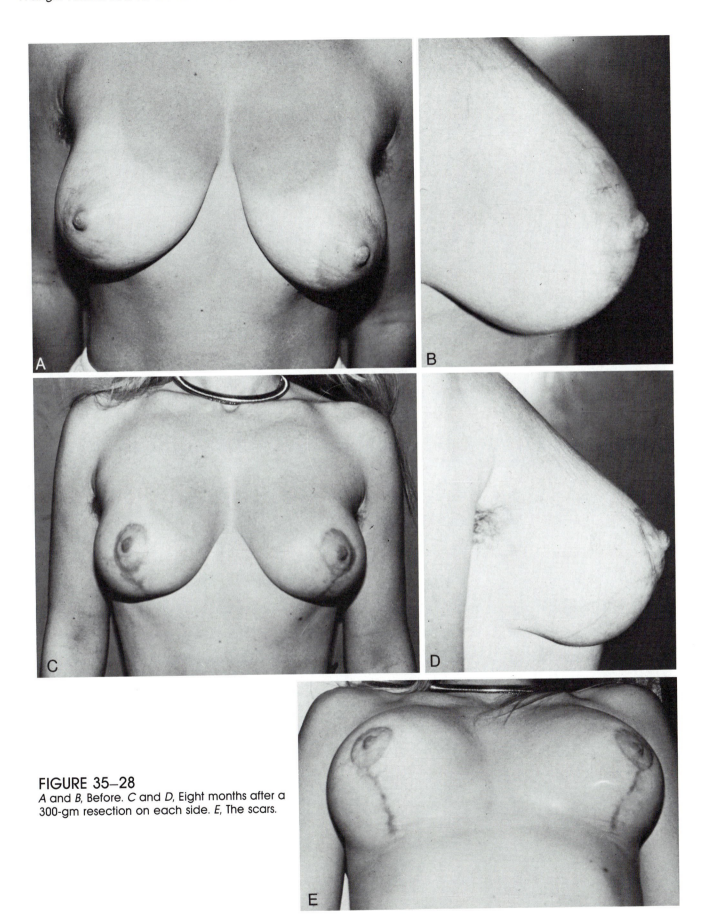

FIGURE 35–28
A and B, Before. C and D, Eight months after a
300-gm resection on each side. E, The scars.

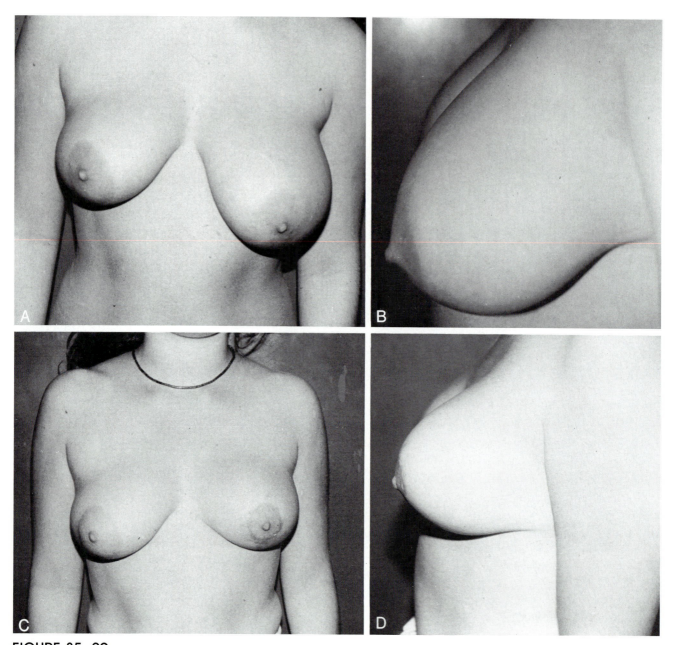

FIGURE 35–29
A and B, Asymmetry, before. C and D, After resection of 400 gm on the left side.

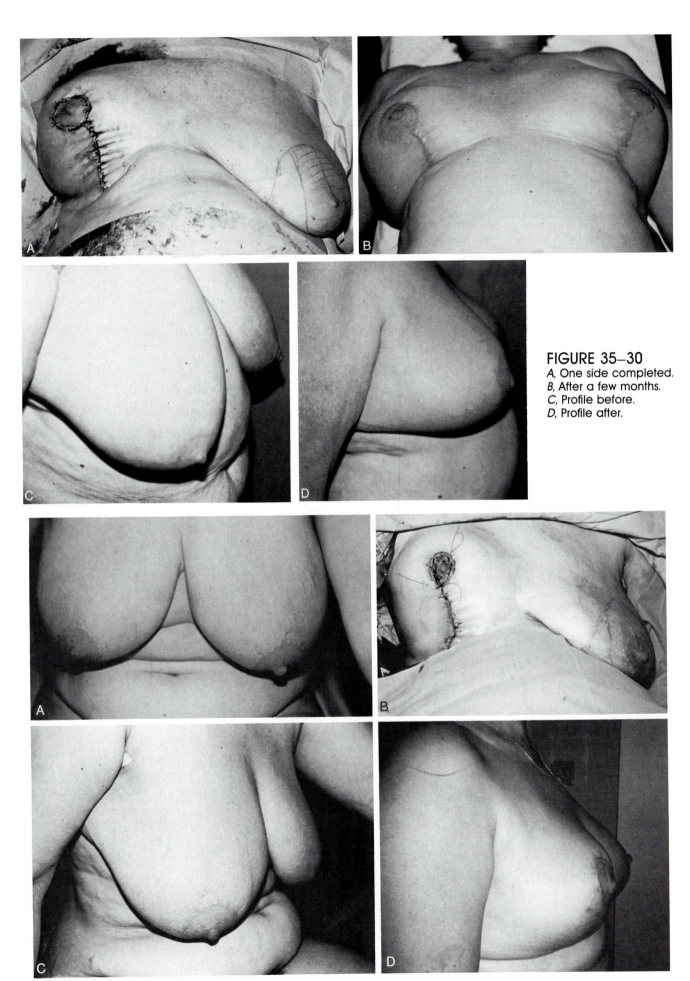

FIGURE 35–30
A, One side completed.
B, After a few months.
C, Profile before.
D, Profile after.

FIGURE 35–31
A, Before. B, One side completed. C, Profile before. D, Profile after.

465

References

Arié, G.: Una nueva técnica de mastoplastia. Rev. Latinoam. Cir. Plast. 3:23, 1957.

Balch, C. R.: The central mound technique for reduction mammoplasty. Plast. Reconstr. Surg. 67:305, 1981.

Bostwick, J., III: *Aesthetic and Reconstructive Breast Surgery.* St. Louis, C. V. Mosby, 1983.

Courtiss, E. H., Goldwyn, R. M.: Reduction mammaplasty by the inferior pedicle technique: An alternative to free nipple and areola grafting for severe macromastia or extreme ptosis. Plast. Reconstr. Surg. 59:500, 1979.

Durston, W.: Sudden and excessive swelling of a woman's breast. Phil. Trans. Royal Soc. London. 4th ed., 1731, p. 78.

Georgiade, N. G., Georgiade, G. S.: Hypermastia and ptosis. In: Georgiade, N. G., Georgiade, G. S., Riefkohl, R., Barwick, W. J. (eds.) *Essentials of Plastic, Maxillofacial and Reconstructive Surgery.* Baltimore, Williams & Wilkins, 1987, p. 694.

Georgiade, N. G., Serafin, D., Morris, R., Georgiade, G.: Reduction mammaplasty utilizing an inferior pedicle nipple-areolar flap. Ann. Plast. Surg. 3:211, 1979.

Georgiade, N. G., Serafin, D., Riefkohl, R., Georgiade, G. S.: Is there a reduction mammaplasty for "all seasons"? Plast. Reconstr. Surg. 63:765, 1979.

Goldwyn, R. M. (ed.): *Plastic and Reconstructive Surgery of the Breast.* Boston, Little, Brown, 1976.

Hallock, G. G., Cusenz, B. J.: Salvage of the congested nipple during reduction mammaplasty. Aesthetic Plast. Surg. 10:143, 1986.

Hauben, D. J.: Experience and refinements with the supero-medial dermal pedicle for nipple-areolar transposition in reduction mammoplasty. Aesthetic Plast. Surg. 8:189, 1984.

Hester, T. R., Jr., Bostwick, J., Miller, L., Cunningham, S. J.: Breast reduction utilizing the maximally vascularized central breast pedicle. Plast. Reconstr. Surg. 76:890, 1985.

Hoffman, S.: Recurrent deformities following reduction mammaplasty and correction of breast asymmetry. Plast. Reconstr. Surg. 78:55, 1986.

Lassus, C.: A technique for breast reduction. Int. Surg. 53:69, 1970.

Lassus, C.: New refinements in vertical mammaplasty. 2nd Congress Asian Section Int. Plast. Reconstr. Surg., Tokyo, 1977.

Lassus, C.: Minimal scarring in mammaplasty. 9 Tag. Ver Deutsch Plast. Chir., Cologne, 1978.

Lassus, C.: New Refinements in Vertical Mammaplasty. Chir. Plast. 6:81, 1981.

Lassus, C.: Treatment of impending nipple necrosis: A technical note. Chir. Plast. 8:117, 1985.

Lassus, C.: An "all season" mammoplasty. Aesthetic Plast. Surg. 10:9, 1986.

Lassus, C.: Breast reduction: Evolution of a technique—A single vertical scar. Aesthetic Plast. Surg. 11:107, 1987.

Marchac, D., de Olarte, G.: Reduction mammoplasty and correction of ptosis with a short inframammary scar. Plast. Reconstr. Surg. 69:45, 1982.

Mathes, S. J., Nahai, F., Hester, T. R.: Avoiding the flat breast in reduction mammaplasty. Plast. Reconstr. Surg. 66:63, 1980.

Moufarrège, R., Beauregard, G., Bosse, J. P., et al.: Reduction mammoplasty by the total dermoglandular pedicle. Aesthetic Plast. Surg. 9:227, 1985.

Peixoto, G.: Reduction mammaplasty: A personal technique. Plast. Reconstr. Surg. 65:217, 1980.

Peixoto, G.: The infra-areolar longitudinal incision in reduction mammoplasty. Aesthetic Plast. Surg. 9:1, 1985.

Pitanguy, I.: Breast hypertrophy. *Transactions of the International Society of Plastic Surgeons, Second Congress, London, 1959.* Edinburgh, Livingstone, 1960, p. 509.

Regnault, P.: Breast reduction: B technique. Plast. Reconstr. Surg. 65:840, 1980.

Skoog, T.: A technique of breast reduction. Acta Chir. Scand. 126:453, 1963.

Strömbeck, J. O.: Mammaplasty: Report of a new technique based on the two-pedicle procedure. Br. J. Plast. Surg. 13:79, 1960.

Strömbeck, J. O.: Reduction mammoplasty: Some observations, and some reflections. Aesthetic Plast. Surg. 7:249, 1983.

36

Gerardo Peixoto

Reduction Mammaplasty: Longitudinal Infra-areolar Incision

Today, in breast reduction surgery, perhaps young patients pay the highest price, in psychologic terms, to see their wishes come true in terms of adjustment in the size of their breasts.

Puberty, along with its various psychosomatic changes, promotes the beginning of breast development. These changes are a constant object of self-evaluation that continues through adolescence. Anomalies may appear during this period (asymmetry, hypertrophy, etc.), which assume a very important role, because the breasts emerge as a source of affirmation of femininity, and their perfection is fundamentally an aesthetic need. A problem is created when hypertrophy that demands surgery appears, for it is in young patients that most techniques do not give the desired results. In addition to large and unaesthetic scars, at times both sensitivity and physiology themselves suffer irreparable damage. The number of young patients, between 15 and 25 years of age, who have small, medium, or large hypertrophy and, at the same time, have skin of absolutely normal texture, is great. In these cases, the skin's elasticity has permitted the growth of mammary volume, preserving its anatomic and physiologic integrity. The observation of these facts led us to develop a method that at the same time uses the capacity of normal skin to contract and results in a smaller scar.

GENERAL CONSIDERATIONS

As we have observed, the amount of skin to be removed in reduction mammaplasty can vary from a considerable to a small amount, or may even be unnecessary (see Figs. 36–3 and 36–7). The circumstance of little or no skin removal occurs when the skin maintains its normal texture, even though the hypertrophy of the mammary gland has stretched it, but still conserves its anatomic and physiologic completeness, consequently maintaining its specific properties of elasticity and contractibility.

Such principles were used by us for decreasing the length of the incision in reduction mammaplasty in young patients (see Figs. 36–5 and 36–10). In these patients (15 to 25 years old) who present turgid breasts and unstriated skin still having a normal texture (see Fig. 36–1), we can remove either a small amount of skin or none at all. After the removal of the excess content,

the skin tends to gradually retract over the remaining framework.

The skin's ability to expand and contract has been widely observed. During gestation, the abdomen stretches amply and, if the structure of the skin is not disrupted, retracts completely, returning to its original state. This also occurs in cases of liposuction carried out on different areas of the human body. The procedure is followed by skin retraction proportional to the quality of the skin. The ever more frequent use of expanders utilizes this property of skin tissue in a very advantageous way.

Our concept takes into account the whole breast and considers the following factors.

Age. The method is indicated most for young, nulliparous patients (between 15 and 25 years of age), when the hypertrophy exists in conjunction with an elastic, normal skin and strong Cooper's ligaments and with the effects of gravity in stable equilibrium.

Skin. It should have normal structure with absence of striae, maintaining all its anatomic and physiologic characteristics, so that it still possesses all its specific properties of contractibility and elasticity, which will permit its later retraction over the remaining framework (see Figs. 36–15 and 36–16).

Content. In these cases, the content is predominantly glandular, and the breasts should have visual and tactile turgidity. Because the breast is similar to the geometric figure of a cone, the amputation of its base permits the obtainment of a cone of smaller proportions (see Fig. 36–12), which will result in an absolutely normal final appearance. The skin will retract over the contents. The retraction of the skin will occur gradually, and its final adaptation will be completed in approximately 1 to 3 months, sometimes a little longer, depending on the size of the breast. The size of the areola also decreases, accompanying the retraction of the cutaneous tissue.

Blood Supply. The blood supply to the breast is furnished principally by the lateral thoracic artery, a branch of the axillary, and by the internal mammary artery, a branch of the subclavian, and secondarily by intercostal penetrating branches and by terminal branches of the thoracoacromial artery. The principal trunks of these arteries, as well as their corresponding veins, are located in the subcutaneous cellular tissues, thus being preserved during the reduction of the content (see Fig. 36–13).

Innervation. Because there is no skin resection at the level of the areola and nipple, and the reduction of the contents is restricted to glandular tissue, there is no possibility of damage to the motor and sensitive innervation of the breast.

Disposition of the Mammary Tissue. The breast has a greater quantity of glandular tissue in its external quadrants (see Fig. 36–11). This disposition should be maintained during the resection of the excess, and we accomplish this by drawing an oblique line with more external tissue (see Fig. 36–13).

Preservation of Mammary Function. The function of the breast is perfectly preserved, because only the base of the gland is amputated (see Fig. 36–14), all of its forward portion remaining intact.

Morphologic Aspect. The amputation of the base of the mammary cone permits the breast to retain all of its individual characteristics of form, having only its volume reduced and the abnormal ptosis eliminated. We say "abnormal" because every breast, because of its weight and means of attachment to the thoracic wall, has a small subsidence that results in a slight bulging of the inferior pole, the natural conformation of the organ.

Breast Placement. The normal placement of the breast in relation to the thorax depends on the stable equilibrium between content and skin (see Fig. 36–2).

Scar. The scar, which follows the markings shown in Figures 36–5 and 36–10, is small and longitudinal, starting at the base of the areola and ending 1 cm above the inframammary fold. It is located completely within the cutaneous area of the gland, which generally produces a good aesthetic result, many times becoming nearly imperceptible with the passing of the years. On the contrary, the horizontal incision frequently results in an unsightly scar (see Fig. 36–18).

SURGICAL TECHNIQUE

Markings

During the first examination of the patient, we normally determine which of the two markings (see Figs. 36–5 and 36–10) will be used. In surgery, with the patient under general anesthesia, through bidigital pinching of the inferior pole, we check whether it will be necessary or not to remove skin tissue. If so, we proceed with the pinching (see Figs. 36–3 and 36–6) and determine two points. From these two points we establish two more internal parallel points, approximately 0.5 cm inward from those first established. These latter

points will furnish the greater transverse diameter of the ellipse, which goes from the areola to a point 1 cm from the inframammary fold. The reason for this 1-cm difference is that when skin must be removed in the inferior pole, it exists above this point (see Fig. 36–4).

Surgical Procedure

With the patient supine and under general anesthesia, we make an incision according to the selected marking. The breast is drawn upward by a strong hook placed in the skin immediately above the areola. The gland is completely separated from the thoracic wall. After hemostasis, with the gland still in the drawn position, we measure the height of the glandular tissue to be preserved. This calculation is made from a point located at the inferior base of the nipple, going downward 5 to 7 cm, according to the wish of the surgeon with respect to the new breast. Once the height of resection has been calculated, the excess glandular tissue is severed in an oblique transverse line that starts at the external median line and goes to the anterior axillary line (see Fig. 36–13). This oblique line permits the maintenance of a greater quantity of glandular tissue in the external quadrants, which preserves the characteristics of the organ and its accommodation on the thorax (see Fig. 36–20B). The complete amputation of the base is executed by obeying a line that, in relation to the skin, gives the aspect of a triangle with an anterior base (see Fig. 36–15). Depending on the type of glandular tissue (whether rigid or malleable), an interior suturing is executed without fixing the gland to the thoracic wall.

At the end of the operation, the breast may have an excellent contour or it may have smaller or greater distortions. These distortions may be more frequent in cases with large resections and will gradually disappear with the evolution of the skin retraction process, which can last from 1 to 3 months, and sometimes longer.

Complications

Our patients have never experienced complications directly attributable to the method. We enumerate, however, some precautions that should be taken in order to prevent any possible minor problems:

1. Seek to avoid excessive trauma to the borders of the skin of the surgical incision during the introduction and removal of compresses during hemostasis. Trauma could produce mini-necrotic areas, which could hinder the quality of the future scar.
2. Observe the quantity and symmetry of the remaining tissue in both breasts with the utmost care in order to ensure perfect postoperative symmetry.
3. Do not fix the gland to the thoracic wall. The gradual skin retraction will place it in its normal position.
4. Internal suturing should only be done when the glandular tissue does not have sufficient turgidity.

Text continued on page 482

FIGURE 36–1

Large hypertrophic breasts with normal skin texture. The specific properties of elasticity and contractibility are preserved. This is an example of an ideal case for this method.

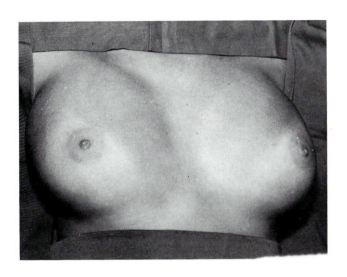

FIGURE 36–2

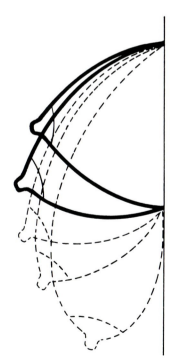

The normal placement of the breast in relation to the thorax depends on the stable content/skin equilibrium. When the breast volume increases and the skin maintains its strength, the equilibrium remains. In this case, when the contents are removed, the skin (black lines) will retract spontaneously. Irreversible progressive ptosis occurs when the skin partially loses its capacity for retraction as a result of breakdown of its elastic fibers.

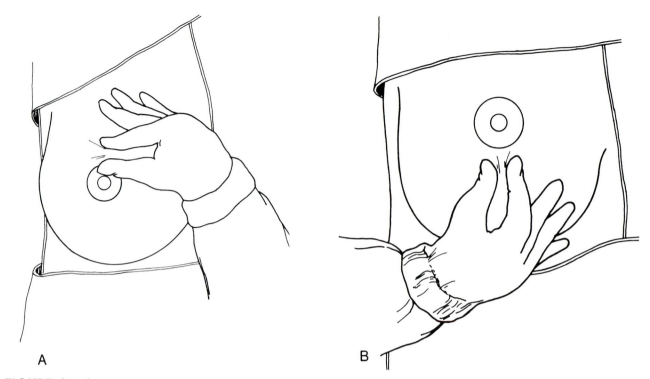

A   B

FIGURE 36–3
A and *B,* Digital pinching in the superior and inferior poles reveals that there is no skin to remove.

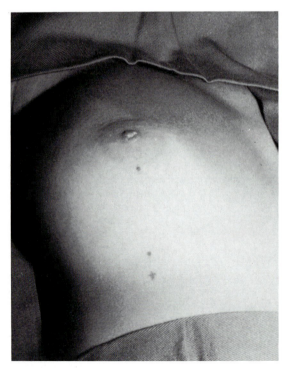

FIGURE 36–4
The superior dot is on the inferior limit of the areola. The inferior dot is on the inframammary fold. The medial dot is 1 cm above the fold.

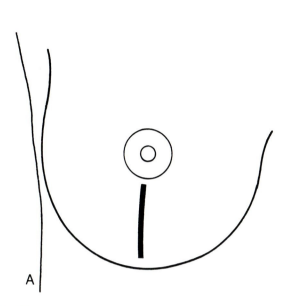

FIGURE 36–5
A and *B*, Diagram and intraoperative markings.

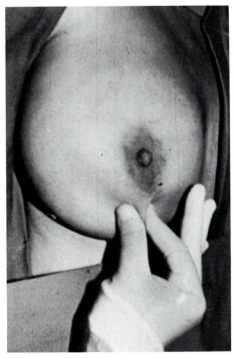

FIGURE 36–6
Bidigital pinching reveals that there is skin to remove.

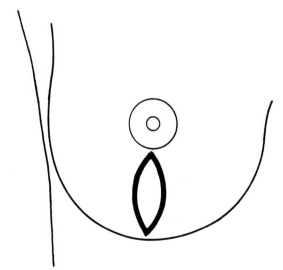

FIGURE 36–7
Design used when there is skin to remove.

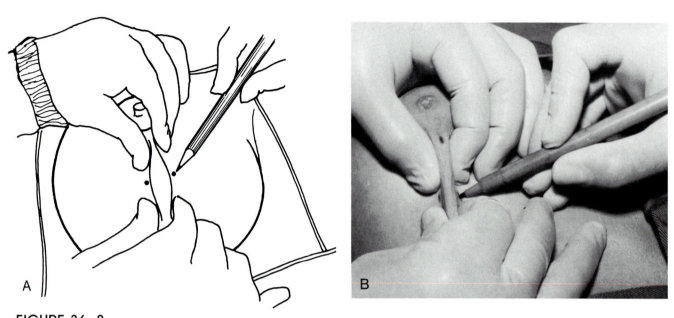

FIGURE 36–8
A and *B,* With bidigital pinching, using two hands, one can determine the amount of excess skin. A dot is placed on each side.

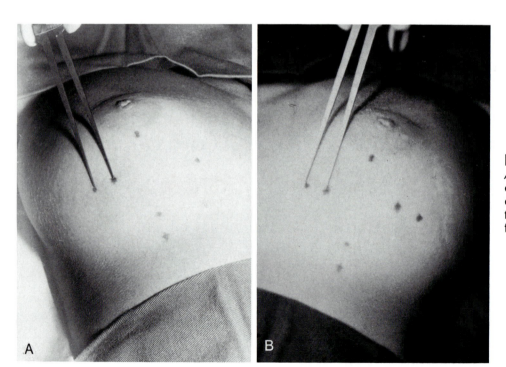

FIGURE 36–9
A and *B,* Using a compass, one can make the internal dots (1 cm inside), to allow for the skin that remains between the fingers.

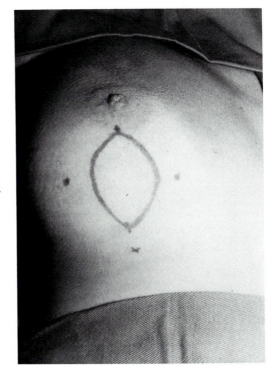

FIGURE 36–10
The dots are connected, forming an ellipse.

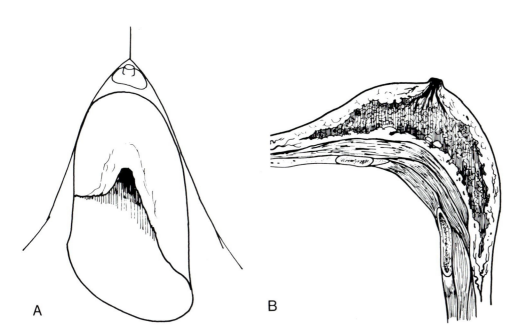

A

B

FIGURE 36–11
A, Diagram showing the normal predominance of adipoglandular tissue in the external quadrants. *B,* Another design showing the natural accommodation on the thoracic wall.

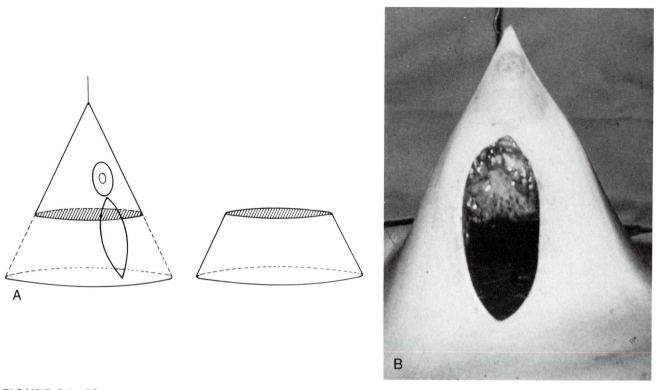

FIGURE 36–12
A and *B*, The mammary gland has a shape that resembles the geometric figure of a cone. The best way to reduce the breast is to amputate the base of the cone.

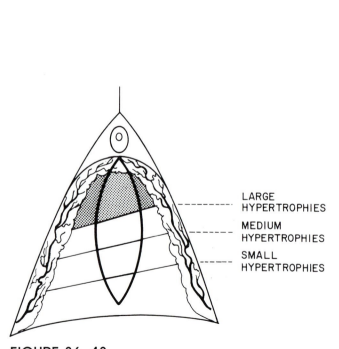

FIGURE 36–13
Diagram showing the levels for resection of the adipoglandular tissue in large, medium, and small hypertrophy. The principal blood supply is preserved. The oblique line of resection can be observed.

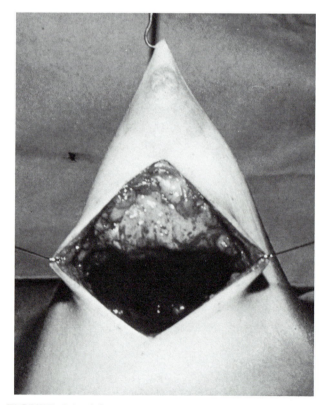

FIGURE 36–14
The skin pulled laterally to show a wide surgical focus, in which there is little difficulty in carrying out resection and hemostasis.

FIGURE 36–15

Skin retraction and fixation of the base on the thoracic wall. A, With amputation of the base and inferior pole. B, With only the base amputated.

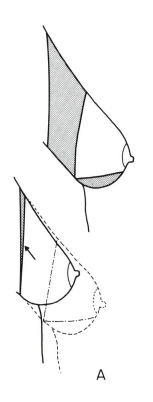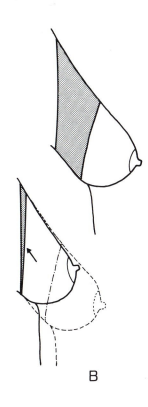

A

B

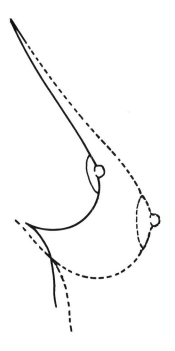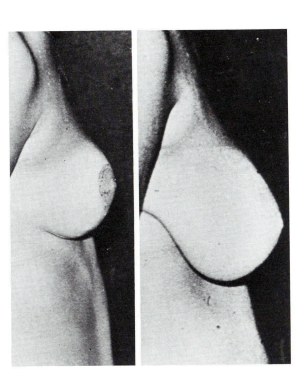

FIGURE 36–16

After the retraction there is a smaller breast with a natural shape.

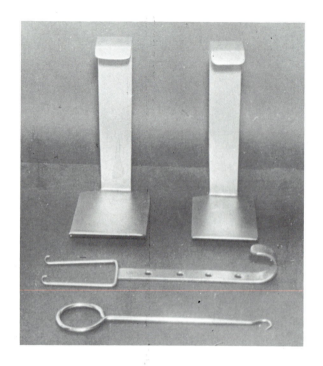

FIGURE 36–17
Set of complementary instruments for the operation. The two spreaders are of our own design. The blade of the smaller one is 7 × 4 cm; the larger one, 8 × 5 cm. A double hook and a "jaw hook," already mentioned in the text, are shown.

FIGURE 36–18
A and *B*, Examples of mammaplasties with inverted-T incisions. In both cases a marked difference can be seen between the longitudinal and the horizontal scar. The longitudinal scar is nearly imperceptible.

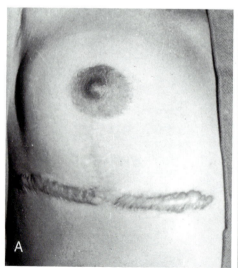

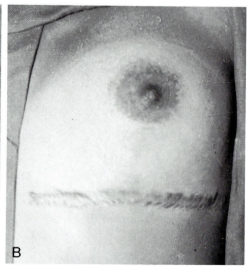

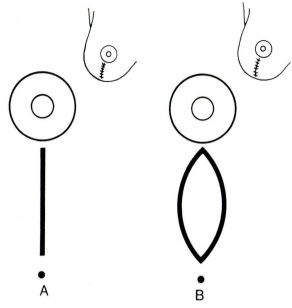

FIGURE 36–19
A and *B,* The design of the markings and the final suture of the incision.

A   B

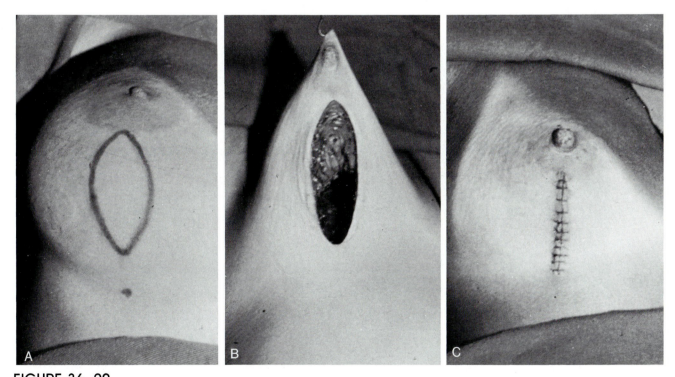

A   B   C

FIGURE 36–20
A, Skin demarcation chosen. *B,* Resection showing the base of the breast amputated following an oblique line, thus leaving more tissue in the gland's external quadrants. *C,* Final result.

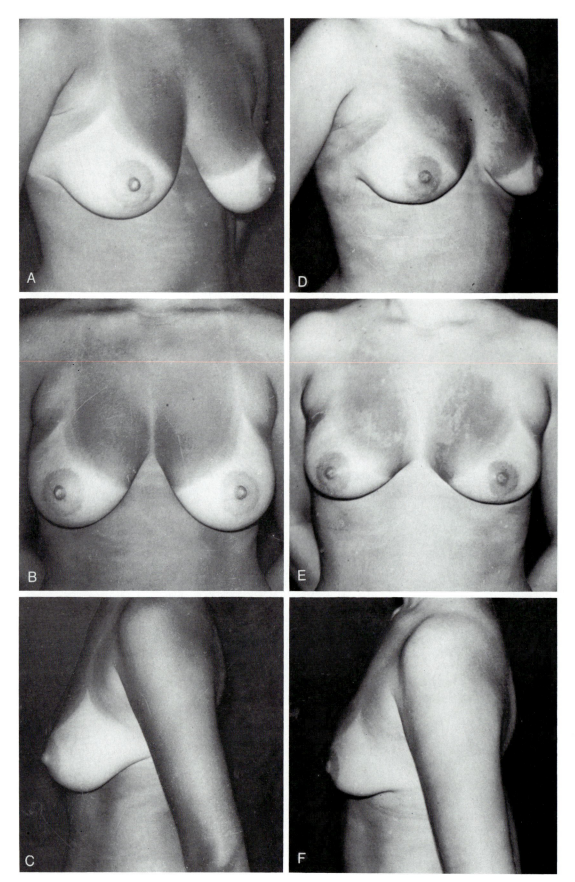

FIGURE 36–21

A to *F*, A 17-year-old patient with medium hypertrophy. Preoperative views and postoperative views, 6 months after surgery.

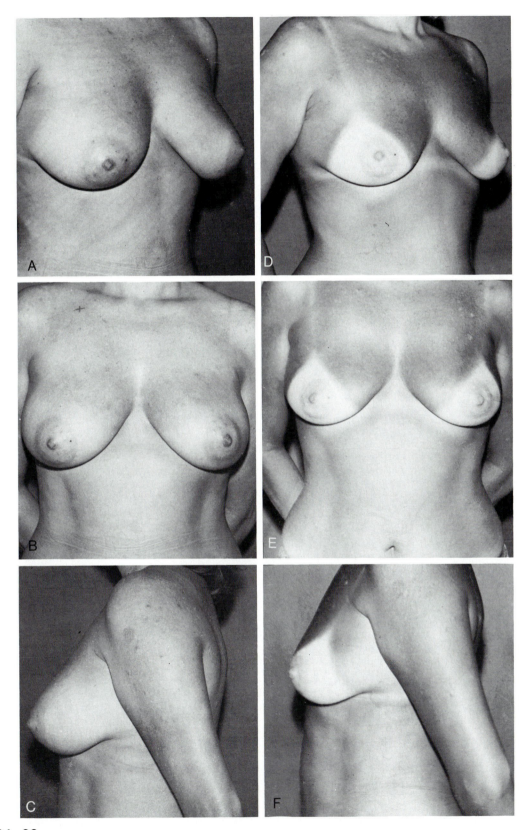

FIGURE 36–22
A to *F,* A 20-year-old patient with medium hypertrophy. Preoperative views and postoperative views, 2 years after surgery.

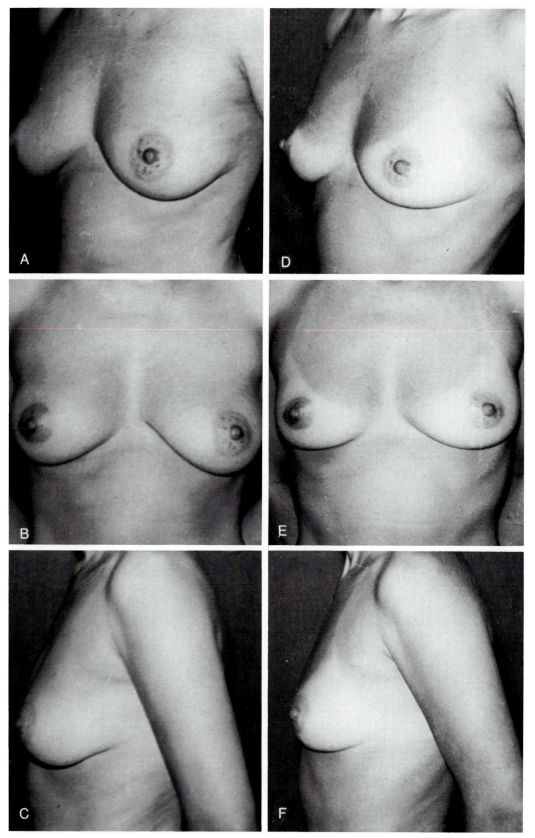

FIGURE 36–23
A to F, A 22-year-old patient with medium hypertrophy. Preoperative views and postoperative views, 3 years after surgery.

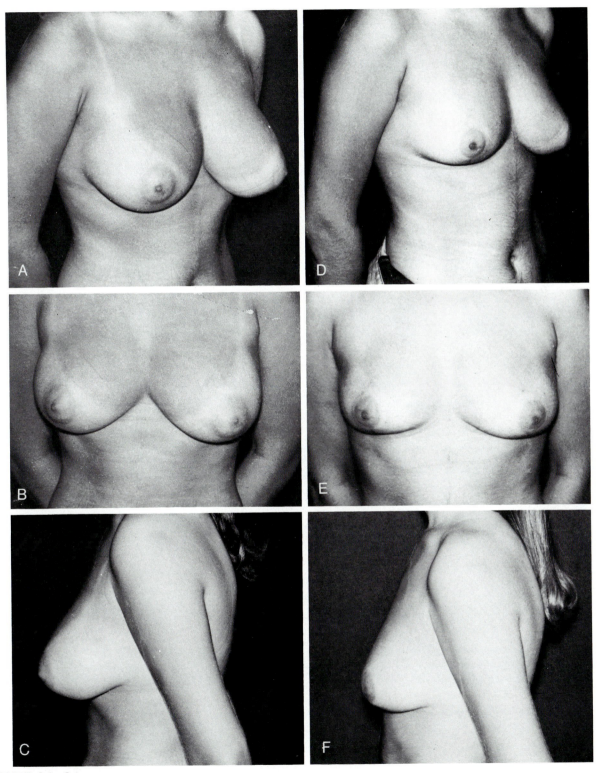

FIGURE 36–24

A to *F,* A 20-year-old patient with large hypertrophy. Preoperative views and postoperative views, 2 years after surgery.

CONCLUSION

We believe that this method is an excellent solution for selected patients. It is important to remember that it is indicated for patients of an age group in which the total functional correction and aesthetic aspect of the organ are of utmost importance. Neither should it be forgotten that it is precisely in these cases that the results obtained by the use of the usual techniques present the greatest problems.

References

Arié, G.: Una nueva técnica de mastoplastia. Rev. Latinoam. Cir. Plast. 3:23, 1957.

Lassus, C.: Breast reduction: Evolution of a technique: A single vertical scar. Aesthetic Plast. Surg. 11:107, 1987.

Longis, E.: Mammaplasty with an L-shaped limited scar and retropectoral dermopexy. Aesthetic Plast. Surg. 10:3, 1986.

Maillard, G. F.: A Z-mammoplasty with minimal scarring. Plast. Reconstr. Surg. 77:66, 1986.

Maliniac, J. W.: Arterial blood supply of the breast. Arch. Surg. 47:329, 1943.

Morestin, H., Guinard, A.: Hypertrophie mammaire traitée par la résection discoide. Bull. et Mém. Soc. de Chir. de Paris 33:649, 1907.

Peixoto, G.: Reduction mammaplasty: A personal technique. Plast. Reconstr. Surg. 65:217, 1980.

Peixoto, G.: Reduction mammaplasty. Aesthetic Plast. Surg. 8:231, 1984.

Peixoto, G.: The infra-areolar longitudinal incision in reduction mammaplasty. Aesthetic Plast. Surg. 9:1, 1985.

Pena, M. T., Barraguer, E. L., Perez, A. R.: Reduction mammaplasty: Personal considerations. Cir. Plast. Ibero-Lat. Am. XIV:3, 1988.

Pitanguy, I.: Breast hypertrophy. *Transactions of the International Society of Plastic Surgeons, Second Congress, London, 1959,* Edinburgh, Livingstone, 1960, p. 509.

Salmon, M.: Les artères de la glande mammaire. Ann. Anat. Pathol. 16:477, 1939.

37

Daniel Marchac

Mammaplasty with a Short Horizontal Scar

Since 1977 I have been using a technique derived from several different techniques in an effort to overcome some of their shortcomings.

In the beginning of my plastic surgery training, in the 1960s, I was first taught by Claude Dufourmentel (1961) to utilize his lateral oblique method. The approach was a large ellipse, starting around the areola medially and going laterally and obliquely downward to the lower part of the axilla.

Through this approach a wide skin dissection was carried out to expose the gland for performing a Biesenberger (1928) type of remodeling, that is, a resection and plication on itself of the gland, the vascularization being obtained through deep vessels from the thoracic wall.

This technique allowed beautiful remodeling of the breast tissue but was dangerous because it compromised the blood supply. I still remember painfully one of my first cases as resident, in which areolar necrosis occurred in a lovely young girl. Dufourmentel abandoned this Biesenberger glandular approach and started to resect a lateral wedge of gland, freeing the gland from the pectoralis fascia, but with no more extensive skin undermining. The procedure was much safer and simpler.

Nevertheless, in my hands, the results were not satisfactory. Too often the breasts were too close to each other and the nipples medially positioned. Some results were excellent, but many were not. There seemed to be no predictability. The only constantly satisfactory results were obtained with pure ptosis, but the lateral scar was often too conspicuous.

After the introduction of Pitanguy's (1967) technique, I started using Pitanguy's technique and obtained good results in terms of consistency, shape, and size. However, I was dissatisfied with the long horizontal scar, especially the medial part.

Lalardrie and Jouglard (1974) presented a new technique based on the preservation of a disk of glandular tissue beneath and centered by the areola, nourished by the superficial subdermal vessels. There was no skin undermining, but a vast de-epithelialization around the areola and a remodeling of the remaining skin with an inverted-T scar. Because a great amount of skin was removed around the areola, the horizontal scar was shorter, but the periareolar scar was not satisfactory in my experience. Too much tension resulted in spreading of the areola and/or a distended scar.

My idea was to utilize the Dufourmentel principle of an elliptical excision, but putting it vertically instead of laterally. It would then go beyond the inframammary fold as in the Arié technique (Arié, 1957). To avoid this, I decided to interrupt the wedge by a horizontal incision, which resulted in an inverted T. By positioning this horizontal incision well above the inframammary line, I was able to achieve a very short horizontal line and to suture the skin, especially around the areola, with limited tension.

This approach has proven satisfactory over the years. Because it was different from the usual methods, and required perhaps more surgical judgment during the operation, it raised initially little interest: "Why bother so much about scars? The important thing is to get a nice shape," was what I heard frequently. Now, the demands evolving, the residual scars have become more of a problem, and a technique minimizing the scars has become more appealing. It is obvious that shape and stability should not be sacrificed for obtaining shorter scars, but experience since 1977 has shown that this technique is able to produce a nice-looking and stable breast with short scars of good quality.

It must be stressed that this technique is especially indicated in ptosis correction and moderate reduction (up to 500 gm per breast).

DESCRIPTION OF THE METHOD

The general principle is that of a vertical wedge excision. The following limits are marked with the patient in a semi-sitting position on the table (Fig. 37–1):

1. The vertical axis of the breast, that is, the line on which one wishes to place the areola and the vertical part of the inverted T. This is determined by lifting the breast by the upper part and placing the areola in the desired position. The vertical axis is usually 9 to 10 cm from the midline.
2. The lateral sides of the wedge. The breast is pushed medially and laterally, gently, and one draws a line in continuity with the axis of the breast line. The width thus obtained is verified by pinching the area between the fingers.

483

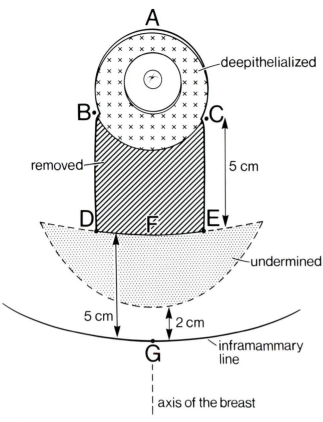

FIGURE 37–1
The width of the excision depends on the laxity and sagging of the breast. The horizontal lower incision is normally 5 cm above the inframammary level (see text), but the hatched area located below it shows the skin area removed at the final adjustment (see Fig. 5), and 2 cm or less is the real elevation of the inframammary fold.

3. The upper limit of the skin incision, a gentle curve passing about 1 cm above the areola.
4. The lower limit, a horizontal line placed well above the inframammary line, usually at 5 cm, or less in the case of small reduction or ptosis correction.

Symmetry is carefully checked. The distances between the midclavicular point and the nipples are compared, and a scale is tattooed on the patient with surgical ink at 18, 16, 14 cm to ensure similar levels on both sides (Fig. 37–2). The areola is marked (3, 4, or 5 cm in diameter), and de-epithelialization is performed around it up to the incision lines.

The skin incision is made on the vertical lines and on the horizontal one. At this lower level a subcutaneous dissection is performed down to the inframammary line and then upward, behind the gland and in front of the pectoralis major. This dissection of the posterior aspect of the gland must be generous, especially superiorly, to allow it to be elevated.

In case of breast hypertrophy, a full-thickness glandular resection is performed along the vertical lines, in continuity with the full-thickness skin incision. About 2 cm below the areola, an incision is performed for about 2 cm deep. The surgeon then excises glandular tissue

below the areola, being careful to keep an even thickness of 1.5 to 2 cm beneath the areola. If necessary, more gland can be excised laterally, at the deep aspect.

Suspension of the gland to the aponeurosis of the pectoralis major is the next step: a 2-0 absorbable suture is placed at the upper limit of the thoracic undermining and at the posterior aspect of the gland, approximately 2 cm above the areola. This suspension stitch should be carefully placed on the axis of the breast. When it is tied, adequate noticeable bulging must be obtained at the upper part of the breast. The areola should not be retracted.

Glandular vertical suturing is very important. It provides a lower buttress that will support the gland and reconstruct a conical breast. The two lateral glandular columns corresponding to the vertical cuts are sutured in several layers, which brings together the attached skin (Fig. 37–3).

In case of pure ptosis, the breast tissue is vertically split up to the areola. The two halves are overlapped, and the lateral is put usually under the medial one.

The dermal layer of skin on the segment BC to CD is then sutured, and the new inframammary line shows itself if the width of the resection was well calculated (Fig. 37–4).

A horizontal incision is performed, slightly longer on the lateral side, 2 to 4 cm medially and 3 to 5 cm laterally. A lower quadrangular skin flap is created (Fig. 37–5). Its base is transected by the shortest possible line between the two ends of the horizontal incision.

The new inframammary line—1 to 2 cm above the previous one—should now be precisely defined by careful subcutaneous defatting and resection of the gland that could slide below the new inframammary line. If the vertical glandular suture has been well done, and with the help of the superior suspension, the breast tissue remains easily above the inframammary fold.

The areola is then adjusted. Sometimes it is possible to suture it to the edges of the de-epithelialized area. If

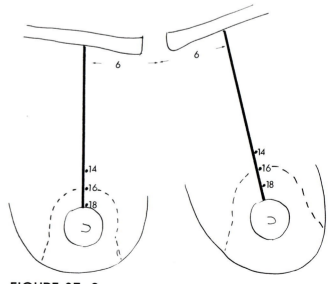

FIGURE 37–2
A tattooed scale is used above the areola to ensure symmetry.

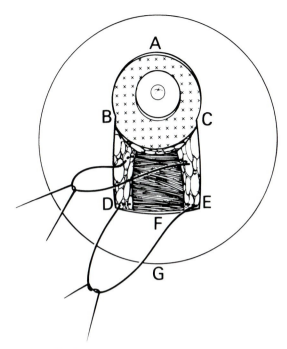

FIGURE 37-3
After suspension to the pectoral fascia has been performed, the suture of the glandular pillars is a fundamental step in reconstructing a glandular cone. This suture should be done with a strong absorbable stitch in several layers and will bring together skin that is not undermined. This suture should be low, bringing points D and E into contact.

one feels that there is a remaining skin excess around the areola, a suture is passed at the limit of the de-epithelialization and tied loosely, as if one is closing a purse, until suitable skin tension is obtained.

A 3.5-cm circle is marked, with 4.5 to 5 cm kept on

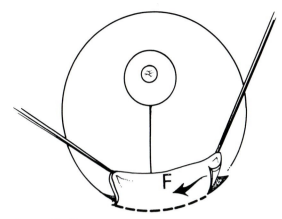

FIGURE 37-5
An incision as short as possible connects, across the lower flap, the two ends of the previous horizontal incision (note point F).

the vertical line; and this area is de-epithelialized. A suction drain is inserted, and the final suturing is performed. We use interrupted absorbable stitches on the dermis and an intradermal 3-0 Prolene for final approximation with generous skin-strip taping.

It is then important to exert pressure on the empty skin pocket existing between the new and the old inframammary folds. A brassiere with a wide lower strip is the best choice. If a brassiere is not available, a pressure dressing is applied for 24 hours, to be replaced by the brassiere. This brassiere will be worn continuously for 2 weeks, until the sutures are removed, and then during the day for another 6 weeks.

RESULTS AND COMPLICATIONS

In a review of 176 patients operated on, with complete data, examined after a minimum of 1 year after surgery, the aesthetic result of the operation has been judged satisfactory in most cases (Table 37–1) (Figs. 37–6 and 37–7). The horizontal scar remains hidden below the breast in the standing patient in most cases; the lateral scar is visible for 2 to 3 cm in some very large reductions (Table 37–2).

The stability, evaluated in 51 cases reviewed 4 years or more after surgery, has been excellent. The result has been maintained or has even improved—in comparison with the first postoperative year—in most cases (Table 37–3; Fig. 37–8). Sensitivity of the areola has been preserved or very moderately diminished.

Complications have been minimal. No areolar or glandular necrosis has been observed. Two hematomas necessitated evacuation.

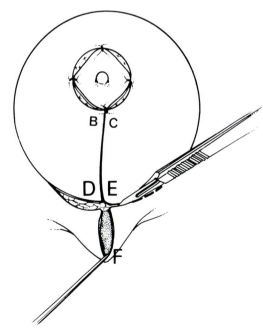

FIGURE 37-4
After dermal suturing of line BC, DE, the new inframammary line shows itself. A horizontal incision is made, 2 to 3 cm medially and 3 to 4 cm laterally.

TABLE 37-1
Evaluation of Aesthetic Results of 176 Patients

| | RESULT | | | |
	Excellent	Good	Mediocre	Bad
Ptosis	44	20	4	—
Moderate hypertrophy	50	20	6	—
Hypertrophy above 500 gm	19	11	2	—

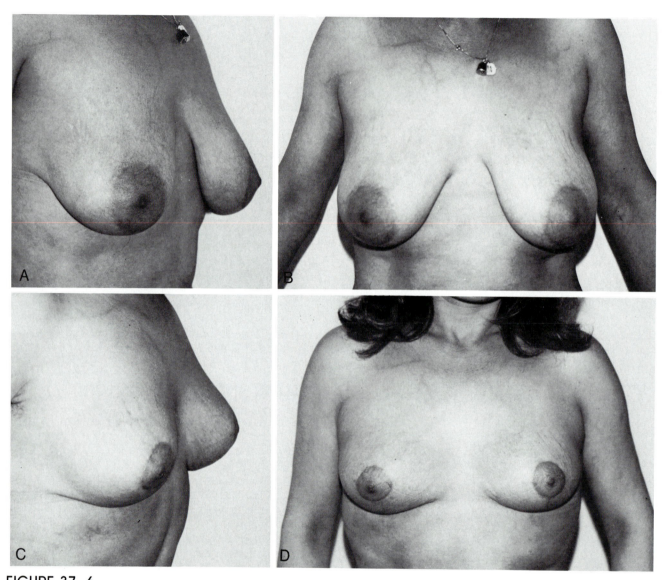

FIGURE 37–6
A and *B,* A 35-year-old patient with moderate hypertrophy and severe ptosis. *C* and *D,* The same patient 10 months after surgery.

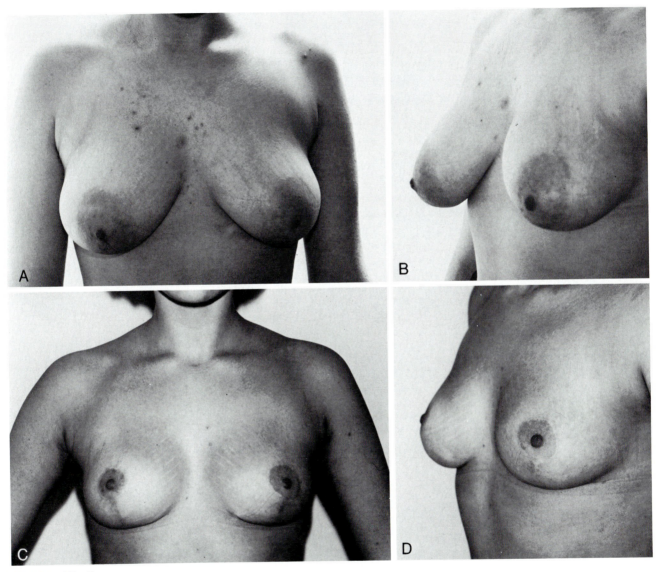

FIGURE 37–7
A and *B*, A 20-year-old patient with medium hypertrophy and severe ptosis. *C* and *D*, The same patient 6 months after operation. The horizontal scar remains hidden under the breast.

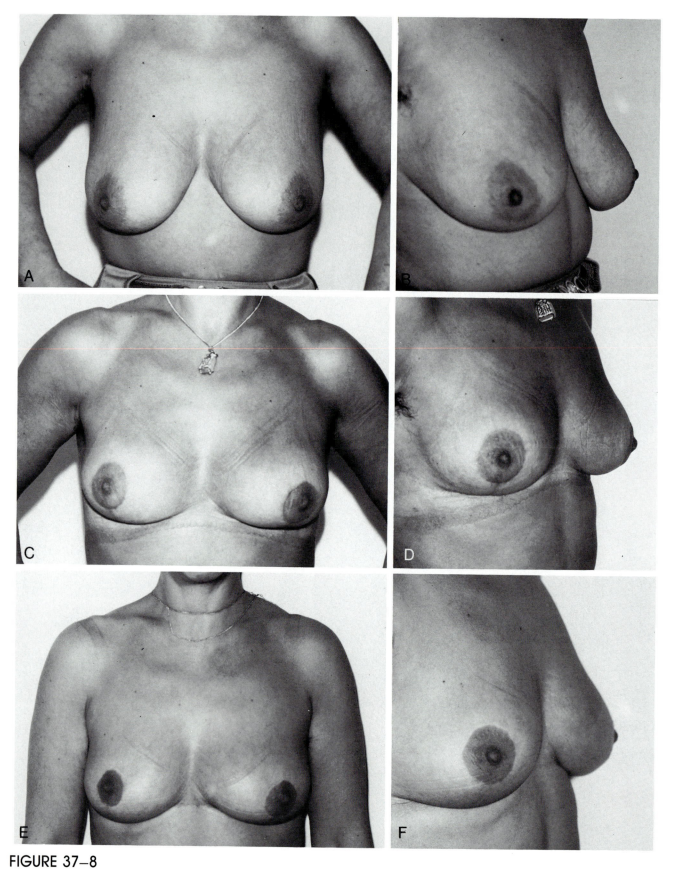

FIGURE 37–8

A and *B*, A 45-year-old woman with moderate hypertrophy and ptosis. *C* and *D*, The same patient 6 months after removal of 200 gm from each breast and ptosis correction. *E* and *F*, The same patient at 12 months, when good stability was achieved.

TABLE 37–2
Average Scar Length of 176 Patients

	SCAR LENGTH (cm)
Ptosis	6.4
Moderate hypertrophy	7.8
Hypertrophy above 500 gm	9.1

A few problems have been encountered that are now avoided by minor modifications in the technique:

1. Asymmetry of the areolas. This is easily corrected by superior half-moon–shaped skin excision, but better avoided by a careful marking of a scale on the midclavicle-areola line.
2. Delayed healing at the junction of the vertical suture and areola. Because this junction is an area of maximum tension, to diminish it, we make a 1-cm indentation 5 cm above points D and E on the vertical line (see Fig. 37–1).
3. Depression at the junction of the vertical and horizontal lines. This can be avoided by a careful glan-

TABLE 37–3
Stability*

	RESULT			
	Excellent	Good	Mediocre	Bad
Ptosis (23)	15	6	2	—
Moderate hypertrophy (19)	12	5	2	—
Hypertrophy above 500 gm (9)	3	4	2	—

*Evaluated after 4 years in 51 patients.

dular apposition on the midline and preservation of some fat under the skin when one is dissecting the lower part of the gland from the inframammary fold.
4. Bulging at the medial part of the inframammary fold. This can be avoided by a careful defatting at this level and easily corrected by liposuction and compression.

Patients are always warned of the possibility of a secondary correction of imperfection, but in fact only 1 of 11 required minor outpatient revision (for areola asymmetry or medial bulging).

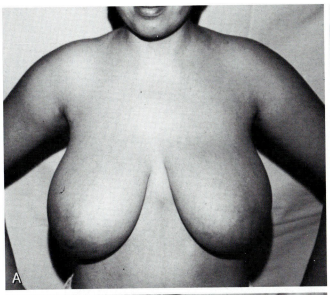

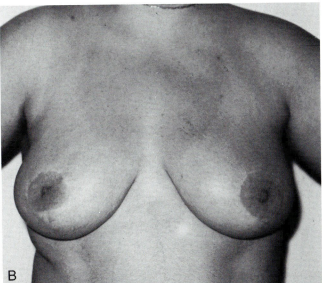

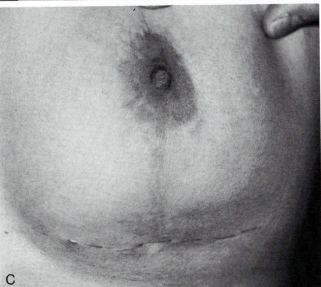

FIGURE 37–9
A, Severe hypertrophy in a 20-year-old woman. *B,* The same patient 6 years after removal of 700 gm from each breast. *C,* The horizontal scar remains very short and well hidden (it has been drawn for emphasis).

INDICATIONS

This operation is especially easily performed and gives satisfactory results in *pure ptosis* and *moderate hypertrophy* (up to 500 gm per side). The same technique can be utilized in large hypertrophy, but its use in such situations is more difficult in execution, especially if the gland is firm and lacks pliability (Fig. 37–9).

In younger patients with firm large breasts, it is especially important to avoid the long visible horizontal scar. We therefore utilize our technique in these cases but with special care to avoid skin tension. Sometimes superior suspension retracts the nipple-areola complex in these firm breasts, and we reduce the suspension after completion of glandular vertical suturing.

References

Arié, G.: Una nueva técnica de mastoplastia. Rev. Latinoam. Cir. Plast. 3:23, 1957.

Biesenberger, H.: Eine neue Methode der Mammaplastik. Zentralbl. Chir. 55:2382, 1928.

Dufourmentel, C., Mouly, R.: Plastie mammaire par la méthode oblique. Ann. Chir. Plast. 6:45, 1961.

Lalardrie, J. P., Jouglard, J. P.: *Chirurgie Plastique du Sein*. Paris, Masson, 1974.

Marchac, D., de Olarte, G.: Reduction mammaplasty and correction of ptosis with a short inframammary scar. Plast. Reconstr. Surg. 69:45, 1982.

Pitanguy, I.: Surgical treatment of breast hypertrophy. Br. J. Plast. Surg. 20:78, 1967.

A Z Reduction Mammaplasty with Minimal Scarring*

A technique is described for reduction mammaplasty utilizing a Z-plasty creating two triangles of skin in the infra-areola area. This technique involves de-epithelialization in the periareola area with repositioning and also glandular resection at the mammary base. The addition of this skin in the vertical inferior portion of the breast cone appears to result in an improved breast contour.

A 6-year follow-up study of our patients appears to indicate that the young women between the ages of 14 and 30 years who are free of striae gravidarum are the best candidates if they are in need of less than 900 gm reduction per breast.

The formation of prominent hypertrophic scars in the inframammary area, particularly in young teenage patients or patients in their early twenties, has been of considerable concern to many plastic surgeons over the years. Even though a satisfactory reduction mammaplasty has been carried out, scars have been particularly noticeable in the inframammary fold.

A change in concept by some surgeons in order to avoid as much as possible these prominent scars was first described by Peixoto (Peixoto, 1980, 1984). He described the technique of decreasing the size of the breast mound by excising various thicknesses at the base of the breast tissue mound, still allowing normal glandular function. The redundant skin appeared largely to redrape over a period of months following the internal reduction. To offset the residual redundancy, Marchac (1983) described his technique of utilizing a short transverse scar and excision of the redundant skin in a vertical plane. The undermined inferior mammary excess skin was allowed to redrape as part of the inframammary thoracic skin.

The development of a Z-type inframammary repair of the breast following these procedures was a further development of the techniques initially developed by Arié (1957); Dufourmentel and Mouly (1961); Elbaz and Verheecke (1972); and Meyer and Kesselring (1975), who made an L-shaped scar. This was similar to the B technique of Regnault (1974). Approximately 6 years ago we described a form of Z-plasty that was developed from the oblique techniques described by

others but with certain advantages in this new configuration.

The vertical displacement of the nipple-areola complex was of concern to us, and this was accomplished by means of a periareolar Schwarzmann (1930) de-epithelialization procedure. However, considerable tension was found to be present around the areola, as in the dermal-vault technique of Lalardrie and Jouglard (1974).

The technique to be described takes advantage of the skin elasticity present in the young patient, as compared with the laxity of the tissue and skin in the more mature female.

The addition of a Z-plasty to the inferior breast mound allows more skin to be added vertically with these two interlocking flaps. The upper medial flap, when advanced medially, reduces the periareolar tension and lessens the tendency for the formation of a widened scar. The lower lateral flap will form the inframammary crease line and reduce the cone width. These two flaps act as rotation advancement flaps, shaping the breast and at the same time minimizing the extent of any postoperative scarring.

TECHNIQUE

The markings are made with the patient in an upright position. The vertical axis of the breast is determined with a line drawn from the inframammary crease line and extended superiorly to the midclavicular line through the areola.

The amount of periareolar de-epithelialization is determined either by gently pinching the areola and superior areola skin as described by Peixoto (Fig. 38–1A) or by gently moving the breast medially and laterally. In this way the "arch gateway" is drawn after the technique by Marchac. The base of this arch is established by drawing a 5-cm horizontal line 5 cm above the inframammary crease. An isosceles triangle is created by joining the base line and the point of the inferior areolar area of de-epithelialization (Figs. 38–1B and 38–2). The breast is then placed under tension by application and tightening of a tourniquet, which is a Penrose rubber drain or sponge drawn around the base. A technique similar to that described by Schwarzmann is

---

*Reproduced in part with permission from Maillard, G. F.: A Z-mammaplasty with minimal scarring. Plast. Reconstr. Surg. 77:66, 1986.

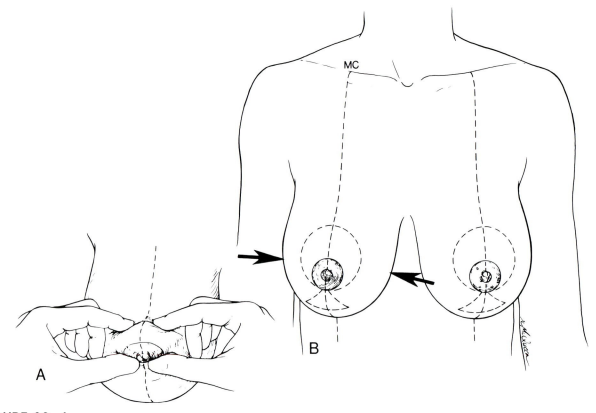

FIGURE 38–1
A, Periareolar de-epithelialization is estimated on the vertical axis of the breast by gently pinching the skin (Peixoto, 1984).
B, A 5 × 5-cm isosceles triangle is drawn, the base of which is 5 cm above the mammary fold.

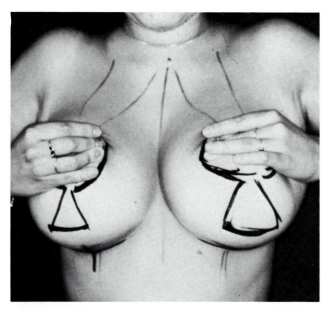

FIGURE 38–2
Ideal candidate for the Z-plasty technique: a 20-year-old patient with firm skin and mammary tissue and no striae. The triangles are marked below the round periareolar de-epithelialization area. (From Maillard, G. F.: A Z-mammaplasty with minimal scarring. Plast. Reconstr. Surg. 77:66, 1986.)

then carried out, de-epithelializing the periareolar area (Fig. 38–3). The skin is then excised over the de-epithelialized area. The isosceles triangle is then incised and remains attached to the breast tissue. By pulling upward on the two Lahey clamps, one extends the dissection to the inframammary fold, which is widely undermined and carried up to the 3 and 9 o'clock positions of the previously de-epithelialized periareolar breast (Fig. 38–4).

The subcutaneous dissection is extended widely inferiorly to the inframammary fold. At this point the mammary tissue is dissected free from the pectoral fascia, care being taken to preserve the perforating branches of the internal mammary artery (see Fig. 38–4). At this point, the previously placed tourniquet is removed. The amount of breast tissue estimated to give the desired eventual breast volume is resected after the technique of Peixoto (Fig. 38–5A) decreasing the size of the pyramid base in height and width (Fig. 38–5B). The breast specimen including the small portion of skin from the isosceles triangle is weighed, and the remaining breast volume is estimated visually and by palpation.

The breast mound characteristically has a flat appearance. With the technique suggested by Marchac, the remaining breast is placed under tension by a suture superior to the areola and also in the pectoral muscle in the region of the infraclavicular area, producing a full-

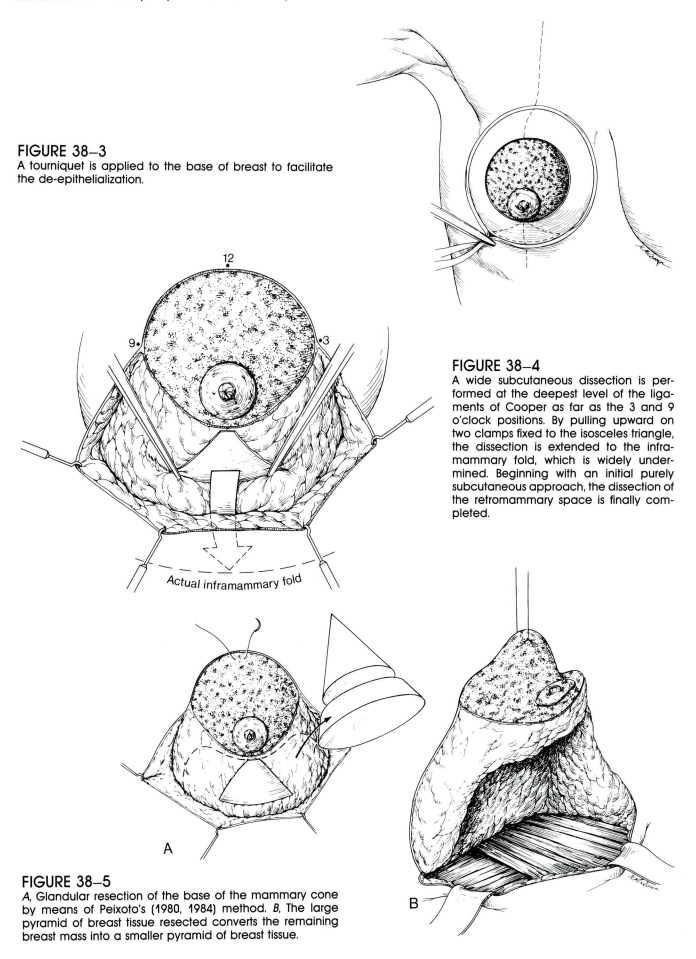

FIGURE 38–3
A tourniquet is applied to the base of breast to facilitate the de-epithelialization.

FIGURE 38–4
A wide subcutaneous dissection is performed at the deepest level of the ligaments of Cooper as far as the 3 and 9 o'clock positions. By pulling upward on two clamps fixed to the isosceles triangle, the dissection is extended to the inframammary fold, which is widely undermined. Beginning with an initial purely subcutaneous approach, the dissection of the retromammary space is finally completed.

Actual inframammary fold

FIGURE 38–5
A, Glandular resection of the base of the mammary cone by means of Peixoto's (1980, 1984) method. B, The large pyramid of breast tissue resected converts the remaining breast mass into a smaller pyramid of breast tissue.

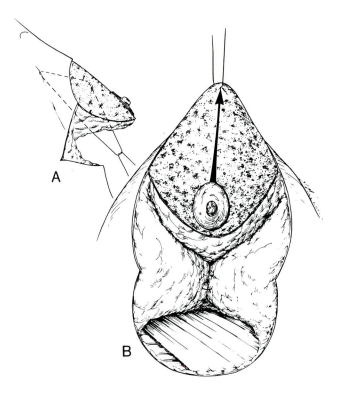

FIGURE 38–6
A, Placing a single suture between the gland just above the areola and the pectoral fascia in the infraclavicular region produces a fullness in the upper quadrant. *B,* The lateral and medial glandular areas are now approximated.

ness in the upper breast quadrant (Fig. 38–6A). This enables the surgeon to approximate the medial and lateral glandular portions with a number of sutures. The areola is then moved to its new position by placing the first suture at 12 o'clock (Fig. 38–6B). The inferior lateral skin triangle is now advanced medially, creating the inframammary fold. Advancing this flap narrows the base of the cone and also increases the horizontal tension. The medial triangular flap is then advanced laterally, which produces a rotation advancement and at

the same time decreases the periareolar tension (Fig. 38–7). A number of inverted sutures and sterile paper sutures are used to approximate the skin edges without tension (Figs. 38–8 and 38–9). A lightly self-adhering dressing is carefully applied and changed weekly for 4 to 6 weeks. This type of dressing is technically important because it assists in the skin redraping and skin retraction. Suction drainage is utilized for 2 days postoperatively.

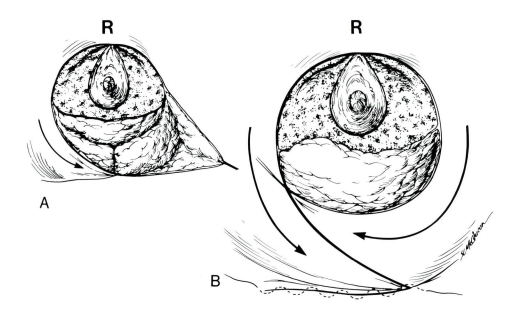

FIGURE 38–7
A, After moving the areola up, the two triangles are interlocked horizontally in the form of a Z-plasty. First, the lateral triangle is sutured into the new inframammary fold. *B,* The medial triangular flap is gently advanced and rotated laterally to diminish the tension around the areola, in a way similar to the action of the diaphragm of a camera, and creates a Z-plasty. This maneuver also adds tissue vertically, giving a better contour to the inferior portion of the breast.

Right

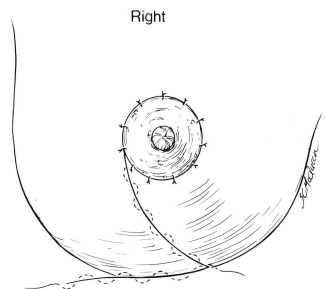

FIGURE 38–8
Result at the end of the procedure.

INDICATIONS

This procedure is indicated for female patients under the age of 30 with thick, elastic skin. The upper limit of breast reduction in these patients is 900 gm per breast. Patients with striae gravidarum, indicating the rupture of elastic fibers, are not considered good candidates for this procedure.

RESULTS

This technique was initially described approximately 6 years ago and has been used in 125 patients (200 breasts). The average age of the patients has been 28 years at surgery. We have now followed these cases for more than 6 years (Figs. 38–10 to 38–18).

Secondary defatting procedures below the new infra-

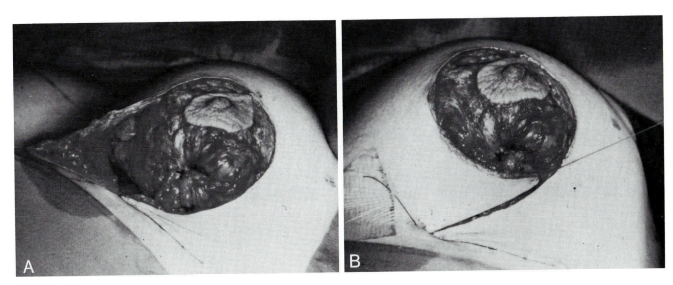

FIGURE 38–9
A and B, The interlocking of the two Z-plasty triangles at surgery, demonstrating the minimal tension on the skin because practically no skin is resected.

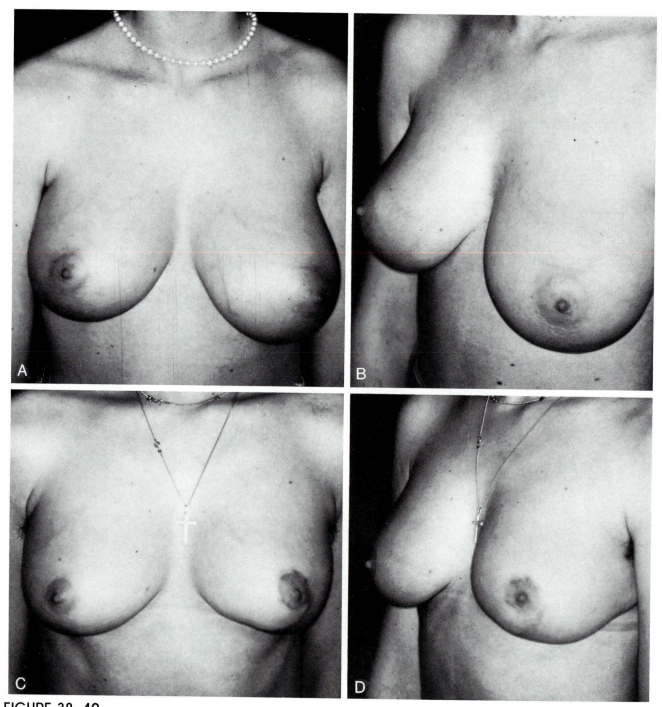

FIGURE 38-10
A and *B*, A young patient with preoperative unilateral hypertrophy. *C* and *D*, The same patient 6 months after reduction, showing the minimal Z-shaped scar.

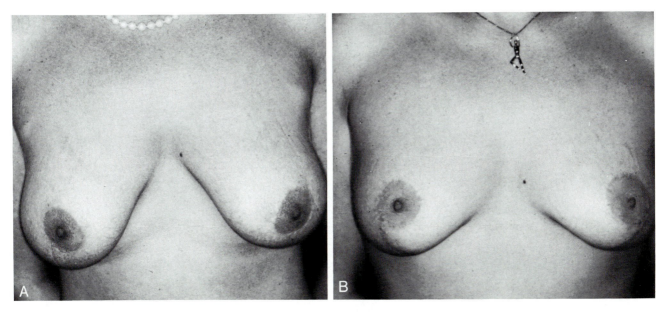

FIGURE 38–11

A, A 20-year-old patient before mastopexy and reduction mammaplasty. *B*, The same patient 1 year after a 250-gm resection on each side. Note the natural-looking breast with minimal scarring.

mammary fold were carried out in three of the earlier patients. The nipple-areola complex was increased in size in the larger reduction mammaplasties (over 600 gm), although less than previously reported by Peixoto and Marchac. Sensitivity of the nipple-areola complex was objectively and subjectively slightly reduced but gradually improved over a 3-year follow-up. No hematomas or skin sloughs were encountered. The ability to lactate satisfactorily for breast-feeding has not been tested; none of this group of patients has become pregnant.

CONCLUSION

The technique of utilizing a Z-plasty configuration in the closure of the inferior breast mound represents a new dimension in continued attempts to minimize post–reduction mammaplasty scars and at the same time attain a satisfactory reduction and coning of the breast with aesthetically acceptable results.

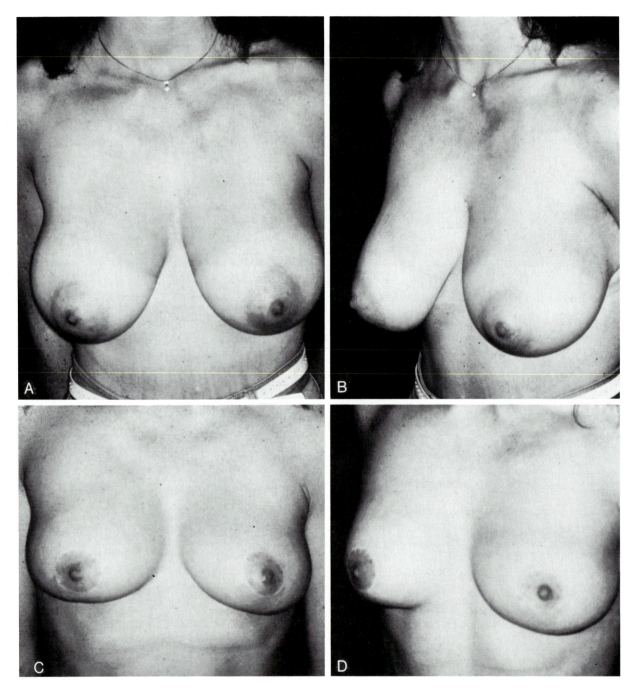

FIGURE 38–12

A and *B*, A 23-year-old patient with hypertrophy and ptosis. *C* and *D*, The same patient 13 months after a 300-gm reduction on each side.

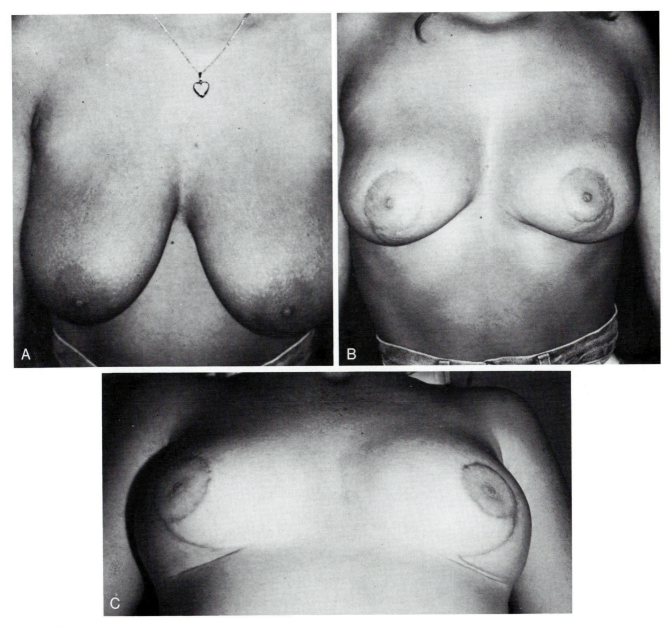

FIGURE 38–13

A, A 19-year-old patient with breast hypertrophy. *B,* The same patient 3 years after a 350-gm reduction on each side. *C,* The same patient, with minimal bilateral Z-shaped scars.

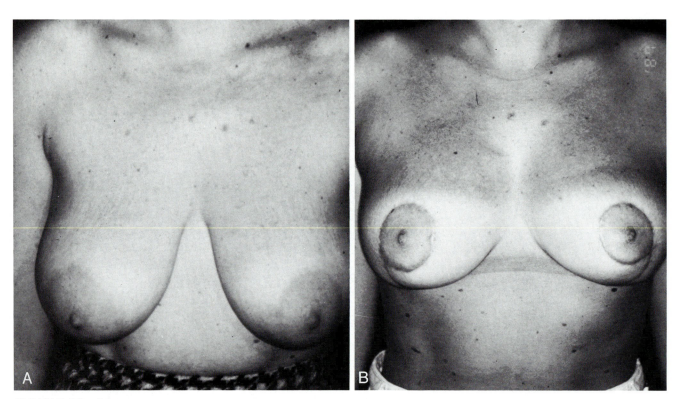

FIGURE 38–14
A, A 20-year-old patient with juvenile hypertrophy. *B,* The same patient 1 year after a 500-gm reduction on each side.

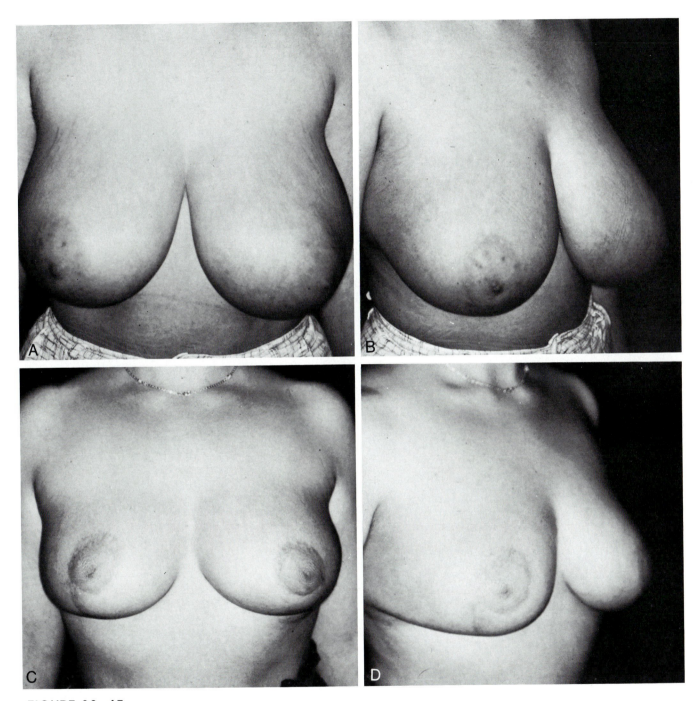

FIGURE 38–15
A and *B,* An 18-year-old patient with massive juvenile hypertrophy. *C* and *D,* The same patient 1 year after 900-gm reduction on each side.

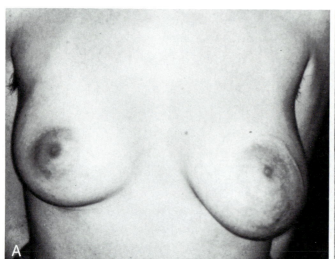
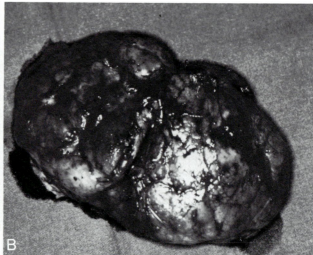
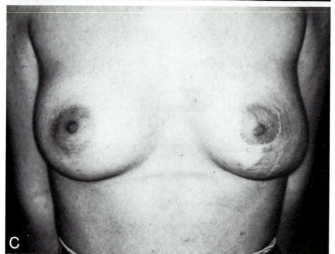

FIGURE 38–16

A, A 14-year-old girl with gross deformity of the left breast caused by a giant fibroadenoma. *B*, Resected 400-gm giant fibroadenoma. *C*, The same patient 1 year after resection, with redraping of the skin by the same Z procedure.

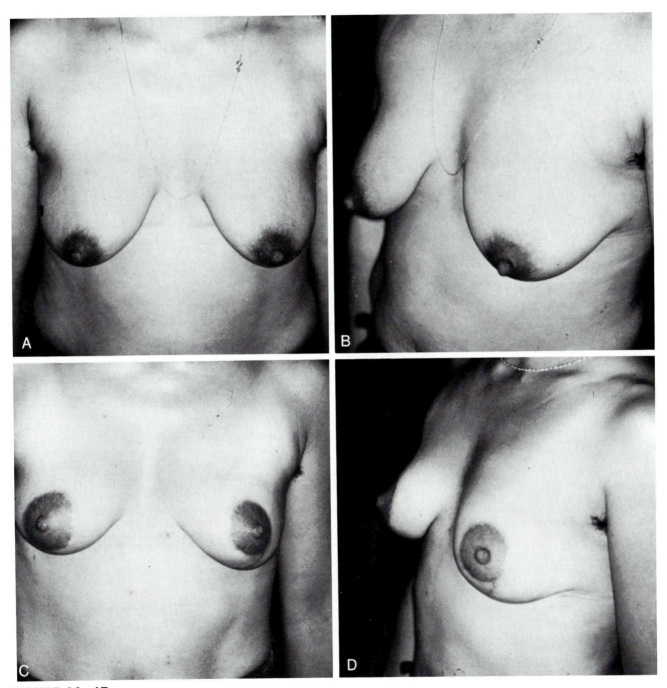

FIGURE 38–17
A and *B*, Ptotic postpartum breasts, but with firm and elastic skin. *C* and *D*, Result 1 year after mastopexy utilizing a Z-plasty technique as described.

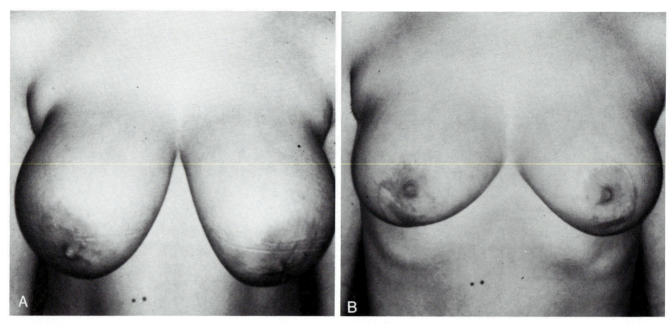

FIGURE 38–18

A, A 16-year-old girl with a distorted upper pole of the breast due to ptosis as a result of juvenile hypertrophy. *B*, The same patient 2 years after the Z procedure and reduction mammaplasty. Note the slight discoloration around the areola but excellent natural shape and a very short scar.

References

Arié, G.: Una nueva técnica de mastoplastia. Rev. Latinoam. Cir. Plast. 3:23, 1957.

Dufourmentel, C., Mouly, R.: Plastie mammaire par la méthode oblique. Ann. Chir. Plast. 6:45, 1961.

Elbaz, J. S., Verheecke, G.: La cicatrice en L dans les plasties mammaires. Ann. Chir. Plast. 17:283, 1972.

Gillies, H., Millard, D. R.: *The Principles and Art of Plastic Surgery.* Boston, Little, Brown, 1957.

Lalardrie, J. P., Jouglard, J. P.: *Chirurgie Plastique du Sein.* Paris, Masson, 1974.

Lassus, C.: A technique for breast reduction. Int. Surg. 53:69, 1970.

Maillard, G. F.: A Z-mammaplasty with minimal scarring. Plast. Reconstr. Surg. 77:66, 1986.

Maillard, G. F., Montandon, D., Goin, J. L.: *Plastic and Reconstructive Breast Surgery.* Paris, Masson, 1983.

Marchac, D.: Mammaplasty with a short transverse scar. In: Williams, H. B. (ed.): *Transactions of the International Congress of Plastic Surgeons. (Montreal).* 1983, p. 765.

McKissock, P. K.: Reduction mammaplasty with a vertical dermal flap. Plast. Reconstr. Surg. 49:245, 1972.

Meyer, R., Kesselring, U. K.: Reduction mammaplasty with an L-shaped suture line. Plast. Reconstr. Surg. 55:139, 1975.

Peixoto, G.: Reduction mammaplasty: A personal technique. Plast. Reconstr. Surg. 65:217, 1980.

Peixoto, G.: Reduction mammaplasty. Aesth. Plast. Surg. 8:231, 1984.

Regnault, P.: Reduction mammaplasty by the "B" technique. Plast. Reconstr. Surg. 53:19, 1974.

Schwarzmann, E.: Die Technik der Mammaplastik. Chirurg 2:932, 1930.

Skoog, T.: A technique of breast reduction: Transposition of the nipple on a cutaneous vascular pedicle. Acta Chir. Scand. 126:453, 1963.

Strömbeck, J. O.: Mammaplasty: Report of a new technique based on the two-pedicle procedure. Br. J. Plast. Surg. 13:79, 1961.

The Massive Hypertrophic Breast: Surgical Treatment

There are many ways to reduce a hypertrophic breast. The massive hypertrophic breast is quite different from the usual large breast and requires a special technique for surgical correction if the surgeon is to avoid nipple slough and wound dehiscence and, most important, to achieve a satisfactory cosmetic result.

MASSIVE HYPERTROPHIC BREAST PROFILE

The massive hypertrophic breast usually is found in a rather obese woman. In the adolescent person, the tissue is firm, with a clublike bulbous end. The breasts are massive, with the fullness distributed throughout them. In the more mature woman and in the elderly, the breasts are very pendent, thin, and flat, with narrow bases and low to flattened nipples. The areolae are very wide and usually blend into the rest of the skin. The base may contain skin and subcutaneous tissue only. Breast tissue present usually is concentrated in the clublike bottom half. The breasts consist primarily of fat. As the breasts become more pendulous, the nipple-areola area retracts with flattening of the nipple. The fourth intercostal nerve, giving sensation to the region, is pulled taut, diminishing sensation, a form of neurapraxia.

The woman with massive hypertrophic breasts is usually of the pyknic type, more often obese than not. The young girl may be curvaceous, but fat distortion occurs early in life. The woman looks squat and prematurely older. Despite constant dieting, the breasts never recede and always remain huge throughout life. Their size is severely aggravated during pregnancy. The past history shows that most of these women begin to develop at the age of 10 years or so, frequently before menstruation starts. By the time adolescence is completed, the breasts are massive and never undergo involution after pregnancy.

These women tend to shun physical exercise because the massive breasts make activity painful. Control of the pendulumlike masses is difficult. Skin irritation is exacerbated as the breasts rub against the chest and abdominal walls, resulting in intertrigo. The special brassieres used to contain the mammae make deep grooves in the shoulders. Back and shoulder pain is common. Cystic disease is commonly seen.

The women have difficulty in fitting clothes and even young women look very pudgy and older. Bathing suits are shunned.

Social contacts create psychologic problems. Boy-girl relationships are difficult because the girl tries to hide her huge breasts, a target for the adolescent boy making his early contacts with the opposite sex. The girl develops psychologic trauma and withdraws from male contact. Her sexual outlook becomes warped, and fantasies are common.

HEREDITY AND ENDOCRINE PREDISPOSITION

Most women with large breasts give family histories of obese, large-breasted women. Most accumulate fat about their buttocks, breasts, and thighs at an early stage.

Breast development is controlled by a complex neurohormone system based in the hypothalamus. Stimuli emitting from this area affect the pituitary, adrenals, and ovaries. An overabundance of estrogen stimulates the breast parenchyma. With the onset of puberty, prolactin from the anterior pituitary, estrogenlike hormones from the adrenals, and estrogen and progesterone from the ovaries stimulate the mammae to swell, causing tenderness and some pain. The congestion is aggravated by aldosterone secretions from the adrenal cortex with sodium and fluids being retained. The menstrual cycle exacerbates the condition. As maturity progresses, cystic breast diseases are common. There is no diminution in size with menopause. Contraceptive pills containing hormones add to the discomfort. Male hormones such as androgen have little to no value in size reduction. Dieting has little effect on the size of these massive breasts.

THE FREE NIPPLE GRAFT PROCEDURE—THE TECHNIQUE OF CHOICE

Most surgeons want to move the nipple-areola complex on a pedicle, hoping to retain some of the erotic nipple-areola sensation. These large breasts are very ptotic, and movement on a pedicle to a proper level may be very dangerous in terms of vascular failure. The danger of slough is very great. The need to mobilize the nipple on a pedicle to get the elevation most often sacrifices the fourth intercostal nerve, thought to be the main sensory branch to the nipple-areola area. This defeats the reason for trying to move the nipple on a pedicle.

In older women, pendulous breasts leave very little more than skin and subcutaneous tissue in the superior flattened, stretched base pedicle. Shaping a breast with this configuration and trying to elevate the nipple on a pedicle jeopardize the blood supply and make for a most unaesthetic breast reconstruction. The solution is partial amputation, breast reshaping (using an inferior flap of breast tissue to fill the upper flat part in older women), and free nipple grafting on the apex of the new mound. The nipple take should be excellent.

The free nipple graft technique is constantly criticized as being inferior to other methods such as the McKissock (1972), Strömbeck (1960), inferior pedicle, superior pedicle, and so forth, for the following reasons:

1. Nipple sensation should be left intact.
2. There should be no nipple distortion.
3. The cosmetic results are better with the other methods.
4. The free graft techniques as were performed left "pancake breasts."

This author has developed his own technique using the free nipple grafts. His findings over the past 20 years have demonstrated the following:

1. We have never lost a free nipple graft.
2. The sensation loss is no greater in the free nipple graft technique as compared with other operations in which the massive hypertrophic breast is reduced. As a matter of fact, in all methods of breast reduction in very large breasts where the nipple-areola complex has to be moved a considerable distance, a pedicle will lose sensation, varying from none to 75%. In free nipple grafting, the loss may be from 25% to 50%. However, reliable persons, such as nurses, report sensation return greater than 50% over ensuing years. The sensation may vary from touch to erotic stimulation. Apparently, sensory nerves grow down from the superior intercostal nerves to reneurotize the nipple, restoring the sensation. Added explanation for the satisfactory sensation with our free nipple graft technique includes the following:
   a. Thinning the areolar circle, but leaving the smooth muscle at the base of the nipple intact.
   b. Inward growth of nerve fibers from the surrounding skin, mostly the superior region.

SURGICAL TECHNIQUE

As shown in Figure 39–1, the Rubin (1976) pattern is a modification of the Wise (1972) pattern. The scale is shown. Comparison is made with the Strömbeck. The angle of the two lines that will become the vertical scar

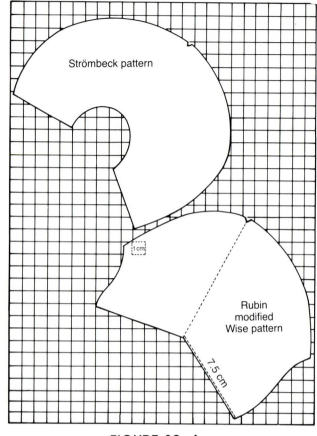

FIGURE 39–1

is less than that of Strömbeck and is more like the McKissock pattern (see Fig. 39–1).

One must consider the quality of the breast tissue. If the patient has firm breast tissue, more skin is needed for the vertical line closure. The angle between the two lines must be made smaller.

As shown in Figure 39–2, the patient is marked in a standing position. The points marked are the sternal notch *(SN)* (Fig. 39–2A) and the midpoint on the clavicle between the notch and acromioclavicular junction *(MC)*. To find the nipple site, one drops a perpendicular line midpoint on the clavicle down on the vertical breast (see Fig. 39–2), and a line from sternal notch will meet the perpendicular line. The junction will be the nipple site. In a short woman, the sternal notch perpendicular line will be about 20 cm. A taller woman may require 22 cm or more. A good check is to note that the nipple center will line up with the arm at the junction of the middle and lower thirds. In Figure 39–2 the nipple site is found in the left breast. Once this is done, the right breast is marked in a similar fashion. The Rubin pattern is placed over the breast so that the apex of the triangle will be at the nipple site. The pattern is rotated until the notch on the superior margin lines up with the sternal notch. The pattern is then marked with an indelible ink pen. Scratches are made with a No. 15 blade at key points to avoid the obliteration of pen markings when the breasts are "prepped" for surgery.

As shown in Figure 39–3A, the upper part of the breast incorporated in the pattern is now separated from

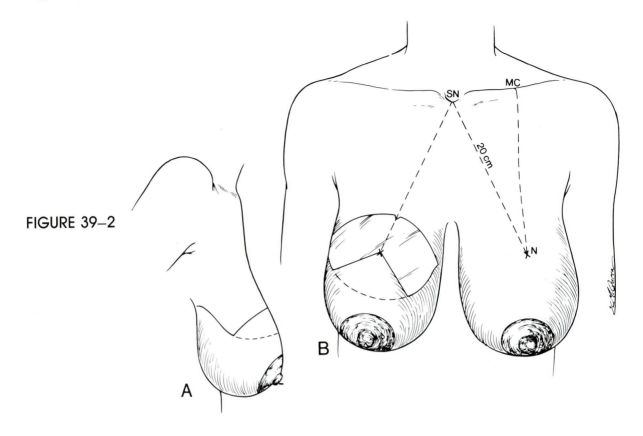

FIGURE 39–2

the excessive inferior portion by cutting along the inferior line. This line will be the new inframammary fold. The inferior part of the breast is left attached to the pectoralis for its blood supply. It will be used as a filler (see Fig. 39–7) if needed for the upper portion of the superior part of the breast.

As shown in Figure 39–3B, the nipple-areola complex *(N)* is excised and stored in a saline sponge. The diameter of the new areola is about 4.5 cm. The areola is thinned to the dermis bed, and the circular nipple muscle is left intact. This thick muscle allows response to erotic stimuli.

As shown in Figure 39–4, the superior breast flap is now being shaped (Fig. 39–4A). The de-epithelialized triangle *(T)* is now inverted to form a "girder." Three temporary black silk sutures close the wound edges. A finger placed under the sutures makes the closure easier. The triangle is closed. The dermal "girder" is pulled down (Fig. 39–4B). The "girder" is sutured with two 2-0 black silk mattress sutures, by means of which the dermis is buried. A triangle *(T)* of epithelium is excised, which leaves dermis. The triangle will be inverted when the skin margins are sutured. The margins become the vertical line of the reconstructed breast.

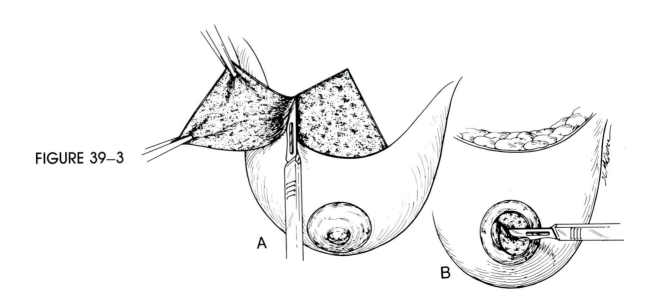

FIGURE 39–3

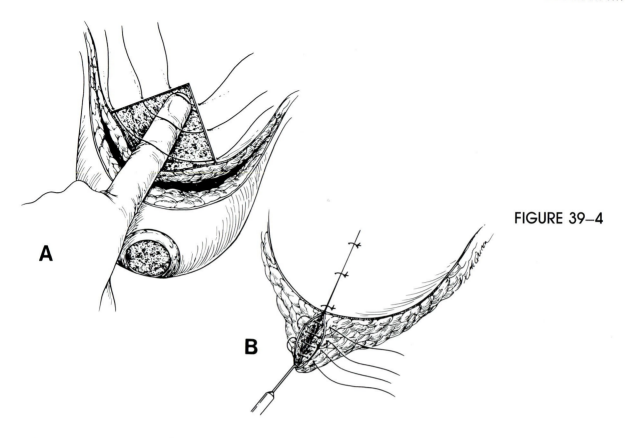

FIGURE 39–4

As shown in Figure 39–5, the breast is coned by placing three black silk No. 2 sutures through the parenchyma (Fig. 39–5A). The coned breast is pulled medially by two black silk No. 2 sutures through the lateral parenchyma and fastened to the perichondrium at the junction of the fourth costal cartilage and the sternum (Fig. 39–5B). If not needed, the excess inferior breast is removed at the inframammary line.

As shown in Figure 39–6, when the breast is very pendulous and the upper portion is merely skin and subcutaneous tissue, breast parenchyma must be brought up to give bulk and shape (Fig. 39–6A). The lower breast flap that is still attached to the pectoralis is now contoured as needed by removing excess paren-

chyma and de-epithelializing the skin (Fig. 39–6B). The attachment to the pectoralis is the conduit for blood vessels to supply this inferior flap, which is brought up and sutured to the pectoralis in the region of the third costal cartilage with 2-0 black silk sutures. Trimming the excess parenchyma can give a pleasant contour (Fig. 39–6C).

As shown in Figure 39–7, the nipple site is remeasured. A 4.5-cm circle is de-epithelialized, leaving a bleeding dermis. The nipple-areola complex is sutured to the site with eight 5-0 black silk sutures acting as tie-overs. The margins of the areola are sutured to the skin with 5-0 nylon subcuticular pullout sutures. Pressure is made over the complex by placing Xeroform gauze and

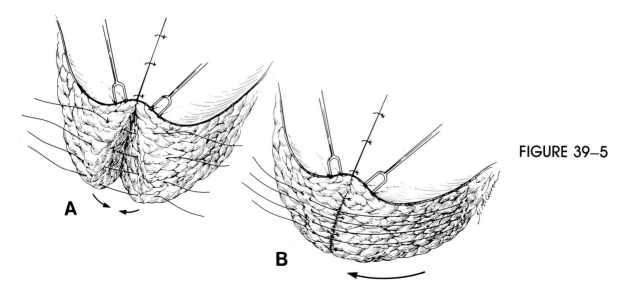

FIGURE 39–5

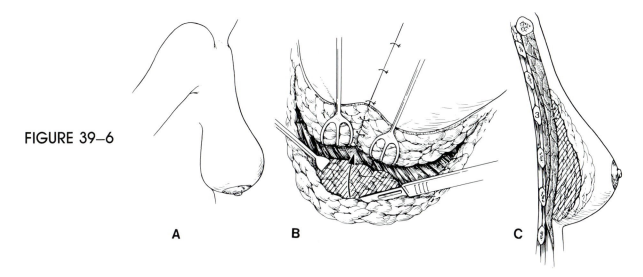

FIGURE 39-6

A   B   C

wet cotton held by the eight 5-0 black silk tie-overs. All skin wounds are closed with 4-0 Dexon for deep sutures and 3-0 nylon for subcuticular pullout sutures.

PITFALLS AND HOW TO AVOID THEM

Uneven Nipple-Areola Location

Breasts must be pattern-marked in a standing position before the operation. This locates the nipple position on the skin only. Pendulous breasts fall laterally even in a standing position. An assistant must gently hold them toward the midline, barely touching; then the position is marked (see Fig. 39-2A).

Unequal Breast Volume

Skin markings are only a gross blueprint of how much parenchyma is to be removed. Surgical removal must be performed by the same surgeon on each side holding the knife or electrocautery at the same angle. After excess parenchyma is removed, the surgeon must palpate the remaining breast for thickness and volume.

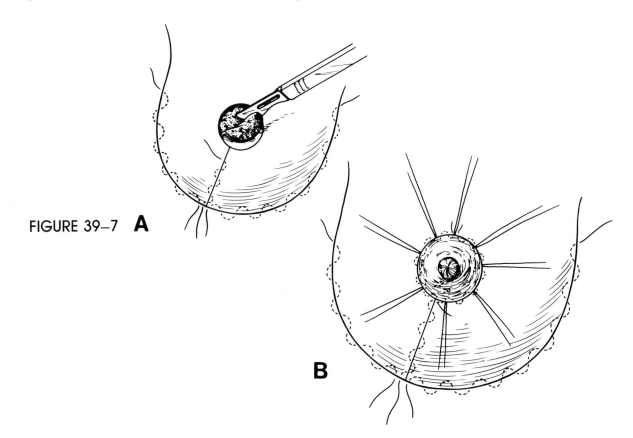

FIGURE 39-7 **A**

B

This is purely approximate. Measuring or weighing each side of the removed parenchyma is incorrect for volume equality, because most breasts have unequal bulk originally.

Unequal Contour

This technique creates contoured breasts. Black silk 2-0 (eventually biodegradable) shapes the breasts and pulls them medially for cleavage (see Fig. 39–6B). The contour can be seen immediately and corrected if necessary. No pressure dressing is used to distort the contour. Four-by-four sponges and a soft stretch nylon bra are all that are needed to maintain the surgical wounds and shape.

Nipple-Areola Take Failure

Carefully removing the epidermis at the designated site with a sharp knife will leave a bleeding dermal bed to receive the nipple-areola complex. The latter is prepared by removing all of the epidermis down to the

dermis while all the muscles of the nipple are left intact. Eight 5-0 silk tie-overs over wet cotton and 6-0 nylon subcuticular sutures can give a firm attachment to the underlying breast (see Fig. 39–7A and B).

Horizontal Skin Line Above the Inframammary Fold

This is a frequent error and is due to misjudgment of the breast density. In the full, tense, firm breast (juvenile and in obese persons), the vertical limbs of the pattern must be increased to 8 cm instead of 7.5 cm, giving a longer reconstructed breast (see Fig. 39–1).

Suture Line Slough

Sloughing can occur at the junction of the vertical and horizontal lines and is due to too much tension. The answer is found in removing excess parenchyma or narrowing the pattern. The full, firm breast must be evaluated before surgery. By removing less of a triangle, more skin will be available.

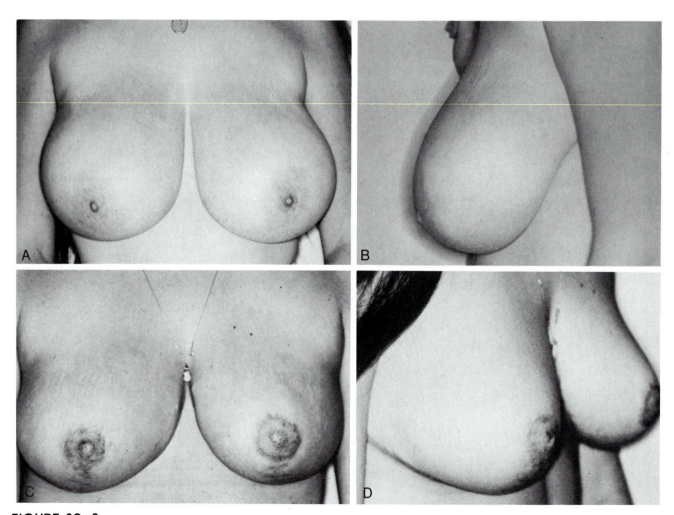

FIGURE 39–8

A and B, Twenty-year-old obese primipara with massive breast hypertrophy of endocrine origin. *C and D,* Postoperative views 6 months after surgery.

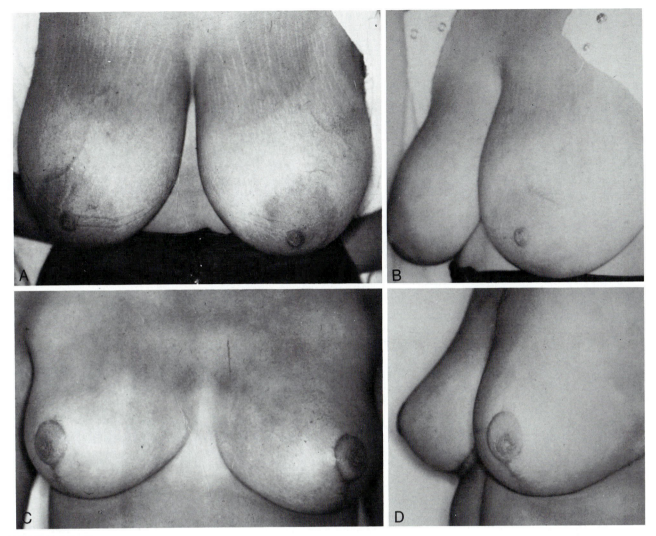

FIGURE 39–9
A and *B,* Eighteen-year-old woman with massive breast hypertrophy of endocrine origin. *C* and *D,* Postoperative views 1 year later.

Dog-Ears Medially and Laterally

Giving a contour to a very large breast creates dog-ears, both medially and laterally. This is caused by the inferior inframammary line being longer than the cut breast line.

The solution is found in curving the pattern as shown in Figure 39–1. At no time should the incisions cross the midline, because this creates a shelf. Instead, the medial incision should curve upward on the breast about 3 cm from the midline. The lateral dog-ear can easily be removed by a triangular incision.

Scars

Scars are unavoidable. However, they can be minimized by suturing with little tension. Deep, nonabsorbable sutures can hold the breast contour without pressure on the skin. All skin wounds are closed with two deep, absorbable suture layers and the skin closed with 3-0 nylon subcuticular sutures, reinforced with Steri-Strips. The subcuticular sutures are removed in 3 weeks. Wearing the stretch nylon brassiere gives support for 6 months. Brassieres are worn day and night during that time to prevent stretching the scars. Some scars hypertrophy despite all of the preceding precautionary measures.

Bottom Sagging after 1 Year

Bottom sagging is the most difficult problem to avoid. Even when the technique is performed correctly, the lower half of the breast may sag after several months, giving the breast an unequal appearance, with the nipples pointing upward.

The cause may be loss of weight, very soft skin, or separation of deep nonabsorbable sutures. Every attempt must be made to have patients with soft skin wear their brassieres during sleep as well as in the daytime.

SUMMARY

A partial amputation-free nipple grafting technique is described that consistently produces cosmetically acceptable breasts in massive hypertrophic mammae, whether in young or older women (Figs. 39–8 to 39–11).

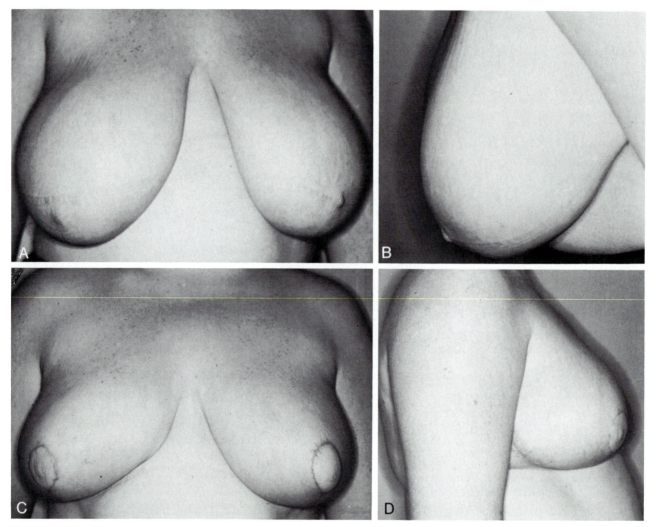

FIGURE 39–10
A and B, Obese multipara with massive firm breasts. C and D, Postoperative views 1 year later.

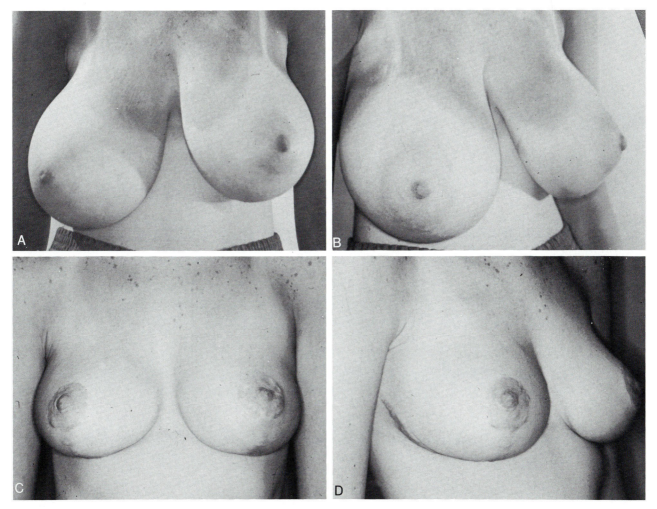

FIGURE 39–11
A and *B*, Massive breast hypertrophy in a 34-year-old woman. *C* and *D*, Postoperative views 2 years later.

References

Conway, H.: Mammaplasty: Analysis of 110 consecutive cases with end results. Plast. Reconstr. Surg. 10:303, 1952.

Lexer, E.: Hypertrophie bei der Mammae. Münch. Med. Wochenschr. 59:2702, 1912.

McKissock, P. K.: Reduction mammaplasty with a vertical dermal flap. Plast. Reconstr. Surg. 49:245, 1972.

Rubin, L. R.: Surgical treatment of the massive hypertrophic breast. In: Georgiade, N. G. (ed.): *Reconstructive Breast Surgery.* St. Louis, C. V. Mosby, 1976, p. 218.

Strömbeck, J. O.: Mammaplasty: Report of a new technique based on the two pedicle procedure. Br. J. Plast. Surg. 13:79, 1960.

Thorek, M.: *Plastic Surgery of the Breast and Abdominal Wall.* Springfield, Ill, Charles C Thomas, 1942.

Wise, R. J.: Surgical management of the hypertrophic breast. In: Masters, F. W., Lewis, J. R.: *Symposium on Aesthetic Surgery of the Face, Eyelid, and Breast, Phoenix, 1970.* St. Louis, C. V. Mosby, 1972, p. 174.

40

Comparison of Various Reduction Mammaplasty Techniques

Cosmetic operations on the nose have a long-standing tradition, going back to the Vedas (about 2500 B.C.) of ancient India and the early work of Gaspare Taglacozzi (1597) in medieval times. Operations on the female breast only started at the turn of the century (Dehner, 1908; Lexer, 1912; Pousson, 1897; Verchère, 1898) and were truly developed after World War I (Aubert, 1923; Axhausen, 1926; Biesenberger, 1928; Holländer, 1924; Joseph, 1925; Kausch, 1916; Kraske, 1923; Kuester, 1926; Lexer, 1931; Lotsch, 1923, 1928; Passot, 1925). In 1928 the famous Viennese surgeon Eiselsberg (cited by Biesenberger [1931]) apologized, when he performed a reduction mammaplasty in front of visitors, that this kind of surgery "would have been condemned" only 10 years before but was now demanded by the public, so that "we had to change our position in order to fulfill the wishes of our patients."

Since that time public and surgical opinion has changed a great deal, so much so that for major deformities even third-party payors (Schmidt-Tintemann, 1974) are amenable to paying the necessary costs.

Five main aims are now recognized by all surgeons concerned with this type of operation as being of outstanding importance:

1. The operation should be a single-stage procedure. All methods using more than one procedure have now only historical interest (Joseph, 1925; Kausch, 1916; Kuester, 1926; Noël, 1928; Schreiber, 1929).
2. It should provide as much margin of safety for the survival of nipple, skin, and gland as possible.
3. The result should approach the classic cone shape of a pretty female breast as closely as is possible (Reich, 1975) with as little scarring as is feasible (Axhausen, 1926; Passot, 1925; Reich, 1975).
4. The result should be long-lasting (Georgiade and Georgiade, 1987; Georgiade et al., 1989; McKissock, 1980), provided that extreme changes in body weight are avoided by the patient.
5. The procedure should basically—or at least not mainly—not depend on the artistic ability of the surgeon, but should follow a principal pattern, which can be taught and learned during a reasonably extended training program (Aufricht, 1949; Georgiade et al., 1979a; McKissock, 1972; Pitanguy, 1967; Strömbeck, 1960, 1964).

Other aims are not quite as uniformly agreed upon:

1. Must a single type of operation be applicable to all sizes and shapes of breasts at all ages and under all general conditions?
2. How much skin undermining is permissible?
3. Should the maintenance of shape rely mainly on the skin (skin brassiere) (Palacin et al., 1988; Penn, 1955; Wise et al., 1963) or on the shaping of a glandular cone (Biesenberger, 1928, 1930; Göbell, 1927; Gillies and McIndoe, 1939; Hester et al., 1985) as such, with the skin a mere cover to be draped over it?
4. How important is lactation today? Should safety and speed of operation be jeopardized by an attempt to secure sensitivity of the nipple and breast-feeding at all costs?
5. How far should a surgeon follow the particular wishes of a patient, especially regarding the size of the resulting breast and the placement of scars?

Before going anywhere further, I shall give my personal position on these questions:

1. In accordance with Georgiade et al. (1979b) and Lupo (1970), I do not believe that there is a technique that can be applied to all patients, with all kinds of breasts and in all imaginable general states of health, without jeopardizing one or another of the basic principles of plastic surgery at least to some degree.
2. Only as much skin undermining as is absolutely necessary is permissible (McKissock, 1985). When in doubt, safety should always take precedence over a further shade of beauty (Gillies and Millard, 1957; McIndoe and Rees, 1958).
3. Neither skin nor gland alone can and will maintain the shape of a breast for any length of time. Both must work together to fight gravity; gravity, as we all know, is directly proportional to weight. A small breast will practically invariably have a better chance of keeping its shape, place, and size than a large one.
4. The importance of lactation depends entirely on the age of the patient. While in a young woman who wants to have children it can play quite an important role, in an elderly person past menopause it has no place for consideration. The possibility of loss of sensitivity, which is unavoidable with some tech-

niques and occurs with all others with varying degrees of probability, should and must be discussed with the patient before operation. To promise too much or to reassure a patient too much may result in a poor doctor-patient relationship.

5. If one has a multitude of options regarding technique at one's disposal, as I believe one should, all details and possibilities should be discussed with the patient before her operation and agreed upon. The more a breast is reduced, the longer and safer the result will last. But an extreme reduction of glandular tissue will at the same time by necessity leave a greater amount of skin behind, which will have to be dealt with—usually with longer scars.

In the last four decades a great multitude of techniques has been developed that can be categorized in four main groups:

1. Techniques whose main aim is skin reduction and which can safely be combined with some augmentation of the breast mass as such (Dufourmentel, 1961; Gläsmer and Amersbach, 1928).

2. Techniques dissecting the mammary gland free of its skin cover, forming the breast tissue as such, and then draping the skin over the new formed mound. Most of these methods result in a suture line imitating an inverted T; some try to get rid of the skin surplus with a lengthy scar toward the side and could be summarized as "oblique" (Dufourmentel and Mouly, 1961; Gläsmer and Amersbach, 1928; Holländer, 1924). All of them depend on the blood vessels from the gland itself (Biesenberger, 1928; Hester et al., 1985; Kraske, 1923; Lexer, 1912, 1931; Marchac and de Olarte, 1982; Regnault, 1974). No skin or dermal attachment is preserved or attempted. A circular strip of dermis immediately around the nipple, however, remains attached to the gland for reasons of safety (Schwarzmann, 1930).

3. Techniques using dermal pedicles (Cardoso et al., 1984; Courtiss and Goldwyn, 1977; Georgiade and Georgiade, 1987; Georgiade et al., 1979a, 1979b; Kaplan, 1978; McKissock, 1972, 1980; Labandter et al., 1982; Pitanguy, 1967; Robbins, 1977; Skoog, 1963; Strömbeck, 1960, 1964; Weiner and Aiache, 1973). They all rely on the fact that a great deal of the blood supply of the nipple is provided by its surrounding dermis. Whether the nourishing vessels do really arise from the fourth intercostal artery (Strömbeck, 1964) or enter the breast mainly in the inframammary area (McKissock, 1980) still remains a matter of argument. All surgeons working for chest wall reconstructions, however, are familiar with the big and safe flaps, which can be developed from the skin cover of the breast (Sauerbruch, 1928); so the question seems slightly academic.

4. Techniques that discard all attachments of the nipple and/or the nipple-areola complex to the mammary gland and skin and transfer the nipple as a free full-thickness skin graft (Adams, 1944, 1947; Robertson, 1963; Thorek, 1922).

Each group of techniques offers certain advantages and certain handicaps. As usual in plastic sur-

gery—which, according to Sir Harold D. Gillies (1957), still remains the "eternal struggle between beauty and blood supply"—each surgeon should be familiar with at least one method in each of the four groups to avoid the classic surgical mistake of adapting a patient to a technique. The opposite should always be the surgeon's aim.

GENERAL PRINCIPLES OF REDUCTION MAMMAPLASTY

Whatever the method used, reduction mammaplasty remains a major operation and should only be undertaken with the necessary general precautions of preoperative analysis. The results of the medical tests obtained will greatly influence the selection of the appropriate technique for each particular patient (see in the descriptions of different techniques).

Because failure in technique or treatment will result in major deformities, which sometimes cannot be completely corrected in secondary endeavors, only reasonably experienced and well-trained surgeons should undertake this kind of operation in a major surgical operating facility.

We perform all reduction mammaplasties with the patient under general anesthesia. Anybody unfit for this for a medical, or any other, reason is a poor candidate for this operation and should be rejected.

After intubation anesthesia has been established, great care must be taken to place the patient in a semirecumbent, absolutely symmetric position on the operating table. The arms must be spread sideways to permit the surgeon and assistant easy approach to the chest, and the placement of the arms must be carefully checked for symmetry as well. Failure to do this preoperatively or allowing someone to lean on one arm and so move it will almost invariably result in asymmetric breasts at the end of the operation. Unfortunately, this fact might only be discovered when all the drapings are removed and the entire patient becomes visible again. Because major asymmetry cannot be tolerated today, the entire procedure of scrubbing and draping of the patient has to be redone, and symmetry must be achieved by opening the sutures on one or even both sides and resuturing all these wounds. This not only involves a very considerable loss of time and adds to the operative stress on the patient but also is usually quite a handicap for the development of good scars, which are difficult to obtain anyway (if nothing else, double suture marks are practically inevitable).

With the exception of minor skin excisions with absolutely no indication of bleeding, we use suction drainage, one on each side, routinely for a day or two, because the avoidance of hematomas is important in these frequently extensive wounds.

After surgery, a careful and properly fitting dry dressing should be applied and left in place for at least 3 days so that wound healing is not disturbed.

A discussion of the four methods used in our unit follows.

Techniques for Which Skin Resection Is the Main Aim

For minor cases, Dufourmentel's "résection oblique" and its variations are very useful, especially in patients in whom otherwise extremely large breasts would be produced if the large skin envelope should be filled by a prosthesis (Figs. 40–1 and 40–2). For major resections of skin, we use the Lexer-Kraske-Gohrbandt technique (Figs. 40–3 and 40–4).

Procedure

In the usual position the sternal notch and the xiphoid process are marked, and from them the desired position of the future nipple is measured and marked.

An oblique incision is made for about 6 to 7 cm from the areola toward the anterior axillary line, slanting downward at an angle of about 45 degrees (see Fig. 40–1A and B). From this the lower half of the breast is undermined, and, if necessary, the augmentation mammaplasty (always retropectoral in our unit) is performed.

Then a semilunar or, if a reduction of the size of the areola seems advisable, a circumareolar incision is performed. All excess skin between the old and the new position of the nipple can now be excised above this cut and a dog-ear avoided by a triangular excision above the primary cut (see Fig. 40–1A and B). A simple skin suture, usually without any need of drainage, completes the operation (see Fig. 40–1C and D). The postoperative treatment is the same as for any augmentation mammaplasty.

Advantages

This is a very minor operation.

It avoids undue enlargement of the breasts when large skin envelopes are combined with little residual glandular tissue (see Fig. 40–2).

There are comparatively short scars for a reduction mammaplasty in an area where they are easily hidden.

Disadvantages

It is applicable for minor skin reductions.

It does leave a lateral scar, which can be visible (see Fig. 40–2B).

It does not significantly improve the shape of breast but mainly eliminates surplus skin.

Setbacks

If the technique is applied in major skin reductions, the lateral scar may become unduly long if a dog-ear is avoided, as it should be.

The resulting breast tends to be somewhat flat (if not augmented at the same time, as in Figure 40–2B).

Indications

This procedure is indicated for (1) small breasts needing augmentation that would become too large if all the skin envelope were to be filled and (2) breasts needing

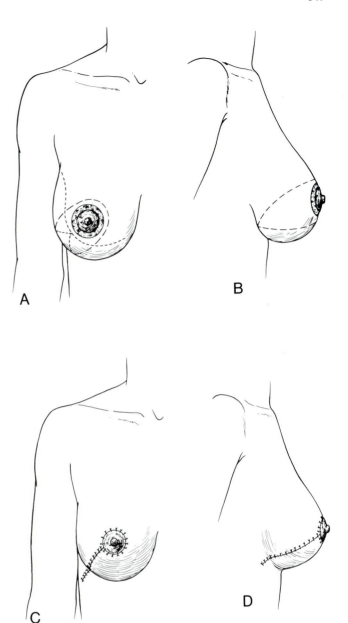

FIGURE 40–1
A and *B*, The dotted lines show the outline of the breast incisions and breast resection using Dufourmentel's "oblique technique." *C* and *D*, The appearance of the breast and the usual location of the lines of closure are shown.

a nipple lift of not more than 3 cm and little or no reduction.

Lexer-Kraske-Gohrbandt Technique

In the Lexer-Kraske-Gohrbandt technique, all of the skin is dissected off the gland, and the mound is formed by shaping the mammary tissue.

Procedure

After careful marking of the sternal notch and the xiphoid process, the desired position of the new nipple

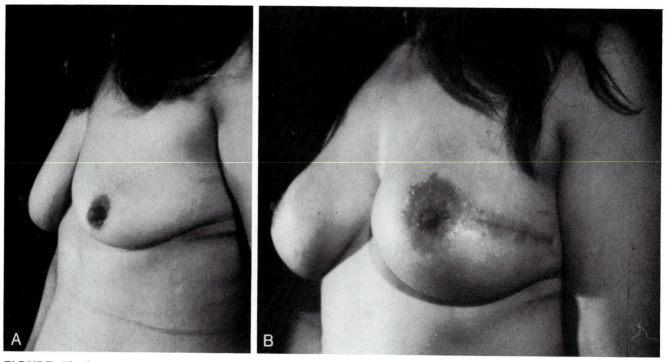

FIGURE 40–2
A, A 29-year-old patient, the mother of five children, is shown preoperatively. *B,* The same patient is shown 3 months after reduction with a long lateral scar.

is marked with ink and the point fixed with a needle prick because it might otherwise be lost and difficult to find again. No further markings are necessary (see Fig. 40–3A).

The nipple is circumcised, which leaves a 5-cm diameter circle of nipple-areola tissue in the center. The cut should be obliquely outward so as not to disturb the

subdermal plexus around the nipple (Schwarzmann, 1930) (see Fig. 40–3A and B).

From this circular hole a vertical cut is made down to the inframammary fold and another one from the upper pole of the nipple hole to about 1 cm below the future nipple position (ink mark). The skin is then dissected free for at least 5 cm above the aforementioned ink

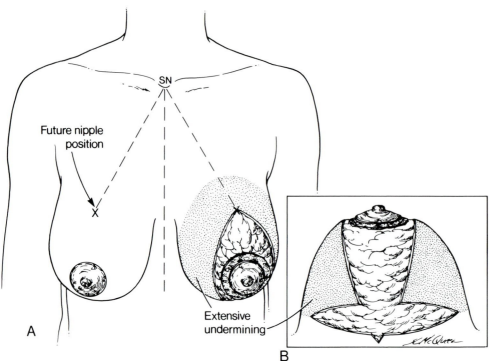

FIGURE 40–3
A and *B,* The new areolar position is marked (SN-X). The nipple-areola complex is incised, and a 1-cm border of dermis is left. The skin is excised in an oblique fashion from the new areolar site to the inframammary fold. The skin is then resected in the incised areas. A wide undermining is then carried out (dotted area).

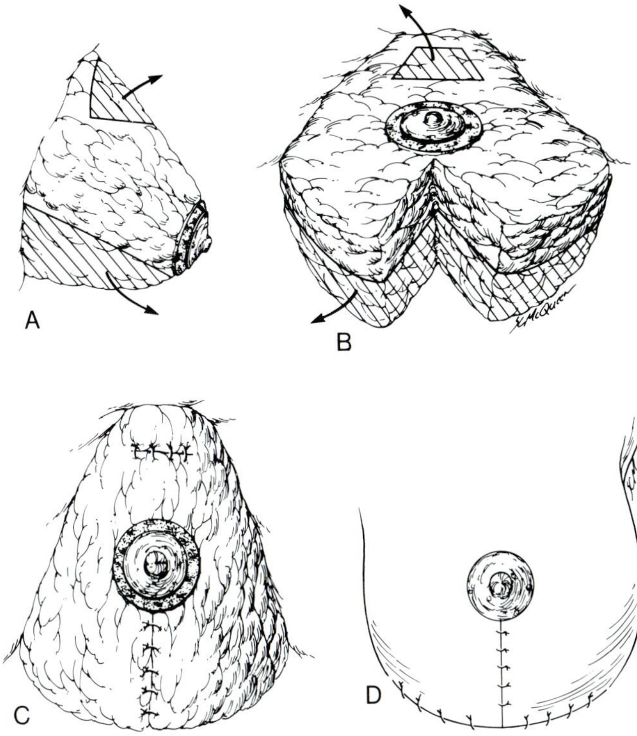

FIGURE 40–4
A and *B*, A square wedge of breast tissue is excised from the superior aspect of the breast and the inferior aspects. *C*, The areas of excision are closed with heavy sutures. *D*, Appearance of breast after reduction and closure.

mark and widely to the sides (see Fig. 40–3B). It has proved expedient to get a wide dissection along the inframammary fold to both sides of the breast toward the midline as well as toward the sides. However, care should be taken never to meet the other breast wound in the midline, because of the well-known poor quality of all scars in the sternal region. By wide undermining, the secondary fitting of the skin over the glandular mound and its tailoring are greatly facilitated.

After careful hemostasis a square piece of mammary tissue is excised above and a wedge-shaped one below the nipple-areola complex (see Fig. 40–4A to C). The amount of resection is a matter of the aesthetic perception of the surgeon but should not exceed 350 to 500 gm on each side, so as not to jeopardize the nutrition of the nipple. Only after another check of the hemostasis is the upper (square) excision sutured horizontally and the nipple lifted almost to its new position. This should never be done before the lower wedge excision is performed, because the two breast tissue pedicles might be kinked by the upper suture line and unintentionally severed by the lower excision. The lower excision is sutured vertically, care being taken to bring especially the lateral extension of the breast sufficiently inward to form a nice mound. The lowest of these stitches should be rather heavy material and take the superficial thoracic fascia in a wide bite, so as to fix the newly formed breast firmly against the chest wall.

If one draws the skin outward and downward, one can visualize the whole surplus easily. A hook is inserted in the uppermost corner of the incision and the whole skin tightened around the newly formed cone with three or more towel clips. The skin excision can be eased considerably if a curved bowel clamp is placed on the skin from both sides and the incision performed along the sides of the clamps. A vertical 7- to 8-cm-long two-layer suture is performed, and the lowest point is fixed with a comparatively heavy suture against the skin of the desired submammary fold. Two large dog-ears result on both sides of this suture and are taken care of in the usual manner. The undermining of the lower part of the incision downward as rejuvenated by Marchac and de Olarte (1982) is of considerable help in keeping the inferior scar as short as possible.

After completing the operation on the other side and once more checking the symmetry of both breast cones, the desirable new nipple position is marked. This mark should be rather close to the original ink mark. If this is not the case, the position of the patient should be carefully checked so that asymmetry, because of a changed placement of the patient on the operating table, is avoided.

An elliptical skin excision, including the upper end of the skin suture line, is then made, and the nipple let out, which should occur with ease and without much pull in any direction. Circular suturing of the nipple concludes the operation after the placement of the usual suction drain (see Fig. 40–4D).

Advantages

This procedure is quick and easy and readily adaptable to any given shape of breast.

The sensibility of the nipple and the possibility of breast-feeding are in no way impeded.

An excellent shape can be obtained by this method, one that will be retained well into the future (Fig. 40–5).

If the procedure is performed as an adjuvant of a breast reconstruction on the other side (to achieve

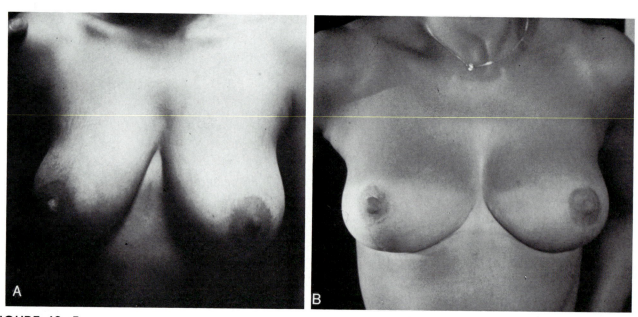

FIGURE 40–5
A, A 25-year-old patient is shown before reduction with the Lexer-Kraske-Gohrbandt technique. *B*, The same patient is shown 2 years after reduction of 290 gm from the right breast and 370 gm from the left breast.

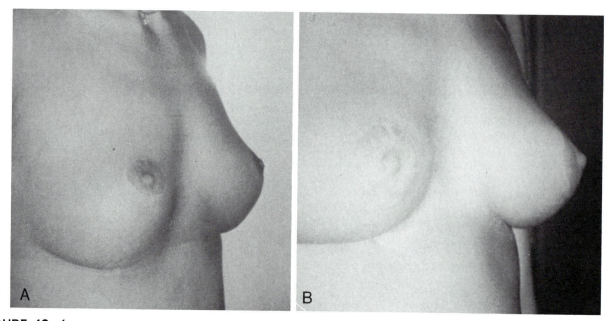

FIGURE 40–6
A, A 22-year-old patient is shown after a mammaplasty performed elsewhere. *B*, The same patient is shown 2 years after secondary reduction with the Lexer-Kraske-Gohrbandt technique. Notice how well the shape has been maintained after 2 years.

symmetry), an epigastric pedicle is possible, because no nutrition is required from the skin below the inframammary fold to any part of the new breast.

The technique is very suitable for secondary corrections after not very successful primary operations, especially when improving the shape and not the size of the breast is the patient's primary concern (Fig. 40–6).

Disadvantages

The method is not safe for major excisions of glandular tissue. The blood supply to the nipple might be insufficient.

Wide skin undermining is necessary, and the resulting skin flaps are of considerable length. No tension whatsoever should be permitted on the vertical suture line below the nipple and in any case is not necessary, because the shaping of the breast cone has been performed by modeling the gland. Compromised blood supply at the lower end of the scar because of undue tension might result in a considerable lengthening of the healing period and unsightly scar areas where the two branches of the T meet.

The technique does not follow a given pattern. It is therefore not easy to teach or learn and relies a great deal on the artistic ability of the surgeon. In experienced hands it is still very much worthwhile. When in doubt, one should choose the more reliable dermis pedicle techniques.

Setbacks and Complications

The vertical scar can widen considerably if the procedure is performed under tension.

Gentle handling of the long skin flaps is mandatory if secondary nutritional problems are to be avoided.

Indications

This procedure is indicated for small, mainly ptotic breasts in the younger age group, especially when breastfeeding is greatly desired by the patient.

In very small breasts with a very loose skin a small, retropectoral augmentation mammaplasty can be easily performed at the same time.

It is first choice among all techniques if an operation to adapt a healthy second breast to its reconstructed counterpart seems desirable.

Techniques Using Dermal Pedicles

Although some doubts were expressed as to whether dermal pedicles really provide all of the blood supply to the nipple in these methods (McKissock), their main principle remains undisputed. Even attempts to de-skin and not to de-epithelialize the pedicles (Crepeau and Klein, 1982; Kaplan, 1978; Kroll, 1988) could not truly disprove the basic idea. Because I strongly believe in safety as a paramount objective in these operations, de-epithelialization seems preferable to de-skinning, especially because we do not find this technique as time-consuming as some other authors (Crepeau, 1982).

All of these techniques and their variations originated in the early 1960s (Strömbeck and Pitanguy published their methods within a few years of each other). The procedure, however, has varied greatly, and almost all possible ways of preserving the blood supply were more or less successfully investigated. Strömbeck (1960) and Pitanguy (1963, 1967) use two dermal strips running horizontally across the breast, and Skoog (1963) even divided one of them, usually the medial one, to ease the positioning of the nipple without tension in its new and desired position. The difficulty in doing so brought the vertical pedicles into the center of attention. Whether the complete vertical pedicle of McKissock (1972) or the inferior vertical one of Robbins (1977) and Georgiade et al. (1979a) is selected remains a question of personal preference. Even three pedicles are sometimes advocated (Cardoso, 1984) but do not seem to be truly necessary. We believe, however, that the central glandular cone behind the vertical inferior pedicle of Georgiade (as mentioned by Kaplan [1978] and others as well) does provide additional safety and have therefore selected this method as the method of choice for most of our cases. On the other hand, a heavy juvenile breast, in which little nipple movement is required, will respond well to the Pitanguy method (Fig. 40–7). We never made a cut through the medial pedicle consciously (Skoog, 1963), and in the one case in which it happened unintentionally there resulted a disaster. So this technique cannot be advocated, and we have found no advantage in the additional upper extension of the dermal pedicle as advocated by McKissock (1972, 1980).

Procedures

All these methods are so well and extensively published in the literature concerned that a detailed description of them can be avoided. Suffice it to say that they, too, should only be done with the use of general anesthesia and in well-equipped units with all surgical and even intensive care facilities at one's disposal should an emergency should arise. Georgiade's description should be followed closely (Fig. 40–8).

Advantages

These techniques have a well-defined pattern to guide any surgeon, which remains sufficiently flexible to serve most of the needs of a particular operation.

Because of the fixed pattern, all these methods can easily be taught and learned in a training program. Even supervising such a procedure is comparatively easy, and the results should be reasonably safe even among the early cases of a trainee.

Even comparatively large breasts in young patients can be operated on with a considerable margin of safety (Fig. 40–9).

These techniques can fairly easily be adapted to the necessities of subcutaneous mastectomy with a considerable amount of superfluous skin, which cannot sensibly be refilled with a prosthesis. In this case, horizontal pedicles are usually the method of choice, because after

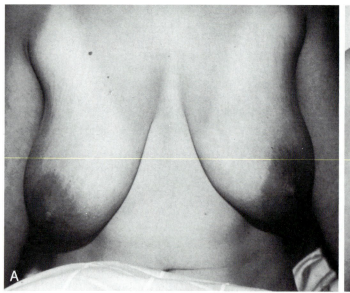
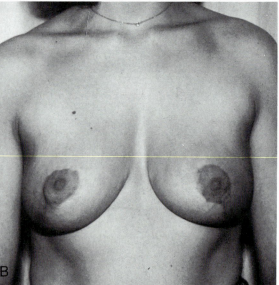

FIGURE 40–7

A, A 29-year-old mother of two children is shown with elongated pendulous breasts. B, The same patient is shown 18 months after undergoing the Pitanguy procedure.

resecting the central part of the breast, the approach to the retropectoral space for augmentation is technically much easier than the somewhat roundabout way from between the pectoralis and the serratus that has to be used in vertical pedicles if one wants to keep as much blood supply intact as possible, as one should.

Disadvantages

Even for an experienced surgeon and his team, the time for de-epithelialization, if done carefully, is considerable; and its performance not always as easy as it sounds.

To obtain a really pleasing form in some cases is more difficult than expected when one reads the literature. There is in more advanced cases usually some difficulty in getting the nipple high enough on the skin cone without the undue—and disfiguring—tension inward and downward that occurs with the use of horizontal pedicles.

In the techniques using a vertical pedicle, its fixation against the chest wall to prevent later sagging of the lower half of the breast because of gravity is another problem frequently encountered, which we resolve by using at least two reasonably heavy and nonresorbable stitches on both sides of the pedicle to keep the inframammary fold where it should be, not only for the inspection on the operating table but also for years to come.

Setbacks and Complications

Because of the prolonged time of operation, the stress on the patient is considerable.

There is usually some marked blood loss, which should be replaced in most cases to ensure smooth healing conditions. We believe that today delayed autotransfusion, which avoids any chance of infection,

whether hepatitis or acquired immunodeficiency syndrome (AIDS), is the method of choice in those cases in which the time of preparing for the actual operation does not play an important role. Five hundred to 1000 ml should be sufficient even in major cases of reduction.

Fixation of the breast mound against the chest wall may be a problem. With some experience and technical attention to detail, the difficulty should, however, be smoothly overcome.

Indications

This technique is indicated in most cases of reduction mammaplasty.

This procedure is also indicated in subcutaneous mastectomy with ample skin that cannot be filled out sensibly with implants.

Techniques Transferring the Nipple as a Free Full-Thickness Graft

These are among the oldest of all reduction techniques (Thorek, 1922; Adams, 1944) and have become more popular again since D. C. Robertson published his well-documented work in 1963 and Pitanguy (in Portuguese) in 1965. We adhere to the Robertson technique because of its ease in design and safety of results.

Procedure

With the patient under general anesthesia and in the usual semiprone position, a curved incision is outlined on the upper half of the breast, its apex at the site of the future nipple (Fig. 40–10A). Then a U-shaped flap is designed centrally, exactly below the position of the

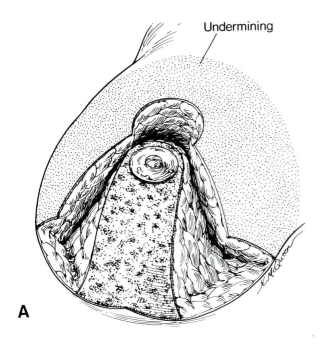

Undermining

A

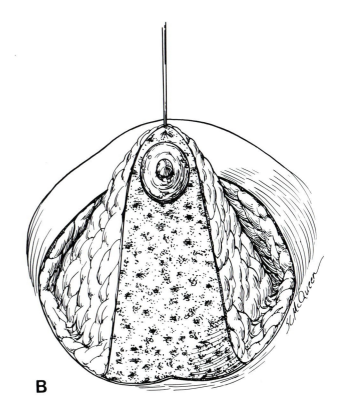

B

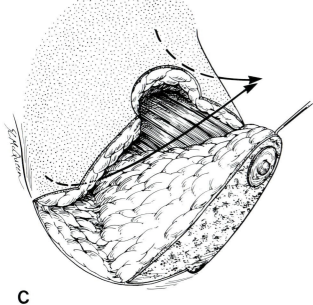

C

FIGURE 40-8

A, The inferior pedicle technique (Georgiade) is shown. Note the wide base and cone of breast tissue. *B*, The length of the dermal pedicle is shown with the underlying wide-based area of breast tissue. *C*, The areas of undermining are shown with the stippling as well as the areas of breast resection, leaving a wide-based cone of breast tissue with excellent blood supply.

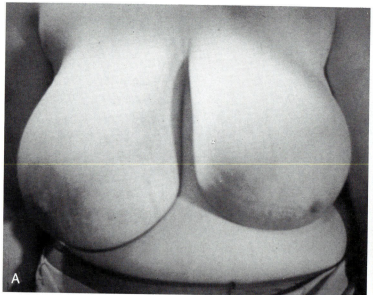
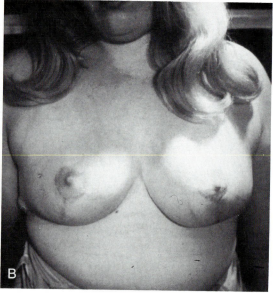

FIGURE 40–9

A, An 18-year-old patient is shown with juvenile breast hypertrophy. *B,* The same patient is shown 1 year after reduction (Georgiade technique). A reduction of 1450 gm of breast tissue from the right breast and 1280 gm from the left breast was performed.

future nipple, about 6 × 6 to 7 × 7 cm in size (as already suggested by May in 1943 for shortening the inframammary scar). Where the ends of this flap meet the inframammary fold, they are united with the upper incision by a slightly curving line medially and laterally (see Fig. 40–10A). Care should be taken that the approximate lengths of the upper and the lower incision are the same.

At this point the nipple is removed as a full-thickness disk 5 cm in diameter and carefully defatted. A semilunar area is then de-epithelialized above the upper incision centrally to receive the free grafted nipple at the end of the resection. This is technically much easier with the breast still intact and the skin reasonably tight, rather than later on, when cutting the epithelium away truly completely might be rather awkward.

The resection of most of the breast tissue is performed with care taken to leave a sufficient wedge of tissue under the lower U flap and not to cut too much out centrally (Fig. 40–10B and C). Medially, close to the sternum, and laterally, in the anterior axillary line, the resection should be quite radical so that dog-ears are avoided in skin closure, still a bit of a problem in these vast resections (more than 2000 gm on each side in most cases).

After hemostasis the tip of the U flap is de-epithelialized for about 1 to 2 cm and united with the previously denuded area on the upper incision, forming the tip of the new cone and the bed for the free nipple graft (see Fig. 40–10A). Then one closes the skin in two or three layers according to the size of the remaining breast, starting medially and laterally to avoid dog-ears in the skin as much as possible (see Fig. 40–10B and C). After skin closure, the free graft is sutured to the tip of the newly formed breast and fixed with a tie-over dressing,

which can be removed after 3 or 4 days (Fig. 40–10D and E). The treatment after surgery is usually very conservative, and the healing process should be uneventful.

Advantages

This is by far the fastest of all reduction mammaplasties. An experienced surgeon with a well-trained team should be able to perform the operation in about an hour.

There is very little stress on the patient, and blood loss is minimal.

The method is extremely safe, and the survival of the nipple practically guaranteed (Fig. 40–11).

Any desired amount of resection is feasible, without any additional time or stress.

Disadvantages

All sensitivity to the nipple is primarily lost, and what is regained later is more skin than nipple sensitivity, especially as far as sexual perception is concerned.

Any chance of breast-feeding is lost forever.

Setbacks and Complications

This is the only technique in which the produced breast can become too small. Resection is so easy and safe that to take out too much becomes a temptation.

There is a double scar on the undersurface of the breast, where in most other methods there is only a single one. This, however, cannot and must not be changed if the main purpose of this technique—its safety—is not to be impeded. If skin flaps are developed

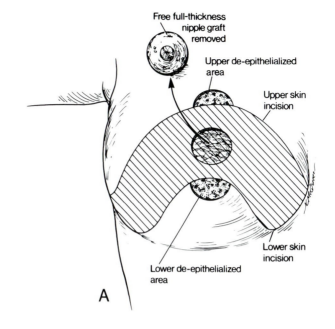

FIGURE 40-10

A, The technique of D. C. Robertson is shown. The areas of excision (oblique lines) and de-epithelialization with a free full-thickness nipple graft removed are shown. *B,* The area of tissue removed is shown. Note the area of de-epithelialization for the new site of the areola. *C,* The inferior flap is now shown, brought superiorly to approximate the superior flap. *D* and *E,* The previously obtained full-thickness nipple-areolar skin graft is shown being reimplanted on the area of de-epithelialization. A tie-over bolus is used to immobilize the graft for 7 days.

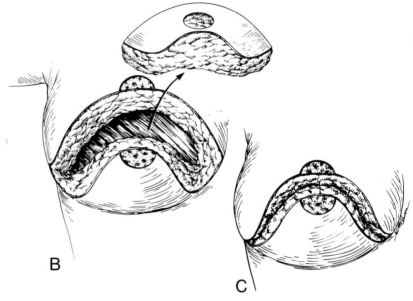

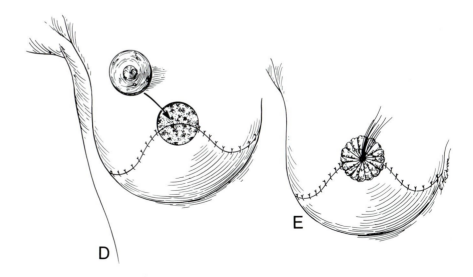

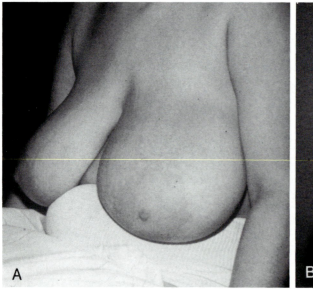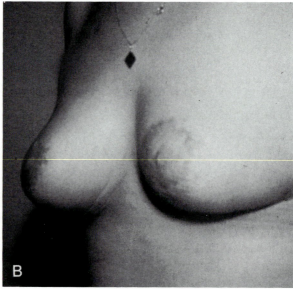

FIGURE 40–11

A, A 49-year-old patient with severe diabetes is shown with large ptotic breasts. *B*, The same patient is shown 2 years after reduction of 1950 gm of breast tissue from the right breast and 2070 gm from the left breast. Note the good coning.

and the essential unity of skin-fat flaps not maintained, the amount of wound surface is multiplied, and complications are likely.

Indications

This technique is indicated when the breasts are extremely heavy and enlarged, with a great distance between the actual and the desirable position of the nipple (more than 15 cm).

It is indicated for elderly women, in whom speed and safety are more important than breast-feeding or nipple sensitivity.

It is indicated in poor-risk cases, in which the reduction of weight is the outstanding reason for operating and not so much pure aesthetic improvement (see Fig. 40–11).

It is indicated for subcutaneous mastectomies with an abundance of skin and the necessity to limit time and stress on the patient.

It is also indicated in some cases of extreme gynecomastia in young men, where a normal positioning of the nipple after removing all its underlying tissue would otherwise result in considerable contour defects.

SUMMARY

Four techniques of reduction mammaplasty have been discussed, and their various merits outlined. The selection of the method to be used should depend mainly on the basic advantages of each technique. Problems and complications inherent in all methods should and must be discussed with the patient preoperatively for selection of the best possible means of achieving satisfaction for patient and surgeon alike.

References

Adams, W. M.: Free transplantation of the nipples and areolae. Surgery 15:186, 1944.

Adams, W. M.: Free composite grafts of nipples in mammaplasty. South. Surg. 13:715, 1947.

Aubert, V.: Hypertrophie mammaire de la puberté: Résection partielle restauratrice. Arch. Franco-Belges Clin. 26:284, 1923.

Aufricht, G.: Mammaplasty for pendulous breasts: empiric and geometric planning. Plast. Reconstr. Surg. 4:13, 1949.

Axhausen, G.: Über mammaplastik. Med. Klin. 22:1437, 1926.

Biesenberger, H.: Eine neue Methode der Mammaplastik. Zentralbe. Chir. 55:2382, 1928.

Biesenberger, H.: Eine neue Methode der Mammaplastik. Erganzung zum Gleichnamigen Aufsatz im Zbl. Chir. 1928. Zentralbl. Chir. 57:2971, 1930.

Biesenberger, H.: *Deformitaten und Kosmetische Operationen der Weiblichen Brust.* Wien, Wilhelm Maudrich, 1931.

Cardoso, A. D., Cardoso, A. D., Pessanha, M. C., Peralta, J. M.: Three dermal pedicles for nipple areola complex movement in reduction of gigantomastia. Ann. Plast. Surg. 12:419, 1984.

Courtiss, E. H., Goldwyn, R. M.: Reduction mammaplasty by the inferior pedicle technique. Plast. Reconstr. Surg. 59:500, 1977.

Crepeau, R., Klein, H. W.: Reduction mammaplasty with inferiorly based glandular pedicle flap. Ann. Plast. Surg. 9:463, 1982.

Dehner, H.: Mastopexie zur Beseitigung der Hängebrust. Münch. Med. Wochenschr. 55:1878, 1908.

Dufourmentel, C., Mouly, R.: Plastie mammaire par la méthode oblique. Ann. Chir. Plast. 6:45, 1961.

Georgiade, N. G., Georgiade, G. S.: Hypermastia and ptosis. In: Georgiade, N. G., Georgiade, G. S., Riefkohl, R., Barwick, W. J. (eds.): *Essentials of Plastic, Maxillofacial and Reconstructive Surgery.* Baltimore, Williams & Wilkins, 1987, p. 694.

Georgiade, N., Serafin, D., Morris, R., Georgiade, G.: Reduction mammaplasty utilizing an inferior pedicle nipple-areolar flap. Ann. Plast. Surg. 3:211, 1979a.

Georgiade, N. G., Serafin, D., Riefkohl, R., Georgiade, G. S.: Is there a reduction mammaplasty for "all seasons"? Plast. Reconstr. Surg. 63:765, 1979b.

Georgiade, G., Riefkohl, R., Georgiade, N.: The inferior dermal-pyramidal type breast reduction: Long-term evaluation. Ann. Plast. Surg. 23:203, 1989.

Gillies, H. D., McIndoe, A. H.: The technique of mammaplasty in conditions of hypertrophy of the breast. Surg. Gynecol. Obstet. 68:658, 1939.

Gillies, H., Millard, R. D.: *The Principles and Art of Plastic Surgery.* London, Butterworths, 1957.

Gläsmer, E., Amersbach, R.: Zur feineren Technik der Hängebrust-Operation. Münch. Med. Wochenschr. 75:1547, 1928.

Göbell, R.: Über Autoplastische Freie Fascien und Aponeurosentransplantation nach Martin Kirschner. Arch. Klin. Chir. 146:462, 1927.

Gohrbandt, E.: Personal communication.

Hester, T. R., Bostwick, J., Miller, L., Cunningham, S. J.: Breast reduction utilizing the maximally vascularized central breast pedicle. Plast. Reconstr. Surg. 76:890, 1985.

Holländer, E.: Die Operation der Mammahypertrophie und der Hängebrust. Dtsch. Med. Wochenschr. 50:1400, 1924.

Joseph, J.: Zur Operation der Hypertrophischen Hängebrust (Mastomiopexie). Dtsch. Med. Wochenschr. 51:1103, 1925.

Kaplan, I.: Reduction mammaplasty: Nipple-areola survival in a single breast quadrant. Plast. Reconstr. Surg. 61:27, 1978.

Kausch, W.: Die Operation der Mammahypertrophie. Zentralbl. Chir. 43:713, 1916.

Kraske, H.: Die Operation der Atrophischen und Hypertrophischen Hängebrust. Münch. Med. Wochenshr. 70:672, 1923.

Kroll, S. S.: A comparison of de-epithelialization and deskinning in inferior pedicle breast reduction. Plast. Reconstr. Surg. 81:913, 1988.

Kuester, H.: Operationen bei Hängebrust und Hängeleib. Monschr. Geburth. Gynak. 73:316, 1926.

Labandter, H. P., Dowden, R. V., Dinner, M. I.: The inferior segment technique for breast reduction. Ann. Plast. Surg. 8:493, 1982.

Lexer, E.: Hypertrophie bei der Mammae Demonstration in der Naturwissenschaftlichen Medizinischen Gesellschaft Jena. Münch. Med. Wochenschr. 59:2702, 1912.

Lexer, E.: *Die Gesamte Wiederherstellungschirurgie.* Vol. 2. Leipzig, J. A. Barth Verlag, 1931, p. 553.

Lotsch, F.: Über Hängebrustplastik. Zentralbl. Chir. 50:1241, 1923.

Lotsch, F.: Über Hängebrustplastik. Klin. Wochenschr. 7:603, 1928.

Lupo, G., Boggio-Robotti, G.: *Chirurgia Plastica del Seno e Delle Regione Mammaria.* Editione Minerva Medica, 1970.

Marchac, D., de Olarte, G.: Reduction mammaplasty and correction of ptosis with a short inframammary scar. Plast. Reconstr. Surg. 69:45, 1982.

May, H.: Reconstruction of breast deformities. Surg. Gynecol. Obstet. 77:523, 1943.

McIndoe, A.H., Rees T.D.: Mammaplasty: Indications, technique and complications. Br. J. Plast. Surg. 10:307, 1958.

McKissock, P. K.: Reduction mammaplasty with a vertical dermal flap. Plast. Reconstr. Surg. 49:245, 1972.

McKissock, P. K.: Reduction mammaplasty. In: Barron, J. N., Saad, M. N. (eds.): *Operative Plastic and Reconstructive Surgery.* New York, Churchill Livingstone, 1980, p. 799.

McKissock, P. K.: Discussion of Hester breast reduction utilizing the maximally vascularized central breast pedicle. Plast. Reconstr. Surg. 76:899, 1985.

Noël, A.: Asthetische Chirurgie der weiblichen Brust: Ein neues Verfahren zur Korrektur der Hängebrust. Med. Welt. 2:51, 1928.

Palacin, J. M., del Cacho, C., Johnson, D., Planas, J.: Reduction mammoplasty with the Peixoto technique. Eur. J. Plast. Surg. 11:132, 1988.

Passot, R.: La correction esthétique du prolapsus mammaire par la procédé de transposition du mamelon. Presse Med. 33:317, 1925.

Penn, J.: Breast reduction. Br. J. Plast. Surg. 7:357, 1955.

Pitanguy, I.: Contribution to the technique of free grafting for the repair of the large mammary hypertrophies. Rev. Latin. Am. Cir. Plast. 7:75, 1963.

Pitanguy, I.: Surgical treatment of breast hypertrophy. Br. J. Plast. Surg. 20:78, 1967.

Pousson, A.: De la mastopexie. Bull. Soc. Chir. 23:507, 1897.

Rahm, H.: Riesenmammae, eine plastische Verkleinerung. Demonstr. in der Breslauer Gesellschft für Chirurgie 1929. Zentralbl. Chir. 57:491, 1930.

Regnault, P.: Reduction mammaplasty by the "B" technique. Plast. Reconstr. Surg. 53:19, 1974.

Reich, J.: The advantages of a lower central breast segment in reduction mammaplasty. Aesthetic Plast. Surg. 3:47, 1979.

Robertson, D. C.: Reduction mammaplasty using a large inferior flap technique. In: *Transactions Third International Congress Plastic Surgery.* Amsterdam, Excerpta Medica Foundation, 1963, p. 81.

Robbins, T. H.: A reduction mammaplasty with the areola-nipple based on an inferior dermal pedicle. Plast. Reconstr. Surg. 59:64, 1977.

Sauerbruch, F.: Die Chirurgie der Brustorgane. 3. Auf, Bd 2. Berlin, Springer-Verlag, 1928.

Schmidt-Tintemann, U.: Mammaplasty: Indication and preoperative considerations. Chir. Plast. 2:105, 1974.

Schreiber, F.: Operation der Hängebrust. Bruns Beitr. Klin. Chir. 147:56, 1929.

Schwarzmann, E.: Die Technik der Mammaplastik. Chirurg 2:932, 1930.

Skoog, T.: A technique of breast reduction: Transposition of the nipple on a cutaneous vascular pedicle. Acta Chir. Scand. 126:453, 1963.

Strömbeck, J. O.: Mammaplasty: Report of a new technique based on the two-pedicle procedure. Br. J. Plast. Surg. 13:79, 1960.

Strömbeck, J. O.: Macromastia in women and its surgical treatment. Acta Chir. Scand. Suppl. 341, 1964.

Thorek, M.: Possibilities in reconstruction of the human form. N.Y. Med. J. 116:572, 1922.

Verchère, P.: Mastopexie latérale contre la mastoptose hypertrophique. Méd. Mod. 9:540, 1898.

Weiner, D. L., Aiache, A. E.: A single dermal pedicle for nipple transposition in subcutaneous mastectomy, reduction mammaplasty and mastopexy. Plast. Reconstr. Surg. 51:115, 1973.

Wise, R. J., Gannon, J. P., Hill, J. R.: Further experience with reduction mammaplasty. Plast. Reconstr. Surg. 32:12, 1963.

PTOSIS

41

Maxine Schurter
Gordon Letterman

A History of the Treatment of Sagging Breasts (Mastopexy)

The term "mastopexy" is derived from the Greek *"mastos"* ("breast") and *"pexi"* ("fixation"). Historically, in an effort to correct ptosis, the mammary gland was elevated and fixed to the pectoral fascia, periosteum of the rib, pectoralis major muscle, or a loop of catgut or fascia lata encircling a rib. The breast has been fixed internally by approximating two of its cut edges or by superimposition. Fixation was also accomplished by the creation of a new "skin brassiere" or solely by skin resection. The Committee on Nomenclature (Letterman and Schurter, 1985) of the American Society for Aesthetic Plastic Surgery has suggested a diagnostic and procedural nomenclature for ptosis and mastopexy.

The earliest publications on aesthetic surgery of the female breast were concerned with the elevation of the ptotic gland. These papers were in the form of case reports written primarily by surgeons of France and Germany. The procedures had usually been carried out on patients who had hypertrophic breasts, because reduction mammaplasty had not as yet been described.

Pousson's article on mastopexy (1897) concerned a young woman whose breasts rested on her thighs when she was seated. He resected an ellipse of skin and fatty tissue over the upper part of each breast. The gland was then elevated and sutured to the aponeurosis of the pectoralis major muscle (Fig. 41–1).

Early in the postoperative period, Michel (1897) presented Pousson's patient at a meeting of the Societé d'Anatomie de Bordeaux. She was healed, free of pain, and very satisfied with the operation.

Verchère's (1898) early case report told of an opera singer whose breasts were hanging by long pedicles to the hypogastric region. Because of her occupation, a scar on the upper part of the breast was not acceptable. Therefore, Verchère resected a large triangle of skin and subcutaneous tissue on the lateral aspect of the

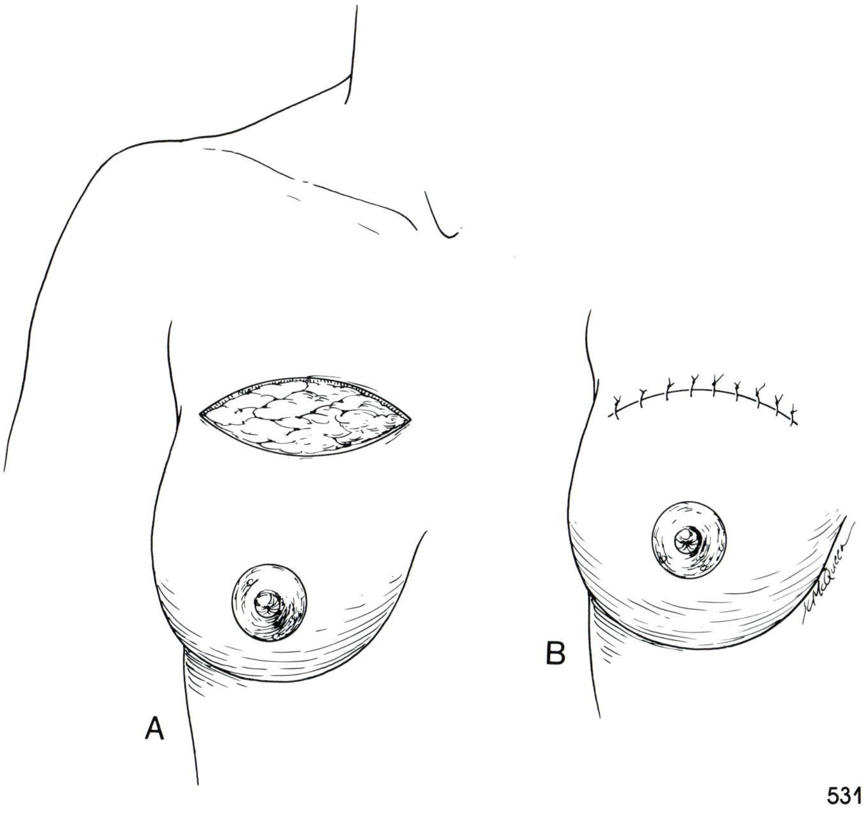

FIGURE 41–1
A and *B*, Pousson's excision of skin and fatty tissue from the upper part of the breast.

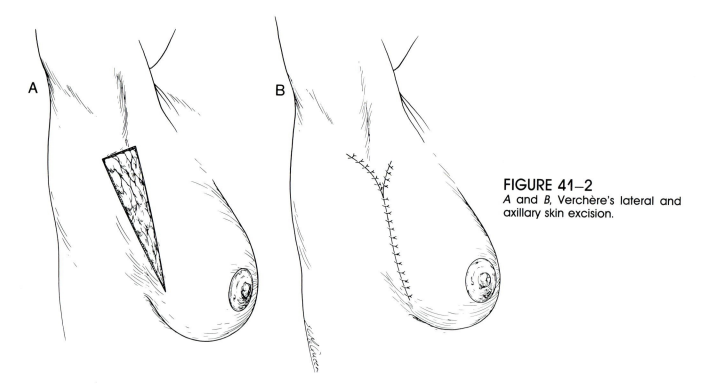

FIGURE 41–2

A and *B*, Verchère's lateral and axillary skin excision.

breast. The defect was closed in the shape of a Y on the lateral aspect of the breast and axilla (Fig. 41–2).

Dehner (1908), in Ludwigshafen, described his case of a 30-year-old woman whose breasts had greatly increased in size over the previous 5-year period. He excised an ellipse of skin and fat on the upper part of the breast, as Pousson had done, but he fixed the gland to the periosteum of the third rib with catgut sutures.

Girard (1910), in Berlin, stated that instead of making the incision above the nipple and areola, he used the inframammary incision of Gaillard Thomas (1882). The breast was then elevated off the chest wall to the level of the second rib. A heavy catgut suture was passed from the upper pole of the breast around the rib. Four sling loops then were passed from the posterior aspect of the breast at different levels through the sling that encircled the rib. For added support, the posterior

surface of the gland was sutured to the pectoralis major fascia with multiple sutures (Fig. 41–3).

Göbell (1914), in Kiel, wrote a two-line report outlining a mastopexy procedure. His exposure was the same as Girard's, but he attached the posterior aspect of the gland to the third rib with fascia lata. He gave a detailed explanation of the procedure 13 years later (1927).

Lotsch (1923) described his method before the Berlin Surgical Society. It was unique in several ways: the nipple was transposed upward on the gland to a higher opening; the skin was widely undermined; skin was excised below the nipple and areola; and the skin closure was primarily vertical. Many later forms of mastopexy and breast reduction utilized some or all of the features of Lotsch's operation (Fig. 41–4).

In the same year Eckstein (1923) gave yet another case report concerning the surgical correction of ptosis

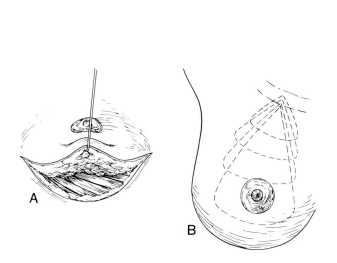

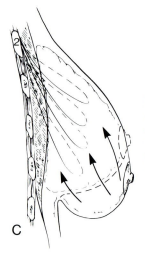

FIGURE 41–3

A to *C*, Inframammary excision of Gaillard Thomas with catgut slings from the second rib to the posterior aspect of the breast, as done by Girard.

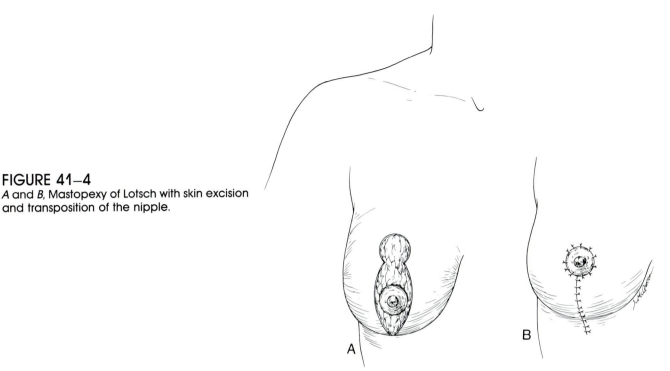

FIGURE 41–4
A and *B*, Mastopexy of Lotsch with skin excision and transposition of the nipple.

of the breast. He circumscribed the areola and widely undermined the skin. The nipple and areola were elevated about a hand's breadth higher and brought out through a small incision at that level, where it was sutured in place. There was postoperative inversion of the nipple, which Eckstein attributed to the enormous weight of the gland. This procedure is not greatly different from what is done today to form a new skin brassiere.

Dartigues (1924), a renowned French professor of surgery, wrote extensively on the subject of aesthetic surgery of the breast. He described four degrees of prolapse. The first was corrected by excision of a semilunar segment of axillary skin and fixation of the axillary tail of the breast to the lateral border of the pectoralis major muscle. For the second, he removed a vertical segment of skin between the areola and inframammary fold. He then sutured the lower pole of the gland to the pectoralis major muscle. Marchac's (1982) description published 60 years later is not greatly different. The third and fourth degrees of ptosis really belong to reduction mammaplasty, since they require glandular resection.

Weinhold (1926) spoke of his mastopexy operation before the Gynecologic Society of Breslau. Skin was excised superiorly around the areola for its elevation, and a compensatory lunar skin excision was made below the areola.

Joseph (1927) proposed a method for elevating the pendulous breast. A diamond-shaped segment of skin was excised between the lateral border of the breast and the anterior axillary line. The anterior skin edge was then sutured to a point 13 cm or so higher on the axillary skin edge. Wound closure resulted in superior and inferior dog-ears. These were excised, and the resulting defects closed. Finally a supra-areolar area was excised, and the nipple and areola were elevated and sutured

into position (Fig. 41–5). Joseph's axillary skin excision is reminiscent of Verchère's procedure.

A procedure consisting of several staged supra-areolar skin excisions was presented by Gläsmer and Amersbach (1928). They described lateral extension of the periareolar excision after the method of Holländer. Noël described a series of supra-areolar excisions. Her student Cesari modified these excisions with compensatory triangular excisions (Fig. 41–6). Further modifications were suggested by a second student, López-Martinez, who used medial and lateral extensions to enhance the superior transposition of the nipple (Fig. 41–7).

Prior to the beginning of the fourth decade of this century, no significant article had appeared in the American literature. Owing in large part to the multilingual capabilities, international reputations, and surgical achievements of Thorek, Maliniac, and Bames, as well as the extensive travels of the distinguished South American surgeons Malbec and Marino, these concepts were brought to the United States and to South America.

Bames' article (1930) published in the *American Journal of Surgery* was a logical progression of the operations of Girard (1910) and Göbell (1914, 1927).

Gillies and Marino (1958) described the "periwinkle-shell" rotation of breast tissue for the correction of the small ptotic breast. This was a form of internal fixation but was never widely accepted, probably because it was a big operation for a small problem.

Regnault (1966), of Canada, pointed out that mastopexy could be performed simultaneously with augmentation with the use of a Silastic prosthesis.

Kahn et al. (1968) showed that mastopexy could be accomplished by skin excision using the Strömbeck pattern. Indeed, as new reduction mammaplasty procedures became available, the techniques were also used for mastopexy.

Another breast fixation procedure was presented by

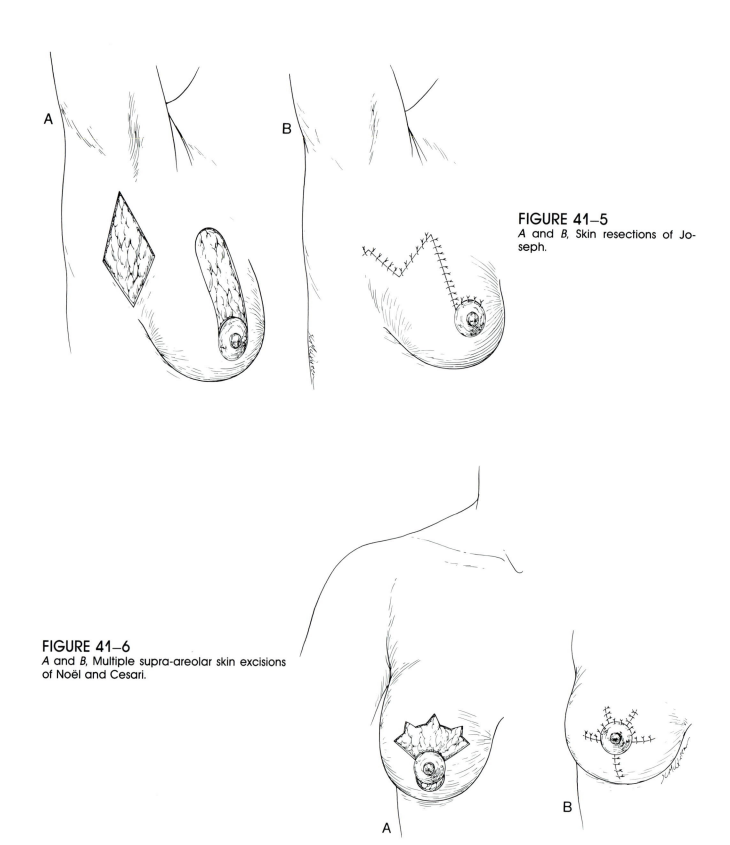

FIGURE 41–5
A and *B*, Skin resections of Joseph.

FIGURE 41–6
A and *B*, Multiple supra-areolar skin excisions of Noël and Cesari.

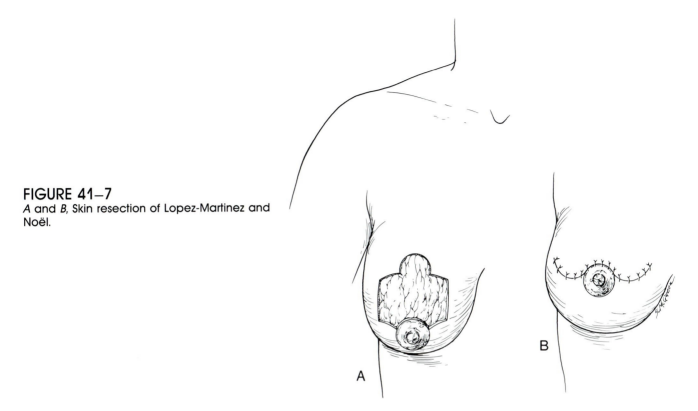

FIGURE 41-7
A and *B*, Skin resection of Lopez-Martinez and Noël.

Dufourmentel and Mouly (1968). The breast fixation was a modified "periwinkleshell" operation, and the skin excision was adopted from their reduction procedure (Fig. 41–8).

Goulian (1971) believed that neither augmentation nor reduction was necessary and described his measurements for preparing a new skin envelope.

Hinderer (1976) attached the elevated mammary gland to tissues in the retromammary area with dermal strips prepared from the skin of the breast itself.

Bartels et al. (1976) demonstrated the use of a vertically oriented periareolar oval skin excision (Fig. 41–9).

Regnault (1978) enlarged upon her original surgical interventions and classified the deformity as minor, moderate, or major ptosis; pseudoptosis; or partial ptosis. These gradations were based upon the relationship of the nipple to the submammary fold. For minor ptosis she excises periareolar skin with a vertical extension down to the submammary fold (Fig. 41–10). Whidden (1978) presented a maneuver for delineating the

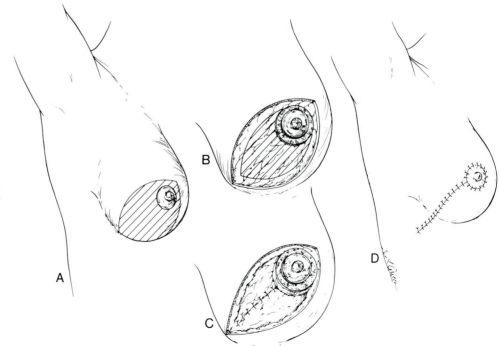

FIGURE 41-8
A to *D*, Dufourmentel and Mouly's lateral skin excision and overlapping of the gland upon itself.

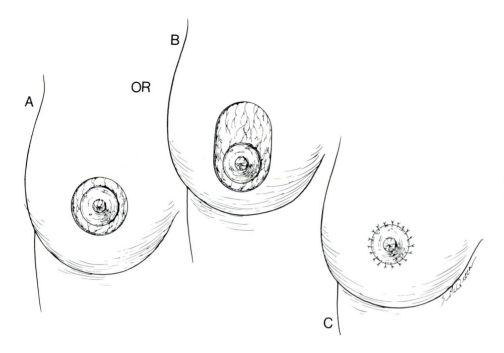

FIGURE 41–9
A to *C*, Circumareolar masto-pexy of Bartels and associates.

area of skin to be excised in order to form a new skin brassiere; he used tailor's tacks for this purpose.

Gruber and Jones (1980), in an effort to minimize scars, described a circular excision of skin around the areola for elevation of the breast. Time showed that the scars stretched and that the gland had a flattened appearance.

Marchac and de Olarte (1982) advocate skin resection, largely in a vertical direction, so that the final scar cannot be seen either medially or laterally and is part of the inframammary crease.

Lassus (1988) describes the same technique for mastopexy as for reduction, resulting in a vertical scar from the areola to or below the inframammary crease.

SUMMARY

Fixation procedures described in the late nineteenth and early twentieth century are no longer generally acceptable techniques. Procedures based on the skin excisions and upon the creation of a new skin brassiere have not produced permanent results; skin continues to stretch. Currently, dermal mastopexy with breast augmentation as well as expansion techniques are subjects of discussion.

References

Bames, H. O.: The correction of pendulous breasts. Am. J. Surg. 10:80, 1930.

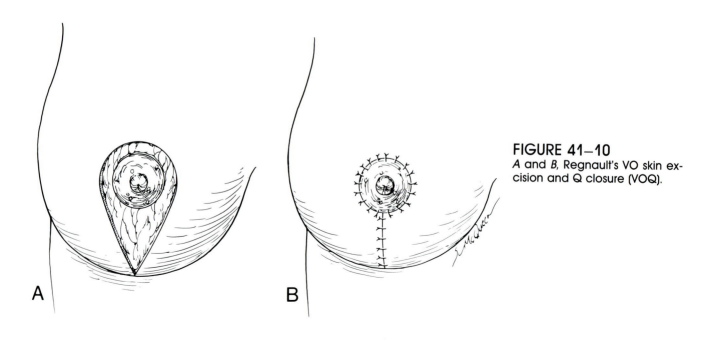

FIGURE 41–10
A and *B*, Regnault's VO skin excision and Q closure (VOQ).

Bartels, R. J., Strickland, D. M., Douglas, W. M.: A new mastopexy operation for mild or moderate breast ptosis. Plast. Reconstr. Surg. 57:687, 1976.

Dartigues, L.: Traitement chirurgical du prolapsus mammaire: Suspension et mastopexie par voie axillotomique (cicatrice cachée dans la région pileuse de l'aisselle). Paris Chir. 16:145, 1924.

Dartigues, L.: Traitement chirurgical du prolapsus mammaire. Arch. Franco-Belg. Chir. 28:313, 1925.

Dehner, M.: Mastopexie zur Beseitigung der Hängebrust. Münch. Med. Wochenschr. 55:1878, 1908.

Dufourmentel, C., Mouly, R.: Modification of "periwinkleshell operation" for small ptotic breast. Plast. Reconstr. Surg. 41:523, 1968.

Eckstein, L.: Discussion of F. Lotsch: Über Hängebrustplastik. Zentralbl. Chir. 50:1333, 1923.

Gillies, H., Marino, H.: The "periwinkleshell" principle in the treatment of the small ptotic breast. Plast. Reconstr. Surg. 21:1, 1958.

Girard, C.: Über Mastoptose und Mastopexie. Arch. Klin. Chir. 92:829, 1910.

Gläsmer, E., Amersbach, R.: Zur feineren Technik der Hängebrustoperation. Münch. Med. Wochenschr. 75:1547, 1928.

Göbell, R.: Mamma pendula und heftiger Mastodynie. Münch. Med. Wochenschr. 61:1760, 1914.

Göbell, R.: Über Autoplastische freie Fascien und Aponeurosentransplantation nach Martin Kirschner. Arch. Klin. Chir. 146:463, 1927.

Goulian, D., Jr.: Dermal mastopexy. Plast. Reconstr. Surg. 47:105, 1971.

Gruber, R. P., Jones, H. W., Jr.: The "donut" mastopexy: Indications and complications. Plast. Reconstr. Surg. 65:34, 1980.

Hinderer, U. T.: The dermal brassiere mammaplasty. Clin. Plast. Surg. 3:349, 1976.

Holländer, E.: Die Operation der Mammahypertrophie und der Hängebrust. Dtsch. Med. Wochenschr. 50:1400, 1924.

Joseph, J.: Zur Beseitigung der Einfachen und der hypertrophischen Hängebrust. Dtsch. Med. Wochenschr. 53:1853, 1927.

Kahn, S., Hoffman, S., Simon, B. E.: Correction of nonhypertrophic ptosis of the breasts. Plast. Reconstr. Surg. 41:244, 1968.

Lassus, C.: The short incision. Presented at the PSEF/ASAPS Third Annual Plastic Surgery of the Breast Symposium, Santa Fe, September 1988.

Letterman, G., Schurter, M.: History of the surgical correction of mammary ptosis. In: Owsley, J. Q., Peterson, R. A. (eds.): *Symposium on Aesthetic Surgery of the Breast.* St. Louis, C. V. Mosby, 1978.

Letterman, G., Schurter, M.: Suggested nomenclature of aesthetic and reconstructive surgery of the breast: Part II. Augmentation mammoplasty and mastopexy. Aesthetic Plast. Surg. 9:293, 1985.

Lotsch, F.: Über Hängebrustplastik. Zentralbl. Chir. 50:1241, 1923.

Marchac, D., de Olarte, G.: Reduction mammaplasty and correction of ptosis with a short inframammary scar. Plast. Reconstr. Surg. 69:45, 1982.

Michel, M.: Sur un cas de mastopexie. J. Med. Bordeaux 27:495, 1897.

Noël, A.: Aesthetische Chirurgie der Weiblichen Brust: Ein Neues Verfahren Zur Korektur der Hängebrust. Med. Welt. 2:51, 1928.

Noël, A., López-Martinez: Nouveaux procédés chirurgicaux de correction du prolapsus mammaire. Arch. Franco-Belg. Chir. 31:138, 1928.

Pousson, M.: De la mastopexie. Bull. Mem. Soc. Chir. Paris 23:507, 1897.

Regnault, P.: The hypoplastic and ptotic breast: A combined operation with prosthetic augmentation. Plast. Reconstr. Surg. 37:31, 1966.

Regnault, P.: Ptosis, asymmetry, tubular breast, and congenital anomalies. In: Owsley, J. Q., Peterson, R. A. (eds.): *Symposium on Aesthetic Surgery of the Breast.* St. Louis, C. V. Mosby, 1978.

Thomas, T. G.: On the removal of benign tumors of the mamma without mutilation of the organ. N.Y. Med. J. Obstet. Rev. 35:337, 1882.

Verchère, F.: Mastopexie laterale contre la mastoptose hypertrophique. Méd. Mod. (Paris) 9:540, 1898.

Weinhold, E.: Discussion zum Vortrag Kuster: Operation bei Hängebauch. Zentralbl. Gynakol. 50:2581, 1926.

Whidden, P. G.: The tailor-tack mastopexy. Plast. Reconstr. Surg. 62:347, 1978.

42

R. C. A. Weatherley-White
Linda C. Huang

The Management of Ptosis

In this chapter, ptosis, or drooping, of the female breast will be considered as a separate entity from breast hypertrophy, although the surgical measures to correct both conditions are in many respects similar. Almost a universal situation in the middle-aged woman, a degree of moderate ptosis is a normal characteristic of the mature breast. When exaggerated by either the effects of breast-feeding or the loss of skin tone accompanying aging, it can mar an otherwise youthful figure and limit, to a distressing degree, the available options for selection and wearing of attractive clothing. Severely ptotic breasts are generally regarded as less sexually appealing than a firmer and more youthful bosom, and a combination of these practical and emotional issues may prompt the female patient to seek surgical correction.

Ptosis generally occurs as a result of two processes: (1) loss of elasticity in the dermis due either to age or the repeated cycle of engorgement and depletion accompanying multiple births and (2) loss of mass resulting from postpartum atrophy, age, or dramatic weight loss.

The object of ptosis correction is to achieve a firmer and more youthful-appearing breast, positioned both higher and with more anterior projection relative to the chest wall. Thus, the surgical procedure will necessarily include resection of excess skin (tightening of the "skin brassiere"), upward transposition of the nipple to a more appropriate location, and plication of the breast tissue to itself and the chest wall to minimize subsequent secondary ptosis. In cases of severe atrophy and loss of bulk, it may be necessary to augment the contour by means of a prosthetic implant. Finally, because this is an entirely cosmetic procedure (as opposed to breast reduction, which has a strong functional component), these goals should be accomplished in such a way as to minimize visible scarring and to preserve, as far as possible, the functions of sensation and successful lactation.

HISTORY

To a great extent, early techniques of mastopexy parallel those of reduction mammaplasty. While certain techniques better satisfy the greater aesthetic consideration demanded by the patient with unattractive, droopy breasts as compared with those individuals with massive pendulous breasts, the basic principles for both were established in the last few decades.

Although early attempts at treating hypermastia can be traced to the sixth century, these techniques were basically subtotal amputations designed to eliminate painfully massive amounts of breast tissue and not restore cosmesis (Letterman and Schurter, 1974). In 1922, Thorek popularized a technique of lower pole amputation with a free nipple graft on the residual nipple pole (Lexer, 1919). Modifications of this technique are still useful today in cases of extreme hypermastia and can produce excellent aesthetic results, but at the loss of nipple sensation and lactation (Gradinger, 1988). Axhausen and Biesenberger each pioneered techniques that involved extensive undermining of skin flaps: inferior and lateral breast tissue resection, followed by 180-degree rotation of the breast parenchymal flap for coning, and completion by insetting and trimming of redundant skin. Compromise of the nipple transposed on such an undermined breast parenchymal flap was a frequent complication (Maliniac, 1950; Gillies and McIndoe, 1939) that was to plague large reductions until the concept of transposing the nipple on a dermal pedicle (Schwarzmann, 1930) was popularized by Strömbeck in 1960.

Many more contributed to our greater understanding of breast ptosis. Notable among these was Aufricht's concept of the "skin brassiere." The overlying skin determines the final breast shape by forcing the soft semifluid underlying breast parenchyma to conform to its contour. This forms the basis of most modern reduction patterns, but is also best illustrated in the dermis-only mastopexy. Here only reshaping of the overlying skin envelope is performed and this results in improved changes in the underlying breast contour.

Penn further extended Aufricht's (1949) and Bames' (1948) concept of preoperative skin marking by defining points on the ideal breast (Penn, 1955). Penn based his "ideal" measurements on the upright patient. His fixed points of sternal notch and nipples form an equilateral triangle with legs 18 to 21 cm long; these points remain fixed in the "ideal breast" despite individual differences in height and weight. Penn also proposed a mammaplasty technique that stressed limited skin undermining and nipple preservation on a dermal patch atop a central breast mound. Hester and others subsequently reaffirmed Penn's technique by examining the vascular supply to the central breast parenchyma (Hester, 1985; Climo and Alexander, 1980).

The relationship between the inframammary fold and the nipple was used by Regnault not only to classify and define breast ptosis but also to distinguish between pseudoptosis and true ptosis (Regnault, 1976). When the nipple is at the level of or lower than the inframammary fold, the breast was defined as ptotic. Regnault described three degrees, ranging from minimal to severe. In first-degree or minor ptosis, the nipple lies at the level of the inframammary fold above the gland. With second-degree or moderate ptosis, the nipple lies below the level of fold. Finally, third-degree or major ptosis is where the nipple lies below the fold level and at the lower contour of the breast and skin brassiere. Pseudoptosis exists when the nipple is above the inframammary fold but the skin brassiere and glandular tissue have descended beneath the inframammary fold (Fig. 42–1).

Thus, according to strict definition, mastopexy involves elevation of the nipple-areola complex. In fact, minor changes in breast volume may be necessary to obtain the ideal nipple-areola complex resting firmly atop the central breast mound. Gonzalez-Ulloa in 1960 described correction of the hypoplastic breast with minimal ptosis by a single-stage mastopexy-augmentation. In cases of pseudoptosis, augmentation alone may provide correction (Regnault, 1976).

In cases of adequate breast volume, Goulian championed dermal mastopexy alone. Goulian felt that the strength of the dermis-to-dermis healing contributed to the long-lasting improvement in contour attained by such dermal mastopexy techniques (Goulian, 1971). In his technique, two triangles of skin lateral to the areola are de-epithelialized, and the nipple is transposed on a superior wide-based dermal pedicle (Fig. 42–2). Removal of the dog-ears occurs in the inframammary fold. Difficulties in redraping the skin, tethered by dermal pedicles, have probably made this procedure of historical interest only. For minimal ptosis, simpler periareolar skin excisions with or without an associated inferior V excision and/or breast augmentation may be used (Fig. 42–3).

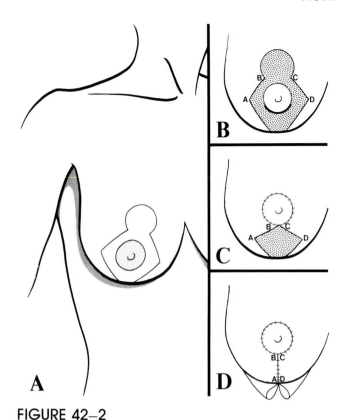

FIGURE 42–2

A, Dermal mastopexy for moderate ptosis with adequate breast volume (Goulian, 1971). *B,* Periareolar de-epithelialization. *C,* Nipple elevated. *D,* Closure after excision of dog-ears in the inframammary fold.

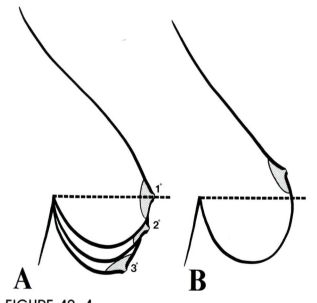

FIGURE 42–1

A, Classification of breast ptosis (Regnault, 1976). *B,* Pseudoptosis.

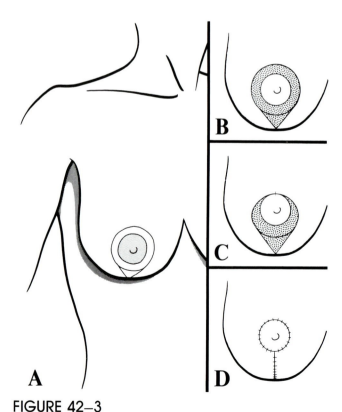

FIGURE 42–3

A, Dermal mastopexy for minimal ptosis using the V excision (Regnault, 1976). *B,* Area de-epithelialized. *C,* Nipple elevated. *D,* Closure with a short vertical limb.

For greater degrees of ptosis or those associated with slight excess of breast tissue, several reduction patterns associated with minimal scarring may be useful. Arié and Pitanguy described removing a redundant wedge of skin and breast tissue from the inferior pole, basing nipple viability on the central breast mound (Arié, 1957; Pitanguy, 1967). An inverted-T scar resulted (Fig. 42–4).

Marchac described a mammaplasty with a short horizontal scar 6 to 9 cm long. A resection of breast tissue inferior and posterior to the nipple is performed, followed by suspension of the parenchyma to the chest wall. Excess skin is removed in a vertical fashion. The final horizontal scar is shorter because some of the excess skin of the lower part of the breast is transferred onto the thorax as the inframammary fold is raised 2 to 3 cm (Fig. 42–5). Long-term results have demonstrated maintenance of ptosis correction (Marchac, 1988).

Maillard's Z-plasty principle utilizes resection of the base of the gland to reduce the size of the mammary cone (Maillard, 1986). The nipple is transposed on a dermal flap, the lateral limb of the Z is used to tighten the inframammary fold, and the medial flap is used to reduce tension around the areola. This results in an oblique scar with a short horizontal component (Fig. 42–6).

Dufourmentel and Mouly described an oblique wedge mammaplasty that is widely used in Europe. The nipple

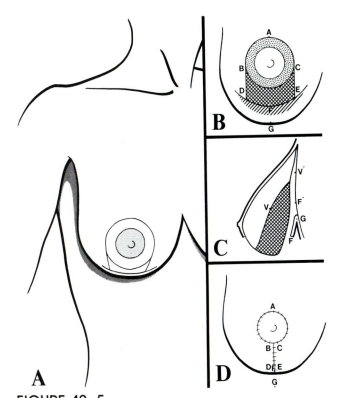

FIGURE 42–5
A, Mammaplasty with a short horizontal scar (Marchac, 1982). *B,* F is the new inframammary fold, above the previous inframammary fold, G. *C,* Gland resected posteroinferiorly. *D,* Short horizontal scar.

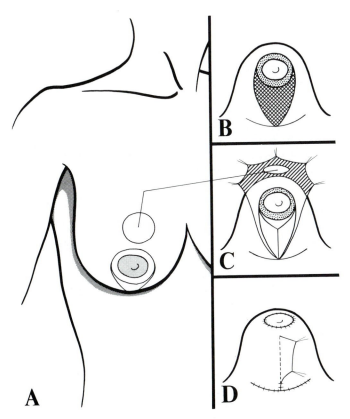

FIGURE 42–4
A, Arié-Pitanguy mammaplasty. *B,* Inferior wedge of skin and breast tissue resected. *C,* Superior flap undermined, demonstrating the new nipple site. *D,* Insetting and trimming of redundant tissue.

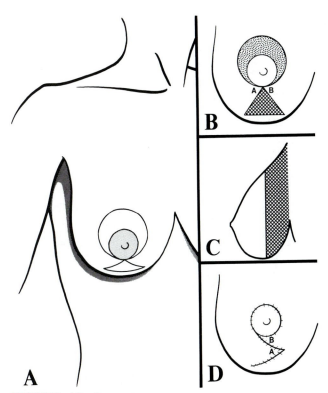

FIGURE 42–6
A, Z mammaplasty (Maillard, 1986). *B,* Circumferential de-epithelialization. *C,* Base of the gland resected. *D,* Closure with the lateral triangular limb of the Z to the inframammary fold.

is transposed on a superior medial dermal pedicle with a single oblique scar (Fig. 42–7). Several factors limit its usefulness (Meyer and Kesselring, 1975; Cramer and Chong, 1976). First, the scar may extend beyond the breast and on to the wall itself. On minor reductions excellent results may be obtained, but there is also a tendency to place the nipples too high and too medially—the "upward squint"—a condition that may be difficult to correct secondarily (Weatherley-White, 1980).

Regnault provides an elegant solution to the problem of scars extending on to the chest wall with the lateral B mammaplasty. Here the flaps are drawn in a rather freehand manner with the patient in a supine position, and the nipple is based on a superior dermal flap. Breast tissue is removed inferiorly and laterally as the infero-lateral flap is drawn medially. A curvilinear scar results with only a lateral horizontal component (Fig. 42–8). Regnault has extended its use to a "minus-plus" mastopexy, in which a reduction of the ptotic lower-pole breast volume is combined with a prosthetic augmentation of the superior pole (Regnault, 1988).

THE AUTHORS' PREFERRED TECHNIQUE

As described in the foregoing section, most surgical procedures to correct ptosis employ either a keyhole-shaped incision with resection of the redundant inferior and central breast skin to achieve tightening of the

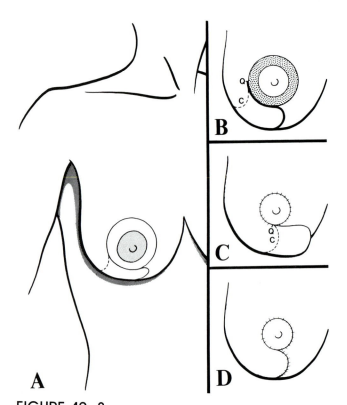

FIGURE 42–8
A, Lateral B mammaplasty (Regnault, 1976). *B,* The upper portion of the "B" is circumferentially de-epithelialized. Full-thickness resection proceeds along the lower portion of the "B." *C,* Lateral flap C brought medially. *D,* Skin gathered around the areola for final closure.

breast and upward repositioning of the nipple or an oblique ellipse of the lateral and inferior skin to achieve the same result. The latter procedure, described by Dufourmentel, achieves a most elegant shape and is widely used in Europe. However, it is the authors' opinion that the scar, extending as it does laterally and inferiorly beyond the territory of the breast, is less cosmetically satisfactory than that afforded by the keyhole plan in which the inverted-T closure limits scarring to the breast and the inframammary fold. The incisions are thus all within the confines of a brassiere or the top half of a two-piece swimsuit.

Initially, the Strömbeck procedure, exactly as described in his pivotal 1960 paper, was employed, with templates cut from x-ray film for planning the sites of the incisions in the breast skin (Strömbeck, 1960). This operation, while generally affording extremely satisfying results, appears to have certain aesthetic limitations, producing in many instances a "squarish" breast, with tugging and even retraction upon the nipple, tethered by its horizontal pedicle. When exposed to the operation of Penn, who clearly showed that nipple circulation did not depend on discrete vascular pedicles but would survive if the nipple were attached to a "patch" of dermis with a diameter about 5 cm greater than that of the areola (Penn, 1955), Weatherley-White devised an operation combining the best features of both procedures, permitting both greater mobility of the nipple and more creative sculpturing of the breast mound (Weatherley-White, 1980).

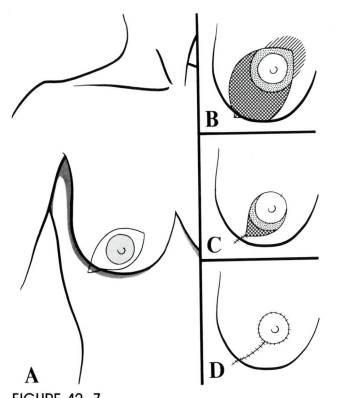

FIGURE 42–7
A, Dufourmentel-Mouly oblique mammaplasty. *B,* Superomedial dermal pedicle. *C,* Lateral oblique glandular resection. *D,* Completed closure.

A further improvement, which permits flexibility in the design of the incisions to accommodate differing body habitus, involved the design of an adjustable metal template to replace the fixed dimensions of the pattern cut from x-ray film. This device, manufactured by the Storz Surgical Instrument Company, consists of a metal loop 5 cm in diameter to which are attached metal arms whose angle in relation to each other can be adjusted. These arms can be locked to ensure the same angle on each breast, and on each arm are notches representing 4, 5, and 6 cm from the inferior edge of the areola (Fig. 42–9).

Because the ultimate result depends in great degree upon the preoperative planning and marking of the incisions, this process will be described in some detail, but an overall picture is presented in Figure 42–10.

The markings are made with the patient awake and in the upright position, both to shorten operative time and to avoid the distortion of landmarks occurring in the supine position. A line is drawn down the midaxis of the breast from midclavicle to the top of the nipple. A central line is drawn from the sternal notch to the xiphoid. The future nipple site is then located, on the midaxis of the breast, at a point opposite the center of the inframammary fold.

There are several checks that should be made to ensure the accuracy of positioning the nipple. The nipple should lie at the same level as the junction of the middle and lower thirds of the humerus. The distance from the clavicle to the center of the future nipple will be, in the short-statured woman, 19 cm; in the woman of average height, 20 cm; and in the taller person, 21 cm or slightly more. The symmetry of nipple placement is checked by measuring the distance from each nipple site to the sternal notch. These measurements must be equal.

The lower incision lies in the inframammary fold, in

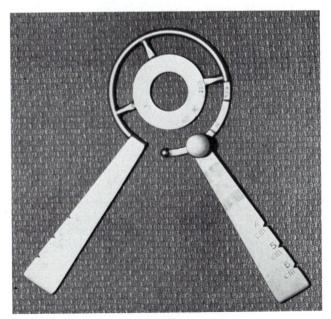

FIGURE 42–9
Adjustable metal template. (From Weatherley-White, R. C. A.: *Plastic Surgery of the Female Breast.* Philadelphia, Harper & Row, 1980.)

the center of which is marked a small equilateral triangle extending superiorly. This triangle is felt to be extremely important, in that not only does it position the union of lateral and medial flaps relative to the inframammary skin but when de-epithelialized, it also supports the tight vertical "three-point closure," which is a frequent source of healing problems.

The template is then placed so that the center of the 5-cm circle lies over the nipple site, and the metal arms are spread symmetrically at the predetermined angle. A 120-degree angle will allow for skin resection producing a B cup; a 90-degree angle will produce a C cup; a 60-degree angle will produce a D cup. The length of the arm of the keyhole is similarly varied: 4 cm for a B cup, 5 cm for a C cup, and 6 cm for a D cup. The length of the vertical incision should never be greater than 6 cm, or the nipple will ride on the upper aspect of the breast with a factitious and preventable ptosis below it (Fig. 42–11).

The horizontal inframammary incisions are initially kept as short as possible and are joined to the upper horizontal incisions within the overhang of the breast. These may be lengthened as the operation progresses for prevention of dog-ears if necessary.

With the markings established (Fig. 42–12), the patient is anesthetized and positioned supine with the table flat and the arms extended 45 degrees from the body (Fig. 42–13A).

Initially a 5-cm diameter circle is marked around the stretched nipple. This is incised, partial thickness, into the dermis; and the adjacent areola and skin are de-epithelialized freehand to a distance 3 to 5 cm from the incision (Fig. 42–13B). This is all the dermis required to maintain vascular support for the nipple; beyond this the skin can be removed full thickness.

The glandular portion of the breast is then dissected from the pectoral fascia and plicated to itself in a vertical fashion for achieving "coning" of the breast (Fig. 42–13 C and D). It is also fixed, with heavy suture material, to the pectoral fascia for ensuring its permanent upward repositioning.

The circumscribed nipple, on its de-epithelialized dermal base, is then moved into position and the flaps approximated with temporary stay sutures (Fig. 42–13E). If all seems satisfactory, the skin is closed in layers under as much tension as will produce adequate lifting without endangering wound healing.

If, on the other hand, it appears that a slight error in planning has been made, it is possible to adjust the situation intraoperatively. If the closure is too loose, producing inadequate uplift, further skin may be resected from the edges of the vertical suture line. If closure can only be achieved under extreme tension (Fig. 42–13F), breast tissue must be removed to protect circulation to the skin edges (Fig. 42–13G). Closure is completed in layers, over suction drains if necessary, and the nipple stretched to a perfect circle, achieved by incising the preoperative markings (Fig. 42–13H).

Suture removal and the appropriate convalescence for preventing undue stretching of the healing incisions proceed according to conventional surgical principles. Representative results of this procedure are shown in Figures 42–14 and 42–15.

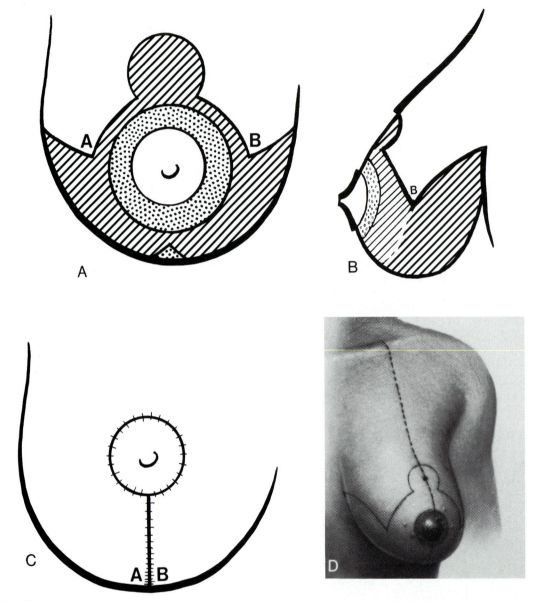

FIGURE 42–10

Authors' preferred technique for ptosis correction. *A,* Areas of de-epithelialization (stippled) and full-thickness skin resection (lined). *B,* Lateral view of full-thickness skin resection. No glandular resection. *C,* Completed closure. *D,* Detailed markings on the breast skin. (From Weatherley-White, R. C. A.: *Plastic Surgery of the Female Breast.* Philadelphia, Harper & Row, 1980.)

occasionally the decreased mass will require augmentation with a prosthetic implant.

Only rarely, however, will a simple augmentation mammaplasty suffice to correct the condition, and the surgeon must be careful not to choose this procedure when the anatomic situation is inappropriate. If the degree of ptosis is more than mild, an augmentation will produce an unsightly "double bubble" contour, with the nipples positioned inferior to the apex of the augmented breast and pointing toward the feet. A useful rule of thumb is *never* to simply perform augmentation mammaplasty when the nipples, in the upright position, lie below the inframammary fold. This situation requires skin resection and upward relocation of the ptosed nipples.

When ptosis is accompanied by severe loss of mass, the mastopexy will require the addition of a prosthetic implant for an optimal result (Fig. 42–16).

After planning the incisions as described in the preceding section, the nipples are circumscribed and de-epithelialized. Skin is resected and the breast gland freed from the pectoral fascia. It is plicated loosely, and the flaps and nipples are approximated with temporary "planning sutures."

A full retromammary pocket is dissected, and an implant is inserted into this location. The inflatable design is uniquely suited to this situation because of the difficulty in preselecting the size of the needed implant. The tension is again tested with stay sutures, and closure is completed as before. This procedure, before and after, is shown in Figure 42–16.

This combined procedure has the drawback of imparting extra pressure upon a closure whose edges are already somewhat compromised by the modest undermining of skin. In this situation, it may be necessary to defer augmentation until survival is ensured.

If a two-stage procedure is inconvenient or undesira-

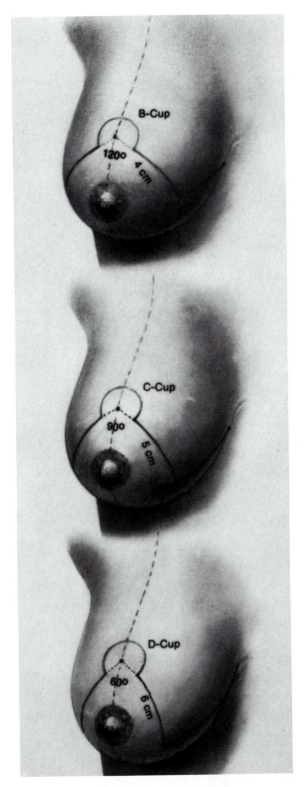

FIGURE 42–11
Varying the angle to achieve a predictable breast size. (From Weatherley-White, R. C. A.: *Plastic Surgery of the Female Breast.* Philadelphia, Harper & Row, 1980.)

PTOSIS WITH LOSS OF BULK

Frequently breast ptosis will be associated with loss of bulk. In most instances, the previous procedure, combining skin resection and plication of the existing breast tissue, will correct the situation adequately, but

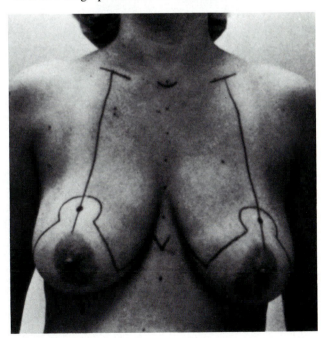

FIGURE 42–12
The markings with the patient in the upright position. (From Weatherley-White, R. C. A.: *Plastic Surgery of the Female Breast.* Philadelphia, Harper & Row, 1980.)

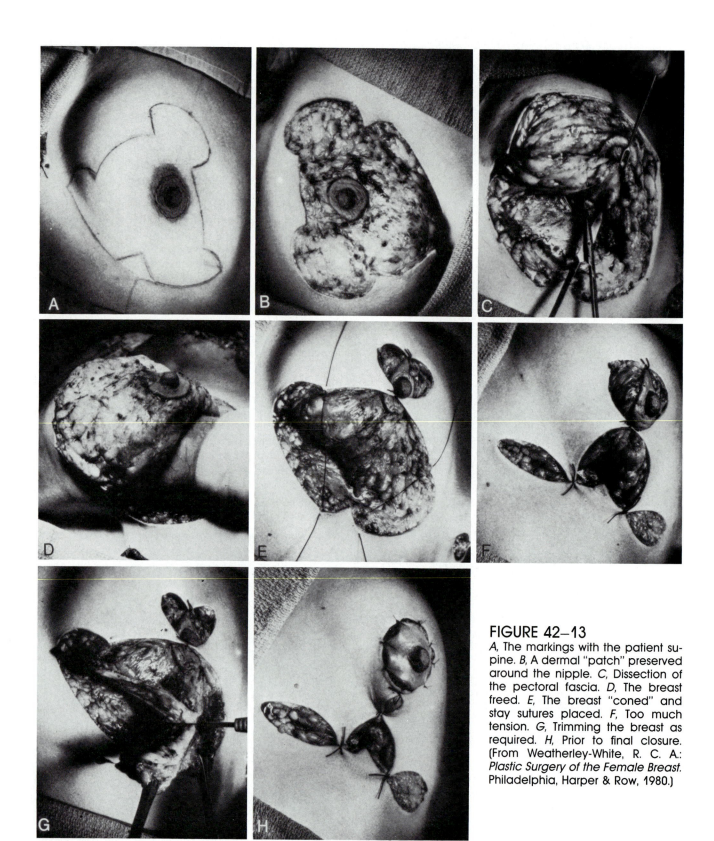

FIGURE 42–13
A, The markings with the patient supine. *B,* A dermal "patch" preserved around the nipple. *C,* Dissection of the pectoral fascia. *D,* The breast freed. *E,* The breast "coned" and stay sutures placed. *F,* Too much tension. *G,* Trimming the breast as required. *H,* Prior to final closure. (From Weatherley-White, R. C. A.: *Plastic Surgery of the Female Breast.* Philadelphia, Harper & Row, 1980.)

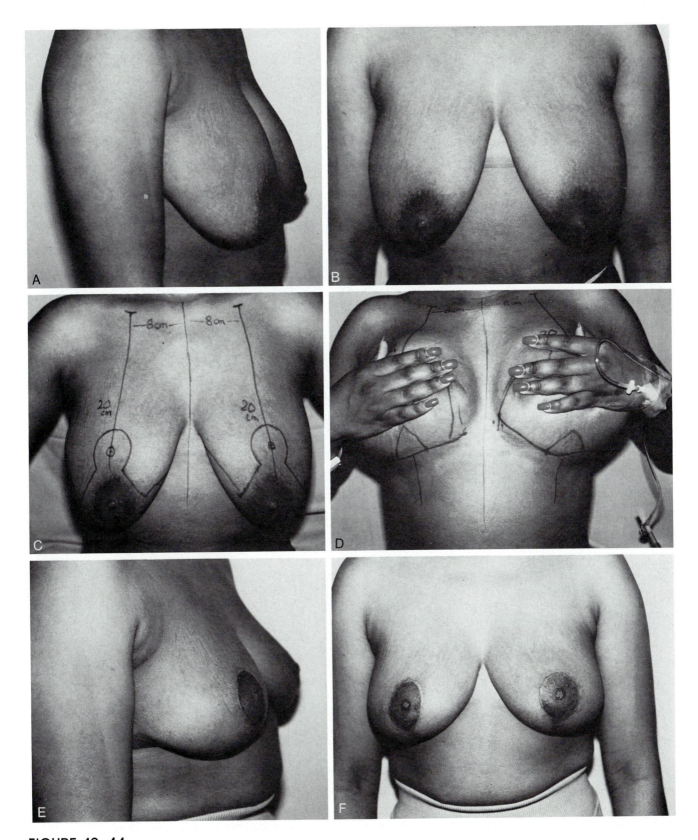

FIGURE 42–14

A and *B,* Third-degree ptosis preoperatively. *C* and *D,* The skin markings. *E* and *F,* Late result. (From Weatherley-White, R. C. A.: *Plastic Surgery of the Female Breast.* Philadelphia, Harper & Row, 1980.)

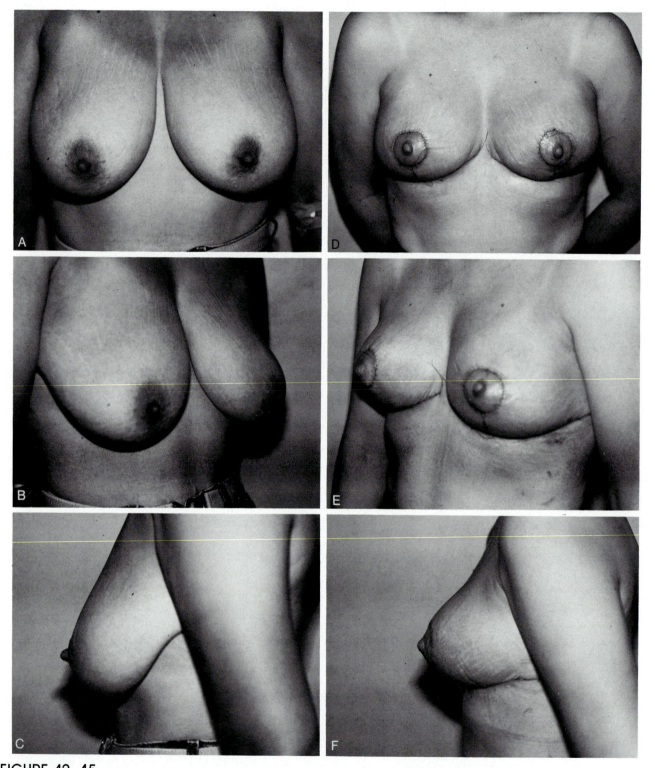

FIGURE 42–15

A to *C*, Second-degree ptosis preoperatively. *D* to *F*, Immediately after mastopexy. (From Weatherley-White, R. C. A.: *Plastic Surgery of the Female Breast.* Philadelphia, Harper & Row, 1980.)

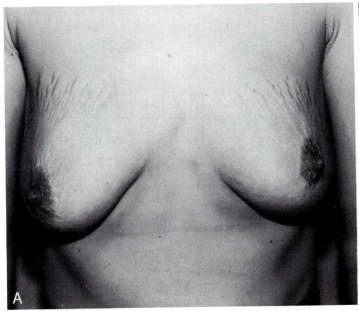
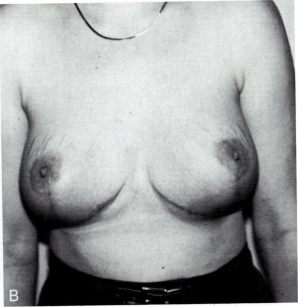

FIGURE 42–16
A, Ptosis with loss of bulk. *B,* Late result after mastopexy and implantation. (From Weatherley-White, R. C. A.: *Plastic Surgery of the Female Breast.* Philadelphia, Harper & Row, 1980.)

ble, a simultaneous submuscular augmentation can be considered. Submuscular placement of the prosthesis may better preserve blood supply to the breast parenchyma and overlying skin, thus providing added security if a large augmentation is anticipated.

SECONDARY PTOSIS

Secondary ptosis is hardly a complication, but rather a recognized, if unfortunate, sequela to any mastopexy procedure. The underlying cause of ptosis, progressive loss of tone and elasticity of the skin, remains unaffected by the initial surgical procedure, and time may well permit ptosis to recur.

Operative correction will depend upon the existing anatomic situation. The entire breast, nipple and all, may again become ptotic. On the other hand, the nipple may remain in its "correct" location while the breast mass sinks, causing the skin of the lower pole of the breast with its attendant scars to stretch.

In the former situation, the distance from the nipple to the sternal notch lengthens, requiring a complete reoperation to elevate the nipple to a more appropriate location (Fig. 42–17).

In the latter, and less common situation, the breast mass descends, causing an increase in the distance between the nipple and the inframammary fold. This can be corrected with excision of a horizontal wedge of tissue in the inframammary fold alone, which may result in some flattening of the breast, or excision of both a vertical and a horizontal wedge of skin, which better preserves nipple projection (Fig. 42–18).

COMPLICATIONS

Asymmetry, improper nipple placement, and generally unacceptable aesthetic results are usually the result of poor planning. Reliance on freehand design with the patient in the supine position, where anatomic landmarks are displaced, will almost inevitably account for this error. Planning should always be undertaken with the patient in the upright position and awake and able to respond to instructions concerning keeping the hips and shoulders level. Enough time should be devoted to this phase of the operation to ensure complete confidence in the location of the incisions; the correct nipple height; and, above all, symmetry of the breasts.

Assuming that there has been correct planning, the most frequent complication is related to wound healing and tension. In order to achieve an effective correction, one must build into the operation a degree of tension,

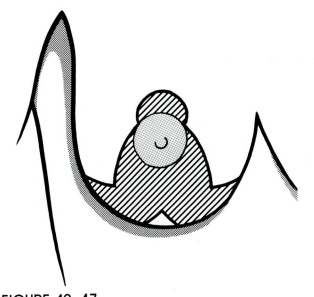

FIGURE 42–17
Correction of secondary ptosis with elevation of the nipple and gland.

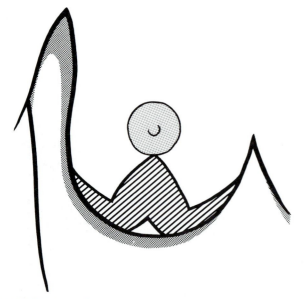

FIGURE 42–18
Correction of secondary ptosis without elevation of the nipple.

which, *if exceeded,* may lead to unsightly scarring or, at worse, wound dehiscence. Such an event is obviously unfortunate but, given the individual variables of wound healing, may occasionally happen even after the most competently performed procedure. The use of temporary stay sutures to test the tension prior to definitive closure, has, in the authors' hands, afforded at least a modicum of security in this regard.

Hematoma is, of course, an ever present possibility when a significant area of tissue is resected. Attention to hemostatic detail and observing the tissue surface for oozing prior to closure are mandatory, and the use of soft suction drains with regular volumetric assessment will alert the surgeon to significant postoperative bleeding. Surgical evacuation of hematomas is important, usually with no adverse impact on the result.

Fat necrosis and infection are rare; and secondary ptosis is hardly a complication, given the fact that the operation does not correct the underlying cause, skin laxity.

In conclusion, reviewing our experience in over 450 cases in which this technique was used, we can state with certainty that it is safe and predictable and yields relatively satisfactory aesthetic results. Complications have been quite rare and patient satisfaction generally high. Based on a combination of two procedures, those of Strömbeck and Penn, it is believed unjustified to claim it as a procedure unique to us. But with the modifications described, in particular the use of the adjustable metal template, it has been a procedure that continues to produce results at least as satisfactory as,

if not superior to, others described in the literature and tested personally.

References

Arié, G: Una nueva tecnica de mastoplastia. Rev. Latinoam. Cir. Plast. 3:23, 1957.

Aufricht, G.: Mammaplasty for pendulous breasts: Empiric and geometric planning. Plast. Reconstr. Surg. 4:13, 1949.

Axhausen, G.: Über Mammaplastik. Med. Klin. 22:1437, 1926.

Bames, H. O.: Reduction of massive breast hypertrophy. Plast. Reconstr. Surg. 3:560, 1948.

Biesenberger, H.: Eine neue methode der mammaplastik. Zentralbl. Chir. 55:2382, 1928.

Climo, M. S., Alexander, J. E.: Intercostothelial circulation: Nipple survival in reduction mammaplasty in the absence of a dermal pedicle. Ann. Plast. Surg. 4:128, 1980.

Cramer, L. M., Chong, J. K.: Oblique mammaplasty. In: Georgiade, N. G. (ed.): *Reconstructive Breast Surgery.* St. Louis, C. V. Mosby, 1976, p. 182.

Dufourmentel, C., Mouly, R.: Modification of "periwinkleshell operation" for small ptotic breast. Plast. Reconstr. Surg. 41:523, 1968.

Dufourmentel, C., Mouly, R.: Plastie mammaire par la méthode oblique. Ann. Chir. Plast. 6:45, 1961.

Gillies, H., McIndoe, A. H.: The technique of mammaplasty in conditions of hypertrophy of the breast. Surg. Gynecol. Obstet. 68:658, 1939.

Gonzalez-Ulloa, M.: Correction of hypotrophy of the breast by means of exogenous material. Plast. Reconstr. Surg. 25:15, 1960.

Goulian, D.: Dermal mastopexy. Plast. Reconstr. Surg. 47:105, 1971.

Gradinger, G. P.: Reduction mammaplasty utilizing nipple areolar transplantation. Clin. Plast. Surg. 15:641, 1988.

Hester, T. R., Bostwick, J., Miller, L., Cunningham, S. J.: Breast reduction utilizing the maximally vascularized central breast pedicle. Plast. Reconstr. Surg. 76:890, 1985.

Letterman, G., Schurter, M.: Will Durston's mammaplasty. Plast. Reconstr. Surg. 53:48, 1974.

Lexer, E.: *Die Freien Transplantation.* Stuttgart, Ferdinand Enke, 1919.

Maillard, G. F.: A Z-mammaplasty with minimal scarring. Plast. Reconstr. Surg. 77:66, 1986.

Maliniac, J. W.: *Breast Deformities and Their Repair.* New York, Grune & Stratton, 1950.

Marchac, D., de Olarte, G.: Reduction mammaplasty and correction of ptosis with a short inframammary scar. Plast. Reconstr. Surg. 69:45, 1982.

Marchac, D., Sagher, U.: Mammaplasty with a short horizontal scar: Evaluation and results after 9 years. Clin. Plast. Surg. 15:627, 1988.

Meyer, R., Kesselring, U. K.: Reduction mammaplasty with an L shaped suture line: Development of different techniques. Plast. Reconstr. Surg. 55:139, 1975.

Penn, J.: Breast reduction. Br. J. Plast. Surg. 7:357, 1955.

Pitanguy, I.: Surgical treatment of breast hypertrophy. Br. J. Plast. Surg. 20:78, 1967.

Regnault, P.: Breast ptosis: Definition and treatment. Clin. Plast. Surg. 3:193, 1976.

Regnault, P., Daniel, R. K., Tirkanits, B.: The minus-plus mastopexy. Clin. Plast. Surg. 15:595, 1988.

Schwarzmann, E.: Die Technik der Mammaplastik. Chirurg 2:932, 1930.

Strömbeck, J. O.: Mammaplasty: Report of a new technique based on the two-pedicle procedure. Br. J. Plast. Surg. 13:79, 1960.

Thorek, M.: Possibilities in the reconstruction of the human form. N. Y. Med. J. 116:572, 1922.

Weatherley-White, R. C. A.: *Plastic Surgery of the Female Breast.* Philadelphia, Harper & Row, 1980.

Charles L. Puckett

43

Breast Ptosis

Ptosis of the breast may be defined as the naturally occurring condition of descent of the nipple-areola complex and breast tissue on the chest wall. The Greek derivation of the word "ptosis" literally means "fall." Indeed, as the breast enlarges from an adolescent bud and becomes mature, it begins its inexorable descent; gradually evolving ptosis is the expected course of events.

Usually as this process progresses the nipple and areola descend disproportionately more than the glandular parenchyma does, and the location of the inframammary crease may actually remain unchanged. In other words, not only does the breast mass droop, but also the nipple and areola descend in relationship to the breast mound. Interestingly, the distance between the nipple and the inframammary crease may change very little. We can map the progress of the events as the adolescent breast assumes the adult female form by the mild glandular ptosis that occurs, thus deepening and defining the inframammary fold (Fig. 43–1). Usually the nipple-areola complex remains central on the breast mound at the apex of the breast cone during this phase. Later, however, with subsequent ptosis, the nipple-areola complex usually descends disproportionately more than does the glandular portion (Fig. 43–2), thereby coming to occupy a more and more dependent position on the breast mound. Although this process usually progresses very slowly, it does progress inevitably with time, and there is no naturally occurring mechanism of reversal.

Ptosis commonly results from loss of breast volume, usually in concert with a decrease in skin elasticity and turgor. This type of ptosis frequently results from the increase, and subsequent decrease, in breast volume that occurs with pregnancy and lactation (Fig. 43–3). However, ptosis may also occur independently in response to the atrophy and loss of skin elasticity associated with advancing age. Conversely, ptosis often occurs concomitantly with increased breast volume; indeed, most cases of macromastia are associated with ptosis (Fig. 43–4). Although ptosis of the breast parenchyma may pose little problem (as is commonly seen with heavier breasts), it is the change in breast configuration with the descent of the nipple and areola that is most disturbing aesthetically. For the purposes of this chapter we will concentrate on the ptosis occurring in the absence of excessive breast volume because the care of this type of ptosis is usually properly attended to in the various reduction mammaplasty procedures.

The significance of the degree of ptosis is a matter of subjective interpretation. Mild degrees of ptosis may have minimal aesthetic impact; whereas severe ptosis, as can occur with a major loss in breast volume (even in a relatively young woman), can be very disturbing emotionally. Therefore, a classification of degrees of ptosis is helpful. Regnault (1966, 1976, 1984) has provided us with the most useful and consistent classification system (Table 43–1). Although other authors have offered modifications of this classification system or other systems that have some utility (Bostwick, 1983; Lewis, 1972), some variation of Regnault's system remains our best guide to therapeutic options. In a 1976 paper, Regnault defined first-, second-, and third-degree ptosis (Regnault, 1976). According to her guidelines, in first-degree ptosis (minor) the nipple lies at the level of, or above, the inframammary fold and above the lower contour of the gland (see Fig. 43–3). In other words, the nipple-areola complex remains anterior on the breast mound above the lowest portion of the breast mound and above the inframammary fold. In second-degree ptosis (moderate) the nipple lies below the level of the inframammary fold but remains above the lower contour of the breast (Fig. 43–5). Again, the nipple is anterior on the breast mound and above the lowest portion of the glandular breast but has descended below the level of the inframammary fold. In third-degree ptosis (major) the nipple lies even lower, below the inframammary fold level, and has descended to the lower portion of the contour of the glandular breast (Fig. 43–6). In this configuration the nipple is pointing inferiorly and the nipple-areola complex is in the lowest portion of the breast mound.

For purposes of communication and reproducibility, measurements of ptosis are taken by us with the woman standing, *not sitting,* because some alteration in breast configuration can occur between the standing and sitting position in certain individuals. For Regnault, and for this author, the inframammary fold is the dividing point

TABLE 43–1
Regnault's Grading of Severity of Ptosis*

I	Nipple descent to inframammary crease
II	Nipple lies below inframammary crease but anterior on breast mound
III	Severe descent with nipple inferior on breast mound

*According to the degree of nipple descent.

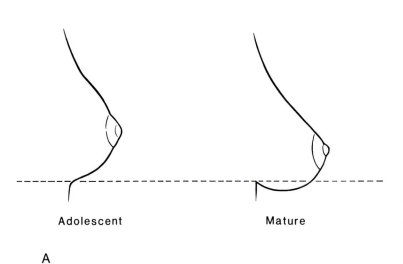

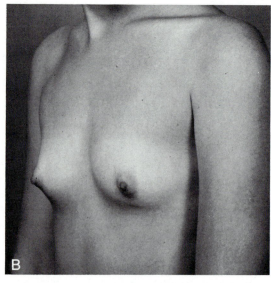

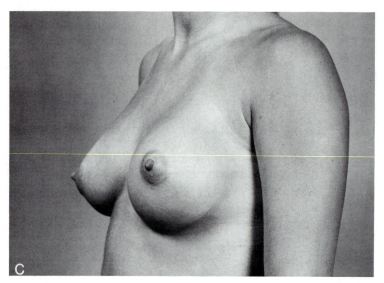

FIGURE 43–1

A, Mild glandular ptosis as the adolescent breast assumes the mature adult form. *B*, Adolescent breasts in the developing stage. Note the lack of inframammary crease definition. *C*, Adult female breasts with a well-defined inframammary crease.

FIGURE 43–2

Advanced ptosis. Note not only the descent of the glandular tissue and the nipple and areola but also the disproportionate descent of the nipple-areola complex as it comes to ride lower and lower on the breast mound.

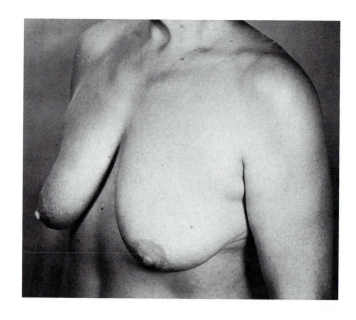

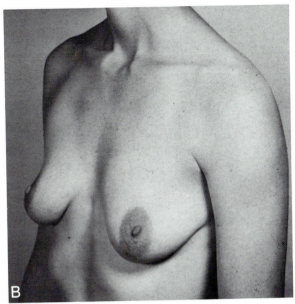

FIGURE 43–3

A and *B,* Mild ptosis resulting from pregnancy and lactation reflects primarily a decrease in breast volume and some loss of skin elasticity.

between first-degree (mild) and second-degree (moderate) ptosis. However, other authors (Bostwick, 1983) have manipulated this definition somewhat and allow the grade I ptosis to include nipple descent somewhat below the inframammary crease. Because of this confusion in definition, and because of the fairly significant impact that nipple position has on the choice of therapeutic options, we have defined this gray zone between grades I and II as grade I½ ptosis (Table 43–2) (see Fig. 43–11A) (Puckett, 1985). We have included in

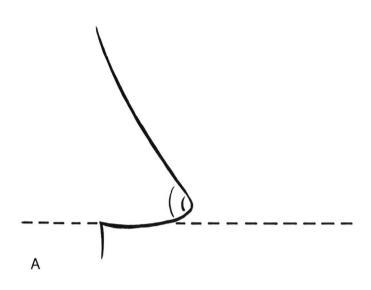

FIGURE 43–4

Ptosis associated with macromastia. This patient subsequently underwent removal of 700 gm of tissue from each breast.

grade I½ those cases in which the nipple position is at, slightly above, or slightly below the inframammary crease. Below this level of nipple descent there seems good agreement that second-degree (moderate) ptosis exists until the nipple has assumed the inferiormost position on the breast mound, at which point most authors would indicate a more severe labeling (third-degree). In Table 43–2 we have designated a grade IIIa, which is the usual expression of severe ptosis, and a IIIb. This is a particularly severe version, occasionally seen, in which the nipple seems almost tethered to the inframammary crease and when viewed in profile appears to "point" directly down or even posteriorly (Fig. 43–7).

For completeness, two other terms need definition. Pseudoptosis has been defined as the appearance of ptosis as a result of decreased breast volume but with the nipple position preserved well above the inframammary crease and anterior on the breast mound. In other words, a true (or measurement-determined) ptosis does not exist, but a visual impression of ptosis does. This

TABLE 43–2
Author's Amended Version of Regnault's Grading of Breast Ptosis

I	Appearance of breast ptosis but with nipple remaining above inframammary crease, breast appearing to have decreased volume
I½	Nipple position at, slightly above, or slightly below inframammary crease; diminished breast volume
II	Nipple lies below inframammary crease but anterior on breast mound
IIIa	Severe ptosis, nipple well below the inframammary crease, and the nipple-areola complex occupying lower portion of breast mound
IIIb	Even greater degree of severity with nipple "pointing" directly inferiorly or posteriorly

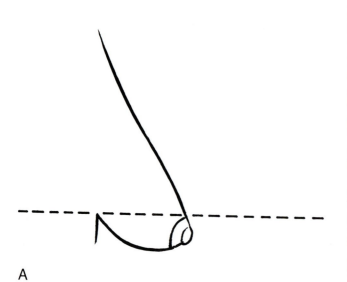

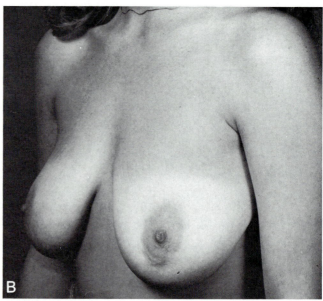

FIGURE 43–5

A and *B*, Grade II ptosis. The nipple is distinctly below the inframammary crease but remains anterior on the breast mound and above the inferiormost portion of the glandular breast.

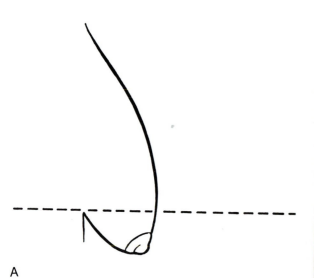

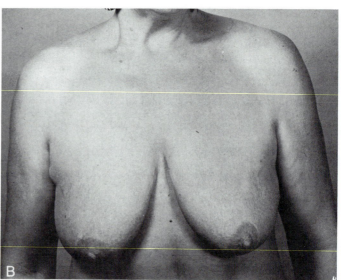

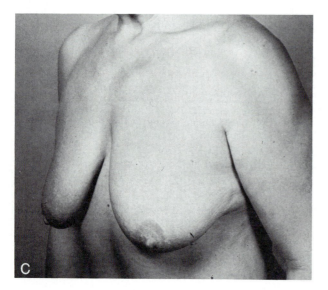

FIGURE 43–6

A, Grade III ptosis. *B*, Note the marked descent of the nipple, now occupying the inferiormost aspect of the breast mound. *C*, Oblique view demonstrating that the nipple now points downward.

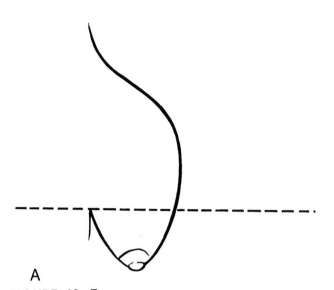
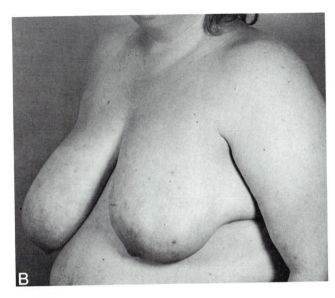

A

B

FIGURE 43–7
A, Severe grade III ptosis. *B,* Note the position of the nipple pointing directly inferiorly or even posteriorly. In this grade III ptosis, the nipple-areola complex seems actually tethered to the inframammary crease.

becomes indistinguishable from grade I ptosis in the author's amended version of Regnault's classification system (see Table 43–2). Finally, glandular ptosis is the condition in which the glandular breast appears to have descended disproportionately in excess of the nipple. In reality this is almost always a contrived condition following overzealous superior surgical repositioning of the nipple-areola complex. This may be seen following overcorrection in a ptosis procedure or with selection of a nipple-areola position too high in the course of a reduction mammaplasty (Fig. 43–8). Presumably this can also occur when there is excessive distance between the nipple and the inframammary fold during reduction mammaplasty. Some authors have referred to this as "bottoming out."

TREATMENT

Because naturally occurring breast ptosis is not physiologically reversible, the surgeon is often called upon for assistance. With the possible exception (conceptually) of hormonal manipulation to gain parenchymal hypertrophy and "refilling" of the volume-depleted breast, and because science has not yet discovered a reliable method of re-establishing the elasticity of overstretched or aged skin, correction of ptosis by other than surgical means is not possible. Frequently, simply repositioning the nipple-areola complex superiorly will restore an aesthetically acceptable breast appearance. Therefore, most breast ptosis procedures concentrate on repositioning the nipple-areola complex at the apex (anteriorly) of the breast cone and do not necessarily attempt to reposition breast tissue on the chest wall. Patient satisfaction is largely related to the accuracy with which this is achieved.

Treatment options can be conceived of as a spectrum, with the complexity of the corrective procedures increasing with the severity of the degree of ptosis (Fig. 43–9).

At one end of the spectrum, the volume-depleted breast with grade I (mild) ptosis or pseudoptosis may be satisfactorily served by simply "refilling" the breast. This most commonly involves an augmentation mammaplasty with insertion of a Silastic prosthesis. Indeed, if no limitations were placed on the degree of augmentation, even moderate ptosis could be so corrected. However, most patients are seeking not larger breasts but rather the achievement of a more youthful contour. Thus, at one end of the spectrum simple augmentation will suffice, and at the other end, severe ptosis, the operation assumes the complexity and incisions com-

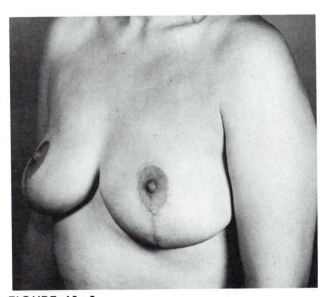

FIGURE 43–8
Glandular ptosis. This condition usually follows either reduction mammaplasty or a ptosis procedure in which the nipple was placed too high on the chest *or* an excessive distance was allowed between the nipple and the inframammary crease.

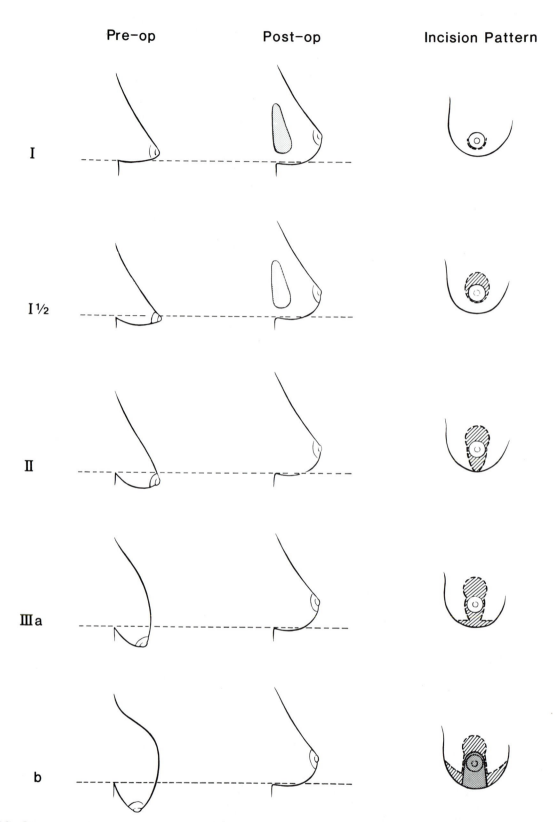

FIGURE 43–9

Ptosis grade related to incision pattern and complexity of surgical correction. Grade I: Augmentation of the breast will often suffice. Circumareolar, inframammary, and transaxillary incisions may be used with equivalent effectiveness. Grade I½ : Mild nipple elevation coupled with breast augmentation is usually effective. Crescent mastopexy and transglandular augmentation are the author's choice. Grade II: Moderate ptosis requires definitive nipple-areola elevation and maintenance. A V excision inferiorly may suffice. Grade IIIa: Severe ptosis will require a V-T correction. Grade IIIb: Correction of the most severe degrees of ptosis will frequently require the construction of a formal Wise pattern for skin reduction and superior repositioning of the nipple-areola complex.

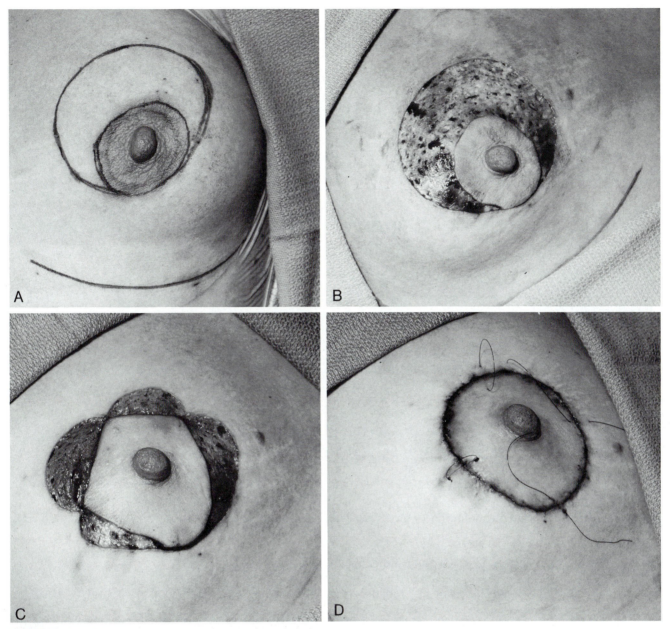

FIGURE 43–10

Crescent mastopexy. *A* and *B*, The crescent mastopexy consists of the de-epithelialization of a crescent-shaped area of skin superior and to either side of the existing areola. *C* and *D*, Approximation with buried dermal sutures is completed with a subcuticular nylon pull-out suture. The "lift" provided for the nipple position is approximately 40% of the superiormost width of the crescent portion.

mensurate with a full reduction mammaplasty. In this author's hands, this would most commonly incorporate a Wise pattern type of reduction with an inferior pedicle developed for nipple transfer. Between these two extremes, however, we have preferred a "cut-as-you-go" approach dictated by the increasing severity of nipple-areola descent.

With nipple descent just beyond that comfortably correctable with moderate augmentation, we would add a nipple-areola "boost," which can often be accomplished with a crescent mastopexy (Fig. 43–10). "Crescent mastopexy" refers to the nipple elevation accomplished by de-epithelialization of a crescent-shaped area of skin above and on either side of the existing areolar

margin with subsequent infolding and approximation of the skin edges (Gasperoni et al., 1988; Puckett et al., 1985).

Crescent mastopexy and augmentation can often provide the small amount of extra assistance that is needed for marginal cases of ptosis between grade I (mild) and grade II (moderate). Generally this refers to those patients with the nipple position slightly above or below the inframammary crease. As noted earlier (Table 43–2), I have conveniently called this grade I½ ptosis to designate this specific entity and therapeutic approach (Fig. 43–11). Failure to appreciate this additional need beyond that corrected by augmentation alone can be an aesthetic disaster. Occasionally in these cases of grade

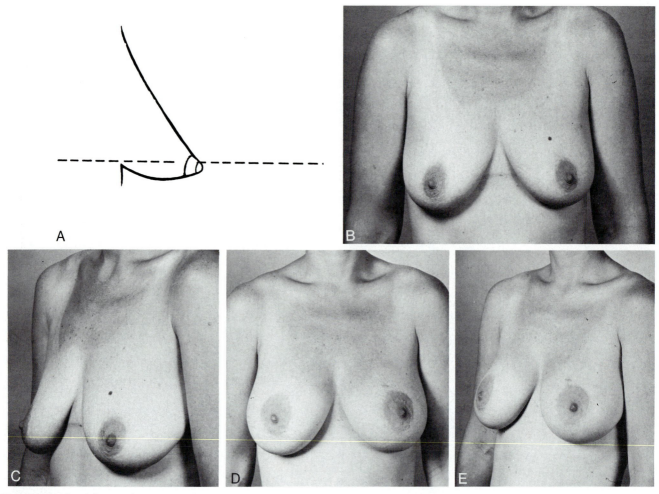

FIGURE 43–11

A, Crescent mastopexy and augmentation for grade I½ ptosis. *B* and *C*, Preoperative views. *D* and *C*, Postoperative views.

I½ ptosis, augmentation alone, while certainly providing a larger breast, would actually accentuate the dependent appearance of the nipple and can "convert" a milder to a more severe ptosis (Fig. 43–12). As one progresses to true moderate ptosis, with the nipple distinctly and significantly below the inframammary crease, a more formal ptosis procedure is necessary (which will be described subsequently) but it is right at this transition point between grades I and II (grade I½) that a little assistance is needed in combination with augmentation. We have found the crescent excision to reliably provide this. However, it only provides a little help and will be inadequate when used for more severe degrees of ptosis.

Practically speaking, the amount of nipple elevation that can be accomplished with a feasibly sized crescent excision is approximately 1.5 cm. This might be the gain with a 3.0- to 3.5-cm-wide crescent excision. Since the inferiormost portion of the areola is tethered, elevation of the nipple is limited to about half, or somewhat less, of the distance between the center of the inner and outer drawn circles (see Fig. 43–10). The de-epithelialized crescent provides a ready access point for transglandular augmentation either subpectorally (my preference) or subglandularly. The crescent excision also provides some tightening of the breast skin, and the net

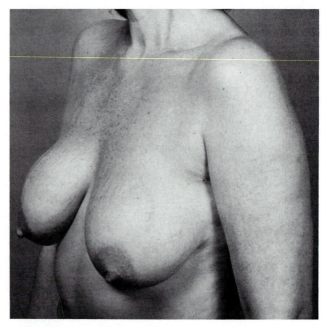

FIGURE 43–12

This patient had grade I½ to II ptosis and received only augmentation with Silastic implants. Without mastopexy, augmentation caused grade III ptosis.

effect is a mild "lift" of the nipple and areola accentuated further by the augmentation (see Fig. 43–11).

There have been criticisms of this procedure because of widening of the circumareolar scars, oval distortion of the areola, and enlargement of the areola. In fact, the scars do widen in about 25% of patients to some degree, but rarely has this been a source of specific patient complaint. Oval distortion of the areola has, similarly, not been a source of complaint; but enlargement of the areola can be if proper attention is not paid. This can usually be prevented by constricting the circumareolar inner circle somewhat in those patients with an initially generous areolar diameter. By discarding some of the outer circumference of the areola, one can significantly limit the final diameter.

We have found this procedure to be predictable and simple to perform, adding only 20 to 30 minutes' operating time to a standard augmentation mammaplasty procedure. We would caution, however, that the additional nipple-areola lift provided is small, and its indication should be strictly limited to candidates with grade I or I½ ptosis.

For ptosis that is more specifically grade II (moderate), the crescent mastopexy (with or without augmentation) will clearly be insufficient. The next step is to incorporate a vertical limb below the circumareolar incision. This more effectively displaces and holds the nipple-areola complex superiorly. Regnault has described this as her VOQ operation (Regnault and Daniel, 1984). We have referred to this spectrum of ptosis procedures as the V-T operation (Fig. 43–13A). If the vertical limb of the V is less than 5 cm in length, its inferiormost point can be tapered without a horizontal

element. This will usually suffice for the lesser versions of grade II ptosis, but as one approaches the grade III level, the vertical length of the V increases. If, in order to close the circumareolar circle, this vertical length is significantly greater than 5 cm, a horizontal limb must be created to absorb the dog-ear, thus converting it to an inverted T (Fig. 43–13B). As one progresses from grade II to grade III ptosis, the horizontal limb will similarly increase in magnitude. The vertical limb is always limited to 5.5 cm or less. Eventually this process will evolve into a pattern that is a precise replica of the classic Wise pattern for reduction mammaplasty (Fig. 43–14D). Many of our grade II ptosis patients, and even some of the lesser versions of grade III, can be successfully managed with a fairly minimal horizontal limb and thus, this cut-as-you-go approach.

With the more severe degrees of grade III ptosis, we actually start with a full Wise pattern and bypass the cut-as-you-go approach in favor of expediency. Therefore, in the most severe ptosis patients (IIIb), we would draw a pattern of the classic Wise type, and the operation would progress in the manner of an inferior pedicle reduction mammaplasty. We simply would remove only a minimal amount of breast tissue and predominantly discard the excess skin (Fig. 43–15). For the position and new shape of the breast to be properly achieved, all of the incisions and dissections for a standard inferior pedicle reduction mammaplasty are done. The superior flaps are undermined at the chest level, but we remove only that breast tissue "in the way" (often less than 100 gm). In the cut-as-you-go approach the need for an inferior pedicle to transfer the nipple and areola gradually emerges as degree and complexity increase. How-

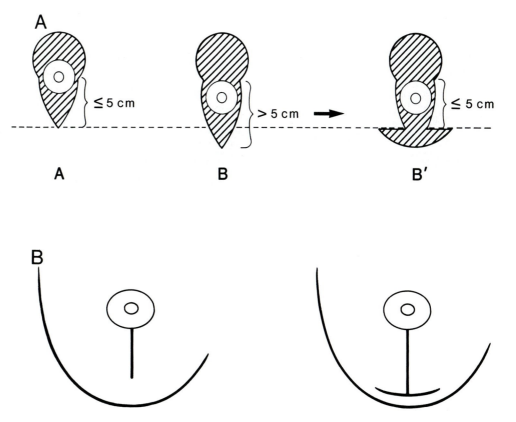

FIGURE 43–13

A, As one exceeds the potential for the crescent mastopexy to provide adequate nipple and areola lift, a V-shaped wedge is added inferiorly. Closure of this V-shaped excision area helps suspend and maintain the lift of the nipple-areola complex. In the milder forms of grade II ptosis, this V can be rather modest (A). However, as greater width and length of the V are required and the vertical length of the limbs of the V exceeds 5 cm (B), a dog-ear must be removed at the inframammary crease level (B'). Excision of this dog-ear at or slightly above the inframammary crease maintains the vertical height of the V limbs at 5 cm. *B*, Closure of the V (A in *A*) results in a vertical line, while closure of the V with dog-ear excision (B' in *A*) results in an inverted-T configuration.

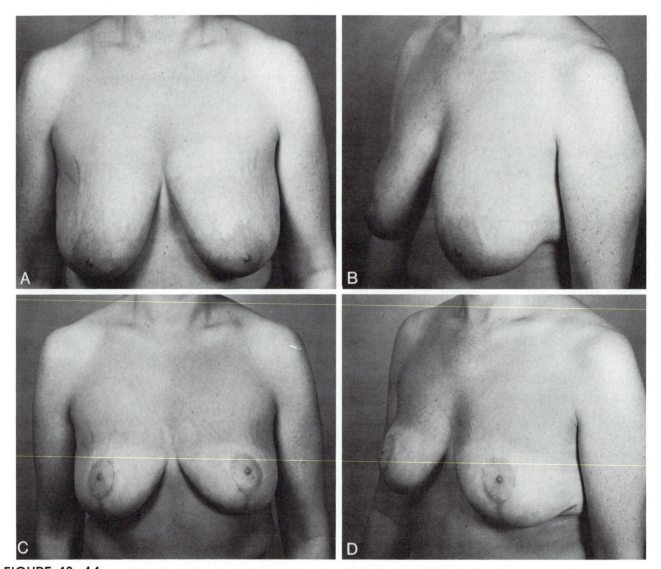

FIGURE 43–14

A and *B*, Preoperative views of a patient with grade II to III ptosis who requested correction without significant volume reduction. *C* and *D*, Postoperative views. Correction used the V-T operation and a limited inferior pedicle dissection for the nipple transfer. Dog-ear correction required a fairly long lateral limb of the horizontal closure of the inverted T. Less than 100 cc of breast tissue was removed.

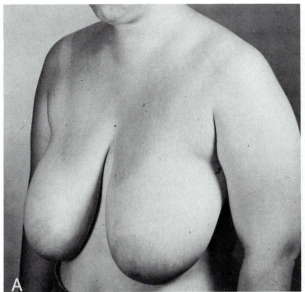 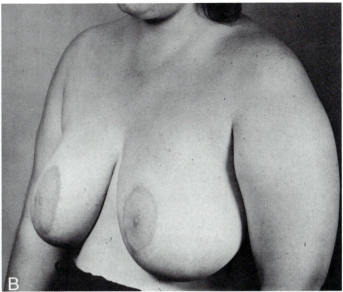

FIGURE 43–15

This plump 19-year-old woman requested correction of grade IIIb ptosis without significant reduction in breast volume. *A,* Preoperative view. *B,* Postoperative view. Correction was achieved with a standard Wise pattern and a formal inferior pedicle dissection for nipple transfer. Approximately 140 cc of breast tissue was removed that was "in the way," to allow superior nipple-areola repositioning.

ever, in the milder versions of the V-T excision, no formal pedicle dissection is performed.

The new nipple position is determined by a variety of techniques, and each surgeon has his or her methods, or "tricks." Ours are the same as in reduction mammaplasty but with the major influence on a balanced final position for the nipple at the apex of the breast cone. The selection of a final resting point for the nipple is usually the result of an amalgam of several different measurements or estimates. Our first and most reliable determinant is actual measurement. This is done by measuring (in the standing position) from the suprasternal notch along a line drawn to the present nipple position (Fig. 43–16). A similar straight line from the midclavicular point to the nipple provides a second point. A distance along these lines is selected at an average of 22 cm inferiorly. This ranges from 21.0 to 22.5 cm, depending upon the individual's height (with 21 cm for the 5-foot individual and 22.5 cm for the 5-foot 8-inch individual). A third point is determined as a reflection of the midhumeral position. A fourth point is determined in reference to the inframammary crease.

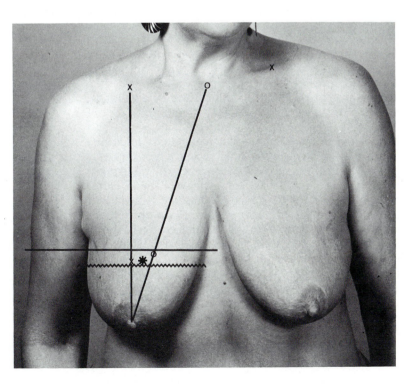

FIGURE 43–16

Technique for determining the new nipple position. Four determinants are selected. In this 5-foot 5-inch individual, the first determinant, ○, is measured 22 cm below the suprasternal notch in the direction of the existing nipple. The second determinant, ×, is measured 22 cm below the midclavicular point. The midhumeral line is noted (solid horizontal line), and the inframammary crease level is noted (wavy line). The final nipple position, *, is an "average" of these points, with greater weight given to the inframammary line. Medial and lateral adjustment may be aided by visual evaluation.

This is usually located by using the thumb and long finger as a caliper. We then select a central point as an average of these four individual sites for our final selection site. We have found the midhumeral line to be of least value, because it is often too high. The inframammary line is most reliable but may be slightly low if used alone. Admittedly, experience is the final determinant, and one occasionally "fudges" this point slightly, because observation may suggest a slightly more harmonious position in some cases than pure measurement alone. This slight alteration is usually concerned with centering on the breast medially and laterally, but vertical determination is predominantly made according to measurement. Errors, if made, should be in favor of too low a position, rather than too high. A slightly low final nipple-areola position is much more aesthetically acceptable by patient *and* physician and is eminently easier to correct than is the "star-gazing" appearance of the excessively elevated nipple (see Fig. 43–8).

Obviously, this represents only one approach to the surgical correction of ptosis, and there are many other effective techniques. Notable among these are the B technique of Regnault (Regnault and Daniel, 1984), which she applies to the moderate or more severe degrees of ptosis; the dermal mastopexy of Goulian (Goulian, 1971) for moderate ptosis; the Dufourmentel-Mouly lateral wedge technique (Dufourmentel and Mouly, 1961, 1965; Weatherly-White, 1980); and the technique of Georgiade (Georgiade, 1976), similar to that described earlier. We have found this spectrum of progression from the crescent, through the V-T approach, to the full Wise pattern for ptosis correction to be reliable, reproducible, and relatively easy to teach. There are, of course, subtleties in technique that only experience can provide, but this concept of progression seems to be one that is relatively easy for the learning plastic surgeon to grasp.

This chapter would not presume to prescribe actual surgical technique, suture choices, and so forth, but will offer a few "points." Though we firmly believe in the value of the holding potential of buried permanent sutures, we use only absorbable suture buried in the breast. The years have taught that buried permanent sutures, particularly in the circumareolar area, will often eventually find their way to the surface. We routinely use an intracuticular nylon pull-out suture and leave it for a very long time, often 3 weeks and more. This provides some longer-term holding potential without the expense of cross marks. Staples are used routinely during the procedure to estimate shape, volume, and so forth, but are always eventually replaced with the intracuticular nylon. When nipple transfer is significant enough to require a pedicle, we always use some modification of the inferior pedicle technique. We have not favored, nor do we advocate, the suspension techniques that reattach breast tissue to the chest wall or pectoral fascia (Errol and Spira, 1980; Hinderer, 1976; Marchac and de Olarte, 1982). Although these might have some applicability with glandular ptosis, the offending agent is usually stretched skin and loss of volume. Skin tightening and reconstruction of a new skin brassiere seem the logical treatment and are the mainstay of ptosis correction. The breast parenchyma can be viewed as nearly fluid in nature and willing to be confined by the reconstructed skin envelope.

The role of augmentation in the form of a Silastic implant in the more severe degrees of ptosis is simply defined by need and patient preference. Many of these patients have adequate volume once the skin brassiere is reconstructed. If needed, or desired, subpectoral or subglandular augmentation can easily and safely be performed during the procedure. For subpectoral placement, we simply split the fibers of the pectoral muscle and make a subpectoral pocket in the standard manner after having entered this space "through" the muscle. The muscle should be completely detached from the sternum and ribs medially and inferiorly to prevent the prosthesis from riding superiorly.

SUMMARY

We have offered a simple strategy for the correction of ptosis of the breast with selection of therapeutic options dictated by carefully determined actual measurement of the severity of the ptosis. The selection of the crescent excision, the V-T pattern, or the full Wise pattern by carefully determined grading of the severity of the ptosis has provided an aesthetically reliable and reproducible technique that has been relatively easy for the learning plastic surgeon to grasp and use. As with any aesthetic surgical procedure, there is no substitute for experience; the nuances of technique that would make this or any other approach fluid can only come with time.

References

Bostwick, J., III: Correction of breast ptosis. In: *Aesthetic and Reconstructive Breast Surgery*. C. V. Mosby Co., St. Louis, 1983, pages 209–249.

Dufourmentel, C., Mouly, R.: Plastie mammaire par la méthode oblique. Ann. Chir. Plast. 6:45, 1961.

Dufourmentel, C., Mouly, R.: Développements récents de la plastie mammaire par la méthode oblique laterale. Ann. Chir. Plast. 10:227, 1965.

Errol, O. O., Spira, M.: Mastopexy technique for mild to moderate ptosis. Plast. Reconstr. Surg. 65:603, 1980.

Gasperoni, C., Salgarello, M., Gargani, G.: Experience in technical refinements in the "donut" mastopexy with augmentation mammaplasty. Aesthetic Plast. Surg. 12:111, 1988.

Georgiade, N. G.: Correction of the ptotic breast. In: *Reconstructive Breast Surgery*. St. Louis, C. V. Mosby, 1976, p. 113.

Georgiade, N. G., Serafin, D., Riefkohl, R., Georgiade, G. S.: Is there a reduction mammaplasty for "all seasons"? Plast. Reconstr. Surg. 63:765, 1979.

Goulian, D.: Dermal mastopexy. Plast. Reconstr. Surg. 47:105, 1971.

Gruber, R. P., Jones, H. W.: The "donut" mastopexy: Indications and complications. Plast. Reconstr. Surg. 65:34, 1980.

Hinderer, U. T.: The dermal brassiere mammaplasty. Clin. Plast. Surg. 3:349, 1976.

Lewis, J. R.: Classification and surgical correction of ptosis of the breast. In: Masters, F. W., Lewis, J. R. (eds.): *Symposium on Aesthetic Surgery of the Face, Eyelids, and Breast*. St. Louis, C. V. Mosby, 1972, p. 183.

Marchac, D., de Olarte, G.: Reduction mammaplasty and correction of ptosis with a short inframammary scar. Plast. Reconstr. Surg. 69:45, 1982.

Puckett, C. L., Meyer, V. H., Reinisch, J. F.: Crescent mastopexy and augmentation. Plast. Reconstr. Surg. 75:533, 1985.

Regnault, P.: Breast ptosis: Definition and treatment. Clin. Plast. Surg. 3:193, 1976.

Regnault, P.: The hypoplastic and ptotic breast: A combined operation with prosthetic augmentation. Plast. Reconstr. Surg. 37:31, 1966.

Regnault, P., Daniel, R. K.: Breast ptosis. In: *Aesthetic Plastic Surgery*. Boston, Little, Brown, 1984, p. 539.

Weatherly-White, R. C. A.: Breast ptosis. In: Weatherly-White, R. C. A. (ed.): *Plastic Surgery of the Female Breast: A Surgical Atlas*. Philadelphia, J. B. Lippincott, 1980, p. 95.

Wise, R. J.: A preliminary report on a method of planning the mammaplasty. Plast. Reconstr. Surg. 17:367, 1956.

Wise, R. J.: Surgical management of the hypertrophic breast. In: Masters, F. W., Lewis, J. R.: *Symposium on Aesthetic Surgery of the Face, Eyelid, and Breast*. St. Louis, C. V. Mosby, 1972, p. 174.

Wise, R. J., Gannon, J. P., Hill, J. R.: Further experience with reduction mammaplasty. Plast. Reconstr. Surg. 32:12, 1963.

Development of Concepts in Reduction Mammaplasty and Ptosis

A classification of mammaplasty techniques for hypertrophy and ptosis, based on the historical development of concepts from 1848 to 1988, is presented in this chapter, as are surgical conclusions with regard to safety requirements and aesthetic aims. Breast ptosis is classified according to preoperative evaluation, and techniques for correction are indicated. The additional procedures for prevention of secondary ptosis are mentioned, and my "doughnut" periareolar technique (1969) and dermal brassiere mammaplasty (1971, 1972) are described and discussed.

Mammaplasty for hypertrophy and ptosis developed in stages, based on the concepts prevailing in each period with regard to vascular supply and innervation, the importance of lactation, and aesthetic aims concerning achievement and preservation of a pleasing shape and the location and length of the unavoidable residual scar. Earlier reports can be found that describe techniques initiating new principles that characterize a group of techniques popularized later on. The search still continues today. Probably there will never be the "ideal technique" applicable to every degree of hypertrophy and ptosis.

The requirements for an ideal technique are as follows:

1. Adequate reduction of the gland and safe transposition of the nipple-areola complex with regard to the skin, residual gland, and nipple-areola complex itself.
2. Preservation of sensation and erectility of the nipple-areola complex.
3. Preservation of nursing ability.
4. Achievement of pleasing symmetric breasts with adequate filling of the upper breast hemisphere.
5. A residual scar of minimal length and visibility.
6. Prevention of secondary ptosis (the results should be long-lasting).

The young plastic surgeon interested in mammaplasty is faced with hundreds of publications about old and newer ideas, modifications of techniques, and combinations of procedures, making it difficult to find a comfortable technique, a condition of success mentioned by Lewis (1983). Today there is a vast selection of techniques providing excellent results in the hands of their authors. The result of a particular operation,

however, will depend on the surgeon's experience with the technique chosen, on skillful performance, on the artistic sense of the surgeon, and on careful postoperative treatment. The surgeon who believes he has found a "new" solution should enquire whether there was already a predecessor, for the purpose of both assigning deserved credit and avoiding the repetition of errors.

A review of the historical development of concepts in mammaplasty and of some basic surgical conclusions concerning safety and aesthetic requirements may therefore be useful in the selection of a technique and may also determine whether a new technique represents a pre-existing idea.

THE EVOLUTION OF CONCEPTS IN THE FIRST CENTURY OF MAMMAPLASTY FOR HYPERTROPHY AND PTOSIS

Initial Period: From Dieffenbach (1848) to Lexer (1921) and Thorek (1922)

The first publication on the treatment of breast hypertrophy I found, which is not referred to in textbooks, was by Dieffenbach (1848), who described breast reduction of the lower two-thirds of the inferior circumference and of a posterior segment of the breast, leaving a fine linear scar on the submammary fold. This approach was also used by Theodore Gaillard Thomas (1882); Morestin (1903) published the axillary approach for tumor resection. For augmentation mammaplasty with prosthesis, the axillary approach was suggested to me by Vinas (1968); I subsequently presented it (1969) and published a report on it (1972), as did Höhler (1973). Czerny (1895) performed the first augmentation by transplantation of a lipoma to the breast. Previous publications, mentioned by Hauben (1985), such as Paulo de Aegineta's description of breast resection for gynecomastia, also referred to by Albucasis and Ambroise Paré, who believed that female breast surgery had already been performed by Greek and Arabian surgeons, Durston's (1669) incision of a suddenly developing gigantomastia, investigated by Letterman and Schurter (1974), or breast amputations performed for treatment of tumors, cannot be considered aesthetic surgery of the female breast.

Corresponding to the trend toward voluminous breasts and wasp waists supported by firm corsets, the first operations at the end of the last century and beginning of this century were developed primarily for manifestations of stasis and pain caused by the excessive weight and were therefore devised for treatment of the ptosis by skin and gland excisions and by mastopexy, rather than for aesthetic size reduction.

Excisions of skin and glandular segments were made whether at the submammary fold, at the axillary region, at the upper hemisphere, or at the supra-areolar area and the mastopexy was performed with suture material, as, for example, by Girard (1910), or with fascia lata (Göbell, 1927) both to the pectoral muscle and to the second or third rib.

Reduction Mammaplasty with Free Nipple-Areola Complex Grafting: Thorek (1922)

Predecessor. In 1912 and 1913 Lexer presented at the German Society of Surgery a patient with large, deformed breasts, in whom, instead of performing an amputation, he reduced and remodeled the breast and performed in a second stage an areolar sharing technique.

Mammaplasty based on the concept of reduction with transplantation of the complete nipple-areola complex, however, started after Thorek's (1922) publication, popularized thereafter by Adams (1944). Dartigues (1928) mentioned that he had already used the technique in 1920. It is therefore often described as the Thorek-Dartigues-Adams technique. The procedure has been followed, modified, or improved by many surgeons and is still the technique of choice for gigantomastia (Fig. 44–1). For this purpose only two other techniques of nipple-areola complex transposition may be used: Martins' (1979) "roll in-out mastoplasty" and an inferior-flap technique with a large base like that suggested by Georgiade et al. (1979).

The advantages of nipple-areola complex grafting techniques are that they are simple, requiring less surgical ability and aesthetic sense and that they are less time-consuming. The disadvantages are a loss of nursing ability, which in any case is very poor in gigantomastia. However, a few exceptional cases of lactation have been reported by Clarkson (1957) and by Laing (1972). The erectility of the nipple-areola complex is mostly preserved, and some sensation might return.

Reduction Mammaplasty with Transposition of the Nipple-Areola Complex: Lexer (1921)

After the early 1920s the interest in aesthetic mammaplasty increased. Women become more interested in sports, gymnastics, and swimming. Emancipation started with women increasingly in occupations that previously were exclusively male. In fashion, there was now a desire for the silhouette of a teenager, with a smaller breast (*Knabenbrust*). The combination of these social factors, in addition to a better knowledge of tissue handling achieved by the treatment of mutilations during World War I, increased the request for mammaplasty and facilitated the development of new techniques. Toward the fifth or sixth decade the tendency changed again toward more voluminous breasts due to the influence of show business and magazines, increasing the demand for augmentation mammaplasty.

Predecessors. As mentioned by Dartigues (1925) and by Villandre (1925), it can be assumed that the first reduction mammaplasties with transposition of the nipple-areola complex had already been performed in 1909 by Morestin and by Villandre in 1911.

The first publication, however, which I discovered after several years of research, was made in 1921 by Lexer in Spain. This author was the first not only to perform an open transposition of the nipple-areola complex but also to use a technique with moderate skin and gland dissection, far ahead of the group of techniques based on this principle that became popular in the 1960s. Lexer's technique was then republished by Kraske (1923) and is generally known as the Lexer-Kraske technique.

With Lexer's technique, the glandular resection was performed on the lower pole and on an infra-areolar segment, which became more superficial toward the areola. The nipple-areola complex was transposed upward on the gland after supra-areolar skin excision. A mastopexy to the pectoral muscle was added, and the remaining scar was of the anchor type.

Lexer's technique was used by some surgeons. It is, however, surprising that, in spite of its simplicity, it did not become more popular, perhaps because of a certain limitation in cases of large breast ptosis and hypertrophy. Tamerin (1963) and Marino (1963) reintroduced the technique, adding some modifications (preservation of periareolar dermis and major posterior gland resection).

Reduction Mammaplasty with Transposition of the Nipple-Areola Complex and Wide Skin-Gland Undermining: Aubert and Lotsch (1923)

The next important publication is that of Aubert's (1923) "buttonhole technique" with "closed" transposition of the nipple-areola complex, also proposed independently a few weeks later by Lotsch (1923). Although not the first in transposing the nipple, therefore erroneously considered the author of this "capital moment in the history of mammaplasty," Aubert, and also Lotsch, initiated the era of transposition of the gland and the nipple-areola complex, characterized by a wide skin-gland undermining. The advantage was the absence of an infra-areolar scar; the disadvantages were a large

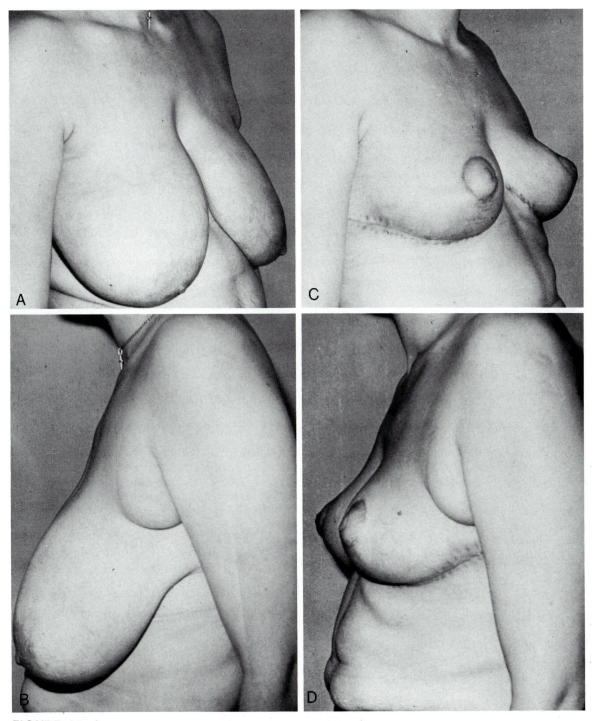

FIGURE 44–1

A to *D*, Gigantomasty treated by free transplantation of the nipple-areola complex using Strömbeck's pattern.

submammary scar, a flattening of the breast (because only the vertical dimension is being reduced), and disregard for the subdermal blood supply.

Another disadvantage of the techniques with wide skin-gland dissection is that the fibrovascular connections of Cooper's ligaments between skin and gland are being transected. These techniques, therefore, rely on a less safe postoperative fixation of the skin on the adequately reduced gland, supposedly acting as a skin brassiere.

Subsequently, multiple one-stage techniques of wide skin-gland dissection followed, with resection of different glandular segments, depending on the authors' opinion with regard to the importance of the vascular pedicles and/or of an inferior oblique or lateral skin segment for achievement of a more pleasing conical shape.

Holländer (1924) and Gläsmer (1930), as well as Prudente (1936), detached the areola from the skin only halfway and were the first to replace the inverted-T scar with an oblique, lateral, or J scar, respectively—one of the characteristics of the techniques developed later on by Marc (1952), by Mir y Mir (1959) for the Biesenberger technique (1928), by Meyer (1971), by Elbaz and Verheecke (1972), and by Regnault (1974). Prudente (1936) also developed an instrument with razor blades for the areolar incision, which he called a halloniotome.

A preoperative geometric planning of the skin resection, to which the glandular resection has to be adapted intraoperatively, was suggested by Bames (1948), by Aufricht (1949), by Galtier (1955), and by Wise (1956), who developed for the first time a pattern, later on modified by Strömbeck (1960). The Biesenberger technique (1928), in which the gland was resected in a lateral S form, gained much popularity and was followed by many surgeons. Gillies and McIndoe (1939) modified the S resection in large ptotic and hypertrophic breasts into a resection in a U form and also of a segment above the areola, preserving both upper pedicles and using the "periwinkle-shell technique" followed by several other surgeons.

In order to reduce the risk of areolar, glandular, or skin damage, some authors recommended two-stage procedures. The most significant defenders were Joseph (1925), Maliniac (1934), and Ragnell (1946); Stark (1980) used Ragnell's technique in one stage.

Transposition of Nipple-Areola Complex with Moderate Skin-Gland Dissection: The Period after 1960

The concept of a moderate skin-gland dissection in mammaplasty is based on consideration of the breast as a modified sudoriparous gland. Being of ectodermal origin, skin and gland should therefore not be treated as separate entities, as stated by Penn (1955). The importance of the subdermal network for the blood supply of both skin and gland was already mentioned by Salmon (1936). Another advantage of a moderate skin undermining is that the fibrovascular connections between skin and gland are respected.

As mentioned before, I consider Lexer's technique (1921) the forerunner.

Another milestone in aesthetic mammaplasty was Schwarzmann's publication (1930). For the first time the nipple-areola complex was transposed on a superomedial dermoglandular flap. The importance of preservation of a periareolar dermis ring was stressed both for the arterial supply and for the venous drainage. Schwarzmann's contribution was of capital importance for the development of most mammaplasty techniques with moderate skin undermining.

The most important techniques based on a limited skin gland dissection were developed by Penn (1955), with certain similarities to Lexer's technique; by Arié (1957), characterized by a vertical infra-areolar scar, trespassing the submammary fold, a technique that served as a basis for Pitanguy's technique of "keel resection" (1960); by Strömbeck (1960); by Dufourmentel and Mouly (1965); by Meyer and Martinoni (1971) (and Meyer and Kesselring [1975]); by McKissock (1972); and by Regnault (1974) (the B technique). Being reliable techniques, easy to perform, they all achieved a deserved wide popularity. I also used Strömbeck's technique from 1964 to 1970 with satisfactory results, except for the fact that in some patients with predominantly ptotic breasts, secondary ptosis occurred, which was the main reason for development of my dermal brassiere mammaplasty.

Some modifications were proposed, such as those of Ribeiro (1973), who proposed the insertion of an inferiorly based "safety flap" for achievement of a better forward projection of the central mass of the breast in Pitanguy's technique, and Piotti (1970, 1972, 1975), who performed with the same purpose a double keel resection with preservation of a wider central mass.

Vogt (1983) published a report on an upper-pedicle nipple-areola complex transposition technique in which the central gland tissue below the nipple-areola complex is used as a superiorly based glandular flap, inverted and attached to the second or third rib to form a "glandular prosthesis." Similar techniques were recommended by Bolivar (1983) and by Ho (1986), as well as by Ramirez (1986), who vertically divides the flap in two. Bragadini (1978) retains the central mammary mass as a glandular prosthesis, resecting the peripheral gland and axillary prolongation with the aim of reducing the possibility of tumor development.

Following Schwarzmann's concept of transposition of the nipple-areola complex on a dermoglandular flap, several different pedicles were developed: by Strömbeck (1960), a transverse pedicle; by McKissock (1972), a vertical pedicle; by Lerner et al. (1972) and Weiner (1973), a superior pedicle. Combinations were proposed by Meyer (1971), by Cardoso (1984) (transverse and inferior pedicle), and by Ramirez (1986) (superior, superolateral, and inferior pedicle).

Figallo (1977) facilitates in the ptotic breast the transposition of the nipple-areola complex on a triangular superior dermal flap by blunt dissection of Cooper's ligaments (usually three on either superior medial or lateral side, containing vessels and nerves, like a mesentery). An inferior dermoglandular flap based on the transposition flap is inserted in the retromammary space and attached to the pectoral plane.

Within the following group of techniques of "dermo-dermal adhesion," the transposition of the nipple-areola complex is performed in my technique (1971, 1972) on a superior dermal flap and a triangular subcutaneous glandular flap with a wide upper base carrying the subdermal blood supply. A similar flap is also used by Elsahy (1982), whereas both Lalardrie (1972) and Garcia Padron (1972) describe a completely circular dermoglandular pedicle. Skoog (1963) transposed the nipple-areola complex on an exclusively dermal flap, which could be considered an intermediate procedure to free transplanting of the nipple-areola complex. Although it is easier to transpose, the nourishment of the nipple-areola complex, however, is only based on the dermal capillaries.

Dermodermal Adhesion Techniques with Transposition of the Nipple-Areola Complex: The Period after 1972

The dermodermal adhesion techniques are characterized by a continuity of skin and residual gland, of skin-dermis, and of subcutaneous tissue–nipple-areola complex. Hence, the blood supply to these structures and also the fibrous connections skin to gland are respected. Moreover, dermodermal adhesions provide an additional means of stabilizing the breast.

Several techniques using the dermopexy principle can be considered precursors: according to Lalardrie and Jouglard (1974), Beare's technique, presented in 1965 but never published; my technique of periareolar dermopexy with retromammary mastopexy (1969); Goulian's technique of dermomastopexy (1971); and Lalardrie and Morel-Fatio's (1971) technique for subcutaneous mastectomy with immediate replacement with a prosthesis.

It was in 1972 when most of the techniques based on the above-mentioned principle were being published: by me, the dermal brassiere mammaplasty, first presented in 1971 (Hinderer, 1971); by Lalardrie, the dermal vault technique; by Schrudde (1972); by Olivari (1972); and by Garcia Padron (1972). They differed in the type of glandular resection: Lalardrie and I resected the deep portion of the breast in a plane parallel to the skin; Schrudde, mainly the superior lateral quadrant; and Garcia Padron, the superficial cone of the gland, maintaining a glandular base. Lalardrie's technique gained several followers, mainly in France.

Inferior Glandular or Dermoglandular Pedicle Techniques: The Period after 1975

In techniques using an inferior glandular or dermoglandular pedicle, the nipple-areola complex is transposed on this pedicle primarily so that the intercostal blood supply will be preserved. The arterial blood supply

and mainly the venous return, this last being descendent, have proved satisfactory, contrary to previous opinions stating that the intercostal perforators are of less importance. Innervation through the lateral intercostal nerves also seems to be adequate. Predecessors were Kohn and Dalrymple (1967), who mentioned that Joseph already used a similar technique in two stages, a report of which was never published. In Kohn and Dalrymple's technique, the lower breast hemisphere is preserved for reconstruction of the glandular cone, which is covered as in Aubert's "buttonhole" technique by the skin of the upper hemisphere, without a vertical infra-areolar scar. Ribeiro (1975), who was next, uses the dermis of the lower flap for fixation of the reconstructed glandular cone to the pectoral fascia.

The spreading of these techniques, which are becoming increasingly popular, began with this last publication and those by Jurado (1976), Robbins (1977), Courtiss and Goldwyn (1977), Climo and Alexander (1978), Reich (1979), and Georgiade et al. (1979), followed by many others. The previous techniques and later modifications differ concerning the inclusion or not of dermis and the width and depth of the base of the glandular pyramid, its eventual attachment to the pectoral plane, and the extent of breast resection medial and lateral to the pedicle and at the superior hemisphere. Georgiade et al. (1979) emphasize the importance of an adequate dimension of the glandular pyramid (8 × 10 cm at its base, and at the nipple-areola complex, of at least 5 cm of depth). The subdermal epigastric and intercostal blood supply then offers greater safety and permits the use of the technique in resections above 1200 gm to substitute for free nipple transplant techniques.

Techniques and Procedures Developed with the Aim of Reducing the Length of the Scar

As the safety and aesthetic result in mammaplasty improved, both patients and surgeons became conscious of the visibility of the residual scar, demanding a development of techniques and procedures to reduce the length of the scars. Obviously this depends largely on the grade of hypertrophy and ptosis and also on the texture of skin and gland. With Erol and Spira (1980) and Bricout et al. (1988), I believe that a shorter scar should never be achieved at the cost of a good shape and stability of the breast.

Procedures to Limit the Length of the Scar in Patients with Severe Hypertrophy and Ptosis

Several procedures have been developed with the aim of reducing the length of the scar, the consequence of the different length of the upper and lower horizontal skin incisions: Regnault (1974) uses B-type skin excisions, with skin displacement toward the areola and laterally, which are similar to the procedures recommended by Prudente (1936) and by Meyer and Martinoni (1971), who emphasize an additional defatting of the medial and lateral lower breast contour. The residual scar is of the J or L type. Similar skin displacements are also used by Jost and Meresse (1974), by Marchac and de Olarte (1982), and by several other authors.

Lassus (1981, 1987) shortened the scar by planning the skin excision above the submammary sulcus, also displacing the skin toward the areola; Faivre and Carissimo (1987), by adding a second dermatopexy.

Penn (1960), Robertson (1963), and Pers and Bretteville-Jensen (1972) avoided a different length of the incisions by means of the insertion of an inferior skin flap. A double, divergent infra-areolar scar resulted that permitted shortening of the inframammary scar, producing a better quality of scar.

A Y-V–plasty of the medial and lateral dog-ears of the inframammary scar, which also produces a better definition of the inferior contour of the breast and adds a stabilizing factor, has been recommended by Galtier (1955), by Piotti (1972), by Georgiade (1979), and by Lewis (1976) and is also used by me (see Fig. 44–22).

Techniques with Short Scars for Juvenile Hypertrophy with Adequate Skin Elasticity: 1980

Cloutier (1978) made the observation that the excision of glandular tissue, leaving the skin intact, permits a spontaneous skin retraction when one is reducing the deep portion of the gland through a submammary incision. It was Peixoto (1980) who first developed a technique in which, through a periareolar incision and after a wide skin-gland undermining, a large glandular pyramid is reduced into a small one. A V excision of the infra-areolar skin is added. The skin envelope is expected to retract within the following postoperative months over both the thorax and the reduced gland. Required, however, is a good cutaneous elasticity, as present in most juvenile hypertrophy with moderate ptosis. This technique has gained increasing interest, mainly among Iberolatinoamerican surgeons, and has been modified by Combescure and Lamarche (1987) and by Tafalla Peña (1988). This author uses the Strömbeck pattern and transposes the areola with an inferior flap technique. Bustos (1988) covers the glandular stump in its lower two-thirds of circumference up to the border of the areola, which is undermined for a few millimeters, with a silicone sheet. The sheet is attached to the pectoral plane.

Felicio (1986) modifies the Peixoto technique by means of a superior and inferior resection of a glandular segment through an exclusively periareolar approach; Cerizola and Fossati (1989) use a posterior keel resection, eventually adding an inferior V skin resection, if needed, or a later liposuction and secondary revision of the scar. These authors accept the disadvantage of a "mature" shape of the breast if a short scar can be obtained.

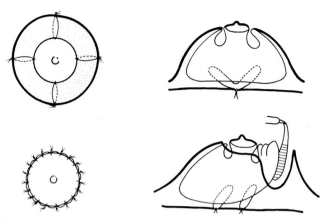

FIGURE 44–2
Original drawing of the author's doughnut technique of periareolar dermopexy with retromammary mastopexy (1969 to 1972). The infra-areolar skin is dissected from the gland toward the retromammary space, and nonabsorbable stitches are used to elevate the gland and to achieve a better forward projection of the breast cone. (From Hinderer, U. T.: Plastia mamaria modelante de dermopexia superficial y retromamaria. Rev. Esp. Cir. Plast. 5:521, 1972.)

"Doughnut" Techniques for Treatment of Normal-Sized Breasts with Minor Ptosis: 1969

The elevation of the areola by supra-areolar excision was reported by Joseph in 1925 and Noël in 1928. As far as I know, I published (1969 and 1972) the first report of a "doughnut" technique, the periareolar dermopexy combined with retromammary mastopexy (Figs. 44–2 and 44–3). An areoloperiareolar epidermis ring is removed so that the nipple-areola complex can be placed on the apex of the breast cone and so that there is tension on the skin, and nonabsorbable retromammary and infra-areolar plication sutures are used for elevating the gland and augmenting the forward projection.

Erol and Spira (1980) use a similar technique, also with superficial plication sutures at the infra-areolar gland, however, without the posterior mastopexy. Doughnut techniques were further reported by several other authors such as Bartels et al. (1976), Williams (1976), Vecchione (1976), Bass (1978), Gruber and Jones (1980), Teimourian and Adham (1983), Saad (1983), Maillard (1986), Puckett et al. (1985), and Gasperoni et al. (1988).

Indicated for treatment of minor breast ptosis, the technique is also useful for hypoplastic and tubular breasts by adding an augmentation with implants.

Rees and Aston (1976) established the differentiation between tubular and tuberous breasts, using in the latter a "telescoping" technique and adding small medial and lateral skin excisions close to the areola.

Techniques of Periareolar and V Skin Excision for Breasts with Moderate Hypertrophy and Ptosis: 1967

Periareolar skin excision combined with the removal of a V segment, whether inferior, oblique, or lateral,

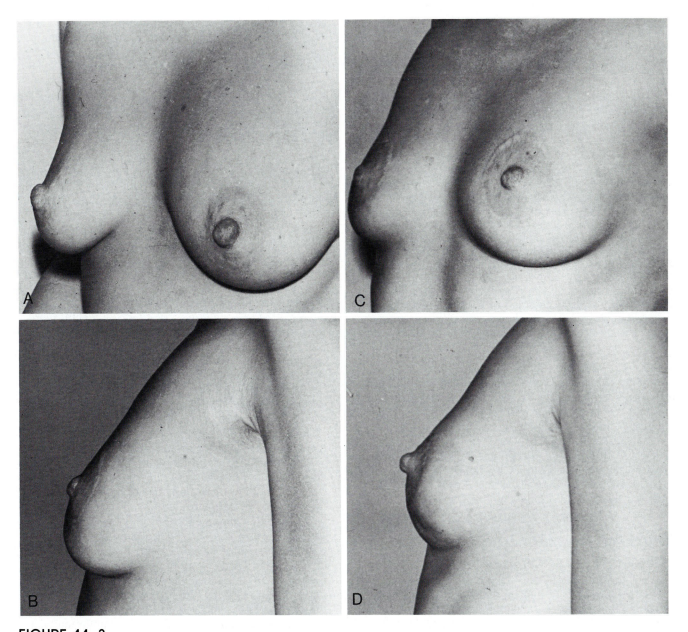

FIGURE 44–3

A and *B,* Preoperative view. *C* and *D,* Postoperative result after use of the doughnut technique, as shown in Figure 44–2. (From Hinderer, U. T.: Plastia mamaria modelante de dermopexia superficial y retromamaria. Rev. Esp. Cir. Plast. 5:521, 1972.)

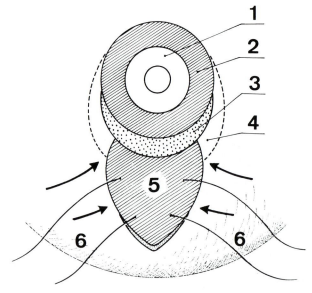

FIGURE 44–4

Technique of periareolar dermopexy with infra-areolar dermopexy in V form, indicated for patients with moderate ptosis, with the aim of avoiding the scar at the submammary fold. *1*, Areola. *2*, Area of periareolar dermopexy. *3*, Dermal incision to permit transposition of the areola. *4*, Area of skin undermining. The excess skin is displaced toward the areola and excised at the upper corners of the infra-areolar dermopexy incision. *5*, Area of infra-areolar dermopexy. *6*, Area of subcutaneous defatting or liposuction to improve the lower contour.

constitutes an intermediate step between doughnut techniques and reduction mammaplasties with moderate skin-gland dissection (Fig. 44–4). The surplus skin to be resected is displaced toward the areola; and the remaining scar is only periareolar, with an infra-areolar, oblique, or lateral extension, however, without surpassing the breast mound (Fig. 44–5).

Several authors have contributed to the development of these techniques, such as Burian (1967); Regnault (1976, 1984), with the B technique; Lewis (1972); Baroudi and Lewis (1976); and Ely (1983).

Dermofat Flaps for Treatment of Ptotic Hypoplastic Breast

The use of dermofat flaps in hypoplastic ptotic breast occasionally achieves an adequate volume replacement without the need for breast implants. Regnault (1966) and other surgeons have insisted that performing mammary augmentation with prosthesis alone is contraindicated whenever the breast is ptotic and the nipple-areola complex is not situated above the level of the submammary fold.

Inverted fat flaps for mammary augmentation for treatment of ptotic breast were first used by Lexer (1921) as a modification of his reduction mammaplasty technique. Lexer was also the first to perform a subcutaneous mastectomy for treatment of fibrocystic mastopathy, performing volume replacement with free fat transplantation from the abdomen or hip (1921). Dermofat flaps

were then proposed by Longacre et al. (1959), by me (Hinderer, 1972), and by many others.

They have also been used in combination with a transposition of the nipple-areola complex and volume replacement with prosthesis. I (Hinderer, 1972) described a technique in which the prosthesis is placed in the subpectoral plane, and a superiorly based dermofat flap is inverted and sutured to the inferior border of the pectoral muscle for reinforcement of the fascia, inferiorly covering a subpectoral implant (Fig. 44–6). Reichert (1972) independently published a technique using a dermofat flap with an inferior pedicle to cover an implant placed in suprapectoral position (Fig. 44–7).

SAFETY REQUIREMENTS IN MAMMAPLASTY

Although most techniques used today offer adequate safety, with the increase of ptosis and hypertrophy, the possibility of vascular complications becomes greater, particularly in breasts that have not suffered functional changes due to previous pregnancies or in breasts with involution after menopause, as stated by Marino (1963).

Based on anatomic studies since Cooper (1840) and mainly on more recent studies, such as those of Weitzel and Bassler (1971) and Mitz (1973), some conclusions with regard to safety can be made:

1. In view of the anatomic unity of skin and gland, undermining should be avoided as far as possible, because it interrupts the anastomotic vessels between skin and gland. Wide dissection may constitute a risk whether for the skin, if it is performed in the subdermal plane, or for the gland, if it is performed along the glandular surface, whenever one of the three vascular pedicles is also removed.

2. Whenever a technique with wide skin-gland dissection and resection of the upper lateral segment is used (Biesenberger techniques), it is advisable, as suggested by Mir y Mir (1977), to perform a previous thermography to determine the magnitude of participation of the internal mammary vessels in the vascular supply of the gland.

3. Both Lalardrie and I prefer to perform breast resection starting at a minimal depth of 2 cm below the areola, in a plane parallel to the skin toward the upper pectoral fascia. The deep glandular tissue is then discarded. This type of resection preserves the blood supply to the skin, to the residual gland, and to the nipple-areola complex. The subdermal network anastomosed with perforators of the internal mammary artery and with the superficial branch of the lateral mammary vessels is preserved, as are the recurrent vessels from the periareolar vascular ring to the nipple-areola complex.

4. In inferior pedicle techniques, Georgiade's suggestion (Georgiade et al., 1979) to preserve a wide and deep dermoglandular pyramid is to be preferred, because both the subdermal epigastric and the intercostal perforator vessels are preserved. If the technique requires a wider skin gland dissection at the upper breast for glandular resection, the undermining

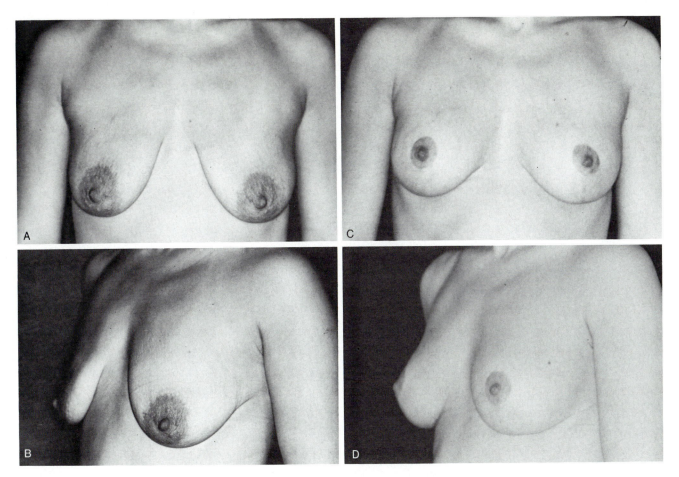

FIGURE 44–5

A and *B*, Patient with moderately ptotic breasts. *C* and *D*, Postoperative result 5 years after surgery with the technique described in Figure 44–4.

FIGURE 44–6

A and *B*, Intraoperative view of mammary augmentation for ptotic breasts with hypoplasia. A superiorly based sub-mammary dermofat flap is being used in combination with nipple transposition on a superior pedicle and infra-areolar dermopexy according to the author's technique (1972).

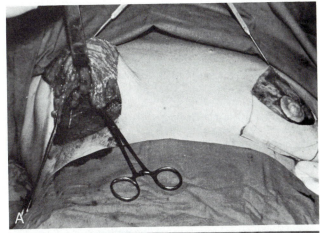

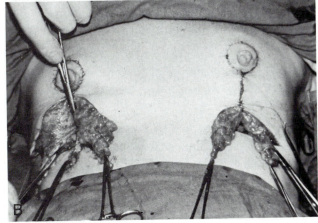

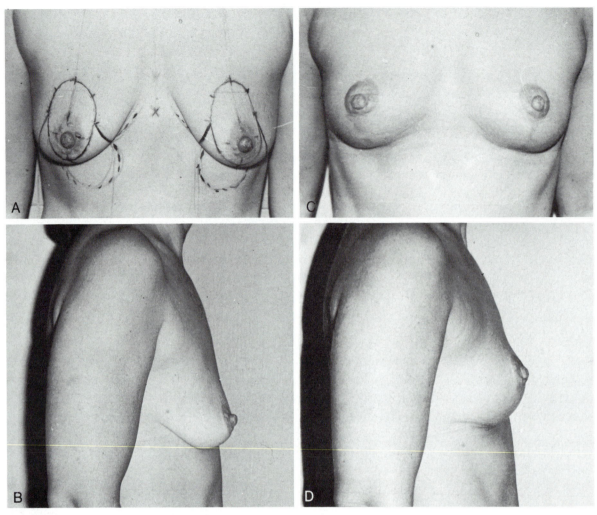

FIGURE 44–7
A to *D*, Preoperative view with markings and postoperative result 2 years after surgery. The hypoplastic breasts were augmented with a superiorly based dermofat flap and the ptosis corrected by nipple-areola complex transposition and infra-areolar dermopexy, as shown in Figure 44–6.

should be done close to the gland in order prevent any risk to the skin.

5. With regard to transposition of the nipple-areola complex, those techniques that respect not only a periareolar dermis ring of at least 6 cm diameter but also the subcutaneous tissue connections with the subdermal network toward the nipple-areola complex are safer. The dermal pedicle itself may be interrupted or minor skin undermining performed more distant to the areola, at the site of the new nipple location, with the purpose of facilitating the transposition. However, undermining should be done at the level of the dermis in order to guarantee the subdermal blood supply toward the nipple-areola complex.

6. From the point of view of the venous return, the same principles apply: preservation of the periareolar dermis ring and continuity of the subcutaneous tissue. As far as possible, a torsion of the nipple-areola complex transposition flap should be avoided. Inferior pedicle techniques have the advantage of favoring the venous return.

7. According to Cooper (1840), Craig and Sikes (1970), Edwards (1976), Courtiss and Goldwyn (1977), and Farina et al. (1980), innervation takes place through the lateral perforators of the fourth and fifth intercostal nerves, through the anterior group of cutaneous branches of the second to fifth intercostal nerve, and through descending cutaneous branches of the superficial cervical plexus. This explains why sensation of the nipple-areola complex, which in large hypertrophy is frequently reduced, may decrease temporarily or definitively in inferolateral dissections or when the upper medial undermining is made more than 2 cm from the sternum. Inferior pedicle techniques with a large base may better preserve the fourth intercostal nerve lateral to the nipple.

PREOPERATIVE AND POSTOPERATIVE EVALUATION OF PTOSIS

Most modern techniques achieve pleasing symmetric breasts of hemispheric or conical shape with a normal weight of 250 to 400 gm. The breast, however, should maintain its shape also beyond the first year after surgery. Before this time has elapsed, it is not possible to judge how much the distensibility of the skin and the stability of the gland will be affected by gravity. Also, the scar needs 1 to 2 years before it can be considered mature. We therefore evaluate the results 1 and 2 years after the operation and, if possible, 5 years after surgery.

The quality of the scar, which depends greatly on unpredictable individual factors, may require secondary surgical correction. We warn our patients of this possibility. In order to avoid additional scars due to interrupted sutures, we use intradermal removable monofilament polyamide on the periareolar and infra-areolar suture line, adding skin adaptation with Steri-Strips. Pressure treatment and monthly intralesional methylprednisolone injection with the Dermojet are used in case of hypertrophy of the scar.

A preoperatively ptotic breast will also tend to secondary ptosis in the postoperative period. Breast ptosis is usually differentiated as predominantly cutaneous or glandular, caused mainly by involution.

The following causes may be involved in breast ptosis:

1. Weight of the breast more than 400 gm, considered by Lalardrie and Jouglard (1974) the maximum of an ideal size.
2. Decreased skin elasticity, which may distend the infra-areolar skin, allowing the gland to be displaced downward around the inframammary fold. In these patients in most techniques the distance from the areola to the submammary fold should be reduced to 4 or 5 cm. An elastic skin, however, may retract postoperatively, pulling the nipple upward, as mentioned by O'Keefe (1983).
3. Decreased tension of the fibrous skin-gland connections. Evaluation may be carried out by judging the mobility and plication of the skin over the gland and also the thickness of the subcutaneous tissue. If these are adequate and no undermining has been performed, the skin may act to some extent as a brassiere, helping to stabilize the gland postoperatively.
4. Distention of the fibrovascular connections of the axillary prolongation along the lateral border of the pectoral muscle, which unites the breast to the fibrous arch of the axilla. As suggested by Dufourmentel and Mouly (1965), evaluation can be made by elevating the arm. Traction through this fibrovascular stabilizing tissue is transmitted to the gland before an elevation by skin tension takes place. This means of fixation should be preserved, or whenever an upper lateral glandular resection is planned, the gland may be suspended again on the stump.
5. Weight reduction. In fatty hypertrophy in an overweight patient, a weight reduction program should therefore be performed before surgery. The most reliable method I have found for weight reduction in a short time is the use of human chorionic gonadotropin in small doses and a low-fat diet, as first proposed by Simeonis and popularized by Vogt (1987).

Lalardrie and Jouglard (1974) classify ptosis with regard to the distance of the lower pole of the breast to the submammary sulcus, whereas Regnault (1966) also takes into account the level of the nipple. I prefer to classify ptosis with regard to the extent of nipple transposition required, in correspondence with the techniques I use.

Minor ptosis (less than 2.5 cm) can be corrected whether by a simple augmentation with implants if the breast is hypoplastic, or by means of a doughnut periareolar dermopexy technique. In hypoplastic breasts with minor ptosis, combined with abdominal lipodystrophy or major skin redundancy due to previous pregnancies, I also use the technique of mammary augmentation with implants through the abdominal approach, which was independently developed by me (Fig. 44–8) (Hinderer, 1968, 1974) and by Planas (1973). It permits the lowering of the inframammary fold to some extent, thus reducing the ptosis (Fig. 44–9).

For moderate ptosis (2.5 to 5 cm) or major ptosis (5 to 10 cm), a V type of skin excision should be added (see Figs. 44–5 and 44–6).

In patients with major ptosis (5 to 10 cm and 10 to 15 cm, respectively) I use my dermal brassiere mammaplasty. In very important ptosis (more than 15 cm), a free nipple transplant technique is to be considered.

For preoperative evaluation of the type of hypertrophy (predominantly fatty, epithelial, or connective tissue) and especially for diagnosis of breast masses, a preoperative mammography should be performed. This is repeated 3 to 6 months postoperatively, because surgery, especially when dermodermal adhesion techniques are being used, may change the image of the breast structure. Postoperative mammography may then be important for comparison in case of any pathologic condition observed later on.

In patients with major hypertrophy and ptosis, for many years, 1 to 2 units of blood have been taken approximately 10 days before surgery to be transfused intraoperatively after hemostasis is obtained. During this time the patient receives hematopoietic treatment.

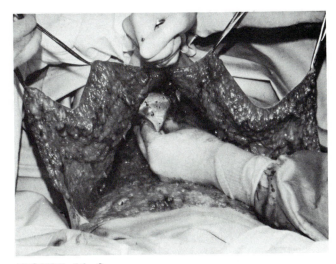

FIGURE 44–8
Intraoperative view of the insertion of a prosthesis by the abdominal approach (Hinderer, 1968 to 1974; Planas, 1973).

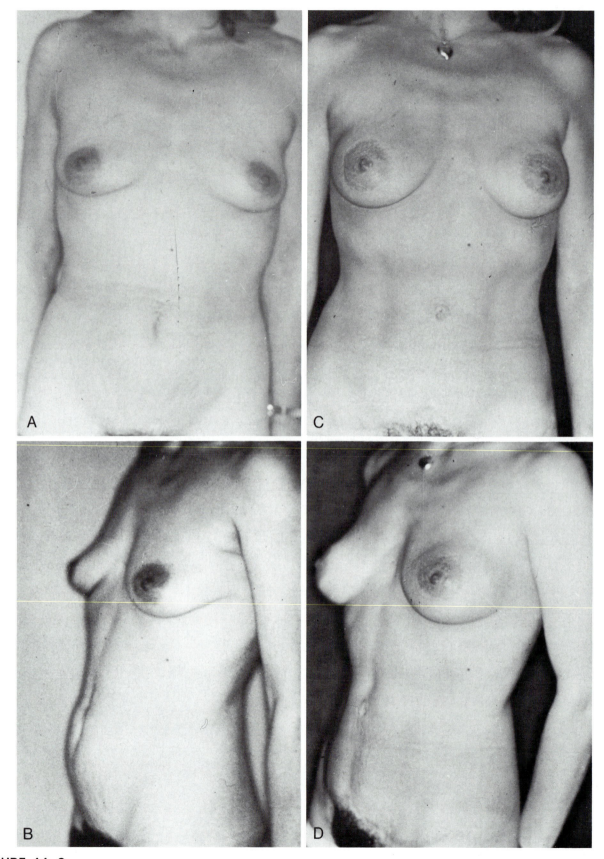

FIGURE 44–9

A to *D*, Preoperative and postoperative views of augmentation mammaplasty by the abdominal approach. This technique can also be used for hypoplastic breasts with moderate ptosis, because it achieves a descent of the submammary sulcus.

ADDITIONAL PROCEDURES FOR PREVENTION OF SECONDARY PTOSIS

For many decades surgeons were concerned about the problem of secondary ptosis after mammaplasty. Several technical details were recommended for additional stabilization of the gland, which can be classified as follows.

Mastomyopexy and Mastocostopexy with Suture Material. Sutures, used already by Dehner (1908) and by Girard (1910), are useful intraoperatively for mounting the breast, for reducing the tension at the skin suture line, and also for immediate postoperative stabilization. A longer-lasting value has, however, been questioned by Schwarzmann (1930) and by Aufricht (1949), who once mentioned that "one cannot suspend the breast only on a suture as it is not possible to suspend a mozzarella cheese on a cord."

Mastopexy by Imbrication of Glandular Flaps. The imbrication of glandular or dermoglandular flaps with eventual additional suture of the dermis to the pectoral plane has been used with the double purpose of achieving a more pleasing breast cone and preventing secondary ptosis. It constitutes an important characteristic of many old and recent techniques.

Mastomyopexy and Mastocostopexy with Autodermal Strips or Alloplastic Material. The use of dermal strips for stabilization of the breast or increasing the forward projection of the central breast mass was initiated by Maliniac (1938, 1950), followed by Lewis (1956) and da Silva (1964). Gillet (1952) suspends the lower breast pole with nylon to the clavicle, Johnson (1981) uses Marlex strips attached to the pectoral muscle, and Bustos (1988) uses a silicone sheet covering the gland.

Mastopexy Technique Using a Muscular or Fascial Pocket. Garcia Padron (1980) presented and, independently, Fontana and Muti (1982) published a technique in which a muscular and/or fascial pocket is dissected above the inframammary sulcus to serve as a lower container of the inferior breast mass, a technique we have used in four patients with a satisfactory result as far as the stabilization of the breast is concerned (Figs. 44–10 and 44–11). In two patients, however, a hematoma occurred in the pocket, with subsequent fat necrosis, probably due to my insufficient experience with the technique.

Dermodermal Adhesion Techniques. These have already been commented upon. Their value as far as stabilization of the breast is concerned has been proved mainly by Lalardrie.

Dermomuscular Fixation. In my (1971, 1972) dermal brassiere mammaplasty an infra-areolar dermal pillar is additionally attached with dermal strips to the pectoral muscle, with the aim of stabilization and achievement of a better filling of the upper breast hemisphere. Strömbeck (1964) already used dermis strips to the pectoral muscle—however, with unfavorable results, probably because the strips served as attachment of the transposition flap and not of an infra-areolar dermal pillar, thus retaining the breast tissue (Fig. 44–12).

PERSONAL TECHNIQUES

The Doughnut Periareolar Dermopexy Technique (1969, 1972)

Indication: Breasts of normal size with minor ptosis and tubular breast.

Advantage: Limited scar (periareolar) (Fig. 44–13).

Disadvantages: The technique produces a flattening of the nipple-areola complex which, on the other hand, might be convenient in tubular breasts. The tendency to the widening of the areola has to be taken into account

Text continued on page 583

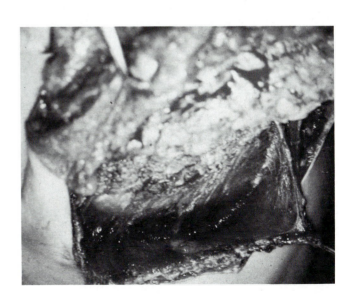

FIGURE 44–10
Intraoperative view of the fascial pocket above the submammary fold in which the reconstructed breast is inserted for prevention of postoperative ptosis (Technique of Garcia Padron [1980] and Fontana and Muti, 1982.)

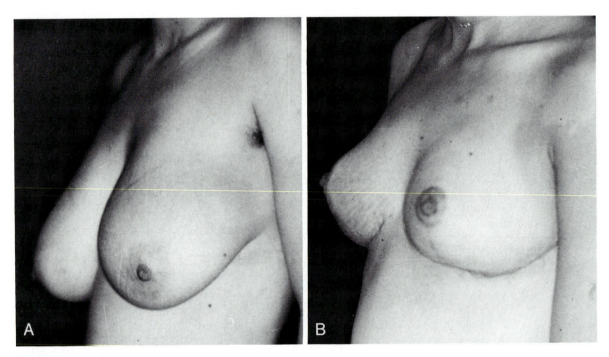

FIGURE 44–11
Preoperative view *(A)* and postoperative view *(B)* 2 years after surgery, showing stabilization of the breast by means of the technique of Garcia Padron and Fontana and Muti.

FIGURE 44–12

Drawing of the author's dermal brassiere technique (1971 to 1972) showing the inferior dermal pillar *(1)* and its fixation to the pectoralis muscle *(2)*. A 60-degree angle between the infra-areolar breast plane and the chest plane is achieved; it depends, however, on the correct fixation of the strips above the submammary sulcus (approximately at the level of the fourth rib). This should be checked intraoperatively with the patient in semi-sitting position.

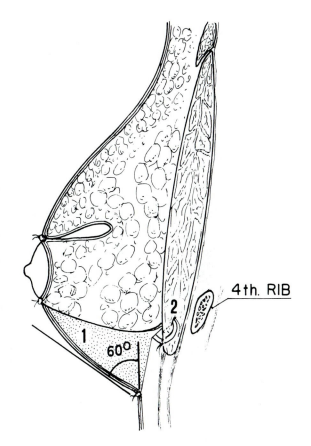

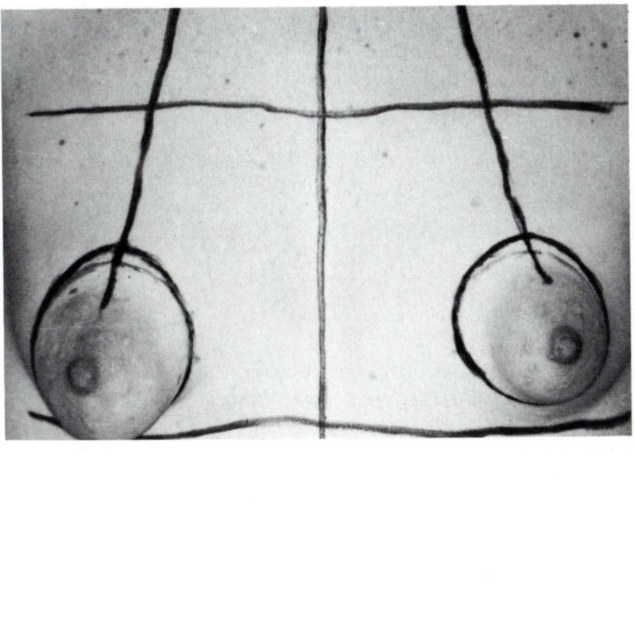

4th. RIB

FIGURE 44–13

The doughnut periareolar dermopexy (Hinderer, 1969 to 1972). The markings are peformed with the patient standing. The apex of the new areola is marked on the intersection of a line 5 cm from the suprasternal notch to the nipple and another connecting the midway points between the acromion and olecranon of both arms. On the upward displaced distended breast, another point is marked 5.5 cm from the submammary fold. These points allow the drawing of an oval, which is medially equidistant from the midsternal line. (From Gonzalez-Ulloa, M., Meyer, R., Smith, J. W., Zaoli, G. (eds.): *Aesthetic Plastic Surgery.* Vol. 4. Padova, Piccin; St. Louis, C. V. Mosby, 1988.)

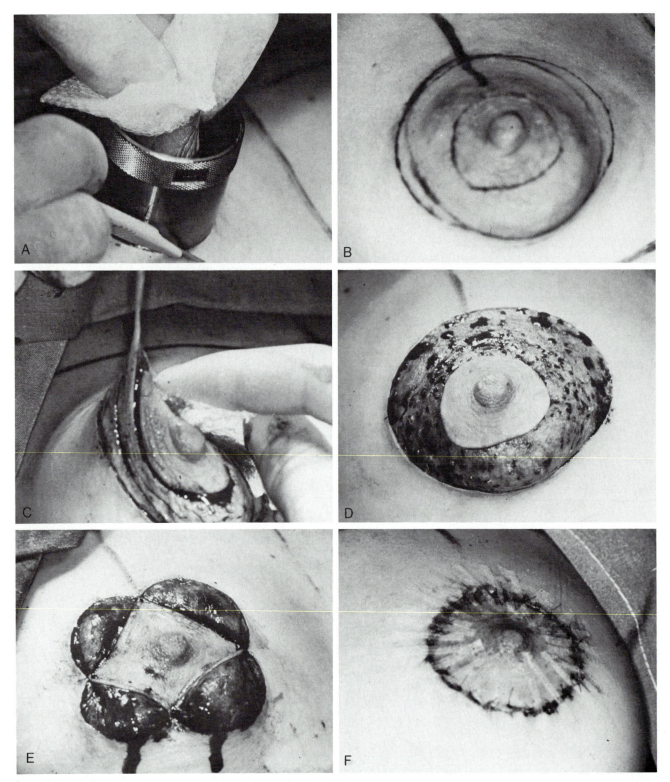

FIGURE 44–14

The doughnut periareolar dermopexy. *A* and *B*, The infra-areolar circular incision is superficially performed on the distended breast. An areolar "cookie cutter" is applied, and strong traction is exerted on the nipple, pulling the areola and periareolar skin through the center of the "cookie cutter." Traction is continued until the skin over the breast is sufficiently taut. The external circle is incised at the border of the instrument. The initial marking, made in the standing position, is used as a guide in order to prevent traction being applied asymmetrically. *C* and *D*, The areolar and periareolar skin between the two circles is incised in small concentric strips, and the epidermis is then stripped away by means of Fournier's maneuver. *E* and *F*, Suturing is completed with interrupted U sutures knotted on the areola, which are passed intradermically to the circumareolar skin. Superficial adaptation is completed with 1/8-inch 3M Steri-Strips.

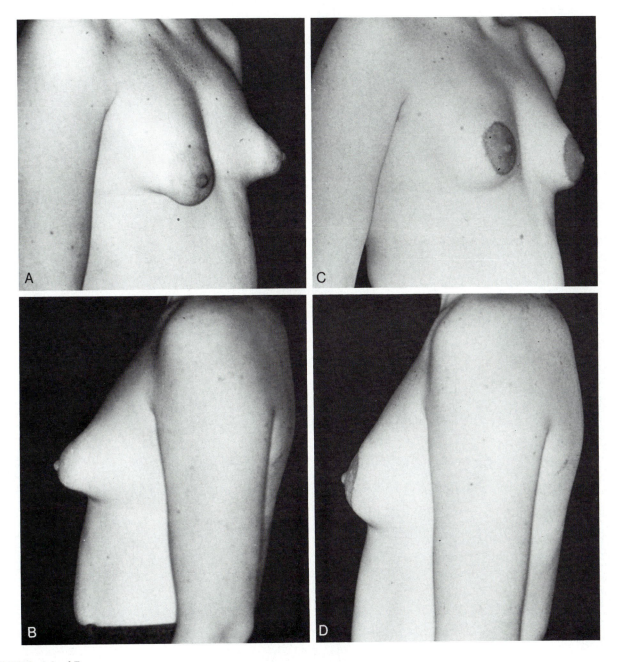

FIGURE 44–15
A to *D,* Preoperative and postoperative views demonstrating the results of the doughnut periareolar dermopexy technique in a patient with ptotic tuberous breasts (see Figs. 44–13 and 44–14). (From Gonzalez-Ulloa, M., Meyer, R., Smith, J. W., Zaoli, G. (eds.): *Aesthetic Plastic Surgery.* Vol. 4. Padova, Piccin; St. Louis, C. V. Mosby, 1988.)

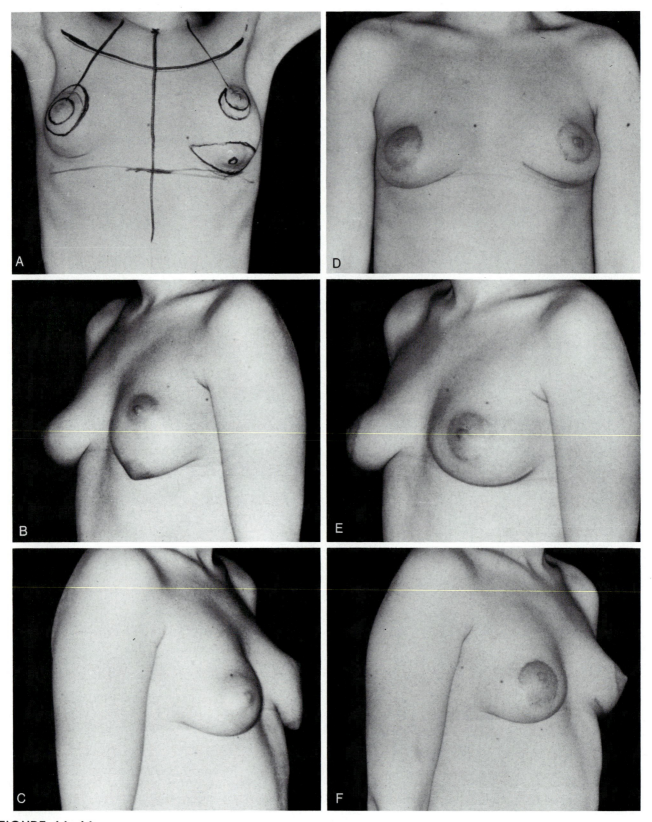

FIGURE 44–16
The doughnut-type periareolar dermopexy technique in a patient with important asymmetry due to polymastia. The markings are modified for removal of a larger periareolar epidermal ring while the areola on the double-breasted side is displaced dowward. The excision of the lower breast is also marked. *A* to *C,* Preoperative views. *D* to *F,* Postoperative result at 6 months.

by reducing the diameter of the areola to approximately 3 cm. The second disadvantage is the widening of the scar, which can be reduced by using Peled's purse-string suture with unabsorbable material (Peled et al., 1985). Otherwise, a secondary revision of the periareolar scar may be required occasionally (Figs. 44–14 to 44–16).

The Doughnut Periareolar Dermopexy Technique with Subpectoral Implantation of Prostheses

Indication: Hypoplastic breasts with minor ptosis.

The advantages and disadvantages of the technique are the same as mentioned before. The insertion of implants increases the base of the breast, which is desirable in tubular breasts (Figs. 44–17 and 44–18).

Hinderer's Dermal Brassiere Mammaplasty (1971, 1972)

Indications: Breast hypertrophy or breasts of normal size with major or important ptosis; secondary mammaplasties. In breasts of normal size with moderate ptosis, only an infra-areolar dermopexy and transposition of the nipple-areola complex may be performed

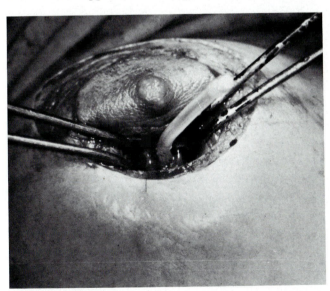

FIGURE 44–17
Intraoperative view of the doughnut periareolar dermopexy technique with subpectoral augmentation with implants. After removal of the circumareolar epidermis, the infra-areolar dermis is incised as well as the breast tissue vertically down to the pectoral muscle. The fibers of the pectoral muscle are bluntly divided to the retropectoral space; and a large enough cavity is dissected, also in a downward subfascial direction, somewhat below the submammary sulcus, for insertion of an implant. In this case an inflatable prosthesis is being used.

with the aim of avoiding the submammary scar, as shown in Figures 44–4 and 44–5 (Figs. 44–19 to 44–23).

Advantages: The technique is reliable and achieves a pleasing shape with adequate filling of the upper breast hemisphere. It provides a long-lasting result, preventing secondary ptosis (Figs. 44–24 to 44–30).

It is safe with regard to skin, gland, and nipple-areola complex survival, and preservation of sensation. The submammary scar usually does not surpass the base of the breast because of a V-Y-plasty, which also defines the lower breast contour better.

Disadvantages: The technique seems more complex; but once understood, is not difficult to perform. It requires a longer operating time than other techniques. The pectoral dermal strip fixation may produce an upward pull at the center of the submammary scar when the patient elevates her arms over the head.

Unfavorable results (estimated on a sample of 500 patients): Postoperative inverted nipple occurred in six patients (1.2%). For repair, Hinderer and del Rio's technique (1983) was used (Fig. 44–31). Occasionally during the first period a somewhat square-looking breast resulted because of a limited postoperative descent of glandular tissue medially and laterally to the infra-areolar dermal pillar. In the last few years this has been corrected by adding an additional fixation at the submammary fold with dermal flaps to the fascia (see Fig. 44–22).

Complications: The complication rate is low; in over 500 patients, there was one partial areolar loss (0.2%) due to an unrecognized hematoma. Major breakdown of the infra-areolar suture line with fat and gland necrosis was found in four breasts (0.8%). Secondary healing was obtained within 6 to 8 weeks, and scar revision was performed 1 year later. Minor breakdown of the suture line occurred in eight breasts (1.6%), requiring scar revision in only five patients.

The Infra-areolar Dermopexy Technique Combined with a Dermofat Flap and Subpectoral Augmentation with Implants

Indication: Hypoplastic breast with major ptosis.

This technique is a further development of two techniques used for ptotic breasts when a subcutaneous adenectomy was performed: volume replacement by an inferiorly based dermofat flap (Hinderer, 1965) or with a superiorly based dermofat flap (Hinderer, 1972) (Figs. 44–32 to 44–34).

The dermofat flap is used to strengthen the inferior part of the musculoaponeurotic wall. It covers the fascia below the inferior border of the pectoralis muscle. Implants are inserted subpectorally. The nipple-areola complex is transposed with the dermal-subdermal pedicle used in the dermal brassiere technique, and an infra-areolar dermopexy pillar is utilized to stabilize the breast, however, without strip fixation (Fig. 44–35).

Text continued on page 601

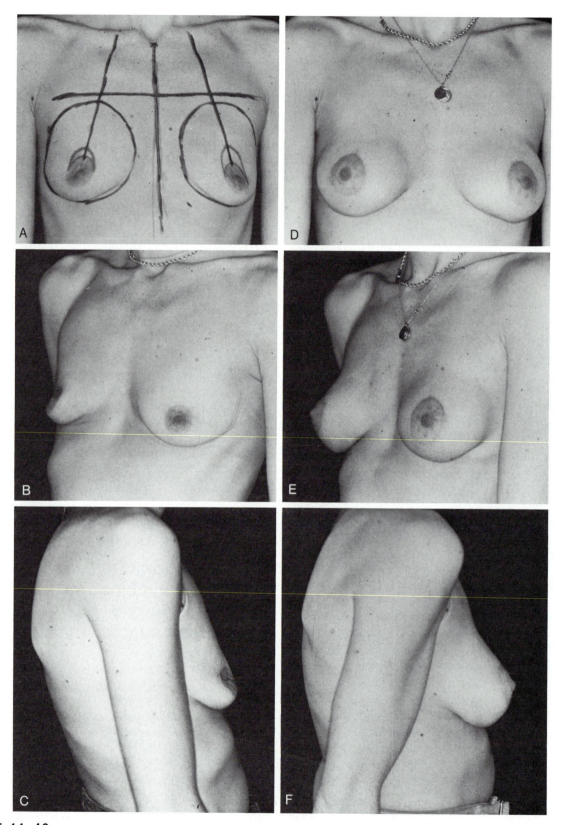

FIGURE 44–18

A to *F*, Preoperative and postoperative views of a patient with hypoplastic breasts and minor ptosis who underwent doughnut periareolar dermopexy with subpectoral insertion of prostheses. In this case inflatable prostheses were used because of the difference in breast size; in the left breast, 10 ml less saline was injected. Notice also the asymmetry, which required a major elevation of the areola on the left side.

FIGURE 44–19

Dermal brassiere mammaplasty: preoperative markings.
The new apex of the areola is marked on the intersection
of a line 5 cm from the suprasternal notch to the nipple
and a line uniting the midpoints between the acromion
and olecranon of each arm. The Strömbeck pattern is
adapted, and the limits of the new areola and the lateral
Strömbeck flaps are checked, approximating the skin between the thumb and index finger of the two hands. If it is
too small or too large for a good breast shape, in line with
the chest shape, the appropriate correction is made. Two
lines drawn from the axilla to the lateral limit of the areola
and from the third intercostal space to the medial limit of
the areola, representing the presumable direction of the
main internal and superficial external mammary vessels,
mark the minimal width of the subcutaneous flap carrying
the subdermal vascularization for transposition of the nipple-areola complex. It is therefore of triangular shape, with
a broad upper base; the dermal upper pedicle of the
nipple-areola transposition flap is narrower. On the submammary fold, a small triangle is marked, at the same
distance to the midline as the apex of the areola. This will
later ease the tension at the inverted-T junction, avoiding
a 90-degree angle. Two vertical lines are drawn from the
ends of the Strömbeck pattern to the submammary fold.

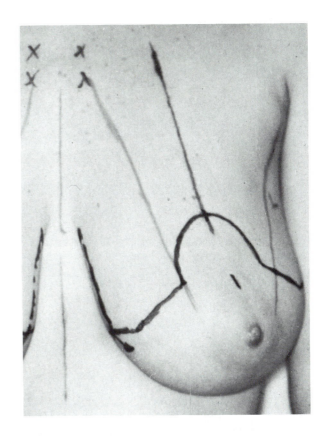

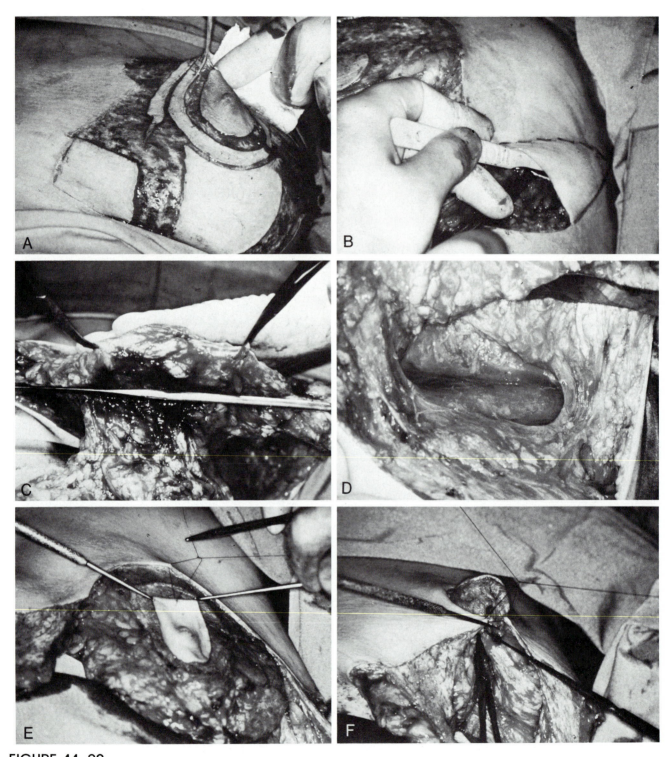

FIGURE 44–20

Dermal brassiere mammaplasty. *A,* The markings are incised, as well as the areola, with a 4-cm "cookie cutter." The epidermis is removed after incision in narrow strips by means of Trabanino's maneuver (1978) of pulling it off with forceps, eventually aided by a scalpel. The area for de-epithelialization includes the nipple-areola transposition flap, two triangles adjacent to the lateral Strömbeck flaps and at the midbreast corner of these, the strips for fixation of the breast. *B,* At the medial and lateral ends of the submammary sulcus, the subcutaneous and glandular tissue is removed for better definition of the lower breast contour. *C,* The breast is divided in an oblique plane, parallel to the skin surface, toward the pectoral fascia in the upper hemisphere, starting at a minimal depth of 2 cm, which should be somewhat thicker at the level of the nipple-areola complex. This splits the breast into two portions, the deeper to be removed from the pectoral fascia. *D,* In the center of the upper hemisphere, the skin and subcutaneous tissues are bluntly dissected from the pectoral plane up to the clavicle. Along the lower lateral border of the pectoral muscle, the fibrous connection to the axilla is preserved because it seems important for the lateral nerve supply to the nipple and will also be used to stabilize the breast and to form the new lower lateral breast contour. *E* and *F,* Whenever the transposition is difficult, the skin at the lower part of the new areolar site and at the upper part of the two triangular flaps for the infra-areolar dermal pillar is undermined close to the dermis.

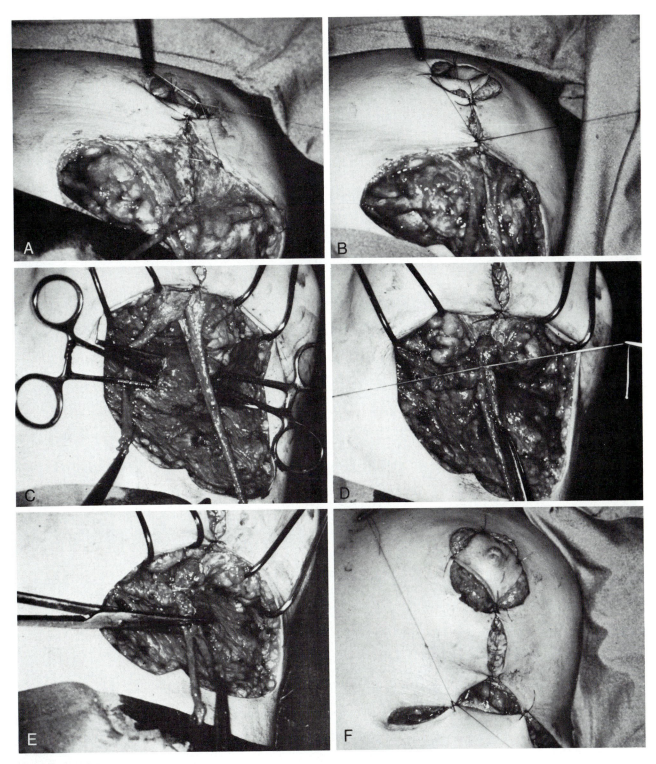

FIGURE 44–21

A, The dermal strips are put under tension and the central border of the triangular flaps is sutured. *B,* The flaps are united face to face with interrupted polyglycolic acid sutures and an Ethilon 3-0 stitch placed at the inferior border. *C,* The patient is put in a semi-sitting position. Two forceps are passed from either side through the pectoral muscle, and the ends of the strips (which are now at the upper border of the infra-areolar pillar) are grasped. *D,* The strips are pulled through the muscle and appropriately tightened, so that the infra-areolar plane adopts a 60-degree angle with the chest plane. Two strong, braided nylon sutures are used to fix the strips together and to the pectoral fascia. *E,* The excess of the strips is then trimmed off. This fixation achieves (1) stabilization of the breast, (2) adequate protrusion of the nipple-areola complex, and (3) good upper breast filling because the remaining gland rests on the upper border of the infra-areolar pillar. *F,* The first pilot stitches are placed at the limit of the small triangular flap. Removable subcuticular sutures are placed at the periareolar and infra-areolar incisions.

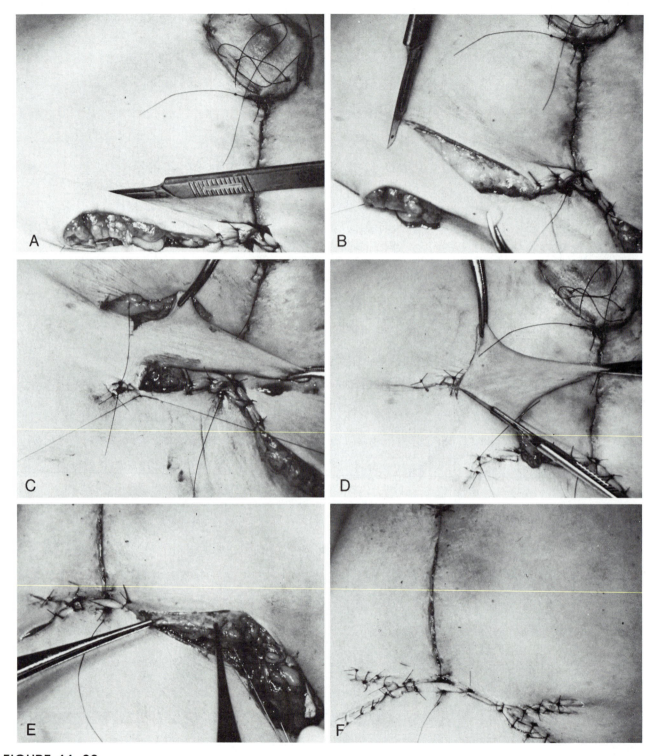

FIGURE 44–22

The dog-ears at the submammary incision are treated by means of a modified V-Y procedure (1) to keep the scar as short as possible and (2) to avoid a square-looking breast, achieving a more round lower contour and stabilization by the Y flap. *A,* An incision is made at the lower breast contour, up to the central level of the submammary incision. *B,* An oblique downward incision relieves the tension at the upper part of the dog-ear. The end of the V flap is grasped with a forceps. *C,* Tension applied on the V flap permits one to start suturing at the ends of both incisions. Adequate removal of subcutaneous tissue is required. *D,* The excess can now be trimmed and the suturing of the Y flap completed. *E,* In order to additionally stabilize the lower breast contour, lately we have added a narrow dermal flap at the upper incision, which is sutured to the fascia. *F,* The inframammary suture lines, completed in Y form, usually are short and remain in the "shadow" of the breast.

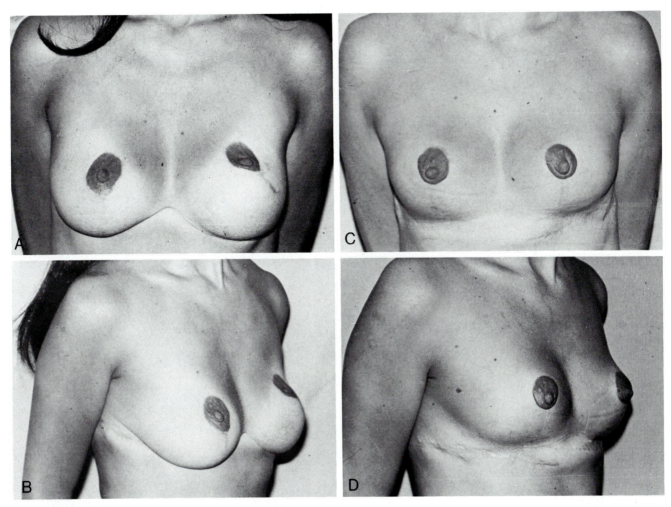

FIGURE 44–23

A to D, The dermal brassiere technique is also useful for secondary ptosis with asymmetry due to an excessively elevated areola because it permits one to displace the whole breast cone to a much higher situation and to center the areola on the breast apex. This patient had undergone an operation elsewhere with the Gillies-McIndoe technique. The distance from the suprasternal notch to the left nipple was 14 cm, and a ptosis of the gland had occurred.

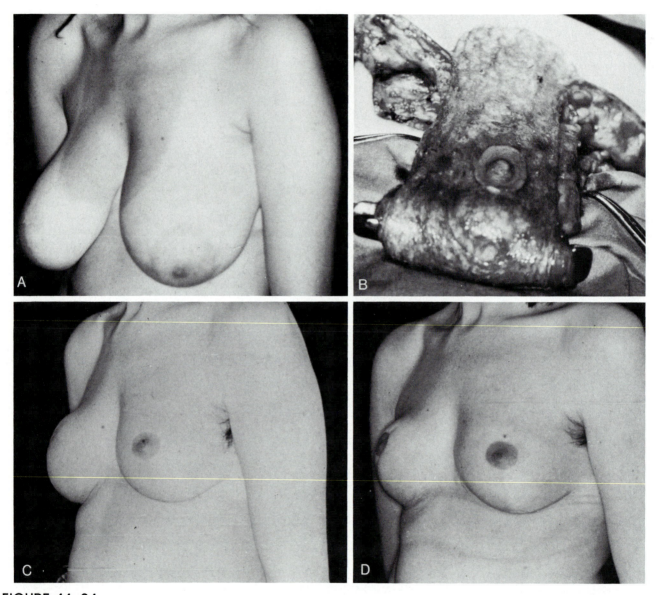

FIGURE 44–24

A, Large hypertrophy, treated on the right side by means of a vertical pedicle technique and on the left side by means of the dermal brassiere technique. *B,* Intraoperative view of the vertical transposition flap used on the right side. *C,* After several months. Secondary ptosis with drooping of the gland has occurred on the right side. *D,* This required a secondary revision of the right side, which was done with an oblique method. Despite this revision, a minor ptosis can be still seen on the right side 3 years after surgery. The left side is still stable.

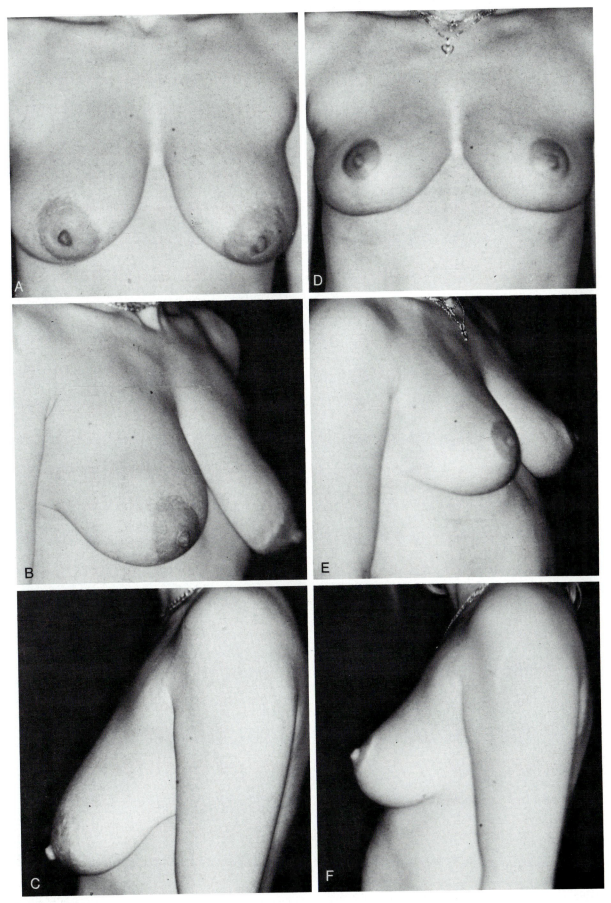

FIGURE 44–25
A to *F,* Patient with ptotic hypertrophic breasts treated by dermal brassiere mammaplasty, preoperatively and 2 years after surgery.

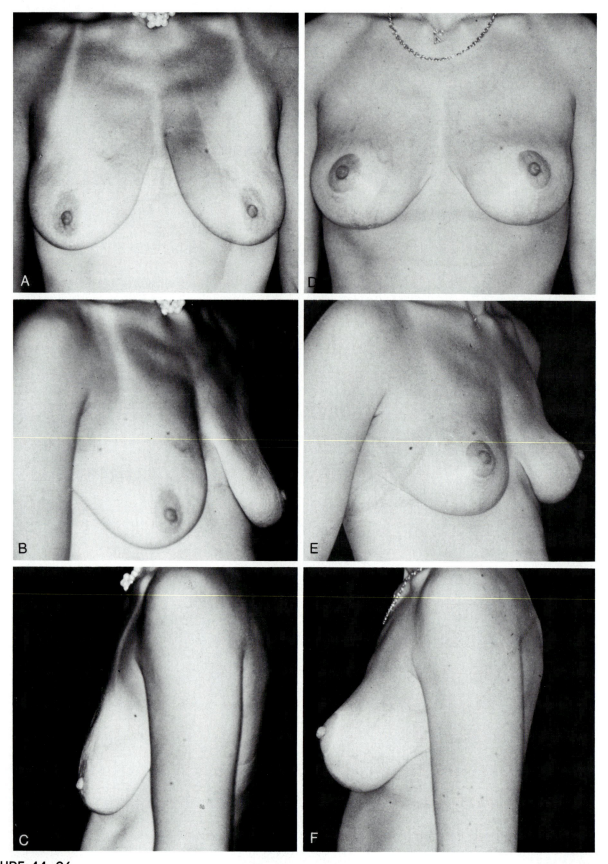

FIGURE 44–26
A to *F*, Patient with ptotic breasts treated by dermal brassiere mammaplasty, preoperatively and 4 years after surgery.

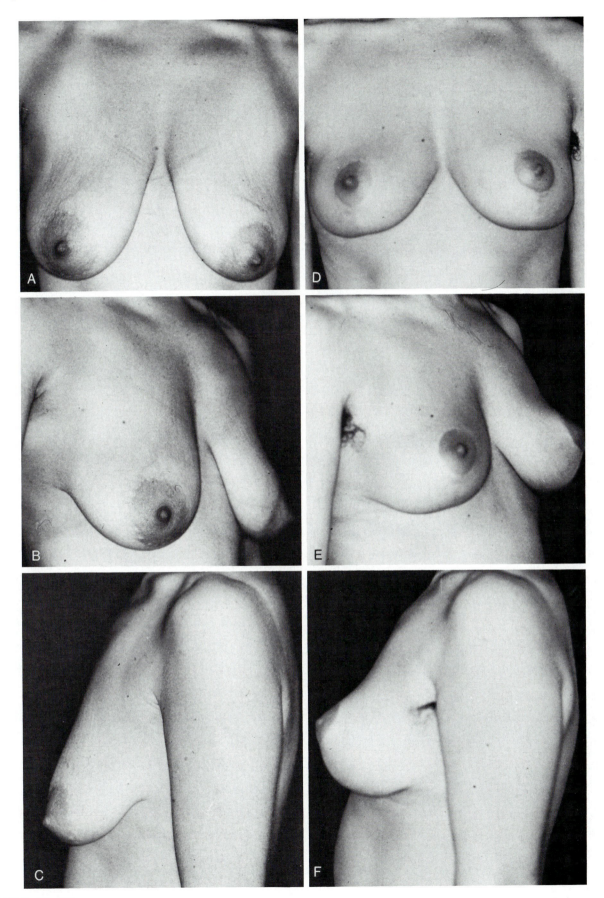

FIGURE 44–27

A to F, Patient with ptotic breasts treated by dermal brassiere mammaplasty preoperatively and 7 years after surgery.

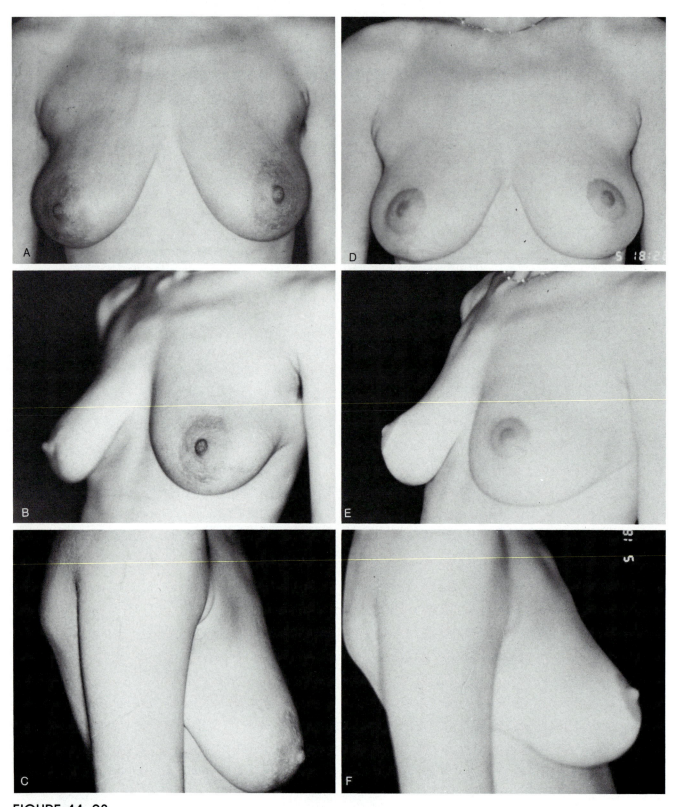

FIGURE 44–28
A to *F*, Patient with ptotic hypertrophic breasts treated by dermal brassiere mammaplasty, preoperatively and 10 years after surgery.

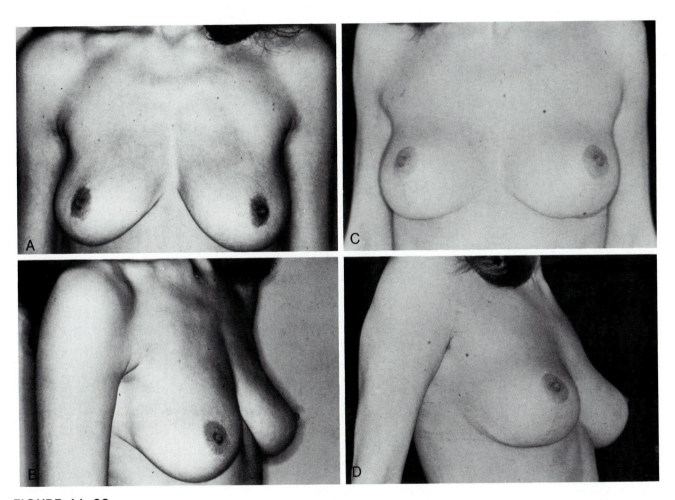

FIGURE 44–29
A to D, Patient with ptotic hypertrophic breasts treated by dermal brassiere mammaplasty preoperatively and 12 years after surgery.

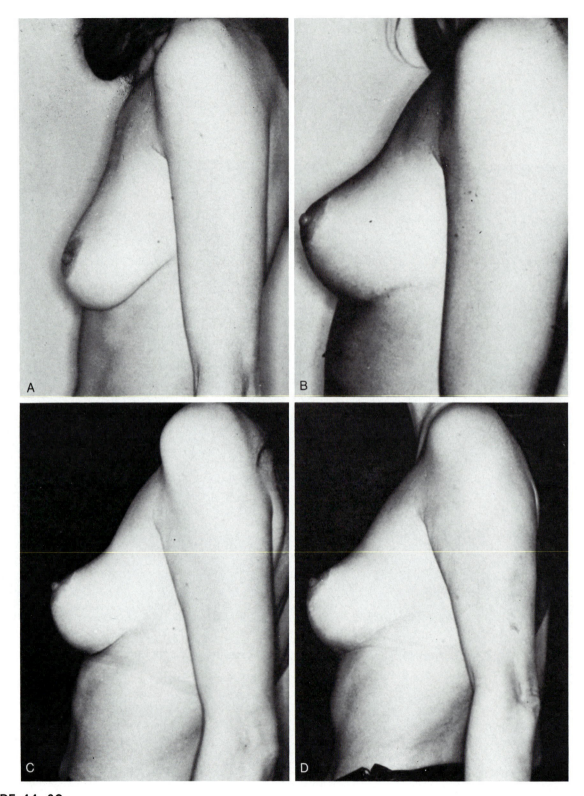

FIGURE 44–30
A to D, Lateral view of the breasts showing the stabilization achieved with the dermal brassiere technique 2 years *(B)*, 8 years *(C)*, and 12 years *(D)* after surgery.

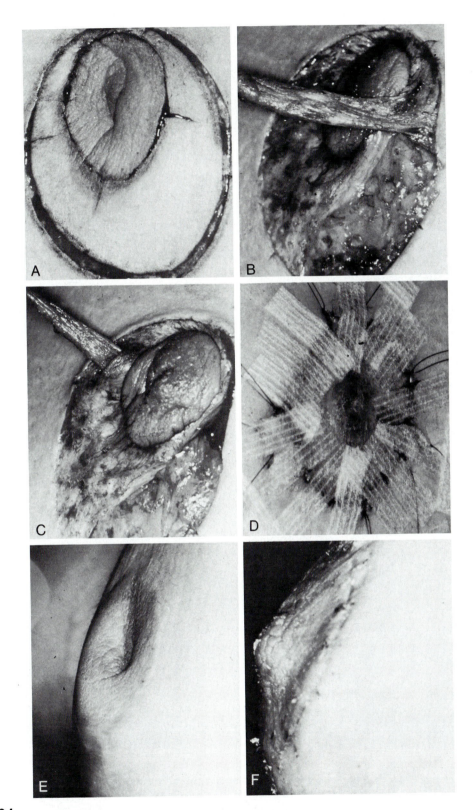

FIGURE 44–31

Hinderer and del Rio's technique (1983) for correction of postoperative inverted nipple and asymmetry or excessive elevation of the areola. *A,* A circular epidermal incision is made on the apex of the cone of the breast, and the epidermis is removed. *B,* A dermal strip is detached. A tunnel is made deep under the nipple, and a purse-string suture applied in the mammary tissue at the base of the nipple. *C,* The dermal strip is passed below the everted nipple and sutured to the opposite side. *D,* Subcuticular continuous suture and adaptation with 3M Steri-Strips completed. *E,* Preoperative and postoperative views of this technique. (From Hinderer, U. T., del Rio, J. L.: Treatment of the postoperative inverted nipple with or without asymmetry of the areola. Aesthetic Plast. Surg. 7:139, 1983.)

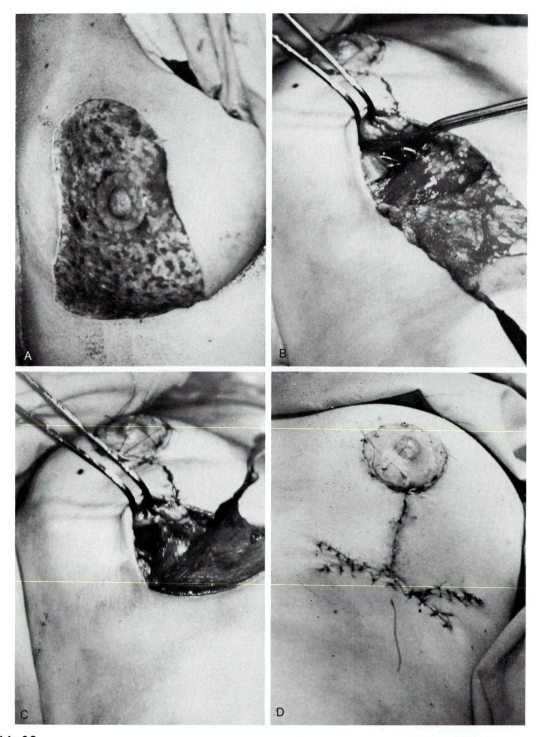

FIGURE 44-32

Intraoperative views of the author's technique for hypoplastic breasts with major ptosis. *A,* After de-epithelialization a dermofat incision below the areola is made for transposition of the nipple-areola complex, which is lifted attached to the gland *(1).* An approximately 2-cm-wide dermofat flap is left attached to the medial and lateral skin flaps to be sutured face to face for infra-areolar dermopexy *(2).* The lower pole of the gland is dissected from the subcutaneous tissue and dissected upward from the pectoral fascia to be displaced upward. The lower dermis and subcutaneous tissue *(3)* are used as an inferiorly based flap. *B,* After transposition of the nipple-areola complex and suturing of the infra-areolar dermopexy flaps, the fibers of the pectoral muscle are bluntly divided and a subpectoral pocket is dissected toward the submammary fold and implants inserted *(1).* The inferior dermofat flap is shown *(2). C,* The inferior dermofat flap is sutured to the inferior border of the pectoralis muscle to strengthen the fascia above the submammary fold, covering the inferior part of the implant. *D,* Suturing is completed by means of the V-Y technique to shorten the submammary scar.

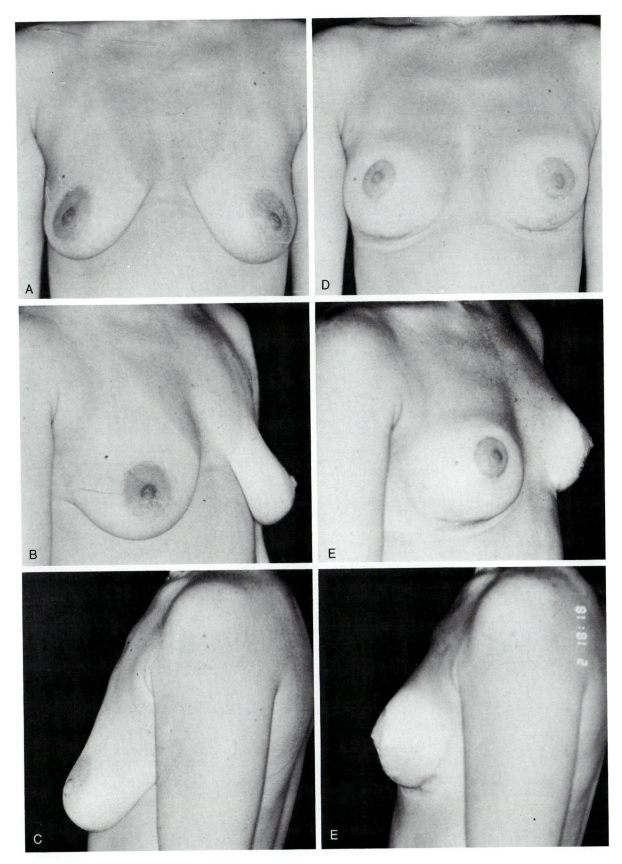

FIGURE 44–33
A to F, Preoperative views and postoperative views 2 months after surgery of the patient shown in Figure 44–32.

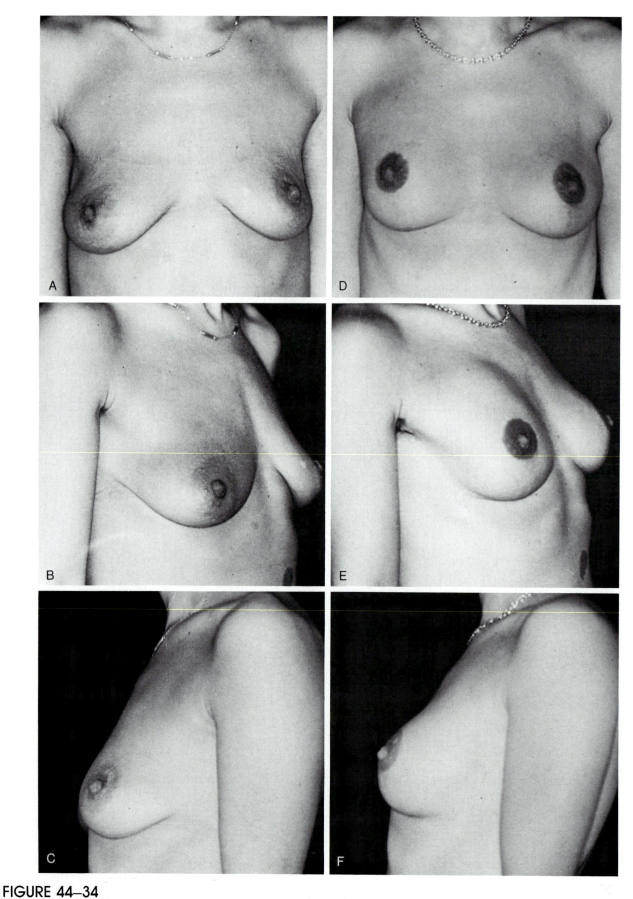

FIGURE 44–34

A to *F,* Preoperative and postoperative views of a patient with hypoplastic ptotic breasts who underwent a variation of the dermal brassiere technique, using an inferiorly based dermofat flap. The postoperative photographs were taken 3 years after surgery.

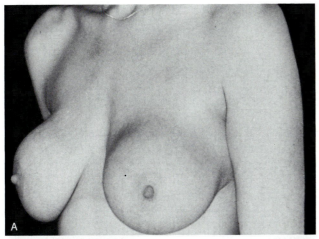
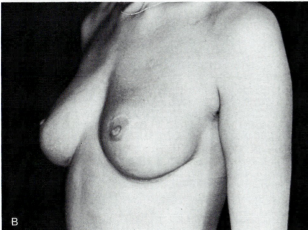

FIGURE 44–35

A and *B*, The insertion of a prosthesis alone is contraindicated whenever the areola is not situated above the level of the submammary sulcus. In this patient, who underwent surgery elsewhere, the submammary implants were removed, new implants were inserted subpectorally, and the author's technique of infra-areolar dermopexy with inferior protection by means of a dermofat flap was used.

References

Adams, W. M.: Free transplantation of the nipples and areolae. Surgery 15:186, 1944.

Arié, G.: Una nueva técnica de mastoplastia. Rev. Latinoamer. Cir. Plast. 3:23, 1957.

Ariyan, S.: Reduction mammaplasty with the nipple-areola carried on a single, narrow inferior pedicle. Ann. Plast. Surg. 5:167, 1978.

Aubert, V.: Hypertrophie mammaire de la puberté: Résection partielle restauratrice. Arch. Franco-Belg. Chir. 3:284, 1923.

Aufricht, G.: Mammaplasty for pendulous breasts: Empiric and geometric planning. Plast. Reconstr. Surg. 4:13, 1949.

Bames, H.O.: Reduction of massive breast hypertrophy. Plast. Reconstr. Surg. 3:560, 1948.

Baroudi, R., Lewis, J. R., Jr.: The augmentation reduction mammaplasty. Clin. Plast. Surg. 3:301, 1976.

Bartels, R. J., Strickland, D. M., Douglas, W. M.: A new mastopexy operation for mild or moderate breast ptosis. Plast. Reconstr. Surg. 57:687, 1976.

Bass, C. B.: Herniated areolar complex. Ann. Plast. Surg. 1:402, 1978.

Biesenberger, H.: Eine neue Methode der Mammaplastik. Zentralbl. Chir. 55:2382, 1928.

Bolivar, E.: Dermadipose and adenadipose flaps in mammoplasty. Aesthetic Plast. Surg. 7:101, 1983.

Bragadini, L. A., Bernardello, E., Margossian, J.: Nuevo enfoque para la reseccion glandular en las hipertrofias mamarias. Cir. Estet. 3:13, 1978.

Bricout, N., Groslieres, D., Servant, J. M., Banzet, P.: Plastie mammaire; La technique utilisée à Saint-Louis. Ann. Chir. Plast. Esthet. 33:7, 1988.

Burian, F.: *The Plastic Surgery Atlas.* New York, Macmillan, 1967, p. 18.

Bustos, R. A.: Mamoplastia reductora con cicatriz periareolar. Transactas VII Congreso Ibero-Latinoamericano de Cirugia Plastica, Cartagena de Indias. 1988.

Cardoso, A. D., Cardosa, A. D., Pessanha, M. C., Peralta, J. M.: Three dermal pedicles for nipple-areola complex: Movements in reduction of gigantomastia. Ann. Plast. Surg. 12:419, 1984.

Cerizola, M., Fossati, G. H.: Plastia mamaria reductora: Tecnica periareolar y periareolar ensanchada. Cir. Plast. Iberolatinoam. 15:57, 1989.

Clarkson, P.: Reduction and aesthetic surgery. In: Gillies, H., Millard, R. (ed.): *The Principles and Art of Plastic Surgery.* Vol. 2. Boston, Little, Brown, 1957, p. 412.

Clarkson, P., Jeffs, J.: Modern mammaplasty. Br. J. Plast. Surg. 20:297, 1967.

Climo, M. S., Alexander, J. E.: Intercostothelial circulation: Nipple survival in reduction mammaplasty in the absence of a dermal pedicle. Ann. Plast. Surg. 4:128, 1978.

Cloutier, A. M.: Volume reduction mammaplasty. Ann. Plast. Surg. 2:475, 1978.

Combescure, Ch., Lamarche, J. P.: Notre technique de Peixoto modifiée pour la correction des hypertrophies mammaires: Indications et resultats. Ann. Chir. Plast. Esthet. 32:30, 1987.

Cooper, A.: *On the Anatomy of the Breast.* London, Longmans, 1840.

Courtiss, E. H., Goldwyn, R. M.: Breast sensation before and after plastic surgery. Plast. Reconstr. Surg. 58:1, 1976.

Courtiss, E. H., Goldwyn, R. M.: Reduction mammaplasty by the inferior pedicle technique. Plast. Reconstr. Surg. 59:500, 1977.

Craig, R. D., Sykes, P. A.: Nipple sensitivity following reduction mammaplasty. Br. J. Plast. Surg. 23:165, 1970.

Czerny, V.: Plastischer ersatz der Brustdruese durch ein Lipom. Zentralbl. Chir. 27:72, 1895.

de Silva, G.: Mastopexy with dermal ribbon for supporting the breast and keeping it in shape. Plast. Reconstr. Surg. 34:403, 1964.

Dartigues, L.: Mammectomie totale et autogreffe libre aréolomamélonnaire: Mammectomie bilatérale esthétique. Bulletin de la Société Chirurgiens 20:739, 1928.

Dehner, J.: Mastopexie zur Beseitigung der Hängebrust. Münch. Med. Wochenschr. 36, 55:1878, 1908.

Dieffenbach, J. F.: *Die Operative Chirurgie.* Vol. 2. Leipzig, Brockhaus, 1848, p. 370.

Dufourmentel, C., Mouly, R.: Developpements recents de la plastie mammaire par la méthode oblique laterale. Ann. Chir. Plast. 10:227, 1965.

Edwards, E. A.: Surgical anatomy of the breast. In: Goldwyn, R. M. (ed.): *Reconstructive Surgery of the Breast.* Boston, Little, Brown, 1976, p. 37.

Elbaz, J. S., Verheecke, G.: La cicatrice en L dans les plasties mammaires. Ann. Chir. Plast. 17:283, 1972.

Elsahy, N. I.: The hexagonal technique for mastopexy and reduction mammoplasty. Aesthetic Plast. Surg. 6:107, 1982.

Ely, F. J.: The devil's incision mammoplasty. Aesthetic Plast. Surg. 7:159, 1983.

Erol, O. O., Spira, M.: Mastopexy technique for mild to moderate ptosis. Plast. Reconstr. Surg. 65:603, 1980.

Faivre, J., Carissimo, A.: La mastoplastica senza resezione cutanea: Una nuova tecnica per il trattamento delle ptosi e ipertrofie mammarie. Riv. Ital. Chir. Plast. 19:269, 1987.

Farina, R.: Reduction mammaplasty with free grafting of the nipple and areola. Br. J. Plast. Surg. 25:393, 1972.

Farina, M. A., Newby, B. G., Alani, H. M.: Innervation of the nipple-areola complex. Plast. Reconstr. Surg. 66:497, 1980.

Felicio, Y.: Mamoplastia de reduccion con solo una incision periareolar. Rev. Iber-latamer. Cir. Plast. 11:245, 1986.

Figallo, E.: Surgical treatment of mammary ptosis without hypertrophy. Plast. Reconstr. Surg. 60:189, 1977.

Fontano, A. M., Muti, E.: Appunti sulla mastoplastica riduttiva (Una tecnica di mastopessi). Riv. Ital. Chir. Plast. 14:139, 1982.

Galtier, M.: *Chirurgie Esthetique Mammaire.* Paris, G. Doin, 1955.

Garcia Padron, J.: Mammareduktionsplastik. Transacta der III Tagung der Vereinigung der Deutschen Plastischen Chirurgen, Köln, 1972, p. 85.

Garcia Padron, J.: Tecnica de sosten muscular en la mastoplastia de reduccion. III Congreso Ibero-Latinoamericano y V Congreso National de Cirugia Plastica, Valencia, 1980.

Gasperoni, C., Salgarello, M., Gargani, G.: Experience and technical refinements in the "donut" mastopexy with augmentation mammaplasty. Aesthetic Plast. Surg. 12:111, 1988.

Georgiade, N. G., Serafin, D., Morris, R., Georgiade, G.: Reduction mammaplasty utilizing an inferior pedicle nipple-areolar flap. Ann. Plast. Surg. 3:211, 1979.

Gillet, G.: Suspension mammaire par prothése sous-cutanée. Presse Med. 60:1325, 1952.

Gillies, H., Marino, H.: The periwinkleshell principle in the treatment of the small ptotic breast. Plast. Reconstr. Surg. 21:1, 1958.

Gillies, H., McIndoe, A.: The technique of mammaplasty in conditions of hypertrophy of the breast. Surg. Gynecol. Obstet. 68:658, 1939.

Girard, C.: Über mastoptose und mastopexie. Langenbecks Arch. Klin. Chir. 92:829, 1910.

Gläsmer, E.: Die Formfehler und die Plastischen Operationen der Weiblichen Brust. Stuttgart, Ferdinand Enke Verlag, 1930.

Göbell, R.: Über Autoplastische freie Fascien und Aponeurosentransplantation nach Martin Kirchner. Arch. Klin. Chir. 146:478, 1927.

Goulian, D., Jr.: Dermal mastopexy. Plast. Reconstr. Surg. 47:105, 1971.

Gruber, R. P., Jones, H. W., Jr.: The "donut" mastopexy: Indications and complications. Plast. Reconstr. Surg. 65:34, 1980.

Hauben, D. J.: The history of mammaplasty. Acta Chir. Plast. 27:71, 1985.

Hinderer, U. T.: Cirugia plastica mamaria de reduccion y aumento. Ann. Acad. Med. Quir. Esp. 50, 1965.

Hinderer, U. T.: Problemas psicologico y psiquiatrico en el paciente de cirugia plastica. Rev. Esp. Psicot. Anal. 4:31, 1968.

Hinderer, U. T.: Brustvergrösserungsplastik. Transacta der VIII Tagung der Deutschen Gesellschaft für Plastische u. Wiederherstellungschirurgie. Hamburg, 1969.

Hinderer, U. T.: Plastia mamaria modelante de dermopexia superficial y retromamaria. Atti Congresso della Societá Italiana di Chirurgia Plastica Ricostruttiva, Pisa, 1971.

Hinderer, U. T.: Plastia mamaria modelante de dermopexia superficial y retromamaria. Rev. Esp. Cir. Plast. 5:521, 1972a.

Hinderer, U. T.: Remodelling mammaplasty with superficial and retromammary dermopexy. Transacta der III Tagung der Vereinigung der Deutschen Plastischen Chirurgen, Köln, 1972, p. 93.

Hinderer, U. T.: Reduction and augmentation mammaplasty: Remodelling mammaplasty with superficial and retromammary mastopexy. Int. Micr. J. Aesthetic Plast. Surg., 1972.

Hinderer, U. T.: Further improvements in the technique of remodelling mammaplasty with superficial and retromammary dermopexy. Int. Micr. J. Aesthetic Plast. Surg., 1974.

Hinderer, U. T.: The dermolipectomy approach for augmentation mammaplasty. Clin. Plast. Surg. 2:359, 1975.

Hinderer, U. T.: The dermal brassiere mammaplasty. Clin. Plast. Surg. 3:349, 1976.

Hinderer, U. T.: Dermal brassiere technique. Transactions IX Instructional Course in Tokyo, International Society of Aesthetic Plastic Surgery, 1977, p. 31.

Hinderer, U. T.: Mammaplasty: The dermal brassiere technique. Aesthetic Plast. Surg. 2:1, 1978.

Hinderer, U. T.: Tratamiento de la hipoplasia mamaria combinado con lipodistrofia abdominal. Ann. Symp. Brazil, 1982.

Hinderer, U. T., del Rio, J. L.: Treatment of the postoperative inverted nipple with or without asymmetry of the areola. Aesthetic Plastic. Surg. 7:139, 1983.

Hinderer, U. T., del Rio, J. L.: Treatment of the hypertrophy and ptosis: dermal brassiere mammaplasty. In: Georgiade, N. G. (ed.): Aesthetic Breast Surgery. Baltimore, Williams & Wilkins, 1983, p. 306.

Hinderer, U. T.: Plastias mamarias de dermopexia. In: Coiffman, F. (ed.): Cirugia Plastica, Reconstructiva y Estetica. Vol. 2. Barcelona, Salvat, 1984, p. 1003.

Hinderer, U. T., del Rio, J. L.: An unusual case of gigantomasty. Aesthetic Plast. Surg. 9:91, 1985.

Hinderer, U. T.: Mammaplasty technique in the treatment of the ptotic breast with hypertrophy, of average size or with hypoplasia. In: Gonzalez-Ulloa, M., Meyer, R., Smith, J. W., Zaoli, G.

(eds.): Aesthetic Plastic Surgery. Vol. 4, Padova, P. Piccin Nuova Libraria, St. Louis, C. V. Mosby, 1988.

Ho, L. C. Y.: The small ptotic breast: Reposition autoaugmentation mammaplasty. Br. J. Plast. Surg. 39:76, 1986.

Höhler, H.: Breast augmentation: The axillary approach. Br. J. Plast. Surg. 26:373, 1973.

Holländer, E.: Die Operation der Mammahypertrophie und der Hängebrust. Dtsch. Med. Wochenschr. 41:1400, 1924.

Hurst, L. N., Evans, H. B., Murray, K. A.: Inferior flap reduction mammaplasty with pedicled nipple. Ann. Plast. Surg. 10:483, 1983.

Johnson, G. W.: Central core reduction mammoplasties and marlex suspension of breast tissue. Aesthetic Plast. Surg. 5:77, 1981.

Joseph, J.: Zur Operation der hypertrophischen Hängebrust. Dtsche Med. Wochenschr. 51:1103, 1925.

Jost, G., Meresse, B.: Choix d'une incision dans les mammaplasties. Ann. Chir. Plast. 19:265, 1974.

Jurado, J.: Plasticas mamarias baseadas em retalho dermico vertical monopediculado. Transactions XIII Congresso Brasileiro de Cirurgia Plastica, Porto Alegre, 1976, p. 29.

Kohn, F., Dalrymple, J.: Plastic reconstruction of the enlarged breast: Report of a new technique. Br. J. Plast. Surg. 20:184, 1967.

Kraske, H.: Die Operation der atrophischen und hypertrophischen Hängebrust. Münch. Med. Wochenschr. 70:672, 1923.

Laing, E.: Un metodo de transplante libre de pezon para la mamoplastia de reduccion. Comunicacion al III Congreso Nacional de Cirugia Plastica, Valencia, 1972.

Lalardrie, J. P., Morel-Fatio, D.: Adjustment after subcutaneous mastectomy. In: Hueston, J. T. (ed.): Transactions of the Fifth International Congress of Plastic and Reconstructive Surgery. Melbourne, Butterworth, 1971, p. 1197.

Lalardrie, J. P.: Reduction mammaplasty for hypertrophy with ptosis. Transact. III Tagung der Vereinigung der Deutschen Plastischen Chirurgen. Koln, 1972, p. 105.

Lalardrie, J. P., Jouglard, J. P.: Chirurgie Plastique du Sein. Paris, Masson, 1974.

Lassus, C.: New refinements in vertical mammaplasty. Chir. Plast. 6:81, 1981.

Lassus, C.: Breast reduction: Evolution of a technique—a single vertical scar. Aesthetic Plast. Surg. 11:107, 1987.

Lerner, S., Tittiranonda, T., Aiache, A. E.: Mastopexy. In: Hinderer, U. (ed.): Abstract Book, First International Congress, International Society of Aesthetic Plastic Surgery. Rio de Janeiro, February 6–11, 1972. Publicaciones Controladas S.A., 1972, p. 30.

Letterman, G., Schurter, M.: Will Durston's mammaplasty. Plast. Reconstr. Surg. 53:48, 1974.

Lewis, G. K.: A method of mastopexy with fascia lata transplants. J. Int. Coll. Surg. 26:346, 1956.

Lewis, J. R., Jr.: Classification and surgical correction of ptosis of the breasts. In: Masters, F. W., Lewis, J. R., Jr. (eds.): Symposium on Aesthetic Surgery of the Face, Eyelid, and Breast. Vol. 4. St. Louis, C. V. Mosby, 1972, 4, p. 183.

Lewis, J. R., Jr.: Reduction mammoplasty: Borrowing the good points of many techniques. Aesthetic Plast. Surg. 1:43, 1976.

Lewis, J. R., Jr.: Mammary ptosis. In: Georgiade, N. G. (ed.): Aesthetic Breast Surgery. Baltimore, Williams & Wilkins, 1983, p. 130.

Lexer, E.: Sitzungsbericht der naturwissenschaftlichen. Medizinischen Gesellschaft Jena. Münch. Med. Wochenschr. 1912, p. 49.

Lexer, E.: Correccion de los pechos pendulos (mastoptose) por medio de la implantacion de grasa. San Sebastian Guipuzcoa Medica 63:213, 1921.

Longacre, J. J., DeStefano, G. A., Holmstrad, K.: Breast reconstruction with local derma and fat pedicle flaps. Plast. Reconstr. Surg. 24:563, 1959.

Lotsch, F.: Über Hängebrustplastik. Zentralbl. Chir. 34:32, 1923.

Maillard, G. F.: A Z-mammaplasty with minimal scarring. Plast. Reconstr. Surg. 77:66, 1986.

Maliniac, J. W.: Deformidades mamarias y su tratamiento. Barcelona, Labor, 1952.

Marc, H.: La plastique mammaire par la méthode oblique. Rev. Port. Obstet. 5:363, 1952.

Marchac, D., de Olarte, G.: Reduction mammaplasty and correction of ptosis with a short inframammary scar. Plast. Reconstr. Surg. 69:45, 1982.

Marino, H.: A review of new trends in corrective mammaplasty. In:

Broadbent, T. R.: Transactions of the Third International Congress of Plastic Surgery. Washington, D.C., October 1963. International Congress Series No. 66, Excerpta Medica Foundation, Amsterdam, 1963, p. 66.

Martins, L. C.: Hipertrofias mamarias. Rev. Fac. Med. Braganca. 1:1, 1979.

McKissock, P. K.: Reduction mammaplasty with a vertical dermal flap. Plast. Reconstr. Surg. 49:245, 1972.

Meyer, R., Martinoni, G.: Mastoplastica di riduzione. In Atti XXI Congresso Naxionale della Societa Italiana di Chirurgia Plastica Ricostruttiva, 1971.

Meyer, R., Kesselring, U. K.: Reduction mammaplasty with an L-shaped suture line. Reconstr. Plast. Surg. 55:139, 1975.

Mir y Mir, L.: Mammaplasty (Film). In: Wallace, A. B. (ed.): Transactions of the International Society of Plastic Surgeons, Second Congress, London, 1959. Edinburgh, E. & S. Livingstone, 1960.

Mir y Mir, L., Brualla Planes, A., Caragol, S.: The value of preoperative thermography in patients undergoing reduction mammaplasty and mastopexy. Ann. Plast. Surg. 3:505, 1979.

Mitz, V., Lassau, J. P.: Etude des rapports entre les vascularisations arterielles glandulaire et cutanee du sein. Arch. Anat. Pathol. 21:365, 1973.

Morestin, H.: De l'ablation esthetique des tumeurs du sein. Paris Bull. Soc. Chir. 29:561, 1903.

O'Keefe, P. J.: Draftmanship for reduction mammaplasty. Ann. Plast. Surg. 10:467, 1983.

Olivari, N.: Probleme der subcutanen Mastektomie aus plastischchirurgischer Sicht. Transacta der III Tagung der Vereinigung der Deutschen Plastischen Chirurgen, Köln, 1972, p. 75.

Peixoto, G.: Reduction mammaplasty: A personal technique. Plast. Reconstr. Surg. 65:217, 1980.

Peled, I., Zagher, U., Wexler, M. R.: Purse-string suture for reduction and closure of skin defects. Ann. Plast. Surg. 14:465, 1985.

Penn, J.: Breast reduction. Br. J. Plast. Surg. 7:357, 1955.

Penn, J.: Breast reduction: In: Wallace, A. B. (ed.): Transactions of the International Society of Plastic Surgeons, Second Congress, London, 1959. Edinburgh, E. & S. Livingstone, 1960, p. 502.

Pers, M., Bretteville-Jensen, G.: Reduction mammaplasty based on vertical vascular bipedicle and "tennis-ball" assembly. Scand. J. Plast. Reconstr. Surg. 6:61, 1972.

Piotti, F.: Considerazioni sulla mastoplastica secondo Pitanguy. Minerva Chir. 1, 1970.

Piotti, F.: Sulla mastoplastica. Minerva Chir. 27:989, 1972.

Piotti, F.: Cause di insuccesso in chirurgia estetica: Mastoplastiche. Riv. Ital. Chir. Plast. 7:447, 1975.

Pitanguy, I.: Breast hypertrophy. In: Wallace, A. B. (ed.): Transactions of the International Society of Plastic Surgeons, Second Congress, London, 1959. Edinburgh, E. & S. Livingstone, 1960, p. 509.

Pitanguy, I.: Mamaplastias: Estudo de 234 casos consecutivos e apresentacoa de tecnica pessoal. Rev. Bras. Cir. October 1961.

Planas, J.: Introduction of breast implants through the abdominal route. Plast. Reconstr. Surg. 57:434, 1973.

Prudente, A.: *Contribucao ao Estudo da Plastica mamaria. Cirurgia Esthetica dos Seios.* Sao Paulo Publicitas, 1936.

Puckett, C. L., Meyer, V. H., Reinisch, J. F.: Crescent mastopexy and augmentation. Plast. Reconstr. Surg. 75:533, 1985.

Ragnell, A.: *Operative correction of hypertrophy and ptosis of the female breast.* Stockholm, I Haeggstroms Boktrycheri, 1946.

Ramirez, M. A.: Correccion de la ptosis mammaria con colgajos cruzados. In: Coiffman, F. (ed.): *Texto de Cirugia Plastica, Reconstructiva y Estetica.* Vol. 2. Barcelona, Salvat Editores, S.A., 1986, p. 1009.

Ramirez, M. A.: Correccion de la macromastia por la tecnica del colgajo tripediculado. In: Coiffman, F. (ed.): *Texto de Cirugia Plastica, Reconstructiva y Estetica.* Vol. 2. Barcelona, Salvat Editores, S.A., 1986, p. 996.

Rees, T. D., Aston, S. J.: The tuberous breast. Clin. Plast. Surg. 3:339, 1976.

Regnault, P.: The hypoplastic and ptotic breast: Combined operation and prosthetic augmentation. Plast. Reconstr. Surg. 37:31, 1966.

Regnault, P.: Reduction mammaplasty by the B technique. Plast. Reconstr. Surg. 53:19, 1974.

Regnault, P.: Reduction mammaplasty by the B technique. In: Goldwyn, R. M. (ed.): *Plastic and Reconstructive Surgery of the Breast.* Boston, Little, Brown, 1976, p. 269.

Regnault, P., Daniel, R. K.: Breast ptosis. In: Regnault, P., Daniel, R. K. (eds.): *Aesthetic Plastic Surgery.* Boston, Little, Brown, 1984, p. 539.

Reich, J.: The advantages of a lower central breast segment in reduction mammaplasty. Aesthetic Plast. Surg. 8:47, 1979.

Reichert, J.: Wiederherstellung der Brustform nach Drusenkorperextirpation wegen Mastopathia cystica unter modifizierter Anwendung der Methode Strömbeck. Transacta der III Tagung der Vereinigung der Deutschen Plastischen Chirurgen, Köln, 1972, p. 79.

Ribeiro, L.: A new technique for reduction mammaplasty. Plast. Reconstr. Surg. 55:330, 1975.

Ribeiro, L. Backer, E.: Mastoplastia con pediculo de seguridad. Rev. Esp. Cir. Plast. 6:223, 1973.

Robbins, T. H.: A reduction mammaplasty with the areola-nipple based on an inferior dermal pedicle. Plast. Reconstr. Surg. 59:64, 1977.

Robertson, D. C.: Reduction mammaplasty using a large inferior flap. Transactions of the III International Congress of Plastic Surgeons, Washington, D.C., Excerpta Medica, 1963, p. 81.

Saad, M. N.: An extended circumareolar incision for breast augmentation and gynecomastia. Aesthetic Plast. Surg. 7:127, 1983.

Salmon, M.: *Les Artéres de la Peau.* Paris, Masson, 1936.

Schrudde, J.: Ein Beitrag zur Rekonstruktion der weiblichen Brust. Transact. III Tagung der Vereinigung der Deutschen Plastischen Chirurgen. Koln, 1972, p. 125.

Skoog, T.: A technique of breast reduction: Transposition of the nipple on a cutaneous vascular pedicle. Acta. Chir. Scand. 126:1, 1963.

Stark, R.: A procedure for mammary reduction and mastopexy: Summary of 100 personally performed operations. Aesthetic Plast. Surg. 1:145, 1977.

Stark, R.: Experience with the modified Ragnell mammaplasty. Scand. J. Plast. Reconstr. Surg. 14:129, 1980.

Strömbeck, J. O.: Mammaplasty: Report of a new technique based on the two pedicle procedure. Br. J. Plast. Surg. 13:79, 1960.

Strömbeck, J. O.: Reduction mammaplasty. In: Gibson, T. (ed.): *Modern Trends in Plastic Surgery*, 1964, p. 237.

Tafalla Pena, M., Lorda Barraguer, E., Rodes Perez, A.: Mastoplastia reductiva: Conceptos personales. Rev. Iberolatinoamer. Cir. Plast. 14:231, 1988.

Tamerin, J. A.: The Lexer-Kraske Mammaplasty: A reaffirmation. Plast. Reconstr. Surg. 31:442, 1963.

Teimourian, B., Adham, M. N.: Surgical correction of the tuberous breast. Ann. Plast. Surg. 10:190, 1983.

Thomas, T. G.: On the removal of benign tumors of the mamma without mutilation of the organ. New York M. & Obstet. Rev., April 1882, p. 337.

Thorek, M.: Possibilities in reconstruction of the human form. New York M. J. & Rec. 116:572, 1922.

Trabanino, R.: The spiral, or string, dissection for "de-epithelization" in reduction mammaplasty. Plast. Reconstr. Surg. 62:806, 1978.

Vecchione, T. R.: A method for recontouring the domend nipple. Plast. Reconstr. Surg. 57:30, 1976.

Villandre: Le traitement chirurgical de prolapsus mammaire. Cited by Dartigues, L.: Archives Franco-Belges de Chirurgie 28:325, 1925.

Vogt, T.: Reduction mammoplasty: Vogt technique. In Georgiade, N. G. (ed.): *Aesthetic Breast Surgery.* Baltimore, Williams & Wilkins, 1983, p. 271.

Vogt, T.: Controversies in plastic surgery: Suction-assisted lipectomy (SAL) and the hCG (human chorionic gonadotropin) protocol for obesity treatment. Aesthetic Plast. Surg. 11:131, 1987.

Weiner, D. L., Aiache, A. E., Siver, L., Tittiranonda, T.: A single dermal pedicle for nipple transposition in subcutaneous mastectomy, reduction mammaplasty or mastopexy. Plast. Reconstr. Surg. 51:115, 1973.

Weitzel, D., Bassler, R.: Beiträge zur Angioarchitektur der weiblichen Brustdrüse. Z. Anat. Entwicklungsgesch. 133:73, 1971.

Williams, J. E.: Augmentation mammoplasty-Inframammary approach. In: Georgiade, N. C. (ed.): *Reconstructive Breast Surgery.* St. Louis, C. V. Mosby, 1976, p. 62.

Wise, R. J.: A preliminary report on a method of planning the mammaplasty. Plast. Reconstr. Surg. 17:367, 1956.

NIPPLE-AREOLA ANOMALIES

45

Bahman Teimourian
Mehdi N. Adham

Congenital Anomalies of the Nipple and Areola

Social progress has made the breast physiologically dispensable, with the milk bottle and baby food products becoming breast substitutes. Women's liberation, sexual liberalism, and body consciousness have changed the social perspective of the breast and its function. As a result, during the past 25 years, cosmetic breast surgery has gained popularity, and a finer and more ideal-looking breast has become desirable.

In the context of breast surgery, the finer points that distinguish an ideal cosmetic result focus on the areola and, to some extent, the nipple. Restoration of an adequate projected nipple, together with an areola, has become an objective in cosmetic surgery.

ANATOMY

The nipple and the areola are located at the fourth intercostal space, slightly lateral to the midclavicular line, with the nipple facing slightly outward and downward. Structurally, the breast is composed of 5 to 25 irregular lobes that terminate as lactiferous ducts in the nipple (Bloom and Fawcett, 1975). The conical nipple is surrounded by the pigmented areola. The nipple and areola vary in size, shape, and color from individual to individual. The average sizes are 1 cm long and 1 cm in diameter for the nipple (Mosley and Miller, 1952; Regnault, 1975), and 3 cm in diameter for the areola (Snyder et al., 1972). The skin of both of these structures is glabrous and contains glands that open either on the surface or into the galactophores (Perkins and Miller, 1926). Both the sebaceous glands and the galactophores contain melanocytes (Montagna and MacPherson, 1974). The epidermis of the nipple and areola contains long dermal papillae that bring the capillary blood network close to the skin surface, giving a pink coloration to the area in fair-skinned individuals (Bloom and Fawcett, 1975). The skin of the areola also contains Montgomery's glands. The lactiferous ducts of the nipple are in close association with smooth muscle and an abundant amount of elastic fibrous tissue. The smooth circular muscle of the nipple runs parallel to the ducts. The areola, like the nipple, contains circular and radial smooth muscle fibers (Snyder et al., 1972) (see Fig. 45-4). With the use of the microscope, Schwager et al. (1974) showed that the dense connective tissue beneath the normal nipple is greater than that seen in the surrounding subareolar area. By means of dissection, Marcus (1934) and Maliniac (1943) showed that the blood supply of the nipple and areola arises from the internal lateral thoracic and intercostal arteries, which form a deep plexus around the base of the nipple and areola in three different patterns (Fig. 45-1). From these plexes, smaller arterioles supply the nipple and areola.

There are also some direct blood vessels from the internal mammary artery that penetrate through the entire thickness of the breast to terminate in the nipple (Serafin, 1976).

The classic work of Cooper (1840) revealed that the nipple and areola received sensory innervation from the anterior cutaneous nerves of the third, fourth, and fifth intercostal nerves and from branches of the lateral cutaneous nerves of the fourth, fifth, and occasionally the third intercostal nerves (Serafin, 1979) (Fig. 45-2). The anterior branch of the lateral rami of the fourth intercostal nerve was discovered by Sir Ashley Cooper (1840) to be a special nerve to the nipple. Later, Craig and Sykes (1970), Courtiss and Goldwyn (1976), and Edwards (1976) emphasized the importance of the role of the fourth intercostal nerve in the innervation of the nipple (Fig. 45-3). The smooth muscle of the nipple and areola also received sympathetic innervation involved in the nipple erection.

From this description of the nerve and blood supply to the nipple and areola, it is evident that the safest plane for surgery of the nipple with minimal sequelae is the superficial superior-inferior plane.

ANOMALIES OF THE NIPPLE

Congenital anomalies of the nipple are classified as shown in Table 45-1.

Polythelia

Polythelia, or the presence of supernumerary nipples, has been recognized since antiquity, but the anomaly was not studied scientifically until the last century (Edwards, 1976; Williams, 1894). Deaver and McFarland

607

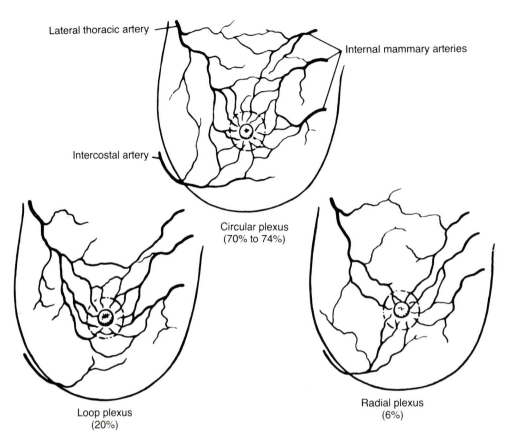

Lateral thoracic artery

Internal mammary arteries

Intercostal artery

Circular plexus
(70% to 74%)

Loop plexus
(20%)

Radial plexus
(6%)

FIGURE 45–1
The blood supply of the nipple and areola with various patterns of periareolar plexus was originally described by Maliniac (1934). (Reproduced with permission from Serafin, D.: Anatomy of the breast. In: Georgiade, N. (ed.): *Reconstructive Breast Surgery.* St. Louis, C. V. Mosby, 1976.)

FIGURE 45–2
Innervation of the breast. (Reproduced with permission from Serafin, D.: Surgical anatomy of the breast. In: Georgiade, N. (ed.): *Breast Reconstruction Following Mastectomy.* St. Louis, C. V. Mosby, 1979.)

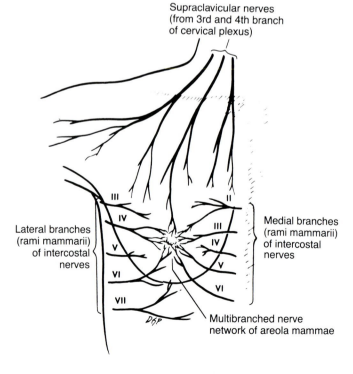

Supraclavicular nerves
(from 3rd and 4th branch
of cervical plexus)

Lateral branches
(rami mammarii)
of intercostal
nerves

Medial branches
(rami mammarii)
of intercostal
nerves

Multibranched nerve
network of areola mammae

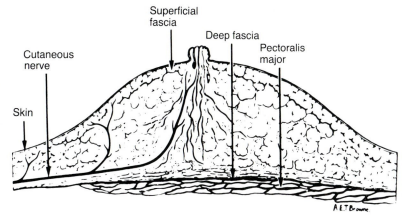

FIGURE 45–3

The anterior branch of the lateral cutaneous branch of the fourth intercostal nerve innervating the nipple. (From Craig, R. D. P., Sykes, P. A.: Nipple sensitivity following reduction mammoplasty. Br. J. Plast. Surg. 23:165, 1970.)

(1917) studied polythelia extensively and summarized the reported cases to that date (Table 45–2). Later, De Cholnoky (1939) extended that study, reporting new cases.

Polythelia, one of the most common congenital anomalies of the nipple, and having a racial variation, occurs in about 5% of the population (Castano, 1969). It is more common in males than in females and occurs more frequently on the left side of the body than on the right. In males, it is sometimes associated with gynecomastia. A supernumerary nipple may appear anywhere along the milk line, either alone or in association with areolar and mammary glandular tissue. Approximately 95% of such nipples occur in the thoracic region, 90% of these having an inframammary location. Supernumerary nipples can also develop in ectopic regions (De Cholnoky, 1939).

Surgical treatment of polythelia depends on the circumstances of the patient. For female patients, who may eventually want to breast-feed a baby, supernumerary nipples located on the breast should be saved, because these nipples may be associated with glandular tissue in the breast. However, extramammary supernumerary nipples can be excised without difficulty, together with any glandular tissue that accompanies them. The best time for complete excision of such nipples is during pregnancy, when the glandular tissue undergoes hyperplasia and becomes more easily palpable.

In female patients who are not interested in breastfeeding, or with males, both intramammary and extramammary supernumerary nipples can be excised with safety at any age.

TABLE 45–1
Classification of Nipple Deformity

Polythelia
Athelia
Flat
Depressed
Inverted
Bifid
Fissured
Imperforate
Hypertrophy

TABLE 45–2
Polythelia

Intra-areolar polythelia
Bilateral
Unilateral
Extra-areolar polythelia
Unilateral
With an areola about each nipple
Without an areola about the supernumerary nipple
Bilateral
With an areola about each nipple
Without an areola about one or all of the supernumerary nipples
Intra- and extra-areolar polythelia
Ectopic

Athelia

Athelia, or the absence of nipples, is a rare anomaly. Athelia is usually, but not always, associated with amastia, an exceedingly rare congenital malformation. In cases of athelia associated with an absence of breast tissue, the pectoral muscle may also be deficient (Fodor and Khoury, 1980).

Trier (1965) reported complete breast absence and reviewed 43 cases in the literature. He categorized the cases into three groups: (1) bilateral absence of breast with congenital ectodermal defect (7 cases); (2) unilateral absence (20 cases); and (3) bilateral absence of the breast (16 cases) with variable associated defects. Later, Tawill and Najjar (1968), Goldenring and Crelin (1961), Kowlessar and Orti (1968), Nelson and Cooper (1982), and Hosokawa et al. (1987) all reported cases with variable degrees of athelia.

Surgical treatmeent of athelia after correction of asymmetry or mound reconstruction can be dealt with in the same way as postmastectomy nipple reconstruction (Gruber, 1979; Muruci et al., 1978), that is, by using a composite graft from the other nipple or by using multiple local flaps in a variety of ways to give nipple projection (Hartrampf and Culbertson, 1984; Cronin et al., 1988). A modification of our technique for correction of an inverted nipple has been used for nipple reconstruction.

Flat, Depressed, and Inverted Nipple

Birkett (1850) discussed the inverted nipple from the point of view of breast-feeding, without consideration for the cause of the anomaly. He recommended avoidance of pressure on the nipple during pregnancy and the use of a special apparatus for eversion of the nipple. He also recommended the technique of using an older child to suck on the breast to evert the nipple. Bryant (1887) devoted a chapter in his book *Diseases of the Breast* to morbid conditions of the nipples. In discussing the acquired inverted nipple, he emphasized that various conditions, either malignant or benign, could give rise to the anomaly. He also recognized that the inverted nipple can be a congenital condition but did not suggest any methods of treatment. Surgical approaches to the inverted nipple started with Kehrer (1879) and, since that time, have undergone many changes.

Etiology and Histology

Inverted nipples are more common unilaterally than bilaterally and, as pointed out by Bryant (1887), may be congenital or acquired. Their classification is shown in Table 45–3.

Although various surgical techniques have been introduced for the correction of the anomaly during the last 100 years, there is no accurate record of its incidence or prevalence. Schwager et al. (1974) reported an incidence of 1 in 57 in an examination of 339 breast specimens, of which 144 were postmortem and the rest mastectomy specimens.

Hereditary factors may play a part in congenital nipple inversion. Skoog (1965) reported a 50% familial tendency among cases he studied. LaMont (1973) reported a set of identical twins with inverted nipples. Hara et al. (1974) described a woman with a chromosome complement of 48,XXXX who had bilateral inverted nipples. Goodman et al. (1979) found 16 members of one family affected with inverted nipples (15 females and 1 male), but the mode of inheritance was not established.

Developmentally, the inverted nipple is believed to be caused by the arrest of growth of the ductal system at an early stage in development (James, 1981). This creates tension on the nipple, the anomaly becoming

more apparent with subcutaneous accumulation of fat. Basch (1893) discovered that the inverted nipple lacked the smooth muscle fibers that grow at a later stage from the areola. Therefore, in the case of nipple inversion, the nipple and areola are somewhat dissociated, being joined only by a soft neck. Normally, when the nipple and areola contract, the interlocking of the radial and circular fibers makes the nipple hard and erect. The absence of musculature in the nipple makes the areolar contraction independent of the nipple, and the outcome of the contraction depends on the position of the nipple. As a result of the hypoplastic development of the ductal system and fibrous bands that prevent eversion of the nipple, the areolar contraction makes the invagination even deeper (Fig. 45–4). In mild cases, pregnancy (LaMont, 1973) and obesity with subcutaneous fat accumulation (Robbins, 1974) cause inversion. In the past, infection was one of the major causes of acquired nipple inversion. Ductal mastitis with fibrous formation and scar retraction interferes with normal development and causes nipple retraction.

Inversion of the nipple that is associated with malignancy has different implications, which are outside the purview of this discussion. Xeromammography can be helpful in questionable cases of inverted nipple.

Surgical procedures of the breast also can cause nipple inversion (Goldwyn, 1972; Gupta, 1965). Reduction mammaplasty in which a pedicle dermal flap is used has produced nipple inversion as a result of the associated tension and scar retraction.

Histologically, the inverted nipple is very different from the normal nipple. Schwager and his associates (1974) established by means of microscopic study that both inverted and normal nipples have normal subareolar tissue but that the dense fibrous tissue beneath the inverted nipple has the same depth as the surrounding subareolar region, whereas the thickness under the normal nipple has almost twice the depth of the subareolar region. The maximum thickness of this fibrous connective tissue in the normal nipple is about 0.8 cm, whereas in the inverted nipple it is about 0.4 to 0.6 cm.

Phases of Surgical Correction of the Inverted Nipple

To correct the inverted nipple, the surgical technique should interrupt all fibrous and ductal systems that hold the nipple down and should provide good body contour, structural stability, and bulk to the nipple to prevent the inversion. Techniques for correcting the inverted nipple have gone through three different phases. The choice of operation today depends on the patient's objective. If the patient wants to breast-feed, and if all available nonsurgical therapies (Gangal and Gangal, 1978; Otte, 1975) have failed, any of the operations in the second phase might be appropriate. If the patient is not interested in breast-feeding, any operation in the third phase might be used.

FIRST PHASE: AREOLAR SKIN SHORTENING OR AREOLAR MYOTOMY

Kehrer (1888) classified the different forms of inverted nipple and as early as 1873 published his technique for

TABLE 45–3
The Principal Causes of Inverted Nipple

Congenital
Depressed
Invaginated
Acquired
Macromastia
Ductal mastitis
Carcinoma
Breast surgery
Mastopexy
Reduction mammoplasty
Other breast surgery
Pregnancy

From Schwager, R. G., Smith, J. W., Gray, G. F., et al.: Inversion of the human female nipple, with a simple method of treatment. Plast. Reconstr. Surg. 54:564, 1974.

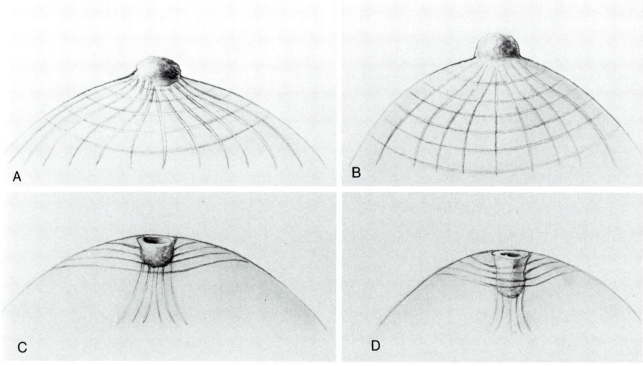

FIGURE 45–4

Contraction of the normal and inverted nipple and areola. *A,* Normal nipple and areola in the relaxed state. *B,* Contraction of the radial and circular muscle with projection of the complex. *C,* Inverted nipple and areola in the relaxed state. *D,* Contraction of the circular muscle, deepening the inversion, with narrowing of the neck, prevents eversion. If the nipple was everted before contraction, it may stay out temporarily.

correcting the anomaly. His operation was used for patients in which the nipple is present but located in a cavity and not accessible to a nursing baby. His operation required the excision of a ring of skin or two crescent-shaped pieces of skin from the surrounding nipple in a manner such that when healed, the depression around the nipple would flatten out, causing the nipple to improve. This technique, not applicable to stunted or malformed nipples, represented the first phase of operations for nipple inversion or, more correctly, for depressed or umbilicated nipple. Later Herman (1889), Williams (1894), and Deaver and McFarland (1917) described the same technique.

A better surgical approach to the correction of the inverted nipple required a scientific understanding of the anomaly. Basch (1893), describing in some detail the embryology and anatomy of deformed nipples, related the cause of inversion to arrest at an earlier stage. He also pointed out that the muscle fibers are absent in the inverted nipple. Therefore, not only is the nipple inverted, but during an areolar contraction, the development of a tight neck prevents the nipple from appearing on the surface. He recommended a double subcutaneous myotomy of the areolar muscle with stretching of the nipple or suture fixation in the everted position. This technique, however, like others of the same period, was applicable to the depressed nipple but not to the truly inverted nipple.

SECOND PHASE: CREATION OF A TIGHT NIPPLE NECK WITHOUT DISTURBANCE OF THE DUCTAL SYSTEM

The next phase of surgical correction of the inverted nipple involved creating a tight neck for the nipple that permanently prevented its retraction and inversion. This approach was the first really appropriate technique for correction of the inverted nipple.

Axford (1889), with the help of Norcom, developed a procedure for this anomaly referred to as mamilliplasty. He excised three 2.5-inch elliptical pieces of skin radially about 0.5 inch from the apex of the nipple. Then, using a catgut purse-string suture in the fascia around the nipple, he created a tight neck. The closure of the epithelialized area also provided additional support for the inverted nipple. This patient was able to breast-feed without difficulty. D'Assumpção and Rosa (1977), Dufourmentel (1950), Schwager et al. (1974), and Skoog (1953, 1965) all reported similar techniques. D'Assumpção (1977) used a quadrilateral skin incision without using the purse-string suture; in addition, he cut the ducts and fibrous bands. Hayes (1980) used the D'Assumpção technique along with augmentation mammaplasty. In the same year, Teimourian and Adham (1980) reported the use of their technique for simultaneous correction of inverted nipple and hypoplastic breast.

Sellheim (1917) introduced a new technique for correction of inverted nipples that remained the procedure of choice for a long period of time. He everted the nipple and made a circular skin incision at its base until the nipple was freed. To prevent its reinversion, he cut several small triangular pieces of skin to create a neck for the nipple. Then he sutured the base of the nipple to the areola. He also performed areolar myotomy. Although this technique was successful in most cases, it did have shortcomings. One was that the effect of narrowing the base of the nipple by removing the triangular pieces of skin was counteracted when the new base was sutured to the outer old areolar skin without modification of its circumference. When the sutures were removed, the nipple gradually retracted because of the continuous peripheral stretching of the scars (Skoog, 1953). To prevent this problem, surgeons designed a variety of operations.

Skoog (1953) described an operation in which he everted the nipple and made a circular incision around its base. Then skin was excised from the areola and the side of·the nipple so as to create two smaller matched circles, which created a tight neck. His operation is based on the same principle as that of Axford (1889). If the inner circle is turned one-eighth of the circumference of the base of the nipple, the de-epithelialized area turns into four quadrilateral areas. Axford, in contrast, used three elliptical skin incisions. Skoog's operation was successful in lactating females and remains the procedure of choice in such women.

Spina (1957) pointed out the advantages of Sellheim's procedure, especially with respect to reducing the size of the areola Spina used a doughnut-shaped piece from the labia to replace or reconstruct an areola. This produced a satisfactory result; however, labial skin has the disadvantage of undergoing pigmentation when exposed to the sun. The better choice if needed would be skin from the inner thigh.

Grodsky (1937) discussed the treatment of nipple deformities with special emphasis on the flat nipple. He described Dieffenbach's technique and also used two techniques of his own for correction. He used four de-epithelialized triangles with the base on the nipple margin and the apex toward the areola. By closing these areas, he produced some nipple projection. This particular form of triangular skin incision was used later by Elsahy (1977) and by Teimourian and Adham (1980) as part of their procedures.

LaMont (1973) used a circumareolar skin incision to free the adhesive bands that kept the nipple in the inverted position. Then a purse-string suture was used to keep the nipple in its new position.

Wolfort (1979) reported a technique for correction of inverted nipples that allows for the preservation of function. This method is a reverse of the V-Y technique of Dieffenbach for the flat nipple (Grodsky, 1937). Wolfort et al. freed the nipple through four triangular skin flaps, each with its apex toward the nipple. Then the muscular ring around the nipple neck was tightened by excising the four pieces of muscle. To add projection, they closed the skin flaps in a V-Y manner (Fig. 45–5). This operation requires extensive skin incision, and it

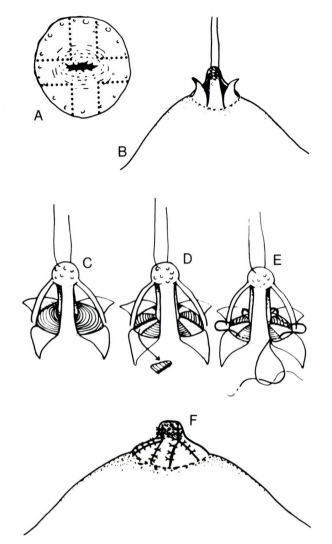

FIGURE 45–5

Wolfort's technique (1978). *A,* Circumferentially based triangles are outlined on each quadrant of the areola. *B,* The triangular flaps as outlined are elevated. *C,* The areolomuscular tissue surrounding the nipple base is exposed through the triangular "windows," and myotomy incisions are designed. *D,* Radial myotomies extend from the nipple base to the areolocutaneous margins. The nipple base and major ducts are not divided. *E,* A purse-string suture gathers the muscle bundles at the nipple base for nipple support. *F,* The nipple is advanced by closing the 4 triangular flaps with the V-Y procedure. (From Wolfort, E. G., Marshall, K. A., Cochran, T. C.: Correction of the inverted nipple. Ann. Plast. Surg. 1:294, 1978.)

seems doubtful that it is any better than the technique of Skoog (Letterman and Schurter, 1967).

Hauben and Mahler (1988) described another technique. It involved outward traction of the nipple with suture, then circumferential incision around the base of the nipple and undermining beneath the areola to free the nipple. After the creation of a 1- to 2-cm nipple base, a purse-string suture was used around the new base. The new defect in the nipple base was covered with freed areolar tissue. The dog-ears were corrected in the four quadrants (Fig. 45–6A to C).

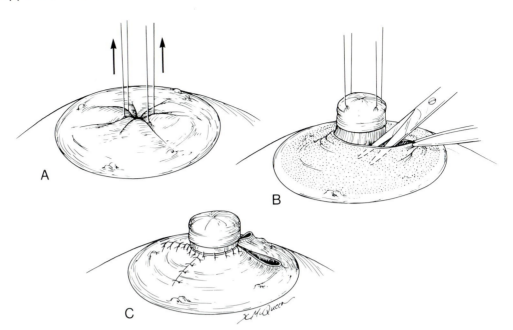

FIGURE 45–6
Hauben and Mahler technique (1988). *A*, Inversion of nipple with a traction suture. *B*, Incision of the base of the nipple and undermining of the areola. *C*, Excision of the redundant areolar skin with four radial incisions and placement of a purse-string suture at the base of the nipple.

THIRD PHASE: PROVISION OF STRUCTURAL BULK WITH DISTURBANCE OF DUCTAL SYSTEMS

Because aesthetic surgery of the breast, especially reduction mammaplasty, has caused nipple inversion in some patients, and because many patients desire correction of inverted nipples for purely cosmetic reasons, surgical approaches to the nipple have been broadened and now even include transection of the lactiferous ducts.

Dufourmentel (1950), expressing dissatisfaction with techniques previously designed for the preservation of nipple function, introduced a technique for attaining cosmetic objectives only. He made a small incision at the inferior base of the nipple. Then he created a cone under the nipple through a V incision by cutting all of the fibrous bands without cutting the ducts. After the nipple was freed, the defect was closed in the Y manner. Although he claimed that none of the mammary ducts were cut, the plane of the incision endangered the continuity of the ductal system, and it is most likely that some of the ducts were cut during the procedure. Nevertheless, he obtained a satisfactory result with this technique.

Until Schwager et al. reported their work, the pathology of the inverted nipple had not been studied microscopically since Basch's (1893) original paper. Schwager et al. (1974) established that the fibrous tissue under the inverted nipple was about the same thickness as that under the areola, whereas in the normal nipple the thickness is twice that amount. This discovery, together with the change in attitude toward breastfeeding, was the foundation for a new phase of breast surgery for the inverted nipple: the addition of structural bulk as well as stability became a regular part of operations designed to prevent nipple inversion.

Schwager et al. (1974) used a technique similar to that of LaMont, but in one congenital form of inverted nipple he had to cut the duct to evert the nipple. This maneuver brought up a new point, that the optimum

result requires transection of the fibrous band as well as the lactiferous ducts. When Hartrampf and Schneider (1976) originally described their direct method of correction of the inverted nipple, they pointed out the necessity of cutting all structures behind the nipple that produce inversion, including the most important structure, the lactiferous duct. These authors also used a bolstered suture to keep the nipple in its new position. They now use a technique described in Figure 45–14. The nipples maintained normal sensation and erectile power. Instead of using a bolstered suture, one can achieve the same goal by placing a suture through the nipple and attaching it to a stabilizing external device, such as a plastic cup, for several weeks.

Broadbent and Woolf (1976), after expressing dissatisfaction with most surgical techniques, including the use of alloplastic material, used a trans–nipple-areola approach to cut the short and hypoplastic ducts to obtain structural fibrous and collagenous bulk for the nipple (Figs. 45–7 and 45–8). Later, Rayner (1980) described a similar technique. The shortcoming of this technique is the inability to obtain a fully projected nipple. Hamilton (1980), Morris and Lamont (1980), and Crestinu (1987) all reported methods for the correction of nipple inversion that are similar to the Dufourmentel technique. The Crestinu (1987) technique involves making an incision radially in the areola near the base of the nipple after eversion of the nipple. Ducts and fibrous bands under the nipple are cut; and after freeing the nipple, one closes the defect in breast soft tissue with a V-Y flap (Fig. 45–9).

Elsahy (1977) designed an operation based on the Schwager findings on the inverted nipple. He used a circular skin incision around the base of the nipple and developed two de-epithelialized triangular dermal flaps at the 3 and 9 o'clock positions. After releasing the fibrous band without cutting the lactiferous ducts, he crossed the flaps through the base of the nipple and sutured them to the opposite side. He closed the skin

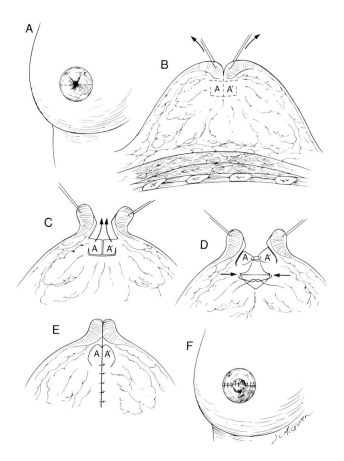

FIGURE 45–7

Broadbent and Woolf technique (1976). *A* and *B*, Schematic drawing of the inverted nipple with traction sutures splitting the nipple. *C*, Midline splitting of the nipple and extending incision into breast parenchyma for approximately 2 cm and then extending the incision laterally and superiorly (*A*, *A'*). *D*, Space is created by advancing *A* and *A'* superiorly is then closed with 5-0 Dexon or Vicryl sutures. *A* and *A'* points are then approximated at a level 2 cm higher than the original position. *E*, The remainder of the nipple is approximated in the newly elevated position. *F*, Final appearance.

defect and sutured the nipple to its base. Elsahy (1977) thus brought up the concept of a dermal sling to prevent inversion.

This procedure had several disadvantages. First, it was unnecessary to carry a skin incision at the base of the nipple completely around it. Second, Elsahy did not interrupt the lactiferous ducts, but passed the sling through them. This maneuver produced fibrosis and strangulation of the ducts and made them functionless. Third, not cutting those tight and hypoplastic ducts compromised the optimal result. Finally, if the flaps had been made at the 12 and 6 o'clock positions, rather than at the 3 and 9 o'clock positions, there would have been less interference with the blood and nerve supply of the nipple.

Haeseker (1984) used a procedure similar to that of Teimourian and Adham, except that he used three dermal flaps, rather than the two that we recommend. Thus, more scar tissue may develop in the nipple and the areola. Because Haeseker did not present photographs of his cases, one cannot judge the results of his technique. Hyakusoku et al. (1988) described a square flap method and the dermal sling to correct inverted nipples, but they appear to have introduced a difficult solution for a simple problem.

THE TEIMOURIAN TECHNIQUE

To achieve more satisfactory results, we (Teimourian and Adham, 1980) modified Elsahy's technique by developing superior and inferior dermal flaps by not cutting the nipple base all the way around, but cutting all of

the lactiferous ducts, and by finally suturing the flaps in the tunnel, rather than crossing them. The operating procedure is as follows.

The nipple is pulled outward by traction suture. The skin around the nipple is marked, and two triangular extensions are made at the 12 o'clock and 6 o'clock positions (Fig. 45–10A to C). The base of each triangle is about 1.0 to 1.2 cm, and the length of the sides of the triangles is about 1.2 cm (of course, exact measurements depend on the size of the nipple). These two triangles are de-epithelialized, and dermal flaps are developed and raised (Fig. 45–10D and E). A tunnel is made starting through the upper or lower incision by cutting all ductal channels, as well as fibrous tissue bands, that keep the nipple inverted (Fig. 45–10F). The flaps are turned under 180 degrees and are sutured together in the tunnel under the nipple with 5-0 Vicryl fine suture (Fig. 45–10G and H). The donor sites are closed with fine material, such as nylon (Fig. 45–10I). The end result is a normal looking nipple with two very fine scars, measuring about 1.0 to 1.2 cm at the 12 and 6 o'clock positions (Figs. 45–11 to 45–13). This method has been used in 13 patients over a 5-year period without complications or recurrence.

If one follows the technique meticulously, the rate of success should be extremely high. However, if the flaps are not of adequate size or thickness, if all the lactiferous ducts and fibrous bands are not totally cut, or if the tunnel is too long, one may have less than satisfactory results.

One of the main advantages of this procedure is that

Text continued on page 620

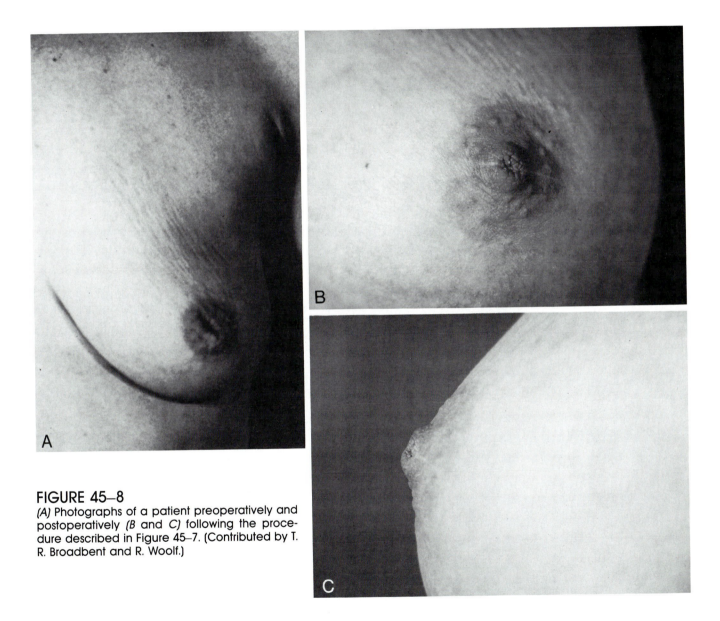

FIGURE 45–8
(A) Photographs of a patient preoperatively and postoperatively *(B* and *C)* following the procedure described in Figure 45–7. (Contributed by T. R. Broadbent and R. Woolf.)

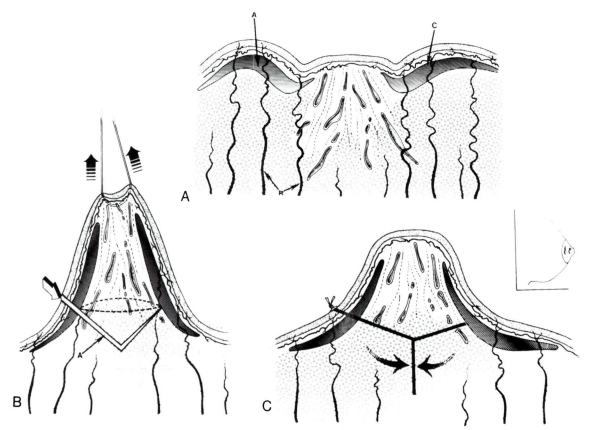

FIGURE 45–9

Crestinu's technique (1987). *A,* Cross section of an inverted nipple. A, Nipple and areola muscle. B, Intraglandular vessels. C. Superficial vessels. *B,* Eversion of the nipple with a traction suture. A, Transection of fibrous band and lactiferous ducts. *C,* Closure of the intraglandular defect with a V-Y advancement flap. (From Crestinu, J. M.: The inverted nipple: A blind method of correction. Plast. Reconstr. Surg. 79:127, 1987.)

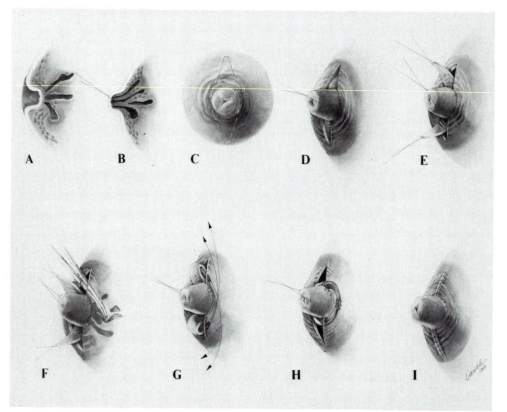

FIGURE 45–10

Teimourian and Adham technique (1980). *A,* Preoperative view of the inverted nipple. *B,* Nipple is everted with traction suture. *C,* The skin around the nipple is marked, and two triangular extensions are made at the 12 and 6 o'clock positions. *D,* The triangles are de-epithelialized. *E,* Development and elevation of dermal flaps. *F,* Development of the tunnel and transection of ductal channels and fibrous bands. *G and H,* The flaps are turned under and sutured together. *I,* The donor sites are closed.

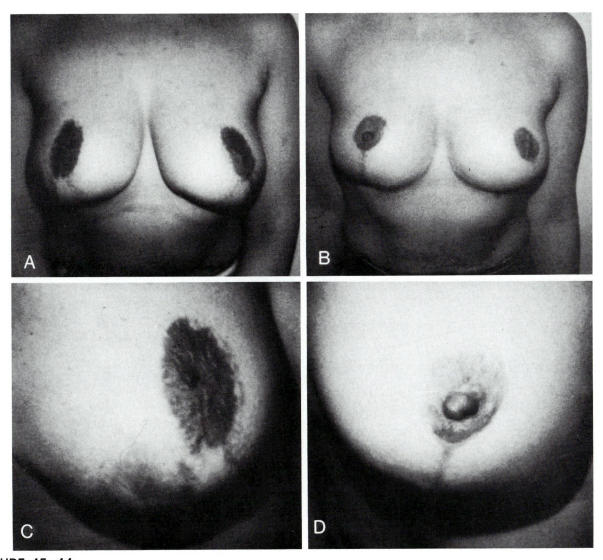

FIGURE 45-11
A and *B*, Bilateral inversion of the nipple secondary to reduction mammaplasty, which was done elsewhere. *C* and *D*,
Appearance after correction of inverted nipples.

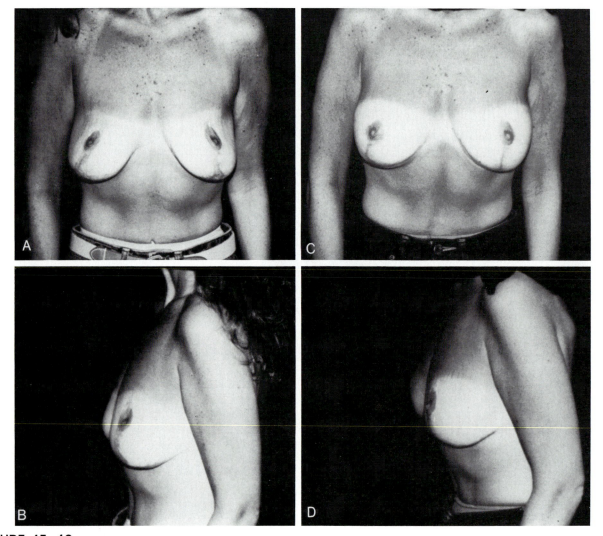

FIGURE 45–12
A and *B*, Bilateral inversion of the nipple secondary to reduction mammaplasty, which was done elsewhere. *C* and *D*,
Appearance after correction of inverted nipples.

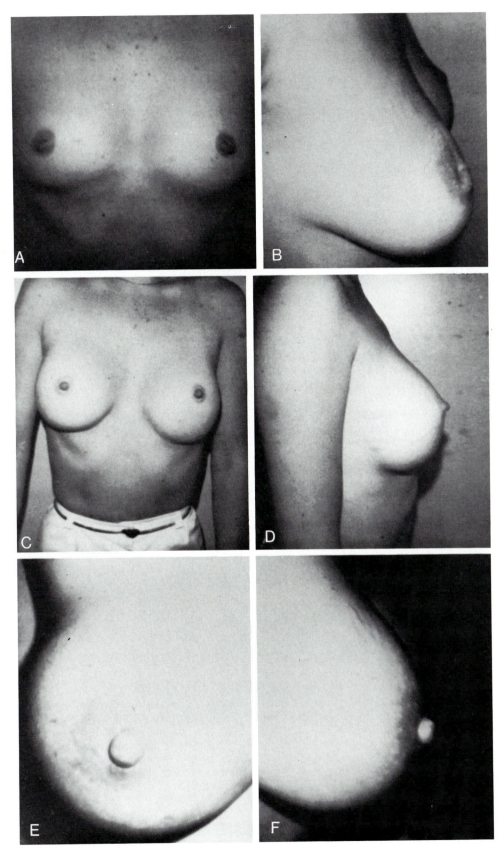

FIGURE 45–13
A and *B*, Bilateral congenital inversion of nipples. *C* to *F*, Appearance after correction of inverted nipples and subpectoral augmentation.

it can be repeated, the flaps being cut at different orientations, such as 1 and 7 o'clock or at 5 and 11 o'clock.

Delorenzi and Halls (1988) reported the use of a nipple splint to maintain the results. A splint may be useful for cases in which the ducts must be maintained; but when the ducts are interrupted, a splint is not required. For some of our earlier cases, we used the splint, but with the development of our present techniques we found its use to be unnecessary.

A simple and direct technique for correction of the inverted nipple has been described by Pitanguy (1981) (Fig. 45–14) and has been used successfully with some modifications by others (Hartrampf and Schneider, 1976) (Figs. 45–15 and 45–16).

Bifid, Fissured, and Imperforate Nipple

Bifid, fissured, and imperforate nipples are very rare and do not appear to adversely affect function. The bifid, or duplicated, nipple is a form of intra-areolar polythelia. In one of two reported cases, the duct opened between the nipples and the patient was not able to breast-feed (Bonnet-Laborderie, 1905). An aesthetic surgical result could be obtained by excision of one of the two nipples (Snyder et al., 1972).

Fissured nipple is possibly a milder form of polythelia. The nipple is usually hypertrophied and can irritate the palate and cause vomiting in a baby. Grodsky (1937) described an operation for this condition that involved flattening of the nipple by cutting the skin from the superior and inferior borders. If the nipple was still enlarged, he recommended areolar myotomy.

The imperforate nipple has no cosmetic significance. The nipple is otherwise normal, but breast-feeding is impossible (Bouffe de Saint Blaise, 1904).

Nipple Hypertrophy

Nipple hypertrophy is also a rare condition. It appears to be a familial defect that becomes more apparent after pregnancy. It is always bilateral and becomes more outstanding when the nipple and areola contract. In 16 cases that were reported by Regnault (1975), 12 were associated with breast hypomastia and 2 with hypermastia.

In 1971 Pitanguy and Cansanção reported a technique by which they divided the nipple horizontally, removing the lower half of it and folding the upper half by suturing the nipple tip to the base of the removed half. Their result was pleasing and caused no disturbances of localization (Stephenson et al., 1975) (Fig. 45–17).

Speall (1974) described an operation in which the skin of the proximal half of the hypertrophied nipple was removed. Three additional wedge-shaped pieces of skin from the distal half were then removed, leaving the 5-mm diameter of the top of the nipple intact. In closing these gaps, the nipple becomes shorter and thinner.

Regnault (1975) used two parallel incisions, the proximal one about 5 mm distal to the base of the nipple. She removed the skin between the two incisions and closed the gap without disturbing the ductal system (Fig. 45–18). She used this technique in augmentation and reduction with good results. Snyder et al. (1976) used a similar method.

Finally, the distal half of the nipple can be amputated by the same technique as that used for nipple sharing

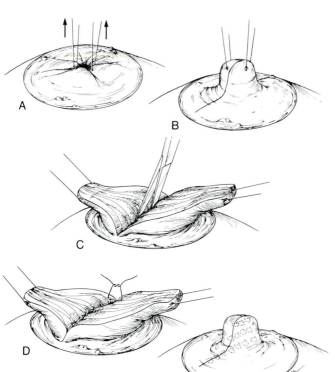

FIGURE 45–14

Pitanguy's technique (1981). *A* and *B*, Inverted nipple advanced with traction utilizing two 3-0 silk sutures. *C*, The nipple is evenly split with sharp dissection, and all the fibrous bands, including the short lactiferous ducts, are released. *D*, The released halves of the nipple are then approximated with 5-0 Dexon or Vicryl sutures. *E*, The final appearance of the protruding nipple is shown.

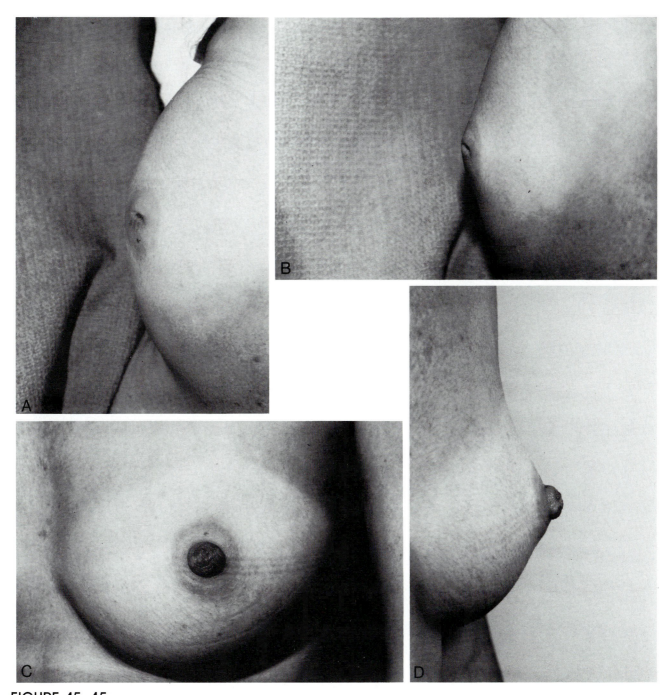

FIGURE 45–15
A and *B*, Preoperative appearance of inverted nipples. *C* and *D*, Postoperative appearance 1 year later by the technique as described in Figure 45–14. (Contributed by Carl R. Hartrampf, M.D.)

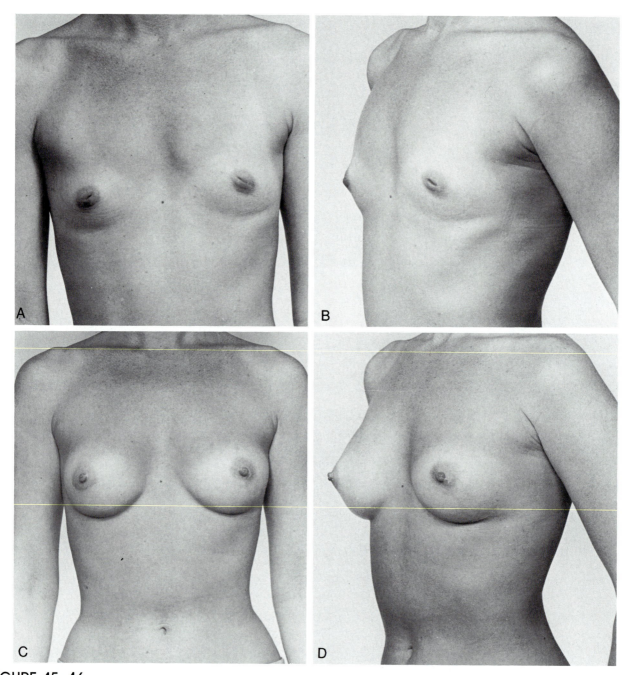

FIGURE 45–16

A and *B*, A 30-year-old patient is shown preoperatively with small breasts and inverted nipples. *C* and *D*, The same patient shown 1 year after augmentation mammaplasty with 165-cc gel prostheses inserted and correction of inverted nipples by Pitanguy's technique. (Contributed by Gregory S. Georgiade, M.D.)

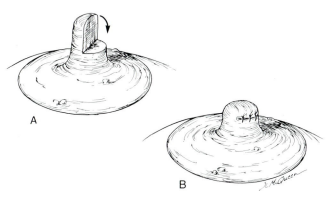

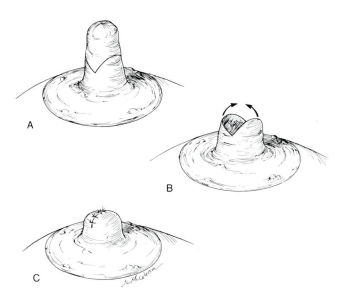

FIGURE 45–17
Pitanguy and Cansancao (1971) technique. *A,* The hypertrophied nipple is divided as shown. *B,* After removal of a portion of the nipple, the nipple is folded on itself, and the tip is sutured to the base.

FIGURE 45–19
A, A wedge of hypertrophied nipple to be excised is shown. *B,* V excision of the nipple. *C,* Approximation with multiple interrupted nylon sutures.

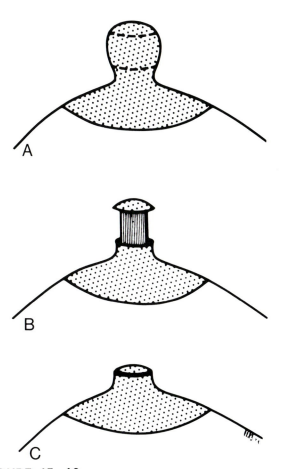

FIGURE 45–18
Regnault's (1975) technique of nipple reduction and nipple circumcision is shown. *A,* Parallel incisions are made, with the lowest incision about 5 mm above the level of the areola and the upper incision around the tip of the nipple. *B,* The entire skin and hypodermis are removed between the two incisions, together with some superficial muscles if necessary. *C,* The two edges are approximated by subcuticular running suture. (From Regnault, P.: Hypertrophy: A physiological reduction by circumcision. Clin. Plast. Surg. 2:391, 1975.)

during breast reconstruction. However, this operation may lead to loss of sensation in the nipple and erectile ability. Quite often a wedge excision can be carried out, minimizing loss of sensation (Fig. 45–19).

ANOMALIES OF THE AREOLA

The anomalies of the areola can be categorized from an aesthetic point of view into three different groups: (1) deficiency of areolar tissue, (2) excess of areolar tissue, and (3) size of presentation of the nipple and areola in relation to the rest of the breast.

Deficiency of the Areola

A deficiency in the size of the areola, as long as it is bilateral, has very little cosmetic consequence. However, a deficiency that is associated with a hypoplastic breast gives the appearance of a masculinized breast. If the condition is treated with augmentation mammaplasty, the overall result improves, and there is generally no need for areola augmentation.

Unilateral deficiency associated with a hypoplastic breast can be corrected by reduction of the contralateral areola, by grafting from the opposite side, or by areola tattooing (Hilton, 1988). In the case of Poland's syndrome, Argenta et al. (1985), in their classic work, showed that the areola can be stretched and relocated so that it covers the normal areola by means of a tissue expander; this procedure can be done as the child grows so as to reduce the psychologic effect of breast deficiency in one's female patients.

Areola Excess

Areola excess rarely accompanies normal breast development. Areola excess is usually associated with hypertrophic or atrophic breast and with ptosis or tuberous breasts. Techniques of breast reduction and mastopexy for third-degree ptosis are discussed in separate chapters. Of special interest to us here is doughnut mastopexy. Davidson (1979), Bartels and Mara (1975), and Gruber and Jones (1980) all described the use of doughnut mastopexy; but Puckett et al. (1985) modified the technique slightly and described crescent mastopexy. In doughnut mastopexy the excess areola is reduced by removal of a doughnut-shaped piece of skin from the areola, whereas in crescent mastopexy a crescent-shaped piece of areola from the superior part is removed to elevate the new areola. To prevent circumareolar scar widening, Williams (1976) and Rees and Aston (1976) recommended excision of a dog-ear medially and laterally. It is our experience that neither doughnut mastopexy nor its various modifications are of much benefit in lifting the breast or reducing areola size. The shortcomings of the technique are that it may result in (1) a globular shaped breast, (2) areola spreading, (3) widening of the scar, or (4) the recurrence of ptosis.

Tuberous Breast

Of the spatial anomalies of the nipple and areola, the most common and challenging is the "herniated areolar complex," also known as "tuberous breast" (Rees and Aston, 1976; Williams, 1976) or "domed nipple" (Vecchione, 1976). Such breasts characteristically have three deformities: (1) herniation of breast tissue into the nipple and areola with a cylindrical projection, accompanied by a relatively large areola; (2) deficiency of the diameter of the base of the breast in both vertical and horizontal axes; and (3) hypoplasia of the breast. The surgical goal should be correction of all three deficiencies. Augmentation of the breast without correction of the herniated areolar complex may lead to a more recognizable abnormality—"Snoopy's nose" deformity (Fig. 45–20).

Surgical correction of the tuberous breast depends on the degree of deformity and associated ptosis and on the relative size of the areola. For mild deformity with no ptosis, the techniques of Williams (1976), Rees and

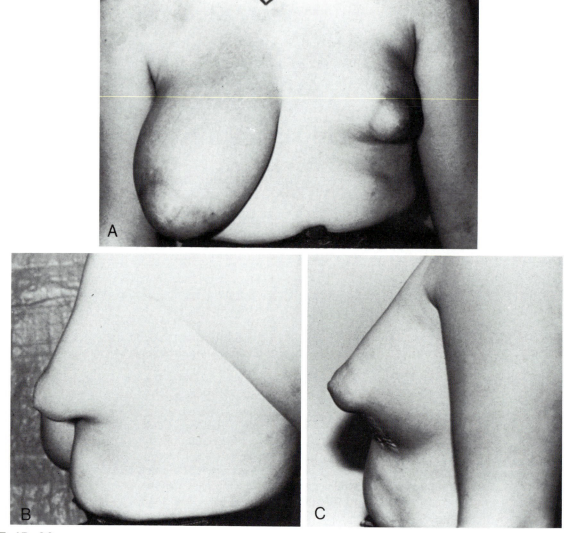

FIGURE 45–20

"Snoopy's nose" deformity. A, Frontal view of a patient with a tuberous breast. B, Left lateral view of a patient with a tuberous breast. C, Left lateral view of the same patient after subglandular augmentation mammaplasty, revealing the "Snoopy's nose" breast deformity.

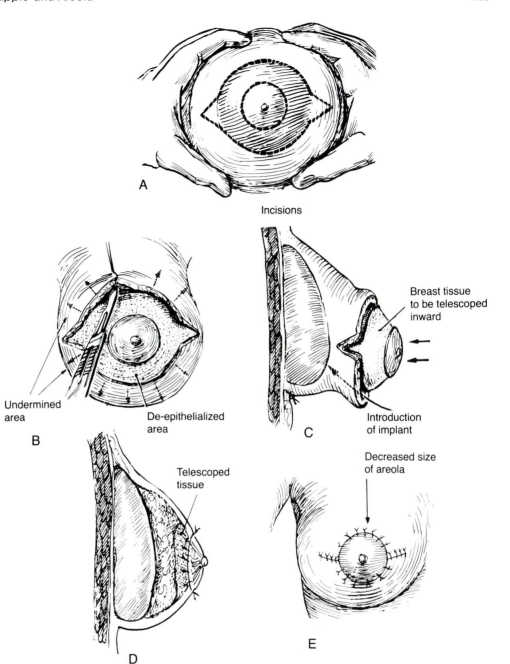

FIGURE 45–21
Rees and Aston (1976) telescoping technique for herniated nipple deformity. *A,* New nipple size and skin incisions are outlined. *B,* Breast tissue is denuded in the subcutaneous plane. *C,* Prostheses are placed under breast tissue on the prepectoral fascia. *D* and *E,* Breast tissue is telescoped into the new skin brassiere and the incisions are sutured. (From Rees, T. D., Aston, S. J.: The tuberous breast. Clin. Plast. Surg. 3:339, 1976.)

Aston (1976), Bass (1978), and Vecchione (1976) may be effective. Williams (1976) corrected this deformity with augmentation mammaplasty and reduction of the areola by excising a doughnut-shaped piece of skin with two triangular extensions on either side. He obtained satisfactory results with this technique.

Rees and Aston (1976) used a similar approach (Fig. 45–21F), except that for breasts with a deficiency in the base in the vertical axis, they made radial incisions in the breast from underneath through an inframammary incision. This had the effect of unfolding the breast and reducing the projection after augmentation (Fig. 45–22).

Base (1978) reduced the areola and augmented the breast through an inferior circumareolar skin incision. He first de-epithelialized a doughnut-shaped piece of skin from the areola to reduce the size. Then he carried the outer incision through the dermal tissue and undermined the skin over the breast tissue to the same extent as the width of the de-epithelialized segment. Through the lower outer skin incision he augmented the breast subglandularly and closed the skin gap by overlapping the outer skin over the de-epithelialized portion. The final result was satisfactory (Fig. 45–23).

Vecchione (1976) corrected domed nipple by excising a doughnut of areolar tissue, mammary ducts, and muscle tissue. Then he sutured the areolocutaneous junction to the edge of the new areola (Fig. 45–24). The final result was a globular breast.

This technique has the same disadvantage as doughnut

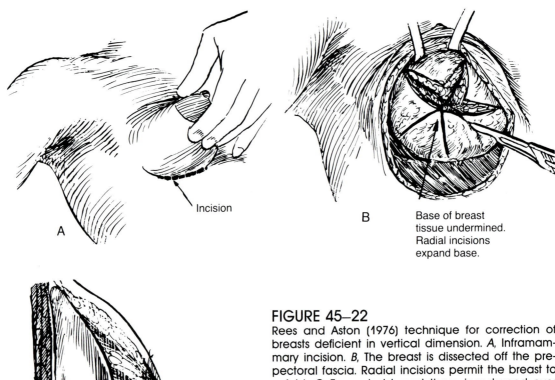

A

Incision

B

Base of breast
tissue undermined.
Radial incisions
expand base.

Size of areola
may be reduced.

C

FIGURE 45–22

Rees and Aston (1976) technique for correction of
breasts deficient in vertical dimension. *A,* Inframammary incision. *B,* The breast is dissected off the prepectoral fascia. Radial incisions permit the breast to
unfold. *C,* Expanded breast tissue is redraped over
the prosthesis. (From Rees, T. D., Aston, S. J.: The
tuberous breast. Clin. Plast. Surg. 3:339, 1976.)

mastopexy. For example, the technique of Bass was
used in one patient, and the result (see Fig. 45–25) was
a wide stretch of areolar scar and a globular breast. To
prevent widening of the scar and to release the breast
constriction, McKinney et al. (1988) described a new
technique for correction of tubular breasts. They
reduced the areola to the shape of a diamond in the
peri-nipple area and augmented the breast by dissection through breast parenchyma down to the prepectoral fascia. They had satisfactory results with this
technique.

Teimourian and Adham (1980), dissatisfied with the
existing techniques, developed a modified version of the
Williams technique. First, the subpectoral augmentation
is done through an inframammary skin incision (Fig.
45–26A). Two circles are drawn on the areola to reduce
it to the appropriate size, the outer circle being at the
areolocutaneous junction. The skin between the two
circles is de-epithelialized (Fig. 45–26B). The new areola
is undermined to about 1 cm from the base of the nipple.
Four wedges of breast tissue are removed from four
quadrants beneath the new areola (see Fig. 45–26B).
The four gaps are closed. This maneuver can be adjusted
to reduce the projection to an acceptable level. Then
the new areola is stretched over the de-epithelialized

area and closed to the old areolocutaneous junction with
interrupted sutures (Fig. 45–26C). The wound is drained
with a small drain. If the condition is unilateral, the
other breast may need augmentation to achieve symmetry (Figs. 45–27 to 45–29).

For severe cases of tuberous breast with ptosis and
atrophy, we recommend standard mastopexy with augmentation completed either in one stage or in several
stages, as done by Toranto (1981) (Fig. 45–30). (See
Chapter 48, Cases 1 and 2.)

Dinner and Dowden (1987) used another modification
for severe cases. They released the breast skin envelope
after augmentation mammaplasty and covered the skin
gap with a medially based skin flap from a new inframammary skin fold. The areola was also reduced with
doughnut mastopexy (Fig. 45–31). Elliott (1988) used a
similar technique, except that he included the serratus-
anterior muscle in the flap. Although these surgeons
obtained excellent results, we believe that these techniques are rather difficult to carry out and in the hands
of an inexperienced surgeon could lead to additional
deformities. We recommend that in such cases of extreme constriction with ptosis the areola be reduced first
and a tissue expander be used for correction of the
breast constriction.

Text continued on page 634

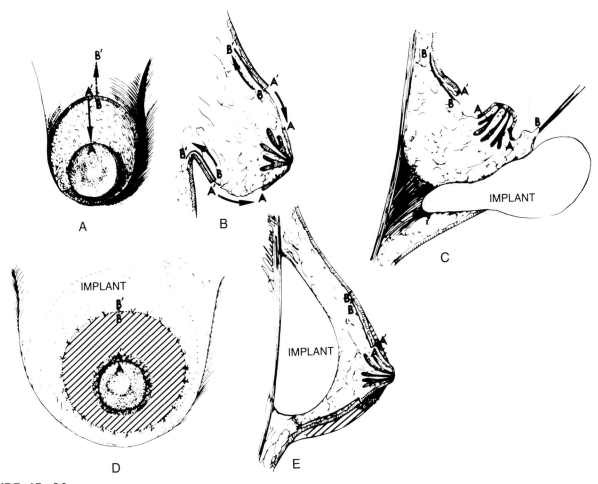

FIGURE 45–23

Bass's (1978) technique of correction of a herniated areolar complex. *A,* De-epithelialization between two concentric circles (A and A'). *B,* A 360-degree subcutaneous dissection is made from B to B'. *C,* Standard augmentation is made by the areolar approach. *D,* The outer edge of the de-epithelialized areola (B) is advanced to the subcutaneous dissection and sutured. *E,* Lateral view. Note that the central ductal elements have not been exposed or transected. (From Bass, C. B.: Herniated areolar complex. Ann. Plast. Surg. 1:402, 1978.)

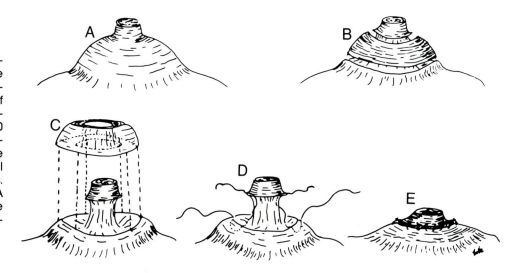

FIGURE 45–24

Vecchione's (1976) technique of recontouring the domed nipple. *A to C,* Excision of the doughnut of areolar tissue is shown. *D,* Anchoring sutures placed 90 degrees apart are responsible for the recession of the central ductal core. *E,* Final closure with 6-0 nylon sutures. (From Vecchione, T. R.: A method for recontouring the domed nipple. Plast. Reconstr. Surg. 57:30, 1976.)

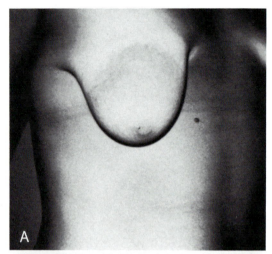

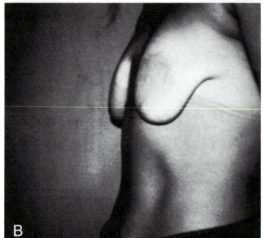

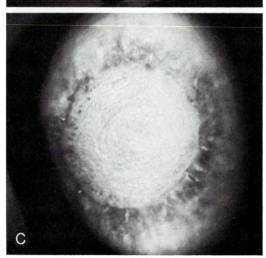

FIGURE 45–25
A, Frontal view of the right breast of a patient with tuberous breasts and ptosis. *B,* Lateral view of the same patient. *C,* Postoperative view of the nipple and areola after correction by Bass's technique. Notice the wide scar and flat nipple.

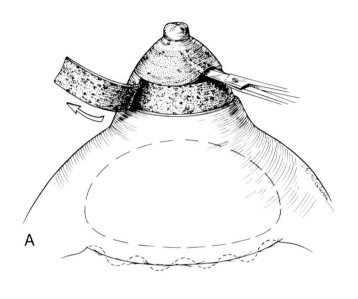

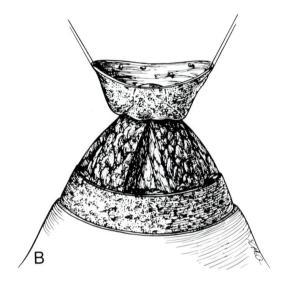

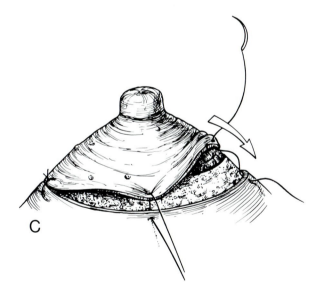

FIGURE 45–26

Teimourian and Adham technique. *A*, Appearance after subpectoral augmentation—the "Snoopy's nose" deformity. A horizontal strip of areolar skin is de-epithelialized. *B*, The skin of the new areola is undermined to within about 1 cm of the base of the nipple. Four wedges of breast tissue are removed from four quadrants beneath the new areola. *C*, The gaps are closed with Vicryl sutures. The new areola is stretched over the de-epithelialized area and closed to the old areolocutaneous junction.

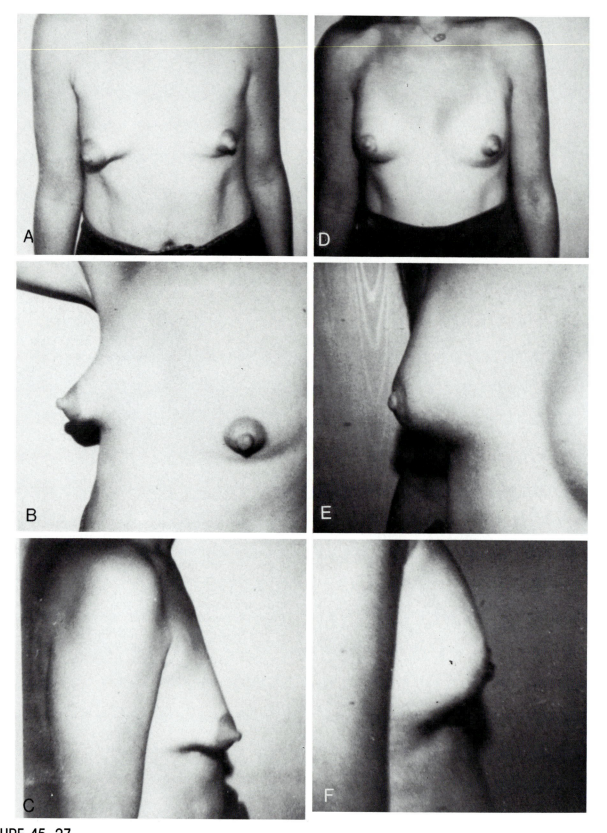

FIGURE 45–27
Preoperative and posterior views of patient with tuberous breasts. *A to C,* Preoperative views of the tuberous breast on the right side. *D to F,* Postoperative views after bilateral subpectoral augmentation and correction of tuberous breasts.

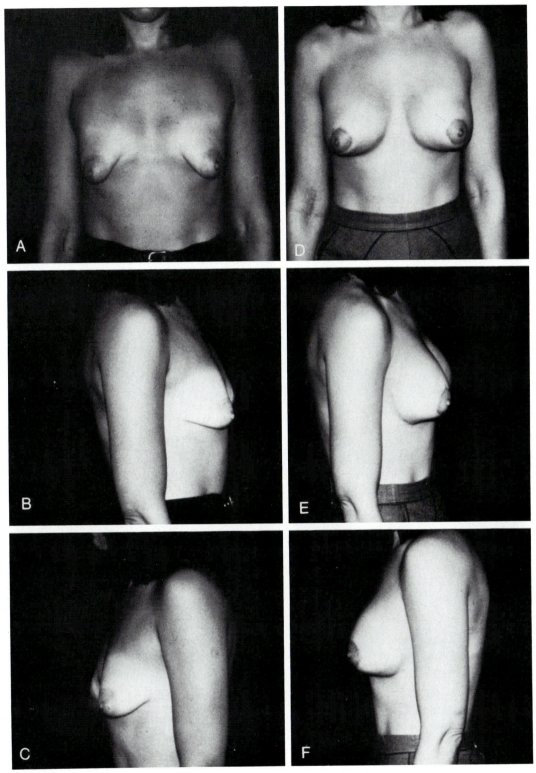

FIGURE 45–28
Patient with tuberous breasts and ptosis. *A* to *C,* Preoperative view. *D* to *F,* Postoperative view after correction by the Teimourian and Adham technique.

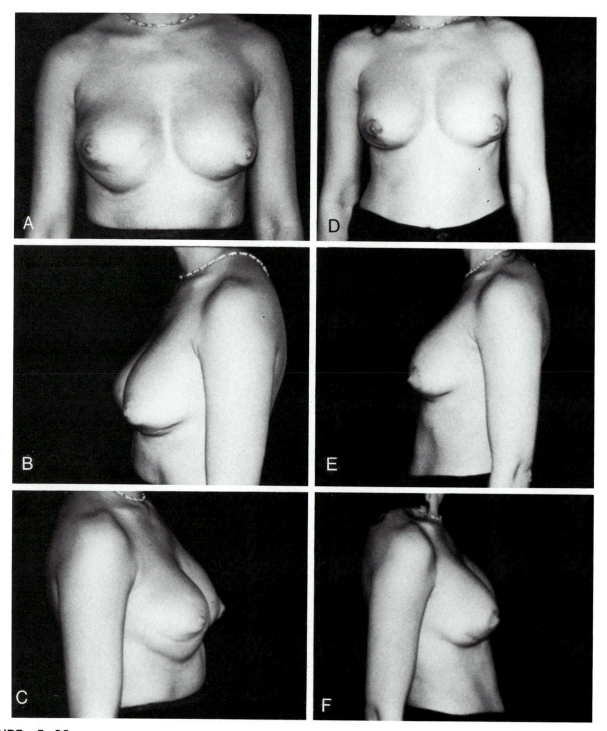

FIGURE 45–29
Patient with "Snoopy's nose" breast deformity. *A* to *C*, Preoperative view. *D* to *F*, Postoperative view after correction by the Teimourian and Adham technique.

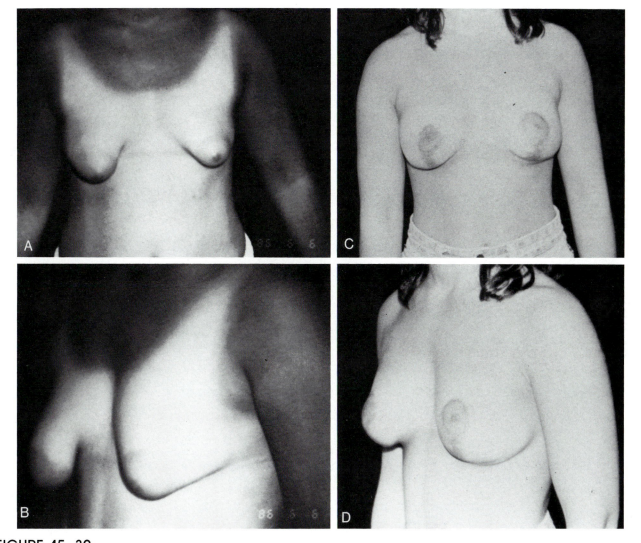

FIGURE 45–30
A and *B*, Preoperative view of a patient with severe tuberous breasts. *C* and *D*, Same patient after correction with mastopexy and augmentation mammaplasty.

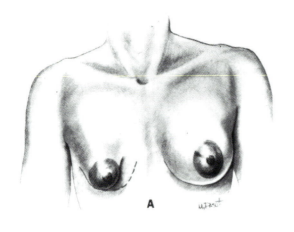

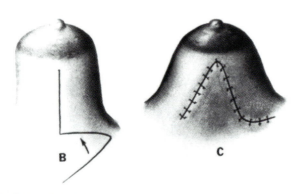

FIGURE 45–31

Dinner and Dowden technique (1987). *A*, Preoperative sketch of a patient with a tuberous breast. *B* and *C*, Breast after correction of the breast constriction with a flap from the new inframammary skin fold. (See Case 3, Chapter 48.)

References

Argenta, L. C., Vanderkolk, C., Friedman, R. J., et al.: Refinements in reconstruction of congenital breast deformities. Plast. Reconstr. Surg. 76:73, 1985.

Axford, W. L.: Mammillaplasty. Ann. Surg. 9:277, 1889.

Bartels, R. J., Mara, M. E.: Simultaneous reduction of areola and an augmentation mammoplasty through a periareolar incision. Plast. Reconstr. Surg. 56:588, 1975.

Basch, K.: Zur Anatomie und Physiologie der Brustwarze. Arch. Gynecol. 44:15, 1893.

Bass, C. B.: Herniated areolar complex. Ann. Plast. Surg. 1:402, 1978.

Birkett, J: *Diseases of Breast and Their Treatment*. London, 1850, p. 208.

Bloom, W., Fawcett, D. W.: *A Textbook of Histology*. Philadelphia, W. B. Saunders, 1975, p. 907.

Bonnet-Laborderie: *Jour. de Science Médicale*. Lille, 1905, II, 5. Cited by Deaver, J. B., McFarland, J: *The Breast: Its Anomalies, Its Diseases, and Their Treatment*. Philadelphia, Blakiston's, 1917, p. 671.

Bouffe de Saint Blaise: *Annales de Gynecologie et d'Obstetrics*, 1904, 25, I, 49. Cited by Deaver, J. B., McFarland, J: *The Breast: Its Anomalies, Its Diseases, and Their Treatment*. Philadelphia, Blakiston's, 1917, p. 671.

Broadbent, T. R., Woolf, R. M.: Benign inverted nipple: Transnipple-areolar correction. Plast. Reconstr. Surg. 58:673, 1976.

Bryant, T.: *Diseases of the Breast*. London, Cassell, 1887.

Castano, M.: Dorsal scapular supernumerary breast in a woman. Plast. Reconstr. Surg. 43:536, 1969.

Cooper, A.: *The Anatomy of the Breast*. London, Longman, 1840.

Courtiss, E. H., Goldwyn, R. M.: Breast sensation before and after plastic surgery. Plast. Reconstr. Surg. 58:1, 1976.

Craig, R. D. P., Sykes, P. A.: Nipple sensitivity following reduction mammoplasty. Br. J. Plast. Surg. 23:165, 1970.

Crestinu, J. M.: The inverted nipple: A blind method of correction. Plast. Reconstr. Surg. 79:127, 1987.

Cronin, E. D., Humphreys, D. H., Ruiz-Razura, A.: Nipple reconstruction: The S flap. Plast. Reconstr. Surg. 81:783, 1988.

D'Assumpção, E. A., Rosa, E. M.: Correcting the inverted nipple. Br. J. Plast. Surg. 30:249, 1977.

Davidson, B. A.: Convention circle operation for massive gynecomastia. Plast. Reconstr. Surg. 63:350, 1979.

De Cholnoky, T.: Supernumerary breast. Arch. Surg. 39:926, 1939.

Deaver, J. B., McFarland, J.: *The Breast: Its Anomalies, Its Diseases, and Their Treatment*. Philadelphia, Blakiston's, 1917.

Delorenzi, C., Halls, M. J.: A nipple splint. Plast. Reconstr. Surg. 81:959, 1988.

Dinner, M. J., Dowden, R. V.: The tubular tuberous breast syndrome. Ann. Plast. Surg. 19:414, 1987.

Dufourmentel, L.: Chirurgie reparatrice et corrective des teguments et des formes. 2nd ed. Paris, Masson, 1950, p. 370.

Edwards, E. A.: Surgical anatomy of the breast. In: Goldwyn, R. M. (ed): *Plastic and Reconstructive Surgery of the Breast*. Boston, Little, Brown, 1976, p. 53.

Elliott, M. P.: A musculocutaneous transposition flap mammaplasty for correction of the tuberous breast. Ann. Plast. Surg. 20:153, 1988.

Elsahy, N. J.: Correction of deformed areola and nipple. Acta. Chir. Plast. 19:224, 1977.

Ely, J. F.: Personal communication, 1988.

Fodor, P. B., Khoury, F.: Latissimus dorsi muscle flap in reconstruction of congenitally absent breast and pectoral muscle. Ann. Plast. Surg. 4:422, 1980.

Gangal, J. T., Gangal, M. H.: Suction method of correcting flat nipples or inverted nipples. Plast. Reconstr. Surg. 61:294, 1978.

Goldenring, H., Crelin, E. S.: Mother and daughter with bilateral congenital amastia. Yale J. Biol. Med. 33:466, 1961.

Goldwyn, R. M.: *The Unfavorable Result in Plastic Surgery*. Boston, Little, Brown, 1972, p. 380.

Goodman, R. M., Bonne-Tamir, B., Ashbel, S., et al.: Genetic studies in a family with inverted nipples (mammillae invertitia). Clin. Genet. 15:346, 1979.

Gray, S. W., Skandalakis, J. E.: *Embryology for Surgeons: The Embryological Basis for the Treatment of Congenital Defects*. Philadelphia, W. B. Saunders, 1972, p. 405.

Grodsky, M.: Reconstruction des mamelons déformes. Rev. Chir. Struct. June: 126, 1937.

Gruber, R. P.: Nipple-areola reconstruction: A review of techniques. Clin. Plast. Surg. 6:71, 1979.

Gruber, R. P., Jones, H. W.: The "donut" mastopexy: Indications and complications. Plast. Reconstr. Surg. 65:34, 1980.

Gupta, S. C.: A critical review of contemporary procedures for mammary reduction. Br. J. Plast. Surg. 18:328, 1965.

Haeseker, B.: The application of de-epithelialized "turn-over" flaps to the treatment of inverted nipples. Br. J. Plast. Surg. 37:253, 1984.

Hamilton, J. M.: Inverted nipples. Plast. Reconstr. Surg. 65:507, 1980.

Hara, S., Haywood, B. D., Davis, K. K., et al.: A black female with the 48,XXXX chromosome constitution. Am. J. Ment. Defic. 79:464, 1975.

Hartrampf, C. R., Culbertson, J. H.: A dermal fat flap for nipple reconstruction. Plast. Reconstr. Surg. 73:982, 1984.

Hartrampf, C. R., Schneider, W. J.: A simple direct method for correction of inversion of the nipple. Plast. Reconstr. Surg. 58:678, 1976.

Hauben, D. J., Mahler, D.: A simple method for the correction of the inverted nipple. Plast. Reconstr. Surg. 71:556, 1988.

Hayes, H.: Simultaneous augmentation mammaplasty and correction of inverted nipples. Ann. Plast. Surg. 5:401, 1980.

Herman, G. E.: Kehrer's operation for depressed nipple. Lancet 2:12, 1889.

Hilton, B.: Nipple-areola reconstruction using intradermal tattoo. Plast. Reconstr. Surg. 81:450, 1988.

Hosokawa K., Hata, Y., Yano K., et al.: Unilateral athelia with subcutaneous dermoid cyst. Plast. Reconstr. Surg. 80:732, 1987.

Hyakusoku, H., Okubo, M., Fumiini, M.: Combination of the square flap method and the dermal sling to correct flat or inverted nipples. Aesthetic Plast. Surg. 12:107, 1988.

James, T.: Curiosa paediatrica: V. Inverted nipples. S. Afr. Med. J. 60:548, 1981.

Kehrer, F. A.: In Muller, P.: *Handbuch der Gerbürtshülfe.* Vol. III, Part 2. Stuttgart, F. Enke, 1888, p. 450. Cited by T. Skoog.

Kehrer, F. A.: Über Excision des Warzenhofs bei Holwerzen. Beitr. Exp. Gerbürtshülfe Gynaekol Gizessen 43:170, 1879–1880.

Kowlessar, M., Orti, E.: Complete breast absence in siblings. Am. J. Dis. Child. 115:91, 1968.

LaMont, E.: Congenital inversion of the nipple in identical twins. Br. J. Plast. Surg. 26:178, 1973.

Letterman, G., Schurter, M.: The surgical correction of inverted nipples. South. Med. J. 60:724, 1967.

Maliniac, J. W.: Arterial blood supply of the breast: Revised anatomic data relating to reconstructive surgery. Arch. Surg. 47:329, 1943.

Marcus, G. H.: Untersuchungen über die arterielle Blutversorgung der Mamilla. Arch. Klin. Chir. 179:361, 1934.

McKinney, P., Cook, C. Q., Lewis, V. L., Fisher, C.: Correction of the tubular breast. Plastic Surgical Forum 11:190, 1988.

Montagna, W., MacPherson, E.: Some neglected aspects of the anatomy of human breasts. J. Invest. Dermatol. 63:10, 1974.

Morris, A. M., Lamont, P. M.: A method for correcting the inverted nipple. Br. J. Plast. Surg. 33:41, 1980.

Mosley, H. F., Miller, G. G.: *Textbook of Surgery.* St. Louis, C. V. Mosby, 1952, p. 269.

Muruci, A., Dantas, J. J., Noguerira, L. R.: Reconstruction of the nipple-areola complex. Plast. Reconstr. Surg. 61:558, 1978.

Nelson, M. M., Cooper, C. K.: Congenital defects of the breast—An autosomal dominant trait. S. Afr. Med. J. 61:434, 1982.

Otte, M. J.: Correcting inverted nipples—An aid to breast feeding. Am. J. Nurs. 75:454, 1975.

Perkins, C., Miller, A. M.: Sebaceous glands in the human nipple. Am. J. Obstet. Gynecol. 11:789, 1926.

Pitanguy, I, Cansanção, A.: Redução do Mamelo. Rev. Bras. Cir. 61:73, 1971.

Pitanguy, I.: *Aesthetic Plastic Surgery of the Head and Body.* New York, Springer-Verlag, 1981, p. 63.

Puckett, C. L., Vaughn, H. M., Reinisch, J. F.: Crescent mastopexy and augmentation. Plast. Reconstr. Surg. 75:533, 1985.

Rayner, C.: The correction of permanently inverted nipples. Br. J. Plast. Surg. 33:413, 1980.

Rees, T. D., Aston, S. J.: The tuberous breast. Clin. Plast. Surg. 3:339, 1976.

Regnault, P.: Hypertrophy: A physiological reduction by circumcision. Clin. Plast. Surg. 2:391, 1975.

Robbins, S. L.: *Pathologic Basis of Disease.* Philadelphia, W. B. Saunders, 1974, p. 1268.

Schwager, R. G., Smith, J. W., Gray, G. F., et al.: Inversion of the human female nipple, with a simple method of treatment. Plast. Reconstr. Surg. 54:564, 1974.

Sellheim, H.: Brustwarzenplastik bei Holwarzen. Zentralbl. Gynakol. 41:305, 1917.

Serafin, D.: Anatomy of the breast. In: Georgiade, N. G. (ed.): *Reconstructive Breast Surgery.* St. Louis, C. V. Mosby, 1976, p. 23.

Serafin, D.: Surgical anatomy of breast. In: Georgiade, N. G. (ed.): *Breast Reconstruction Following Mastectomy.* St. Louis, C. V. Mosby, 1979, p. 48.

Skoog, T.: An operation for inverted nipples. Br. J. Plast. Surg. 5:65, 1953.

Skoog, T.: Surgical correction of inverted nipples. J. Am. Med. Wom. Assoc. 20:931, 1965.

Snyder, C. C., Pickens, J. E., Slater, P. V.: Surgery of the areola-nipple complex. In: Masters, F. W., Lewis, J. R., Jr. (eds.): *Symposium on Aesthetic Surgery of the Face, Eyelid, and Breast.* St. Louis, C. V. Mosby, 1972, p. 192.

Snyder, C. C., Browne, E. Z., Pickens, J. E.: Reconstructive problems of the nipple and areola. In: Goldwyn, R. M. (ed.): *Plastic and Reconstructive Surgery of the Breast.* Boston, Little, Brown, 1976, p. 411.

Speall, A. E.: Cosmetic reduction of the nipple with functional preservation. Br. J. Plast. Surg. 27:42, 1974.

Spina, V.: Inverted nipple. Plast. Reconstr. Surg. 19:63, 1957.

Stephenson, K., Dingman, R., Gaisford, J., et al.: *Yearbook of Plastic and Reconstructive Surgery, 1974.* Chicago, Year Book Medical Publishers, 1975, p. 114.

Tawill, H. M., Najjar, S. S.: Congenital absence of the breasts. J. Pediatr. 73:751, 1968.

Teimourian, B., Adham, M. N.: Simple technique for correction of inverted nipple. Plast. Reconstr. Surg. 65:504, 1980.

Teimourian, B., Adham, M. N.: Surgical correction of the tuberous breast. Ann. Plast. Surg. 10:190, 1983.

Toranto, J. R.: Two-stage correction of tuberous breast. Plast. Reconstr. Surg. 67:642, 1981.

Trier, W. C.: Complete breast absence. Plast. Reconstr. Surg. 36:430, 1965.

Vecchione, T. R.: A method for recontouring the domed nipple. Plast. Reconstr. Surg. 57:30, 1976.

Williams, J. E.: Augmentation mammaplasty: Inframammary approach. In: Georgiade, N. G. (ed.): *Reconstructive Breast Surgery.* St. Louis, C. V. Mosby, 1976, p. 62.

Williams, W. R.: *A Monograph on Diseases of the Breast.* London, John Bale and Sons, 1894, p. 544.

Wolfort, F. G., Marshall, K. A., Cochran, T. C.: Correction of the inverted nipple. Ann. Plast. Surg. 1:294, 1978.

AESTHETIC BREAST SURGERY IN ORIENTALS

46

Naoyuki Ohtake
Nobuyuki Shioya

Aesthetic Breast Surgery in Orientals

SOCIAL ACCEPTANCE OF AESTHETIC SURGERY IN THE ORIENT

At best, social acceptance of aesthetic surgery in the Orient has been tardy. The area's intellectuals, and even those in the medical profession, once looked upon this branch of surgery with considerable prejudice, assuming that its practitioners were merely catering to the whims of the vain by improving the shape of their body parts. Such condemnation may have been partly due to the lingering influence of Confucian morality, because maintaining the integrity of the body, considered a gift from one's parents, is the first duty of filial piety. This negative view may have been bolstered by an observable fact, for, unlike Caucasians, operative scars that result from tampering with the body are more outstanding in the Asian.

Nevertheless, human anguish being as strong in this region as elsewhere, those with prominent deformities have always sought a way to correct them. Thus, with no approved medical channel to aid them, their need for help often gave rise to corrupt surgeons, who took advantage of their plight. This sorry development, in turn, has contributed to the retardation of legitimate medical advancement in this field.

Social acceptance of aesthetic surgery has come slowly. Only in 1975 was plastic surgery officially recognized as an independent specialty of medical practice. As for aesthetic surgery, similar recognition came even later, in 1978, though in the short time that has passed, our place in the medical world has developed firmly. In a study conducted by Uchinuma et al. (1982), a nationwide questionnaire directed to university and high school students has revealed that the term "cosmetic surgery" was know by 92.5% of all respondees. In sharp contrast, the term "plastic surgery" was known by only 18.6%. This and other encouraging signs of social acceptance have aided the continued development of aesthetic surgery as a legitimate medical discipline.

HISTORICAL CONCEPT OF THE BREAST IN THE ORIENT

The breast is now universally accepted as a symbol of femininity, its pleasing shape also an important stimulus to sex, though in the past there was a wide divergence as to how the breast was regarded in the East and the West. Apart from ancient times, when a large breast in most cultures symbolized fertility, the national costume of the Han people, China's most populous ethnic group, was designed to mask the outline of the feminine body. This flat-chested look carried the implication that a woman should be modest in her appearance, and to accentuate the contours of a woman by means of dress was considered shameful.

This tendency was especially remarkable in Japan. A woman's breast in classic Japanese art is given no emphasis, whereas in classic Western art it is generously depicted with unrestrained passion. Rarely are breasts even glimpsed in old paintings and sculptures. Whenever they are seen, however, they are small and flat (Fig. 46–1A), with little appeal to the contemporary eye as objects of enchanting beauty. Following the traditional belief of the East, the breast in old Japanese art depicts maternity and not beauty or pleasure (Fig. 46–1B).

In the aftermath of World War II, however, the Oriental concept of the breast underwent an abrupt change. This was aided by the increased military presence of the West in the region. Occupied Japan, for instance, came under the influence of American culture, and through this exposure the role of its women began to change.

Long denied an active role in life, Asian women became more assertive; and as they emulated their counterparts in the West, their influence in society began to be felt. Accompanying this, a desire to resemble physically their Caucasian role models also grew, that is, to have a well-defined nose; a clear-cut, double eyelid fold; and larger, more attractive breasts.

Time has brought an even greater identity with the West. Mass communication and international travel have made our globe smaller, spurring this trend. Therefore, it should not come as any surprise that Asian women of today are more conscious of their appearance and desire full, aesthetically attractive breasts.

THE BODY OF THE ASIAN WOMAN

The Oriental woman, as the Asian woman is often called, has diverse types—Mongolians, Southeast Asians, Indians—making it difficult to provide a general description. One thing that they have in common, however, is a body structure smaller than that of Occidental

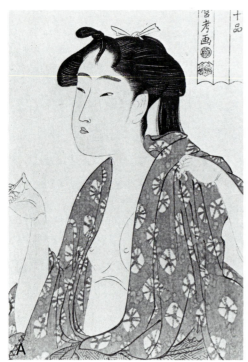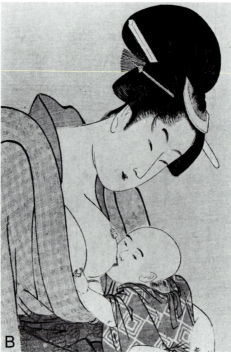

FIGURE 46–1
A, A Japanese lady in ukiyoe. *B,* A nursing mother in ukiyoe. (By Kitagawa Utamaro. Courtesy Tokyo National Museum.)

woman. This is substantiated by data on their average height, weight, chest circumference, girth, and waist measurements (Table 46–1).

Other statistics comparing Japanese and Americans reveal that the height, weight, chest circumference, girth, and waist measurements are much greater in Americans, with the breadth of the chest about the same and the breadth of the shoulders greater in the Japanese. Given these facts, it is apparent that American women have a greater chest and, consequently, larger breasts (Table 46–2) (Yanagisawa, 1976).

Recently, however, the body of the average Japanese woman has been undergoing a change, due to an improvement in both the standard of living and the environment. According to a survey conducted by the Ministry of Education, the height and chest circumference of 2-year-olds have increased by an average of 0.4 cm and 0.2 cm, respectively, this survey covering a 7-year period, from 1975 to 1982 (Table 46–3) (Sakaki, 1985).

Operative Scars

Blacks are said to suffer more often from outstanding operative scars, or keloids (Crikelair, 1977), and whites,

least. Orientals fall between whites and blacks in this respect (Namba, 1984).

Patients are naturally most concerned about operative scars; therefore, skin closures should be done meticulously. Subcuticular stitches should be employed whenever possible, and postoperative treatment to prevent scarring, such as wound taping, should be continued until the scar becomes stable. Even when there is no history of keloid formation, the possibility that a hypertrophic scar or keloid might result should be explained to the patient preoperatively.

AUGMENTATION MAMMAPLASTY

Because Orientals have smaller breasts than Occidentals, aesthetic breast surgery usually is performed for the augmentation of the breast. A survey conducted by Ichida et al. (1983) shows that 13.3% of all cases treated by a department of aesthetic plastic surgery at a Japanese university hospital were related to the breast, and as many as four of five cases involved augmentation mammaplasty (Table 46–4), presumably reflecting an inferiority complex with regard to the size of the breast, due to Western influence.

TABLE 46–1
Measurements of the Japanese Female According to Age Group

	AGE							
	25–29	*30–34*	*35–39*	*40–44*	*45–49*	*50–54*	*55–59*	*60–64*
Body height	154.6	153.1	152.9	152.1	151.5	150.3	149.1	148.5
Chest circumference	82.2	83.2	84.4	86.2	86.6	86.9	87.0	87.2
Waist circumference	65.3	66.6	68.1	70.3	71.9	72.7	73.3	73.8
Girth circumference	88.9	89.6	90.7	92.0	92.6	92.6	92.5	92.0
Body weight	50.1	50.9	52.0	53.5	54.2	53.7	53.1	52.6

From Yanagisawa, S.: *The Study of Japanese Habits.* Tokyo, Koseikan, 1976.

TABLE 46–2
Comparison of Japanese and American Females

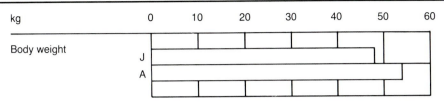

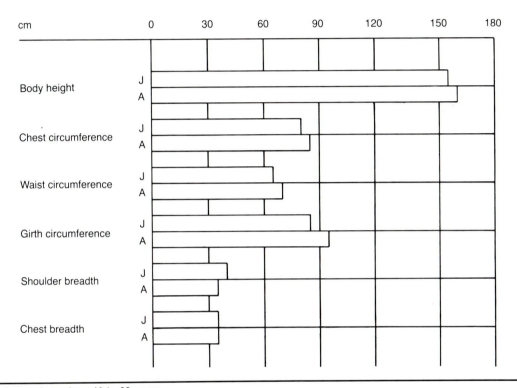

J, Japanese; A, American. Age: 18 to 29 years.
Modified from Yanagisawa, S.: *The Study of Japanese Habits.* Tokyo, Koseikan, 1976.

TABLE 46–3
Changes in the Body Measurements of Women at 20 Years of Age in Japan

	BODY WEIGHT (kg)	BODY HEIGHT (cm)	SITTING HEIGHT (cm)	CHEST CIRCUMFERENCE (cm)
1975	51.1	156.2	83.9	81.7
1978	51.1	157.2	83.4	81.7
1980	50.8	157.3	83.6	81.8
1982	51.1	157.6	83.8	81.9

Data from the Ministry of Education of Japan, 1983.
From Sakaki, K., Kimura, K.: A study in somatometric measurement of freshman students of Tokyo Women's Medical College. Journal of Tokyo Women's Medical College 55:36, 1985.

TABLE 46-4
Aesthetic Plastic Surgery by Type at Japanese University Hospitals

Augmentation rhinoplasty	23.5%
Blepharoplasty	20.2%
Rhytidectomy	13.3%
Reduction rhinoplasty	13.3%
Augmentation mammaplasty	11.6%
Umbilicoplasty	8.3%
Otoplasty	3.3%
Revision of tattoo	3.3%
Reduction mammaplasty	1.7%
Mentoplasty	1.7%

From Ichida, M., Itoh, M., Shroiza, N.: The present state of aesthetic surgery in the university hospitals of Japan. J. J.S.A.P.S. 5:48, 1983.

History of Augmentation Mammaplasty

Period of Foreign-Body Injections

The history of augmentation mammaplasty in the Orient begins with the injection of foreign bodies. Treatment by this injection method allegedly was originated by Gersuny (1900), who injected paraffin to repair a saddle nose in 1899. Because of complications that arose—paraffinoma, thrombosis, postoperative deformities—a few years after operation, this method has since fallen into disuse in both America and Europe (Ortiz-Monasterio and Trigos, 1972).

This method, however, began to be used in the Orient, mainly in Japan and Southeast Asian countries, before any basic studies were done. Little is known of when and how it was introduced into practice here, although some say about 1952, though this is not certain.

Materials that were injected were paraffin and substances of the petrolatum groups, which created complications within a few years similar to those seen in America and Europe (Fumiiri, 1980).

These complications, such as deformities, induration, and even symptoms possibly related to collagen diseases, were reported by Kumagai (1982) and Sonoda et al. (1983). Even death from thrombosis has been reported (Funao and Yanagida, 1965). In addition, another complication, hyperglobulinemia, a systemic reaction to a foreign body, has been reported by Miyoshi et al. (1964), Ohhashi et al. (1978), Ohkubo (1986), and Aoki et al. (1988) as a human adjuvant disease. At present, the concept of a delayed allergic reaction proposed by Chaplin (1969) is widely accepted as explaining these phenomena (Fig. 46-2).

Period of Silicone Injection

In Japan, Akiyama (1958) introduced silicone as augmentation matter (dimethylpolysiloxane, DMPS) in gel form, which was injected into retromammary space by means of a special syringe. Because of its viscosity, this material was thought to be stable in the tissue without dispersion (Mutoch, 1964). The use of silicone fluid supplemented with animal or vegetable oil (Ryh Sakurai's formula) (Kagan, 1963), heat-vulcanized (HV) DMPS, and room temperature-vulcanized (RTV) DMPS (Conway and Goulian, 1963) was reported.

Although silicone purified for medical use was thought to be safe, because it caused less tissue reaction (Narita, 1958), its injection posed problems: a systemic reaction to the foreign material (Fumiiri, 1974) and the migration of this material in the body. Further, there was the danger of this material masking a breast cancer. Another subsequent drawback was discovered, in that its total removal, if necessary, was difficult (Koganei, 1984).

Siliconoma, similar to paraffinoma, was reported by Ben-Hur and Neuman (1965), due to a silicone injection; this also occurred in America and Europe. Even so, our review of the literature (1986) revealed that this method continued to be used in the Orient until about 1970, presumably because of the simplicity of the technique (Ohtake et al., 1988).

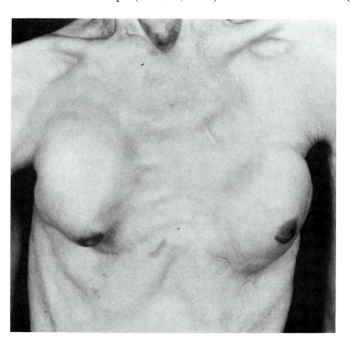

FIGURE 46-2
Severe deformity caused by the injection method of augmentation.

Period of the Bag Prosthesis

The silicone bag prosthesis next was introduced by Cronin and Gerow (1963) and was accepted as being practical and safe. The employment of this bag began a little later in the Orient (Mutoh, 1969), though it often was refused by the patient, not only because it was considered too large for Oriental women but also because its insertion resulted in a long scar. In Japan, an inflatable type requiring a smaller incision for embedding was developed in 1965 (Mutoh, 1987), but interest in the prosthesis soon faded because of the difficulty of injecting viscous silicone and also because of leakage from the injection hole (Fig. 46–3). Thus, a prefilled type in a variety of shapes and sizes is now predominantly used in the Orient.

Indications

The patient's motive for a breast operation should be carefully screened before the operation. Generally, the dominant motive is feeling of inferiority with regard to the size of the breast, but care must be taken because a tendency to paranoia is often detected in some patients. The concept of what constitutes an "ideal breast" varies greatly with age, culture, and personal factors. Unless the surgeon and the patient reach a concrete and full agreement, the surgery should not be performed. In the Orient, it may be wiser to avoid recommending the operation for unmarried women because difficulties may arise at the time of marriage.

Preoperative Evaluation

Type and Selection of the Bag Prosthesis

Various shapes and sizes of bag prosthesis are commercially available, and no one type has been found completely satisfactory in all respects. The double-lumen type, capable of an adjustable capacity, and the low profile type, which supposedly elicits less frequent capsular contracture, are two popular types.

What is essential is to select a type that fits the contours of the patient's thorax. Generally, the low-profile type is selected for a broad thorax; the teardrop type, for a smaller thorax. The round type is usually satisfactory for the average patient.

A wide variety of sizes, from 100 to 350 ml, are available, though a volume between 100 and 200 ml usually is chosen for the Oriental patient. In actual practice, the size is determined during the operation by the use of test bag prostheses (sizers).

Selection of the Skin Incision and Approach

The skin incision selected is largely confined to the following approaches: (1) submammary, (2) transareolar or periareolar (Pitanguy, 1978; Touyama, 1980), and transaxillary (Hoehler, 1973; Watanabe, 1979) (Fig. 46–4).

The submammary incision is commonly used, because it gives the best operative field and is the preferred incision in the case of reoperation.

The transareolar or periareolar incision fails to provide a good operative field.

The transaxillary incision, although normally thought to be the best from an aesthetic point of view, sets off a scar when a sleeveless garment is worn by the patient. Yet with the continuing improvement in operative techniques, this incision is becoming more popular and is now frequently used (see Fig. 46–4).

Selection of the Bag Prosthesis Insertion Site

The site of insertion of a bag prosthesis is behind either the mammary gland or the pectoral major muscle. Which site is better remains controversial; the former has a higher incidence of capsular contracture, although

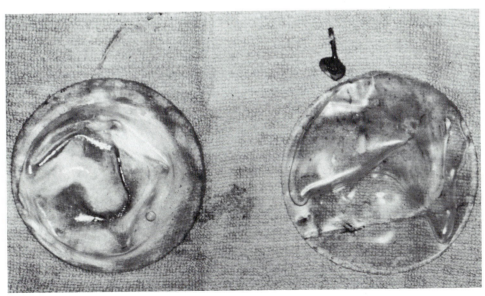

FIGURE 46–3 Leakage of the inflatable bag prosthesis.

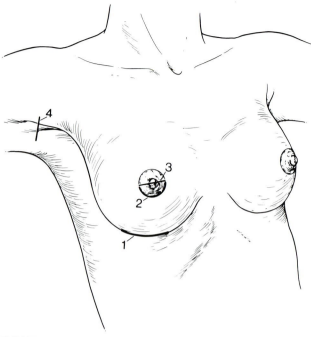

FIGURE 46–4
1, Submammary approach. 2, Periareolar approach. 3, Transareolar approach. 4, Transaxillary approach.

it provides better stability for the prosthesis, whereas the latter has the drawback of a possible movement of the prosthesis caused by the contraction of the muscle (Dempsey and Latham, 1968; Megumi, 1982; Tebbets, 1984).

We still prefer the retromammary placement in primary cases but often employ the retromuscular placement when the patient is lean and has a flat chest or in secondary surgery after removing foreign material injected previously (Ohtake, 1986).

Anesthesia

Although local anesthesia can be used, general anesthesia is preferred for the comfort of the patient. When local anesthesia is used, the pectoral major fascia in the area of the dissection should be well infiltrated with 0.5% lidocaine mixed with epinephrine. In using this procedure, care should be taken to avoid pneumothorax by directing the needle in parallel with the thoracic wall. When general anesthesia is used, epinephrine, diluted 1:200,000, is injected into the site of the incision so as to prevent undue bleeding.

Operative Technique

Design and Incision

SUBMAMMARY APPROACH

The lower margin of the breast is determined and marked with the patient in an upright or sitting position. Then the area in which the bag prosthesis is to be inserted is marked. The patient should not be in a supine position when one is making these determinations, because the breast assumes a different shape in

this position and makes the designing difficult and inaccurate.

The incision is then made one finger's width above the lower margin of the breast and to a length of 3 to 4 cm.

TRANSAREOLAR OR PERIAREOLAR APPROACH

Marking for the pocket is done as for the submammary approach. With the transareolar approach, the design is based on the line traversing the areola, and various modifications are available for expanding this incision (Ezaki, 1980). In the Orient, however, this approach is in disfavor because it causes damage to the mammary gland.

In the periareolar approach, an incision usually is made along the lower margin of the areola. When the expansion of the incision is desired, the authors extend it to both sides by making minor incisions.

TRANSAXILLARY APPROACH

An incision is made on the axillary fold, and it should not exceed the anterior axillary line. It is important to determine accurately the area in the breast to be dissected, particularly in the lower margin.

Dissection

SUBMAMMARY APPROACH

After incision, dissection proceeds basically bluntly, behind the gland and over the pectoral major fascia to secure the space for a bag prosthesis (Fig. 46–5A). For this procedure, a special retractor with lighting has been devised and has proven quite useful (Fig. 46–5B) (Ohtake and Shioya, 1986).

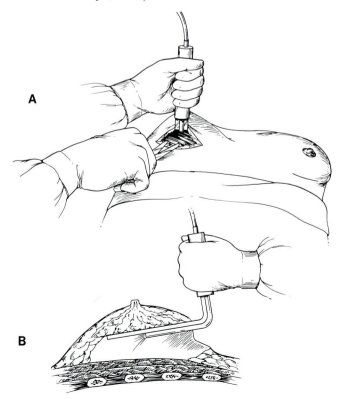

FIGURE 46–5
A, Submammary approach behind the gland. B, A special retractor with lighting is used for examining the pocket.

TRANSAREOLAR OR PERIAREOLAR APPROACH

With the transareolar approach, dissection proceeds vertically, down to the mammary gland; whereas with the periareolar approach the dissection is made around the mammary gland. Care is needed for the hemostasis, because exposure is not adequate with this approach.

TRANSAXILLARY APPROACH

After the skin incision has been made, the dissection progresses along the lateral margin of the greater pectoral muscle. When a pocket is made behind the pectoral muscle major, the lower dissection must be carried out very carefully, because hemostasis is difficult here (Fig. 46–6) (Watanabe et al., 1982).

Insertion of the Bag Prosthesis

Sizers can be used to determine the shape and size, and an appropriate bag prosthesis is inserted. Even when the incision is small, insertion can be achieved by deforming the bag by compression and tucking it in. If a bilateral asymmetry exists between the breasts, it can be corrected by different-sized bag prostheses or differing quantities of saline in the outer lumen of the double-lumen prosthesis.

Drainage

A continuous-suction drain is placed around the bag prosthesis, so that its tube projects through a small separate incision inferior to the lateral portion of the skin incision (Fig. 46–7).

Closure

The connective tissue below the mammary gland is firmly stitched to the thoracic wall with 4-0 synthetic nonabsorbable sutures so as to prevent the bag pros-

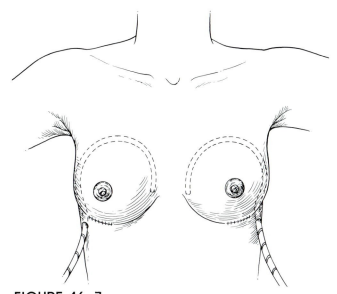

FIGURE 46–7
The preferred position of the suction drain is shown. Note the separate small incision for the drain.

thesis from sagging later. The use of a proper muscle hook or retractor provides protection against possible damage to the bag prosthesis during this procedure. Then intradermal and skin sutures are placed; 4-0 and 5-0 synthetic and nonabsorbable sutures are used, respectively.

Dressing

For the operation involving a bag prosthesis insertion, postoperative dressing is most important; it is virtually an integral part of the operation in terms of controlling bleeding and stabilizing the bag prosthesis.

The operative wound is covered with a gauze dressing and fixed with an elastic adhesive (Fig. 46–8A). This is reinforced by an elastic bandage over the entire chest to give uniform compression to the breast. The dressing is completed when the upper arm is fixed by a bandage that restricts the motion of the shoulder (Fig. 46–8B).

Postoperative Treatment

Rest is most important after the operation; we hospitalize patients for about 2 days. Coughing or vomiting immediately after surgery should be avoided, and patients should be warned that it may cause bleeding. Restricting the movement of the upper arm is important, so as to prevent not only hemorrhage but also a shift in the placement of the bag prosthesis. We make it a rule to have the patient remain at rest for a week.

The drainage tube is removed 48 hours after the operation, but not the dressing, which must continue to exert compression. Sutures are removed on the fourth or fifth postoperative day. On the seventh day all compression is removed, and massage is started. At the same time, the upper arm or arms are freed (Fig. 46–9).

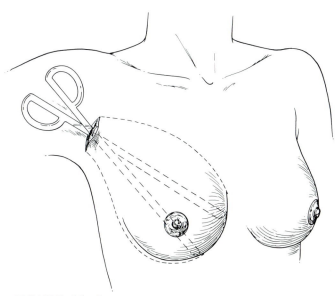

FIGURE 46–6
The transaxillary approach is shown along the lateral margin of the pectoralis major muscle.

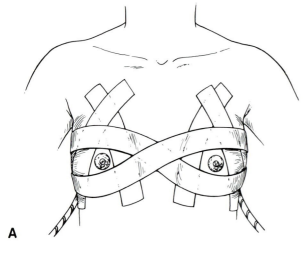

A

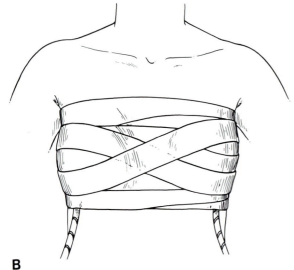

B

FIGURE 46–8
A, Initial gauze dressing fixed with adhesive. B, Elastic bandage applied for uniform compression.

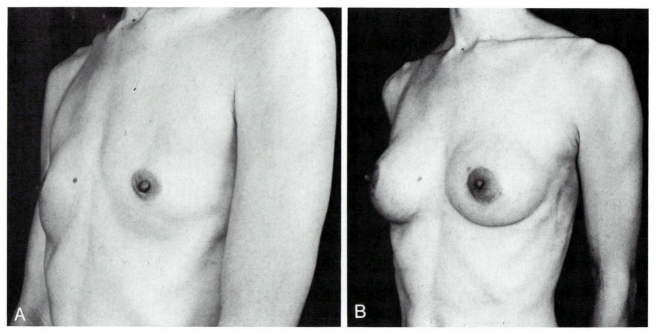

FIGURE 46–9
A, Before augmentation mammaplasty. B, After augmentation mammaplasty.

Complications

Early Complications

HEMORRHAGE AND HEMATOMA

As mentioned previously, adequate hemostasis, good compression, and rest are most important in preventing postoperative bleeding. A drainage tube under the effect of negative pressure may sometimes drain 50 to 100 ml of blood a day in spite of good hemostasis during the operation. No drainage at all suggests the obstruction of the tube; but if there is too much drainage, postoperative hemorrhaging can be strongly suspected. Should a hematoma form, there is no choice but to evacuate the hematoma and stop the bleeding in the operating room.

INFECTION

Precaution against infection cannot be exaggerated when a foreign body is implanted. Prophylactic administration of a broad-spectrum antibiotic is the common practice.

If infection occurs, it is best to remove the bag prosthesis immediately and attempt a second operation 6 months or so after the infection subsides.

Late Complications

AREOLAR DYSESTHESIA

Approximately 15% of all patients reportedly suffer from areolar dysesthesia (Courtiss and Goldwyn, 1976), but this has been said to be resolved in most cases within 6 months (Baker, 1979). This complication, however, is much less common among Orientals.

CAPSULAR CONTRACTURE

Capsular contracture is the most annoying complication associated with augmentation mammaplasty in both Orientals and Occidentals (Fig. 46–10). The thick fibrous capsule around the bag prosthesis contracts and hardens progressively until it becomes markedly deformed. Baker (1979) has classified the severity of the capsular contracture into four grades, and this classification also is used in the Orient. Incidences of this complication have varied with each report, making an analysis difficult.

As to the cause of capsular contracture, several explanations have been proposed. None are considered definitive. One explanation is that a small amount of silicone gel escaping from the bag prosthesis is responsible (Gayon, 1979; Tanino, 1987). Some other authors, however, deny this, pointing out that even with a bag prosthesis with a double lumen, or with a thickened silicone rubber bag that has been developed to prevent leakage, contracture can still occur (Baker et al., 1982).

Infection is blamed in another explanation (Hipps et al., 1978). Infection due to gross contamination is unlikely to occur in a surgical setting, so that what is termed a subclinical infection may pose a problem. Strict sterilization and clean manipulation are a matter of course in every surgical procedure, and systemic prophylactic use of a broad-spectrum antibiotic is also essential because certain organisms like *Staphylococcus*

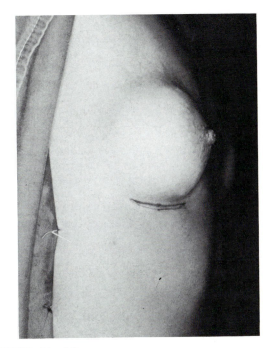

FIGURE 46–10
Capsular contracture.

epidermidis have been found to be present in the mammary glands of healthy women. Another possible cause may be a postoperative hematoma, and every effort should be made to prevent such a development, as has been previously mentioned.

A patient with a keloidal constitution is said to be more apt to suffer capsular contracture, but this has not been proven. We consider postoperative massage helpful in preventing capsular contracture. We begin such treatment about 7 days after the operation and advise the patient to continue this practice for at least 6 months.

Baker's closed capsulotomy (1976) is a popular treatment also in the Orient, and it is performed in outpatient clinics. An open capsulotomy is necessary for severe capsular contracture, and care is needed to prevent injury to a bag prosthesis. To ensure accuracy, a laser knife is sometimes used for cutting the capsule.

Freeman's method (1972) for enlarging the base by cutting along the entire length of the capsule is usually sufficient. Should the case be severe, replacement of the bag prosthesis into the subpectoral space is advisable. The current status of this problem has been summarized by Sugimoto (1987).

EXPOSURE OF THE PROSTHESIS

The exposure of a bag prosthesis is usually caused by a hematoma and/or an infection and sometimes by compression due to the postoperative dressing. If dehiscence due to skin necrosis is noted, early debridement and resuturing could be attempted. If infection is suspected, however, the bag prosthesis had best be removed, and a secondary reconstruction is advised.

UNSIGHTLY SCARS

Any aesthetic operation is not advisable if the patient is found to have a keloidal constitution, although it is not easy to recognize a keloidal tendency preoperatively.

A transaxillar incision may be considered superior in that it provides the least evidence of an operative scar. A transareolar periareolar incision also seems rarely to cause a hypertrophic scar, although a white scar may sometimes be prominent in Orientals with darkly pigmented areolae (Ichida and Shioya, 1982).

ASYMMETRY AND UNNATURAL APPEARANCE

The malpositioning of either or both breast implants is the cause of asymmetry or an unnatural appearance. Improper dissection in making the pocket is usually responsible. Careful designing and a gentle dissection are important. Dressing is also important. The authors make it a rule to apply the dressing after observing the balance between the right and left breasts while the patient is in a semierect position, elevated 45 degrees at the waist (Fig. 46–11).

MASTOPEXY AND REDUCTION MAMMAPLASTY

Although the breast is a symbol of femininity, too large or too pendulous a breast is aesthetically unacceptable, and this may cause mental anguish.

Problems of Reduction Mammaplasty in the Oriental

As has been mentioned, augmentation mammaplasty predominates over reduction mammaplasty among Ori-

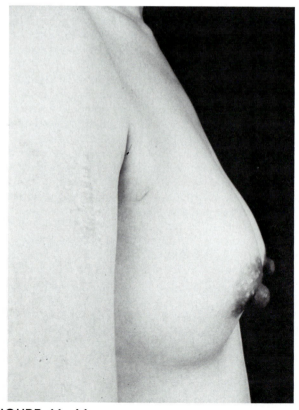

FIGURE 46–11
Malposition.

entals. This is largely due to the small incidence of Asian women with large breasts, as well as to public ignorance of the availability of surgery to remedy this fault.

Most patients who opt to undergo reduction mammaplasty do so not only to achieve aesthetic enhancement but to relieve physical complaints such as intertriginous eczema; stiff shoulders; cervical arthritis; a thoracic deformity; or a brachial, plexus-derived, nerve dysfunction (Uchinuma, 1987). Again, as with other surgery, many patients hesitate to undergo this surgery for fear that it may leave a prominent operative scar, a frequent postoperative occurrence among Orientals (Ichida and Shioya, 1982).

Indications

This operation is not generally indicated at puberty, when the breast is just beginning to develop, together with the rest of the maturing body.

An operation is indicated, however, for cases of giant juvenile hypertrophy, caused by a rare, abnormal reaction of the mammary gland tissue with a hormone; but the decision to operate should be preceded by a full consultation with the patient and her parents, as well as by an examination of the endocrine system.

After adolescence, however, any severe enlargement of the breasts can become an indication for reduction mammaplasty from an aesthetic or functional viewpoint, or both.

Classification

Ptosis and hypertrophy are two separate features, although they often occur combined.

Breast Ptosis (Pendulous Breast)

Breast ptosis (pendulous breast) is defined as the condition of a breast whose nipple is situated at or below the level of the inframammary fold. Regnault's classification (1984) is also applicable to Orientals:

I. The nipple is on the same level of the inframammary fold but above the lower bulge of the breast.
II. The nipple is below the level of the inframammary fold but above the lower bulge of the breast.
III. The nipple is below the level of the inframammary fold and below the lower bulge of the breast.

Breast Hypertrophy

In Occidentals a breast size of 250 to 300 cc is roughly considered best. In Orientals a breast size of about 200 cc would seem appropriate, although no quantitative assessment has been published.

Operative Techniques

Most operative techniques developed by Occidental plastic surgeons for breast surgery are also employed by their Oriental colleagues. Goulian's mastopexy (1971) is

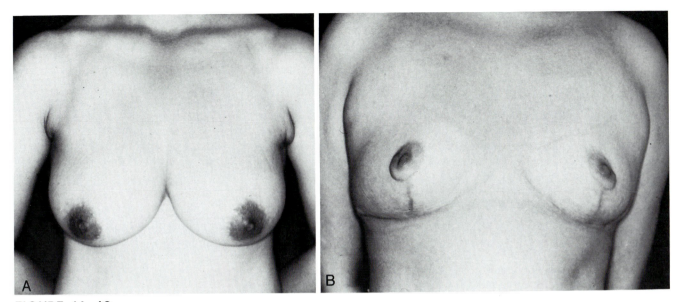

FIGURE 46–12
A, Before reduction mammaplasty. *B*, After reduction mammaplasty.

suitable for a moderate ptosis. McKissock's (1971) or Pitanguy's method (1967) is used for average hypertrophy. Also, in treating some cases of ptotic breasts, augmentation may have to be combined.

Cases where a nipple graft is necessary are less common, and such an operation is rarely performed for Orientals (Fig. 46–12).

Complications

Early Complications

HEMORRHAGE AND HEMATOMA

It must be remembered that adequate precautions to control bleeding during the operation are an important consideration, that care must be taken to secure a good postoperative compression, and that the use of a rather large drainage tube will be required. If the drainage exceeds 100 ml a day, one must reopen the wound to stop bleeding. An unattended hematoma may lead to an impaired blood supply to the nipple and areola, and so early measures are necessary.

INFECTION

To prevent infection, proper prophylaxis is most important. In the Orient, hypertrophic scars resulting from wound complications often mar the primary object of an aesthetic operation. The authors make certain that all patients receive intravenous injection of antibiotics covering a broad spectrum. Intraoperative washing using antibiotics is also important.

CIRCULATORY INSUFFICIENCY AND NECROSIS

Circulatory insufficiency and necrosis have been reported in approximately 1% of all cases (Shirakabe, 1981). The causes include the following: (1) excessive resection of the mammary gland; (2) hematoma; (3) excessive tension of the dermal pedicle; (4) torsion of the dermal pedicle; and (5) excessive tension of the skin brassiere.

Late Complications

DEPRESSION OF THE NIPPLE AND AREOLA

In transposing the nipple and areola, the dermal pedicle is subjected to excessive tension, and the resultant strong force causes the nipple and areola to depress. Further, an excessive resection of the mammary gland produces dead space below the nipple and areola, this also causing a depression.

If the nipple retracts immediately after suturing, a correcting incision is needed, although a slight depression of the areola often only reflects swelling of the adjacent tissue, thus justifying a wait-and-see policy.

OUTSTANDING SCARS

Intradermal sutures should not be placed in the de-epithelialized area, because it is prone to developing cysts. Therefore, scarring becomes highly visible in many cases. This is particularly common among Orientals, and so taping the wound for several months is the recommended procedure.

OTHER COMPLICATIONS

An epidermal inclusion cyst, fat necrosis, and dysesthesia of the nipple are rare complications and quite often are preventable by careful operative manipulation.

INVERTED NIPPLE

A nipple that remains in a constantly retracted state is called an inverted nipple. When it can be reversed by stimulation or by suction, it usually requires no surgical treatment.

Causes of the Inversion

Atrophy or contraction of the bundle of the mammary tracts is the cause, which may be further attributable to one or a combination of the following factors:

1. Impaired development of the mammary tract bundle
2. Scarred adhesion after inflammation of the mammary glands
3. Nipple retraction after reduction mammaplasty
4. Other breast diseases

Degree of Severity

The inverted nipple varies in severity and is generally classified as mild or severe, according to the degree of contraction.

Symptoms and Operative Indications

Surgery is indicated when nonsurgical therapy has had no effect or when prompt treatment is needed (Kami et al., 1985).

This complaint is more common among unmarried patients. Having marriage and pregnancy before them, they are concerned about their appearance and a possible malfunction of lactation. Therefore, a need for not only the preservation of the mammary tracts but also an improvement in the breasts' appearance exists.

Complaints can arise from multiparous women who have experienced difficulty in breast-feeding their first child. In such instances, the preservation of the mammary tracts is more important than the appearance of the breasts.

The depression of the nipple also precipitates deposits, causing repeated inflammation. Many such patients have a history of incisions for drainage. Treatment should be focused on the correction of the depression and a resection of the involved area.

Operative Techniques and Their Selection

A number of operative techniques have been devised and published, including many modifications of each. Only the Japanese literature is reviewed here.

Namba's Method

Namba's technique utilizes Z-plasty, performed around the nipple to tighten the nipple neck and to prevent the nipple from retracting again. During the procedure, the bundle of the mammary tracts must be fully dissected for the nipple to be projected. This method has the advantage of being able to adjust the extent of nipple projection by changing the number, size, and position of the Z-plasty components and is applicable to almost all cases (Fig. 46–13) (Namba and Itoh, 1966).

Sakai's Method

In Sakai's method, the nipple is cut into two skin flaps, with an incision that traverses it. Then the tissue

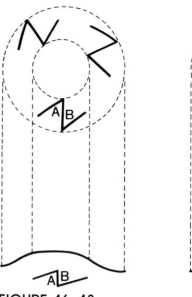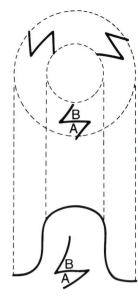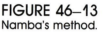

FIGURE 46–13
Namba's method.

surrounding the bundle of the mammary tract is dissected. A spindle-shaped resection of fibrous band characterizes this method. This method is said to allow an adequate resection under direct vision and requires no treatment such as a postoperative suspension. Extension of the lateral walls of the nipple and the tightening of its base are achieved by placing the Z-plasty at the base of the nipple at the time of suture. This method is principally indicated for severe cases, because the preservation of the mammary tract is difficult (Fig. 46–14) (Sakai et al., 1985).

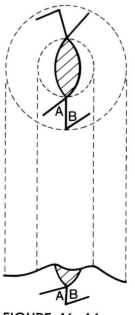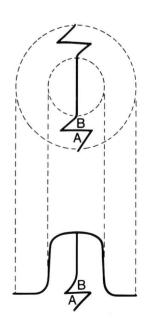

FIGURE 46–14
Sakai's method.

Postoperative Treatment

Suspension

For the nipple to be held in a projected position, it is essential to protect the nipple from compression by using gauze, with an opening in the gauze that matches the nipple size. In cases where retraction or redepression of the nipple is anticipated, its corrected position is secured by using thread passed around the nipple for suspension. Various methods for securing the corrected position have been devised, including the use of dough-nut-shaped gauze (Ichida et al., 1983), a sponge (Kami et al., 1985), and wire and a bolster (Kami and Kim, 1986).

Suction

Continuous use of a suction syringe may be useful in maintaining the nipple in its projected position to prevent a recurrence. The patient is instructed to do this at home.

Complications

Early Complications

An erroneous division of the bundle of the mammary tract, necrosis of a skin flap, and a hematoma are usually preventable by careful manipulation at the time of the operation.

Late Complications

The most frequent complication is a relapse, causing a return of the depression. Should this occur, even after taking the above-mentioned precautions, another operation may be considered. One must always make certain that at the conclusion of the operation the depression has been corrected adequately, so that the nipple will project without the help of a postoperative suspension.

Another late complication is anesthesia, which is usually temporary and is resolved by sensation returning spontaneously in most cases.

GYNECOMASTIA

When a man has large, bulging breasts that resemble those of a woman due to abnormally developed mammary glands, his psychologic pain is great. If he has to bare his chest frequently, he suffers tremendous embarrassment, especially in the Orient, where the daily custom of public bathing still remains. Enduring stares cause him as great a torment as public swimming.

Etiology

Although diseases such as liver cirrhosis and testicular tumors are among the known causes, most cases are idiopathic or related to puberty. It is said that puberty-

TABLE 46–5
Classification of Gynecomastia

Pubertal hypertrophy	7.3%
Endocrine disease	6.8%
Drug-induced hypertrophy	32.3%
Idiopathic hypertrophy	53.7%

From Takatsuka, Y.: Clinical study of 177 cases of gynecomastia. J. Jpn. Surg. Soc. 82:841, 1981.

related gynecomastia usually resolves spontaneously within 2 years.

Classification

Takatsuka (1981) has classified this manifestation according to its etiology and has reported that, generally, gynecomastia caused by an endocrine disturbance shows an effect that is bilateral, whereas gynecomastia that is idiopathic in origin is unilateral (Table 46–5). Because there is no grading classification available in the Oriental literature, the classification proposed by Simon (1976) is used, in which the gynecomastia is graded according to the size of the breast bulge and the amount of excess skin (Table 46–6).

TABLE 46–6
Simon's Classification of Gynecomastia

Grade 1	Small, visible breast enlargement
Grade 2A	Moderate breast enlargement without skin redundancy
Grade 2B	Moderate breast enlargement with skin redundancy
Grade 3	Marked breast enlargement (pendulous female breast)

From Simon, B. E.: Correction of gynecomastia. In: Goldwyn, R. M. (ed.): Plastic and Reconstructive Surgery of the Breast. Boston, Little, Brown, 1976, p. 312.

Operative Indications

Surgery is indicated for an idiopathic type or for a puberty-related hypertrophy that has persisted for 2 or more years. However, some reports justify an operation regardless of the time period, should the patient's mental burden weigh heavily and affect his social life (Tani, 1983).

Some gynecomastia cases have reportedly responded to hormonal therapy (Izumio, 1967). Yamagata (1975), however, denies the effectiveness of hormonal treatment on lesions larger than 5 cm determined by mammography.

Operative Techniques

A mammary gland resection alone by either a periareolar or a transareolar incision suffices for mild cases (grade 2A or less). Recently, treatment by liposuction alone or in combination with surgery has been tried.

Maneuvers of reduction mammaplasty may have to

be employed for moderate to severe cases (grade 2B or more), although with some modification.

Complications

An early postoperative hematoma predominates as a complication, necessitating the insertion of a drainage tube and postoperative compression for good fixation, as well as adequately maintained intraoperative hemostasis.

Complaints of an impaired sensation of the nipple are usually rare.

References

Akiyama, T.: Basic problems of medical use of dimethylpolysiloxane. Jpn. J. Plast. Reconstr. Surg. 1:244, 1958.

Aoki, F., Anze, M., Akao, A.: A case of the so-called human adjuvant's disease which developed after augmentation mammaplasty with DMPS injection. J. J.S.A.P.S. 10:68, 1988.

Baker, J. L.: Augmentation mammaplasty. In: Grabb, W. C., Smith, J. W. (eds.): *Plastic Surgery*. 3rd ed. Boston, Little, Brown, 1979, p. 719.

Baker, J. L., Levier, R. R., Spielvogel, D. E.: Positive identification of silicon in human mammary capsular tissue. Plast. Reconstr. Surg. 69:56, 1982.

Ben-Hur, N., Neuman, Z.: Siliconoma—Another cutaneous response to dimethylpolysiloxane: Experimental study in mice. Plast. Reconstr. Surg. 36:629, 1965.

Chaplin, C. H.: Loss of both breasts from injection of silicone. Plast. Reconstr. Surg. 44:447, 1969.

Conway, H., Goulian, D.: Experience with an injectable Silastic RTV as a subcutaneous prosthetic material. Plast. Reconstr. Surg. 32:294, 1963.

Courtiss, E. H., Goldwyn, R. M.: Breast sensation before and after plastic surgery. Plast. Reconstr. Surg. 58:1, 1976.

Crikelair, G. F.: Scars and keloids. In: Converse, J. M. (ed.): *Reconstructive Plastic Surgery*. Philadelphia, W. B. Saunders, 1987, p. 424.

Cronin, T., Gerow, F.: Augmentation mammaplasty: A new "natural feel" prosthesis. In: Broadbent, T. R. (ed.): *Transactions of the Third International Congress of Plastic Surgery*. Amsterdam, Excerpta Medica Foundation, 1963, p. 41.

Cronin, T. D., Greenberg, R. L.: Our experience with Silastic gel breast prostheses. Plast. Reconstr. Surg. 46:1, 1970.

Dempsey, W., Latham, W.: Subpectoral implants in augmentation mammaplasty. Plast. Reconstr. Surg. 42:515, 1968.

Ezaki, T.: Modified areolar approach. J. J.S.A.P.S. 2:10, 1980.

Freeman, B. S.: Successful treatment of some fibrous envelope contractures around breast implants. Plast. Reconstr. Surg. 50:107, 1972.

Fumiiri, M.: Complications of augmentation mammaplasty using injection material. J. J.S.A.P.S. 2:122, 1980.

Fumiiri, M., Kubota, A., Kobayashi, A.: Postoperative disorders of augmentation mammaplasty by injection method. Jpn. J. Surg. 36:1371, 1974.

Funao, T., Yanagida, J.: Forensic medical study of augmentation mammaplasty. Nihon Iji Shimpo 21:57, 1965.

Gayon, R.: A historical comparison of contracted and noncontracted capsules around silicone breast implants. Plast. Reconstr. Surg. 63:700, 1979.

Gersuny, R.: Über eine subcutane Prosthese. Z. Heilkde. 21:199, 1900.

Goulian, D., Jr.: Dermal mastopexy. Plast. Reconstr. Surg. 47:105, 1971.

Hipps, C. J., Raju, D. R., Straith, R. E.: Influence of some operative and postoperative factors on capsular contracture around breast prostheses. Plast. Reconstr. Surg. 61:3840, 1978.

Höhler, H.: Breast augmentation: The axillary approach. Br. J. Plast. Surg. 26:373, 1973.

Ichida, M., Shioya, N.: Reduction mammaplasty for Japanese women. Jpn. J. Plast. Reconstr. Surg. 23:274, 1980.

Ichida, M., Shioya, N. (eds.): *Atlas of Plastic Surgery 1*. Tokyo, Bunkoudo, 1982.

Ichida, M., Itoh, M., Shioya, N.: The present state of aesthetic surgery in the university hospitals of Japan. J. J.S.A.P.S. 5:48, 1983.

Izumio, M.: Breast tumor of the male. New Medicine 22:2705, 1967.

Kagan, H. D.: Sakurai injectable silicone formula. Arch. Otolaryngol. 78:663, 1963.

Kami, T., Kim, I.: New methods for correction of the inverted nipple. J. J.S.A.P.S. 8:155, 1986.

Kami, T., Nakajima, T., Yoshimura, Y.: Correcting methods of the inverted nipple. J. J.S.A.P.S. 7:192, 1985.

Kumagai, Y.: Scleroderma-like lesion occurrence after augmentation mammaplasty. Clinician 8:2506, 1982.

Koganei, Y., Torikai, K., Uchinuma, E., Shioya, N.: Removal of a foreign body in the breast. Jpn. J. Coll. Surg. 10:42, 1984.

McKissock, P. K.: Reduction mammaplasty with a vertical dermal pedicle. Plast. Reconstr. Surg. 49:245, 1971.

Megumi, Y.: Subglandular and subpectoral insertion of mammary prosthesis. J. J.S.A.P.S. 4:13, 1982.

Miyoshi, K., Miyaoka, T., Kobayashi, Y., et al.: Hypergamma globulinemia by adjuvant reaction in humans. Postoperative disorders after augmentation mammaplasty. Nihon Iji Shimpo 2122:9, 1964.

Mutoh, Y.: Experiences using the injection method. Jpn. J. Plast. Reconstr. Surg. 7:283, 1964.

Mutoh, Y.: Experience with an augmentation mammaplasty using the bag prosthesis. Jpn. J. Plast. Reconstr. Surg. 11:205, 1968.

Mutoh, Y.: Augmentation mammaplasty in Japan. J. J.S.A.P.S. 2:67, 1980.

Mutoh, Y.: Augmentation mammaplasty. In Namba, Y., Shioya, N., Osada, M. (eds.): *Aesthetic Plastic Surgery*. Tokyo, Nankoudo, 1987, p. 625.

Namba, K., Itoh, T.: Some devices for surgical repair of inverted nipple. Jpn. J. Plast. Reconstr. Surg. 9:93, 1966.

Namba, K.: Keloids and hypertrophic scars. Operation 38:257, 1984.

Narita, M.: Basic factors of dimethylpolysiloxane in plastic surgery. Jpn. J. Plast. Reconstr. Surg. 1:299, 1958.

Ohhashi, Y., Kitamura, S., Watanabe, I.: A case of human adjuvant disease after augmentation mammaplasty. Jpn. J. Pathol. 7:383, 1978.

Ohkubo, M.: A histopathological study of complications after augmentation mammaplasty. Jpn. J. Plast. Reconstr. Surg. 6:913, 1986.

Ohsumi, N., Inoue, M., Kitajima, Y., et al.: Therapeutic experience of gynecomastia. J. J. S. A. P. S. 10:57, 1988.

Ohtake, N., Itoh, M., Shioya, N.: Postoperative sequelae of augmentation mammaplasty by injection method in Japan. Aesthetic Plast. Surg. 1988 (In press).

Ohtake, N., Shioya, N.: Augmentation mammaplasty. Operation 40:547, 1986.

Ortiz-Monasterio, F., Trigos, I.: Management of patients with complications from injection of materials into the breast. Plast. Reconstr. Surg. 50:42, 1972.

Pitanguy, I.: Surgical treatment of breast hypertrophy. Br. J. Plast. Surg. 20:78, 1967.

Pitanguy, I. (ed.): *Aesthetic Plastic Surgery of Head and Body*. New York, Springer-Verlag, 1981.

Regnault, P., Daniel, R. K.: Breast reduction. In: Regnault, P., Daniel, R. K. (eds.): *Aesthetic Plastic Surgery*. Boston, Little, Brown, 1984, p. 499.

Sakai, S., Ando, K., Tanabe, H.: Correction of the severely inverted nipple. Jpn. J. Plast. Reconstr. Surg. 28:323, 1985.

Sakaki, K., Kimura, K.: A study in somatometric measurement of the freshman students of Tokyo Women's Medical College. Journal of Tokyo Women's Medical College 55:36, 1985.

Shirakabe, M.: Reduction mammaplasty. J. J.S.A.P.S. 3:1, 1981.

Simon, B. E.: Correction of gynecomastia. In: Goldwyn, R. M. (ed.): *Plastic and Reconstructive Surgery of the Breast*. Boston, Little, Brown, 1976, p. 305.

Sonoda, T., Uchiyama, M., Nakajima, H., Nagai, R.: A case of scleroderma after augmentation mammaplasty by silicon injection. Clin. Dermatol. 5:339, 1983.

Sugimoto, T.: Capsular contracture. In: Shioya, N., Soeda, S., Tsukada, S. (eds.): *Color Atlas of Plastic and Reconstructive Surgery 6*. Tokyo, Medical View, 1987, p. 72.

Takahashi, R., Honda, Y.: Histopathologic study of paraffinoma. Jpn. J. Plast. Reconstr. Surg. 1:73, 1958.

Takatsuka, Y.: Clinical study of 177 cases of gynecomastia. Jpn. J. Surg. 82:841, 1981.

Tani, N., Midera, J., Kondo, S.: Experience with surgical treatment of gynecomastia. J. J.S.A.P.S. 5:75, 1983.

Tanino, R.: Complication of augmentation mammaplasty. In: Namba, K., Shioya, N., Osada, M., (eds.): *Aesthetic Plastic Surgery*. Tokyo, Nankoudo, 1987, p. 644.

Tebbets, J. B.: Transaxillary subpectoral augmentation mammaplasty: Long term follow-up and refinements. Plast. Reconstr. Surg. 74:636, 1984.

Touyama, Y., Touyama, K.: Augmentation mammaplasty by trans-areolar incision. J. J.S.A.P.S. 2:140, 1980.

Uchinuma, E., Itoh, M., Shioya, N.: The attitude of contemporary Japanese to plastic surgery. Jpn. J. Plast. Reconstr. Surg. 25:78, 1982.

Uchinuma, E.: Reduction mammaplasty. In: Shioya, N., Tsukada, S., Soeda, S. (eds.): *Color Atlas of Plastic and Reconstructive Surgery 6*. Tokyo, Medical View, 1987, p. 66.

Watanabe, K.: Transaxillary approach of augmentation mammaplasty. J. J.S.A.P.S. 1:124, 1979.

Watanabe, K., Tsurukiri, K., Fuji, Y.: Subpectoral-transaxillary method of breast augmentation in Orientals. Aesthetic Plast. Surg. 6:231, 1982.

Yamagata, J.: Evaluation of 89 cases of gynecomastia: Diagnosis by mammography and the effect of hormone treatment. Clin. Endocrinol. (Tokyo) 23:801, 1975.

Yanagisawa, S.: The study of Japanese habits. Tokyo, Kobunkan, 1976.

GYNECOMASTIA

Ronald Riefkohl
Eugene H. Courtiss

47

Gynecomastia

Gynecomastia literally means "woman-breast" and refers to an enlargement of the male breast caused by an increase in glandular, stromal, or adipose tissue. Gynecomastia most often is defined simply as any visible or palpable development of mammary contour, despite the fact that 35% of normal men have palpable breast tissue greater than 2 cm in diameter on one or both sides (Ley et al., 1980). Furthermore, an autopsy study of 447 normal male subjects revealed that 40% had histologic evidence of gynecomastia, but only 4 of the subjects had gross enlargement of the breast (Williams, 1963).

Because of these findings, some suggest restricting the term "gynecomastia" to normal pubertal changes taking place in nearly every male individual, and applying the term "macromastia" to a female-like breast (Ley et al., 1980). Uniformity of terminology would be helpful because proper therapy is predicated on specific diagnosis and the recognition of etiologic factors.

INCIDENCE

In a study of 1855 nonobese Boy Scouts, Nydick et al. (1961) observed an overall incidence of gynecomastia of 38.7% in Caucasians and 28.9% in blacks with a peak incidence of 65% occurring in the 14 to 14½-year-old age group. Of 173 boys who were examined for 2 consecutive years, 24% had persistent gynecomastia for 2 years; and of 52 boys examined for 3 consecutive years, 36% had gynecomastia for 3 years. Unfortunately, although the gynecomastia was graded on a scale of 1 to 4, based on size from 0.5 to 2.5 cm, the number of patients in each subcategory was not stated.

The incidence of gynecomastia in older normal men is about 35% (Nuttall, 1979) with a progressive increase in incidence with advancing age if gynecomastia is defined as an asymptomatic, palpable, discrete button of firm, subareolar tissue measuring at least 2 cm in diameter (Carlson, 1980).

There is a wide variation in the reported frequency of bilaterality versus unilaterality, with the majority of series reporting between 25% and 50% incidence of bilaterality (Bannayan, 1972; Hamer, 1975; Von Kessel et al, 1963; Wheeler et al., 1946). The incidence of bilaterality was 75% among the normal young males reported by Nydick et al. (1961).

The occurrence of gynecomastia in prepubertal ages is unusual in the absence of hormonal abnormalities.

Among 23 cases of prepubertal gynecomastia, 5 patients had interstitial cell tumors of the testes (August et al., 1972; Simon and Hoffman, 1976).

ETIOLOGY

Gynecomastia may be associated with a wide variety of dissimilar causative factors (Table 47–1), but the final common pathway usually involves a relative or absolute excess of circulating estrogens, a deficiency of circulating androgens, or a defect in androgen receptors (Carlson, 1980). Although a substantial number of patients with gynecomastia have an underlying disturbance in steroid hormone physiology, the ratio of estrogen to androgen levels is far more important than the absolute level of either hormone (Rodriquez-Rigau and Smith, 1979; Wilson et al., 1980).

Physiologic gynecomastia occurs in newborn male infants because of the action of placental hormones. It persists for only a few weeks (Nuttall, 1979). The specific

TABLE 47–1
Classification

Physiologic
Newborn
Adolescence
Aging (involutional)
Pathologic
Deficient production or action of testosterone
Congenital anorchia
Klinefelter's syndrome
Androgen resistance
Testicular feminization
Reifenstein's syndrome
Defects in testosterone synthesis
Secondary testicular failure
Viral orchitis
Trauma
Increased estrogen production
Excessive estrogen secretion
True hermaphroditism
Testicular tumors
Carcinoma of the lung
Increased substrate for peripheral aromatase
Adrenal disease
Liver disease
Malnutrition
Hyperthyroidism
Increase in peripheral aromatase
Drugs
Familial

cause of physiologic gynecomastia occurring during adolescence has not been precisely defined; however, it is probably caused by an imbalance resulting from free estradiol increasing more rapidly than free androgen (Carlson, 1980). When the serum estrogen/testosterone ratio returns to normal, gynecomastia should recede. Involutional, or senescent, gynecomastia is probably caused by a varying degree of testicular failure and resulting decrease in the total as well as the free androgen level, combined with an increase in luteinizing hormone (LH) (Carlson, 1980). Additionally, obesity favors increased peripheral aromatization of androgens to estrogens (Carlson, 1980). The decreased androgen, increased estrogen, and increased androgen-to-estrogen conversion combine to cause a predominant estrogen effect. There may be as yet unrecognized subtle imbalances in hormone metabolism that may better explain the occurrence of physiologic gynecomastia (Rodriquez-Rigau and Smith, 1979).

A wide variety of pathologic states are associated with gynecomastia. It is convenient to consider them as due to either a deficiency of testosterone or an excess of estrogen. The serum prolactin level is normal in most patients with gynecomastia, and elevated serum prolactin *per se* is not ordinarily associated with gynecomastia (Carlson, 1980).

Gynecomastia is more common in primary testicular failure (congenital anorchia, Klinefelter's and Reifenstein's syndromes) than in secondary testicular failure (pituitary hypothalamic hypogonadism) (Carlson, 1980). Reifenstein's syndrome (hypospadias and gynecomastia) is a form of androgen resistance caused by an abnormality of the cytoplasmic androgen receptor protein (Wilson, 1980).

Increased estrogen production is commonly associated with neoplasm. Feminizing adrenal tumors that secrete estrogen, or estrogen precursors such as androstenedione, are rare malignant tumors usually diagnosed by palpation of an abdominal mass and an increase in urine 17-ketosteroids (Carlson, 1980). Leydig cell tumors are rare and benign tumors that, by producing estradiol, suppress pituitary LH secretion which in turn, decreases testosterone production from normal Leydig cells (Carlson, 1980). These tumors are usually easily palpated, but an occasional small tumor cannot be diagnosed except by spermatic vein catheterization for serum estradiol levels (Carlson, 1980). Rarely, testicular tomography or radioisotope scans may be necessary. Malignant tumors of testicular germinal elements often produce human chorionic gonadotropin, which stimulates Leydig cells to produce excessive estradiol. These tumors also extract steroid hormone precursors and convert them to estrogens (Carlson, 1980). Hepatomas may also produce estrogens by converting estrogen precursors (Carlson, 1980).

The hypogonadism of protein calorie malnutrition occurs primarily on the basis of diminished Leydig cell function (Jacobs, 1948; Smith et al., 1975). Malnutrition impairs the function of both Leydig cells and the pituitary gland, resulting in hypogonadism. When nutrition is restored, gonadotropin secretion and gonadal function return to normal, producing a "second puberty." This "refeeding gynecomastia" is associated with many

TABLE 47–2
Drugs

Estrogenlike effects
Estrogens, heroin, marijuana
Androgens
Gonadotropins
Inhibit testosterone
Spironolactone, cimetidine, cyproterone, flutamide, clofibrate
Refeeding mechanism
Digitalis, isoniazid
CNS agents
Phenothiazines, amphetamines, tricyclic antidepressants, sympathetic modifiers
Cytotoxic agents
Bulsulfan, vincristine, nitrosoureas
Unknown mechanisms
Ethionamide, methyldopa, reserpine, diazepam

chronic debilitating illnesses in which there is a significant weight loss followed by a weight gain, such as congestive heart failure, renal failure, and tuberculosis.

Gynecomastia associated with hepatic disorders, especially alcoholic cirrhosis, is caused by a decreased serum testosterone as well as an excess estrogen conversion from circulating estrogen precursors, plus an increase in the sex-steroid binding globulin, which further reduces free testosterone (Carlson, 1980). About 10% to 40% of patients with hyperthyroidism also have gynecomastia, probably because of an increase in sex-steroid binding globulin and active peripheral tissue conversion of precursors to estrogens (Carlson, 1980).

Gynecomastia may develop when a functioning testis is damaged by an infectious chemical, or physical agent, yet does not develop when the testes are removed altogether (Forbes, 1978). As a general rule, gynecomastia caused by androgen stimulation recedes, whereas that due to estrogen stimulation persists (Paulsen, 1974).

A wide variety of drugs cause gynecomastia (Table 47–2). Ten of the 100 most commonly prescribed drugs, and 16 of the 200 most commonly prescribed drugs have been associated with gynecomastia (Rodriquez-Rigau and Smith, 1979; Smith et al., 1975). Few of the mechanisms whereby drugs induce gynecomastia are clearly understood (Carlson, 1980; Rodriquez-Rigau and Smith, 1979).

Familial gynecomastia is rare. It may be caused by altered end-organ (breast) metabolism, which predisposes the patient to gynecomastia despite normal hormone levels (Rodriquez-Rigau and Smith, 1979). It has been suggested that Tutankhamen and his brothers had familial gynecomastia (Paulschock, 1980).

CLINICAL EVALUATION

The evaluation of the patient with gynecomastia begins with a careful history with particular attention to the use of drugs and possible unknown exposure to estrogens (Table 47–3). The age of onset, the presence of symptoms and their duration, the presence of other systemic diseases and their duration, and a history of recent weight gain or weight loss are particularly rele-

TABLE 47–3
Evaluation of the Patient

History and physical examination
Chest x-ray
Liver enzymes
Urine 17-ketosteroids, 17-hydroxysteroids, estrone, estradiol, estriol, human chorionic gonadotropins
Serum follicle-stimulating hormone, luteinizing hormone
Serum prolactin, lateral skull x-ray
Computed tomographic scan of abdomen
Spermatic vein catheterization
Testicular tomography or radioisotope scan

vant. In most series, only 10% to 20% of patients experience pain, whereas approximately one-third have tenderness. However, there is usually a 4- to 6-month history of pain or tenderness in the pubertal gyneco-

mastia. Probably the most common complaints mentioned to the physician will be embarrassment and anxiety sufficient to prevent participation in activities where the breast abnormality will be evident to others.

On physical examination, the breasts may be well-formed and similar to those seen in the young female (Fig. 47–1); or there may be a small subareolar, discoid plaque having a rubbery consistency, unattached to either skin or underlying tissues. In some patients, the breast enlargement may be indistinguishable from surrounding fat. The breast enlargement is centrally located in over 90% of the patients (Bannayan and Hajdu, 1972). Most patients have bilateral involvement, which may be asymmetric. About 80% of the patients with bilateral involvement have a history of simultaneous enlargement. The projection as well as the diameter should be noted, because excessive projection may be

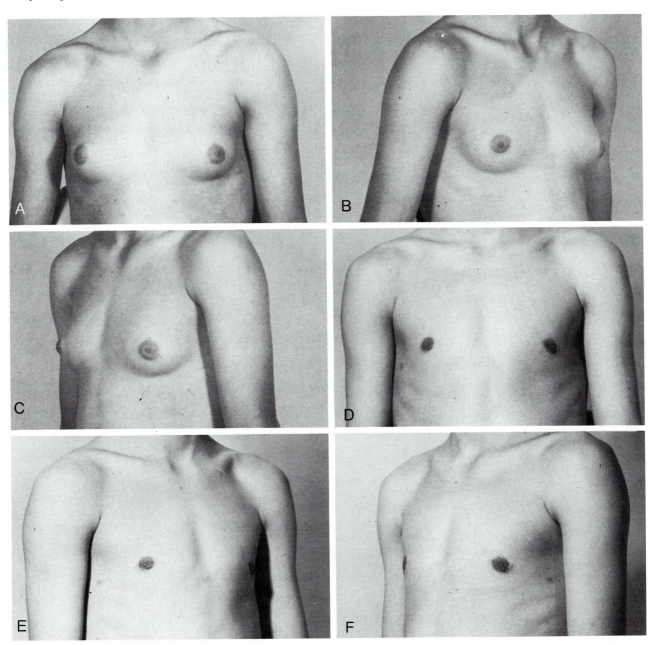

FIGURE 47–1
A to F, Preoperative and postoperative photographs of a 17-year-old boy with moderate gynecomastia corrected through a Webster inferior hemisphere intra-areolar incision.

more disturbing to the patient than an increase in diameter. Nipple hypertrophy associated with gynecomastia is very rare, being found in less than 2% of the patients, and the areola is only rarely enlarged (Bannayan and Hajdu, 1972). A nipple discharge may occur in patients taking androgen medications, those with gynecomastia of long duration, and those with carcinoma of the prostate treated with estrogens (Haagensen, 1971). Also, phenothiazines, reserpine, methyldopa, and other drugs that influence prolactin may be associated with nipple discharge (Haagensen, 1971).

Gynecomastia must be differentiated from carcinoma of the breast. Carcinoma is suspected when there are findings such as a bloody nipple discharge, tumor fixation, skin ulceration, unusual firmness, asymmetry, eccentric location, and adenopathy (Carlson, 1980). It should be noted that gynecomastia does not predispose to carcinoma of the breast, nor is there an association between the two entities, but carcinoma may, on occasion, be found in a male breast with gynecomastia (Fig. 47–2).

The differential diagnosis also includes lipoma, hemangioma, neurofibroma, adipose tissue (pseudogynecomastia), and an enlarged pectoralis major muscle. If no abnormalities are evident on the physical examination, screening tests or more sophisticated studies may be necessary to define the etiology (see Table 47–3).

Mammograms are unnecessary for the diagnosis unless malignancy is suspected; however, malignancy should be easily diagnosed on physical examination. Xeromammograms may be useful to differentiate glandular enlargement from fatty tissue in the older patient. Though there is a report of 40% incidence of microscopic gynecomastia among a series of 97 patients with male breast carcinoma (Heller, 1978), a 40% incidence of microscopic gynecomastia has been reported in an autopsy study of 447 subjects (Williams, 1963). The

intensity of the search for the cause of gynecomastia should be tempered by the clinical setting. An elderly individual with a recent onset of symptomatic gynecomastia should undergo a more thorough evaluation than one with longstanding asymptomatic gynecomastia. The latter is more likely to be physiologic in nature. In one series, 71% of the adults with gynecomastia had a serious underlying disorder (Wheeler et al., 1946); yet in another series, 62% of 68 veterans with recent symptomatic gynecomastia had taken one or more medications known to cause gynecomastia.

PATHOLOGY

There is no clear relationship between the histologic feature and the clinical conditions responsible for gynecomastia. Probably the histologic picture undergoes a progression of changes with time, regardless of the etiology (Rodriquez-Rigau and Smith, 1979). There are three recognized pathologic patterns: florid, fibrous, and intermediate (Bannayan and Hajdu, 1972). In the florid type, there is an increase in the number and length of ducts, proliferation of ductal epithelium, periductal edema, a highly cellular fibroblastic stroma and hypervascularity, and the formation of pseudolobules (Fig. 47–3). In the fibrous type, there are dilated ducts with minimal proliferation of epithelium, absence of periductal edema, and an almost acellular fibrous stroma without adipose tissue (Fig. 47–4). The florid type is most common in gynecomastia of less than 4 months' duration, whereas the fibrous type is most common in gynecomastia of between 4 and 12 months' duration, and the intermediate type is an overlapping pattern of both florid and fibrous types, and apparently seldom regresses. When parenchymal changes predominate (florid type), hormonal imbalances are probably respon-

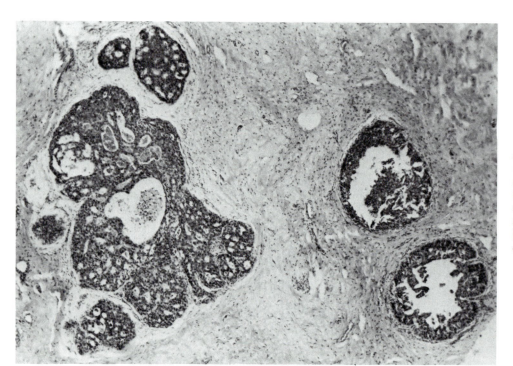

FIGURE 47–2
A 62-year-old man with a long history of alcoholic cirrhosis and testicular atrophy underwent a bilateral gynecomastia excision. Routine sections through the left breast disclosed a small focus of carcinoma.

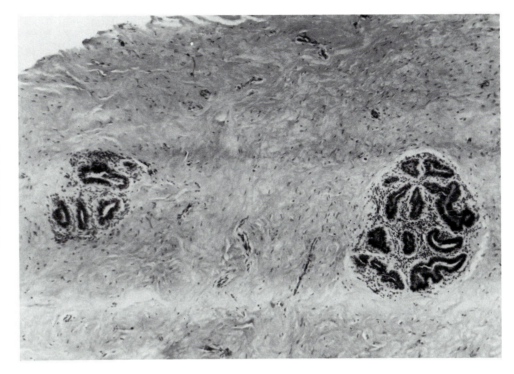

FIGURE 47–3
In the florid type of gynecomastia there is an increase in the number and length of ducts, proliferation of ductal epithelium, periductal edema, a highly cellular fibroblastic stroma and hypervascularity, and the formation of pseudo-lobules.

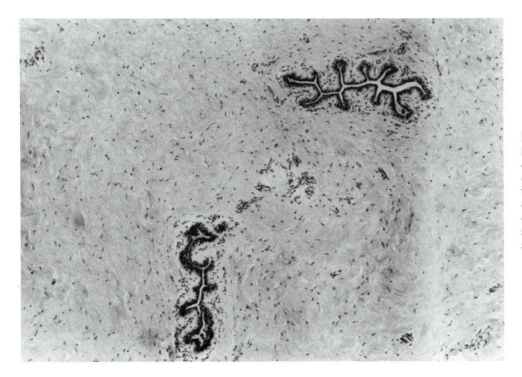

FIGURE 47–4
In the fibrous type of gynecomastia, there are dilated ducts with minimal proliferation of epithelium, absence of periductal edema, and an almost acellular fibrous stroma without adipose tissue.

sible; whereas if stromal changes predominate (fibrous type), unknown factors are probably responsible (Paulsen, 1974).

It should be emphasized that hyperplastic histologic changes indistinguishable from classic gynecomastia may be found in breasts that are not obviously enlarged, with an 8.5% incidence of the florid type and a 31% incidence of the fibrous type (Williams, 1963).

In some patients the cause of the mammary enlargement is fat, indistinguishable from other fat.

TREATMENT

Except for the rare case with disabling pain and tenderness, gynecomastia *per se* does not require specific therapy. However, gynecomastia should not be ignored, because in a substantial number of patients there is an underlying reversible cause.

Most patients seen by the plastic surgeon request treatment for psychologic reasons. The object is to restore a healthy body image. Because transient gynecomastia is common during puberty and adolescence, a simple explanation and reassurance usually suffices, particularly when the enlargement is minimal. However, if there is massive gynecomastia, or excessive projection, treatment may be justified, because these patients may be victimized by their classmates during a critical emotional period, and long-lasting emotional scars may be the result (Rees, 1977). Additionally, gynecomastia of any size that persists beyond an 18- to 24-month period is unlikely to resolve spontaneously. There is controversy regarding treatment in the adolescent age group. Good judgment determines appropriate management; but if there is any question, the advice of a psychiatrist or psychologist should be sought. When gynecomastia is present in an older individual and an underlying cause cannot be identified, the decision for or against treatment will depend on the individual's psychological needs, because in many cases regression will occur spontaneously in 6 to 12 months (Haagensen, 1971).

Pubertal gynecomastia has been successfully treated with several different drugs. Clomiphene, an anti-estrogen, may be used to provide relief and speed regression in a patient with disabling gynecomastia that is self-limited, such as during puberty and "refeeding" gynecomastia, or for the patient with incurable carcinoma. Clomiphene was successful in 65% of a group of patients, all between the ages of 15 and 19, who had gynecomastia for more than 2 years. If there is no response by 3 months, it is unlikely that there will be a response at all (LeRoith et al., 1980). Danazol, a weak androgen that both suppresses gonadotropin secretion and lowers testicular production of testosterone, has been reported to result in a marked reduction of gynecomastia in 60% of the patients treated and a moderate reduction in 25% (Buckle, 1977, 1980; Plano, 1980). Unfortunately, there are side effects, such as weight gain, minor alteration in liver function, acne and increased skin oiliness, and muscle aches. Testosterone is only administered to patients with hypogonadism (Carlson, 1980).

The incidence of estrogen-induced breast enlargement subsequent to diethylstilbestrol administration for carcinoma of the prostate is about 70%, and many of these patients also complain of severe breast pain. If the breasts are irradiated prior to administration of diethylstilbestrol, then breast changes can be prevented or minimized in 90% of the patients. Radiation should be given 2 or more days before estrogen administration by delivering 300 to 500 rads to each breast for 3 alternate or consecutive days (Gagnon et al., 1979; Waterfall and Glaser, 1979). If it is necessary to administer estrogens immediately, 800 rads should be given in one dose to each breast. If the patient already has painful gynecomastia, 500 rads in five fractions may relieve the pain but will not affect the breast enlargement.

Currently, surgical resection is the standard method of treatment. The objectives are resection of the abnormal tissue while restoring the normal male breast contour and minimizing scarring or residual deformity of the breast, nipple, or areola (Simon and Hoffman, 1976). Suction lipectomy is applicable in many patients, either combined with excision or in place of excision (Courtiss, 1987). Suction removes fat; however, glandular tissue cannot be removed by suction. Gynecomastia may be classified by size, for simplifying the choice of surgical technique, into two types: the patient either will or will not require skin reduction in addition to excision of hypertrophic breast tissue. Generally, skin shrinkage is greater in younger than in older individuals; thus, a moderate skin redundancy in an older patient may require excision, whereas in a younger patient the skin will shrink to the reduced breast size (Simon et al., 1973).

There are many different incisions described for the excision of the male breast. Webster (1946) is credited with originating the intra-areolar incision, but it was actually described previously by Dufourmentel in 1928 (Fig. 47–5A). The incision, placed just inside the margin of the areola, extends for a varying length of time along the circumference of the areola. With small areolae, or very large breasts, the infra-areolar incision may be enlarged by lateral and medial extension (Simon et al., 1973) (Fig. 47–5B). The transverse nipple-areola incision is quite popular. However, there is some disadvantage to this approach because of the limited exposure (Forbes, 1978; Simon and Hoffman, 1976) (Fig. 47–5C). Frequently, a distorting infolding of the areola occurs above an inferior areolar incision. This may be prevented by excising a crescent of epithelium above the areola adjacent to a superior areolar incision (Letterman, 1969) (Fig. 47–5D). The technique as described by Ely (1988) utilizing a triple-V incision appears to give maximum exposure (Fig. 47–5D). A transaxillary incision has been recommended because of the advantage of absent scars on the chest wall, but the disadvantage is a more difficult glandular resection (Balch, 1978).

Often, redundant skin must be removed to prevent a postoperative deformity. A crescent of skin may be de-epithelialized above the areola (Letterman and Schurter, 1969) if there is minimal skin redundancy (Fig. 47–5D). However, if there is considerable skin redundancy, other techniques may be necessary. The skin and breast may

FIGURE 47–5

A, Webster intra-areolar incision placed in the inferior hemisphere. *B*, To obtain additional exposure, extensions can be added to the Webster incision. *C*, Transverse nipple-areolar incision. Some surgeons circumscribe the nipple, and others use only the radius, rather than the diameter, for the incision. *D*, Periareolar incision placed in the superior hemisphere of the areola with a crescent of the supra-areolar skin de-epithelialized so that nipple-areolar ptosis can be corrected. *E*, The triple-V incision is used for maximum exposure, as suggested by Ely.

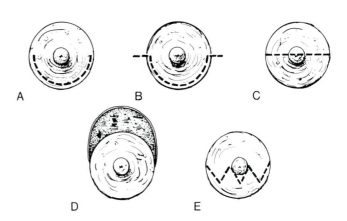

be amputated after removing and replacing the nipple and areola as a free graft (Simon et al., 1973; Simon and Hoffman, 1976). There are numerous techniques for transposing the nipple on a de-epithelialized dermal pedicle. Probably the best method is the laterally based technique (Letterman and Schurter, 1972). Finally, a concentric circle of periareolar skin may be de-epithelialized, which thereby reduces the amount of skin (Fig. 47–6) with moderate reductions. The advantages are a final circular scar, a good blood supply to the nipple and areola, excellent access to the glandular excision, and the possibility of nipple relocation to a higher level if necessary (Eade, 1974).

SURGICAL TECHNIQUE

The Webster intra-areolar incision is employed for patients with small or moderate degrees of gynecomastia (see Fig. 47–1). For larger breasts, the concentric circle technique may provide better exposure for the resection as well as skin reduction (Fig. 47–7). For massive breasts, more skin removal is necessary than the concentric circle technique can provide. In all patients, the extent of the palpable enlargement of the breast tissue is outlined on the skin preoperatively while the patient is standing. Either local or general anesthesia may be chosen. Adolescents who have only excessively projecting "buttons" of breast tissue and others may prefer a local anesthetic.

The thickness of the nipple-areola and that of the breast skin flap are determined by estimating the thickness of the fat on the chest wall outside the breast region; the incision is continued through the fat and underlying breast tissue to this predetermined depth.

The nipple-areola flap and breast skin flaps are elevated at this thickness to the preoperatively outlined extent of the breast with sharp instruments or a suction cannula. If the breast enlargement is due to fat, suction alone may produce the desired result. If not, classic excision is indicated. With accurate estimation of the extent of the hypertrophied tissue and the thickness of the fat on the chest wall, the dissection should reach the pectoralis major muscle fascia very near the preoperatively estimated breast limits (Fig. 47–8). The circumscribed hypertrophic tissue is then excised from the underlying pectoralis major fascia. Contouring by suction lipectomy may be done before or after the excision. Thorough hemostasis is secured; and through a stab wound inferolaterally, a silicone suction catheter is placed within the wound. A few sutures reapproximate the subcutaneous tissues and the transdermal incision (Fig. 47–9).

Gynecomastia in the patient with a large volume of breast tissue can be managed well by means of the triple-V approach as described by Ely and shown in Figure 47–10.

Occasionally, a patient has an extreme degree of skin redundancy that cannot be corrected by the concentric circle technique. Any of the available skin-reduction techniques are acceptable, but the patient should be forewarned about the scars outside the areola.

RESULTS AND COMPLICATIONS

Usually, patients are satisfied with the result. These individuals were ashamed of their transsexual appearance and signs of femininity and were embarrassed about participating in sports or swimming.

The complication rate is low (Table 47–4), and most

Text continued on page 667

FIGURE 47–6

A, The diameter of the concentric circle is determined by adding 0.8 times the radius of the areola to the radius of the areola. For example, if the radius of the areola is 20 mm, the radius of the concentric circle will be 36 mm (20 + 0.8 × 20). *B*, The discrepancy in skin margins is reduced by serially bisecting the closure, thus distributing the redundancy evenly around the areola.

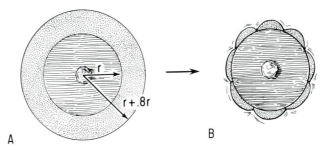

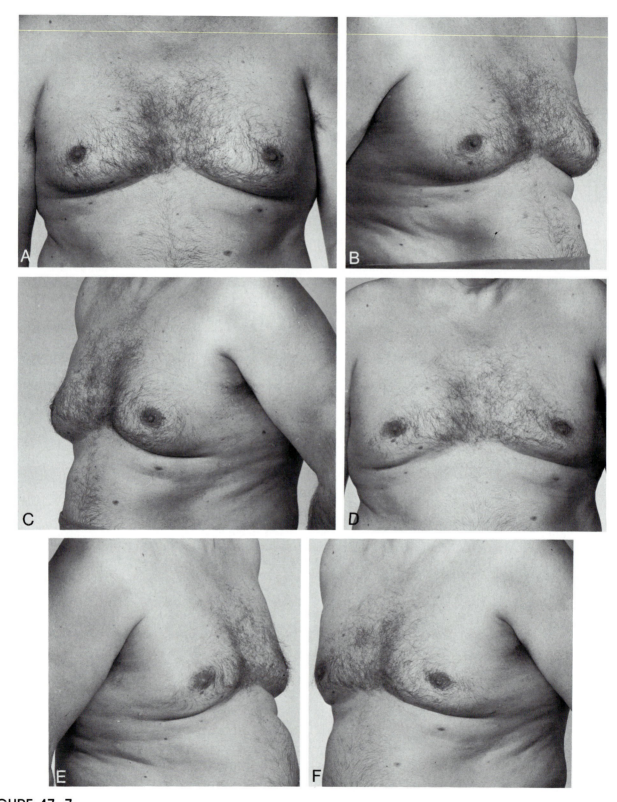

FIGURE 47–7
A to *F*, Preoperative and postoperative photographs of a 48-year-old man with moderate gynecomastia corrected by the concentric-circle technique. Note the faint periareolar scarring.

FIGURE 47–8

A sagittal section depicting development of the skin flap and excision of the hypertrophic breast tissue.

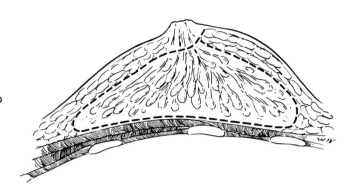

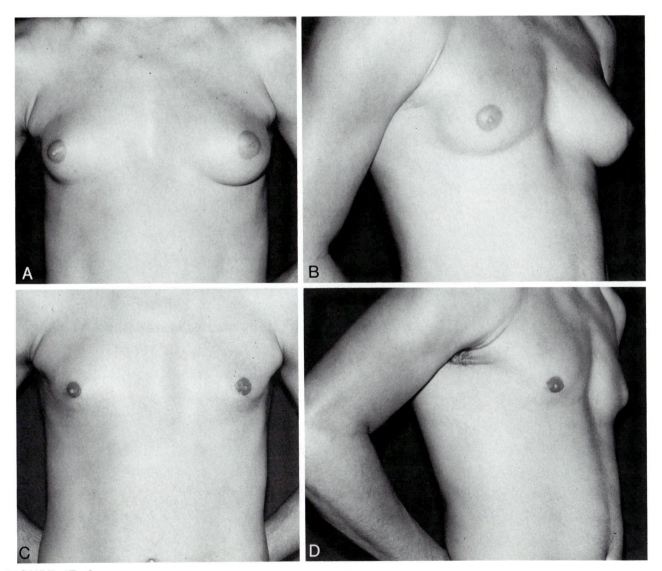

FIGURE 47–9

A and *B,* An 18-year-old male patient is shown prior to correction of gynecomastia. *C* and *D,* The same patient is shown 10 months after parenchymal excision utilizing an intra-areolar incision and suction of fat.

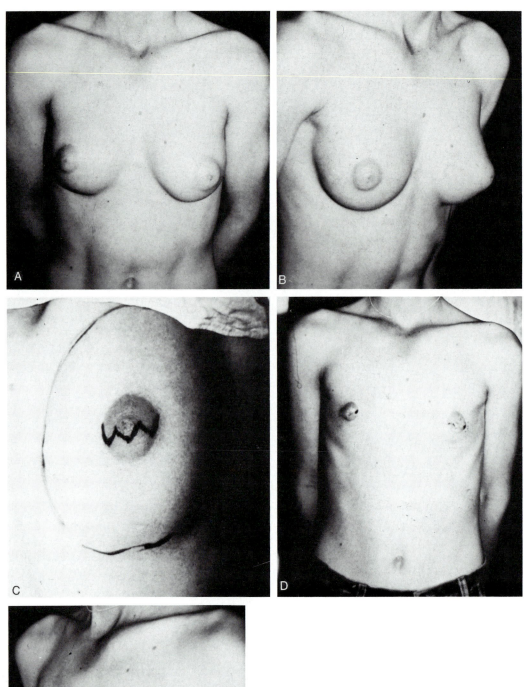

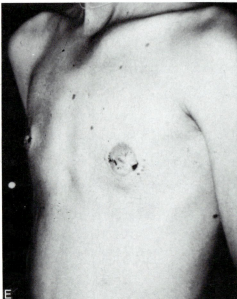

FIGURE 47–10
A and *B*, An 18-year-old male patient is shown with a large volume of breast tissue. *C*, The triple-V incision to be made is shown on this patient intraoperatively. *D* and *E*, Postoperative appearance 1 month after surgery. (Courtesy of J. F. Ely.)

TABLE 47–4
Complications

Inversion of nipple or areola
Nipple or areola necrosis
Contour deformity
Conspicuous scars
Residual skin redundancy
Inadequate breast excision
Breast asymmetry
Hematoma and fluid collection
Infection

complications can be easily prevented. Inversion or folding of the nipple or areola can be prevented by maintaining an adequate thickness of tissue on the nipple-areola flap. Nipple or areola necrosis is unlikely if an adequate dermal circulation is present and the tissues are handled gently. Contour and size asymmetries are prevented by carefully marking the extent of the hypertrophied tissue preoperatively and ensuring the same thickness of tissue on the nipple-areola and skin flaps on both sides. Residual skin redundancy will occur if an insufficient amount of skin was removed. Hematoma or fluid collection is unlikely with secure hemostasis and proper postoperative suction drainage. With the concentric circle operation, the circular scars have been conspicuous in a number of patients, but only a small percentage of patients have requested scar revision. Suction of fat concomitant with excision of the parenchymal tissue has been found to be a very useful addition in the management of gynecomastia.

References

August, G. P., Chandra, R., Hung, W.: Prepubertal male gynecomastia. J. Pediatr. 80:259, 1972.

Balch, C. R.: A transaxillary incision for gynecomastia. Plast. Reconstr. Surg. 61:13, 1978.

Bannayan, G. A., Hajdu, S. I.: Gynecomastia: Clinicopathologic study of 351 cases. Am. J. Clin. Pathol. 57:431, 1972.

Buckle, R.: Studies on the treatment of gynaecomastia with danazol (Danol). J. Int. Med. Res. Suppl. 3:114, 1977.

Buckle, R.: Danazol in the treatment of gynaecomastia. Drugs 19:356, 1980.

Carlson, H. E.: Current concepts gynecomastia. N. Engl. J. Med. 303:795, 1980.

Courtiss, E. H.: Gynecomastia: Analysis of 159 patients and current recommendations for treatment. Plast. Reconstr. Surg. 79:740, 1987.

Davidson, B. A.: Concentric circle operation for massive gynecomastia to excise the redundant skin. Plast. Reconstr. Surg. 63:350, 1979.

Dufourmentel, L.: L'Incision aréolaire dans la chirurgie du sein. Bull. Mem. Soc. Chir. Paris 20:9, 1928.

Eade, G. G.: The radial incision for gynecomastia excision. Plast. Reconstr. Surg. 54:495, 1974.

Ely, J. F.: Personal communication, 1988.

Forbes, A. P.: Chemotherapy, testicular damage and gynecomastia: An endocrine "black hole." N. Engl. J. Med. 299:42, 1978.

Gagnon, J. D., Moss, W. T., Stevens, K. R.: Pre-estrogen breast irridation for patients with carcinoma of the prostate: A critical review. J. Urol. 121:182, 1979.

Haagensen, C. D.: Carcinoma of the male breast. In: *Diseases of the Breast.* Philadelphia, W. B. Saunders, 1971, p. 779.

Haagensen, C. D.: The male breast. In: *Diseases of the Breast.* Philadelphia, W. B. Saunders, 1971, p. 76.

Hamer, D. B.: Gynecomastia. Br. J. Surg. 62:326, 1975.

Heller, K. S., Rosen, P. P., Schottenfeld, D., et al.: Male breast cancer: A clinicopathologic study of 97 cases. Ann. Surg. 188:60, 1978.

Jacobs, E. C.: Effects of starvation of sex hormones in the male. J. Clin. Endocrinol. 8:227, 1948.

LeRoith, D., Sobel, R., Glick, S. M.: The effect of clomiphene citrate on pubertal gynaecomastia. Acta Endocrinol. 95:177, 1980.

Letterman, G., Schurter, M.: The surgical correction of gynecomastia. Am. Surg. 35:322, 1969.

Letterman, G., Schurter, M.: Surgical correction of massive gynecomastia. Plast. Reconstr. Surg. 49:259, 1972.

Ley, S. B., Mozaffarian, G. A., Leonard, J. M., et al.: Palpable breast tissue versus gynecomastia as a normal physical finding (Abstr). Clin. Res. 28:24A, 1980.

Nuttall, F. Q.: Gynecomastia as a physical finding in normal men. J. Clin. Endocrinol. Metab. 48:338, 1979.

Nydick, M., Bustos, J., Dale, J. H., et al.: Gynecomastia in adolescent boys. J.A.M.A. 178:449, 1961.

Paulsen, A.: The testes. In: Williams, R. H.: *Textbook of Endocrinology.* Philadelphia, W. B. Saunders, 1974.

Paulschock, B. Z.: Tutankhamen and his brothers: Familial gynecomastia in the eighteenth dynasty. J.A.M.A. 244:160, 1980.

Plano, V. F.: Danazol: Review of recent studies. J.A.M.A. 79:530, 1980.

Rees, T. D.: Plastic surgery of the breast. In: Converse, J. M.: *Reconstructive Plastic Surgery.* Philadelphia, W. B. Saunders, 1977.

Rodriquez-Rigau, L. J., Smith, K. D.: Gynecomastia. In: Degroot, L. J.: *Endocrinology.* Vol. 3. New York, Grune & Stratton, 1979.

Simon, B. E., Hoffman, S.: Correction of gynecomastia. In: Goldwyn, R. M.: *Plastic and Reconstructive Surgery of the Breast.* Boston, Little, Brown, 1976.

Simon, B. E., Hoffman, S., Kahn, S.: Classification and surgical correction of gynecomastia. Plast. Reconstr. Surg. 51:48, 1973.

Smith, S. R., Chhetri, M. K., Johanson, A. J., et al.: The pituitary-gonadal axis in men with protein-calorie malnutrition. J. Clin. Endocrinol. Metab. 41:60, 1975.

Soyka, L. F., Mattison, D. R.: Drugs and male sexual function. Drug Therapy, August, 1981.

Von Kessel, F., Pickrell, K. L., Huger, W. E., et al.: Surgical treatment of gynecomastia: An analysis of 275 cases. Ann. Surg. 157:142, 1963.

Waterfall, N. B., Glaser, M. G.: A study of the effects of radiation on prevention of gynaecomastia due to estrogen therapy. Clin. Oncol. 5:257, 1979.

Webster, J. P.: Mastectomy for gynecomastia through a semicircular intra-areolar incision. Ann. Surg. 124:556, 1946.

Wheeler, C. E., Cawley, E. P., Gray, H. T., et al.: Gynecomastia: A review and an analysis of 160 cases. Ann. Surg. 124:556, 1946.

Williams, M. J.: Gynecomastia. Am. J. Med. 34:103, 1963.

Wilson, J. D., Aiman, J., MacDonald, P. C.: The pathogenesis of gynecomastia. Adv. Intern. Med. 25:1, 1980.

PROBLEM CASES

48

Ronald Riefkohl
Gregory S. Georgiade
Nicholas G. Georgiade

Problems in Aesthetic Breast Surgery and Their Management

CONTRIBUTORS

Edgar A. Altchek
Louis C. Argenta
Stephan Ariyan
Dale P. Armstrong
Namik K. Baran
Jean-Paul Bossé
T. Ray Broadbent
Cemalettin Celebi

Melvyn I. Dinner
Nabil I. Elsahy
Robert A. Fischl
David W. Furnas
Nicholas G. Georgiade
Kenna S. Given
Robert M. Goldwyn
John H. Hartley, Jr.

Saul Hoffman
Michael E. Jabaley
Carson M. Lewis
William R. N. Lindsay
Malcolm W. Marks
D. Ralph Millard, Jr.
Richard A. Mladick
Walter R. Mullin

Henry W. Neale
John Q. Owsley
Liacyr Ribeiro
Ronald Riefkohl
O. Gordon Robinson, Jr.
Richard C. Schultz
Gilbert B. Snyder
I. Richard Toranto

CASE 1   (Contributed by I. Richard Toranto, M.D.)

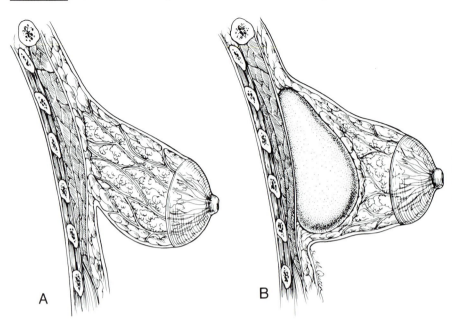

FIGURE 48–1
A and *B*, The author's concept of the appearance of the tuberous breast is shown before and after augmentation mammaplasty.

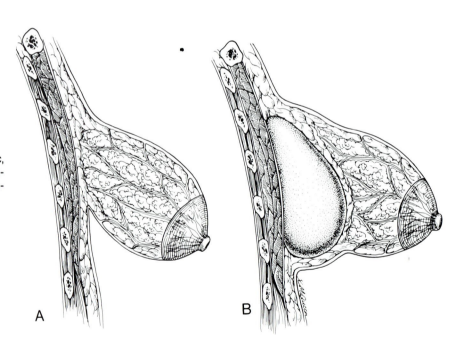

FIGURE 48–2
A and *B*, The appearance of a ptotic, tuberous breast before and after augmentation mammaplasty (author's concept).

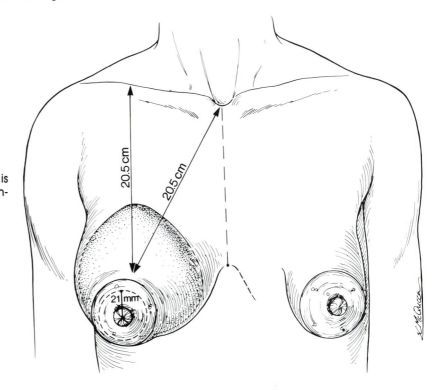

FIGURE 48–3
The planned new position of the areola is shown, following the first stage of augmentation of the tuberous breast.

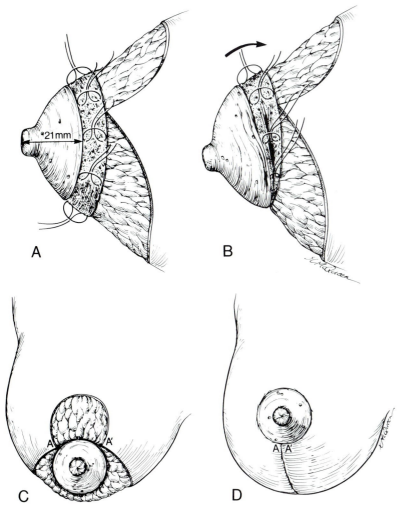

FIGURE 48–4
A and B, The area of areola de-epithelialization is shown, as is the technique of advancement of the new areola position. Notice the collapsing technique created, utilizing 4-0 clear nylon sutures. C and D, The newly positioned areola is shown before and after upward repositioning.

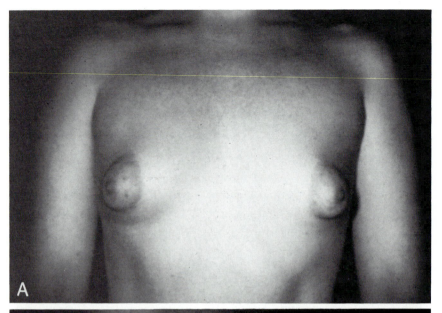

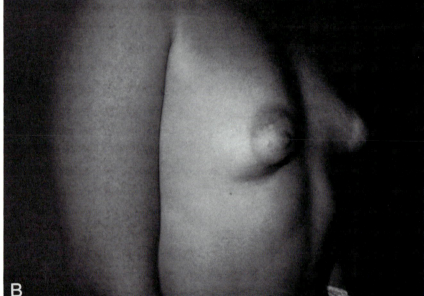

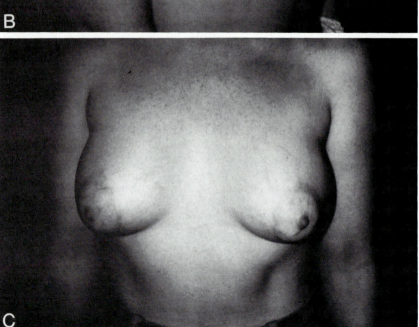

FIGURE 48–5

A and *B*, A 22-year-old woman is shown with moderately severe tuberous breasts. Notice the prominence of the areolae. *C* and *D*, This patient is now shown 4 weeks after a mammary periareola augmentation mammaplasty with 230-cc teardrop gel prostheses. *E* and *F*, The patient is now shown 10 years after correction of ptosis and nipple-areola deformity, having undergone a modified Arié-Pitanguy ptosis procedure with telescoping of the protuberant breast tissue. (See also Fig. 4.)

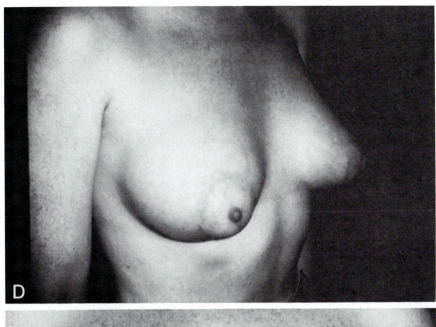

FIGURE 48–5 *Continued*

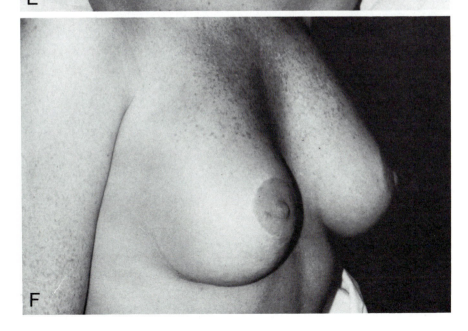

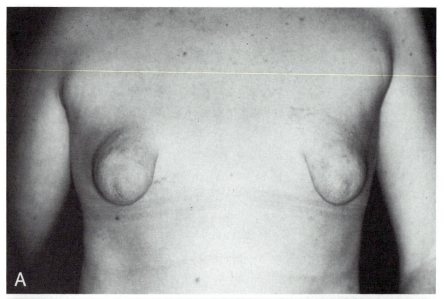

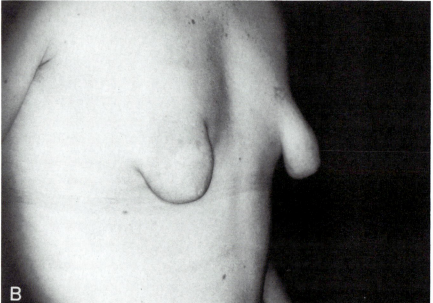

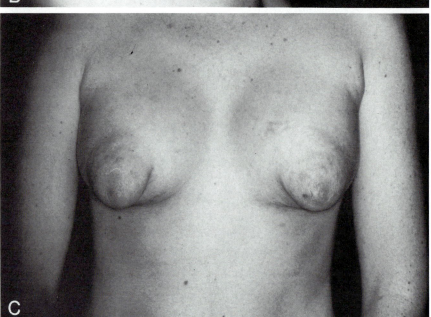

FIGURE 48–6

A and *B*, A 34-year-old patient is shown with severe tuberous breasts, with excess development of nipple and areola area and a marked deficiency of the breast mounds. *C* and *D*, The patient is shown after circumareolar augmentation mammaplasty with a 265-cc teardrop gel prosthesis in the right breast and a 230-cc teardrop gel prosthesis in the left breast. Note the lack of correction of the tuberous deformity. *E* and *F*, The patient is shown 1 year after areola reduction and mastopexy as described in Case 1, Figure 48–1.

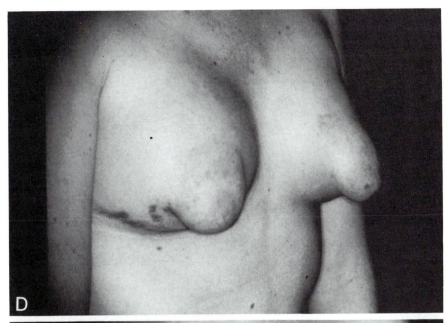

FIGURE 48–6 *Continued*

Editor's Note. Dr. Toranto prefers a two-stage procedure for what he considers to be a sustained correction with maintenance of satisfactory shape and contour.

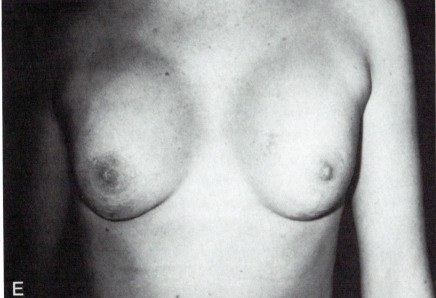

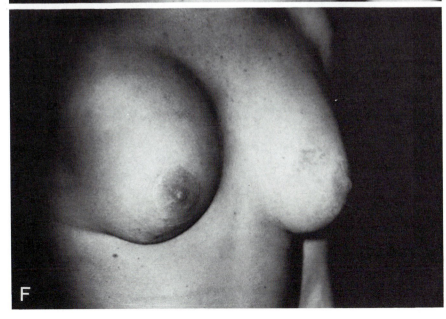

CASE 3 (Contributed by Melvyn I. Dinner, M.D.)

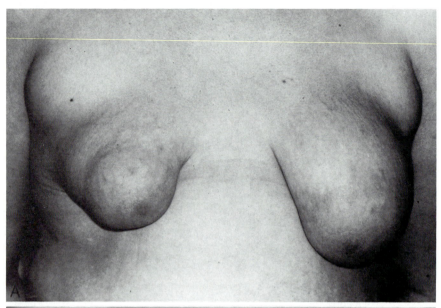

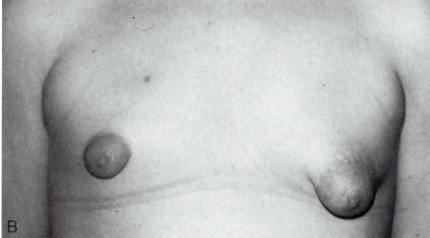

FIGURE 48–7
A, A 28-year-old woman with a tubulo-tuberous breast deformity consisting of underdevelopment of the breast, ptosis, areola hypertrophy with pseudo-herniation of the breast into the areola, and an associated skin envelope deficiency. *B,* An 18-year-old patient is shown with a similar deformity.

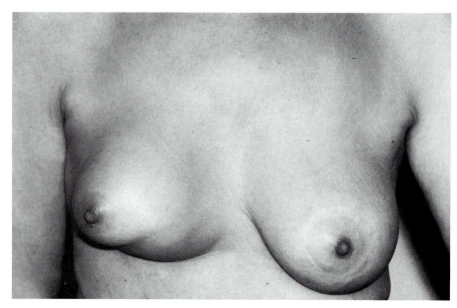

FIGURE 48–8
Augmentation without correction of the skin deformity, exaggerating a constriction band effect in the tuberous breast.

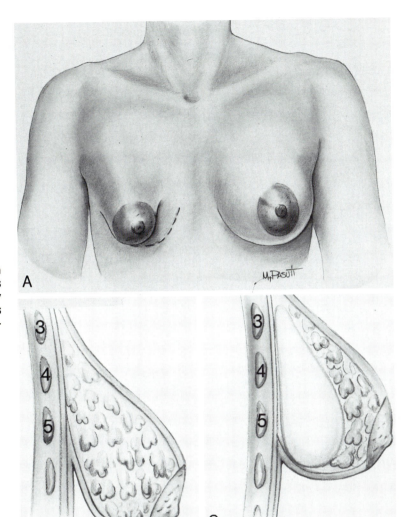

FIGURE 48–9

The normal breast will span the second to sixth intercostal spaces, whereas in this tubulotuberous breast deformity, the vertical breast height may be limited to only two intercostal spaces. This hypoplastic element is improved by a subglandular augmentation.

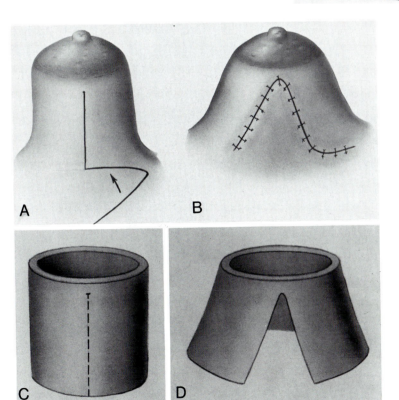

FIGURE 48–10

The initial step is to correct the skin envelope deficiency and convert the tubular shape of the breast into its natural conical shape. This will necessitate release of the constriction band via a full-thickness incision through the skin, subcutaneous tissue, and underlying breast (A), extending from the level of the submammary fold upward almost to the areola. This will declare the extent of the deficiency of skin and size of skin replacement. A medially based full-thickness skin and subcutaneous flap is then transferred to correct the deficit. The deficit created in the submammary fold is repaired by undermining an advancement of the abdominal wall to the level of the submammary fold (B). The artist's representation of the release of the constriction bands, establishing a cone, is shown in C and D.

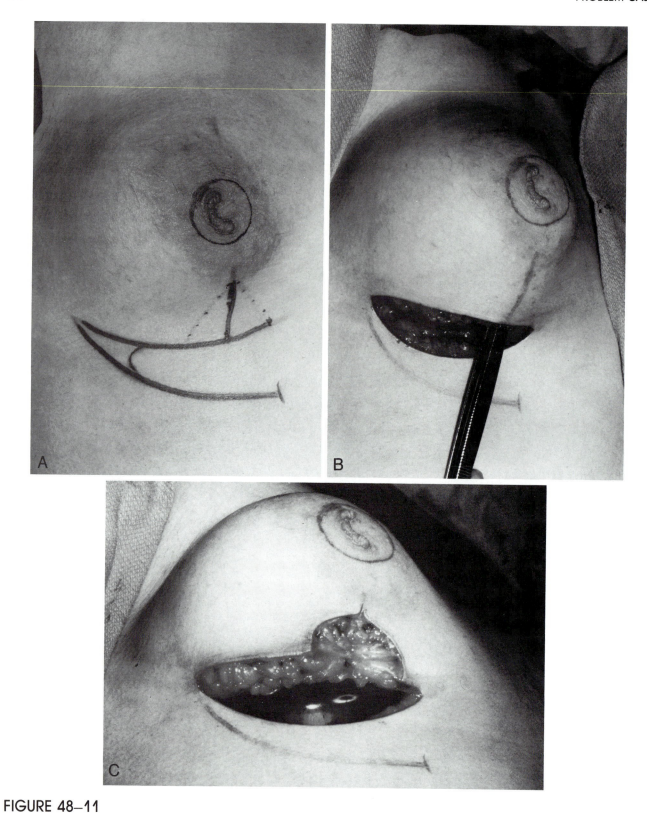

FIGURE 48–11

A to *F*, The technical aspects are shown after the marking, elevation, and transfer of a tailored, medially based flap. Notice how well the flap fits into the infra-areola defect after an augmentation mammaplasty through the same incision.

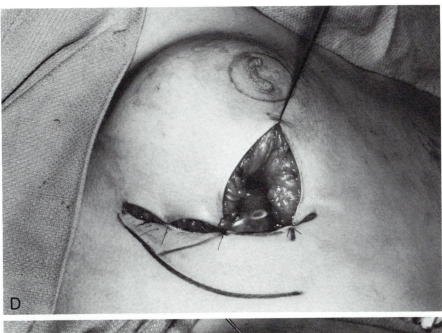

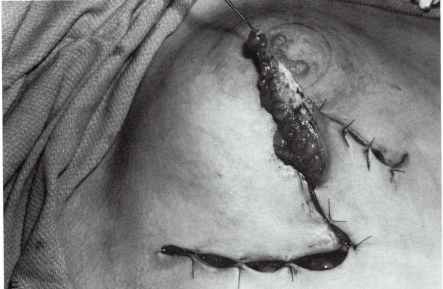

FIGURE 48-11 Continued

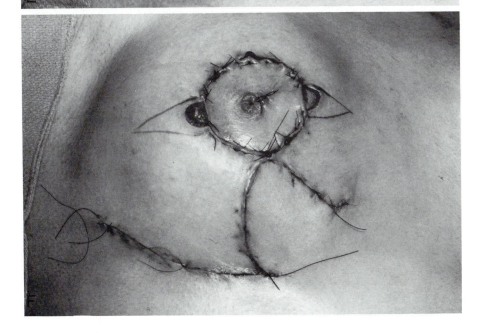

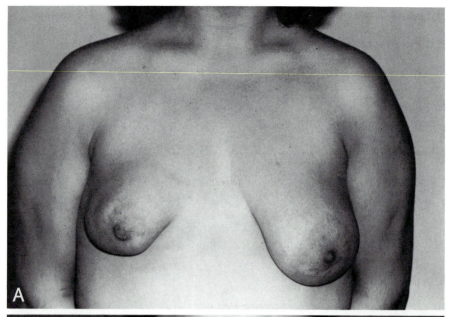

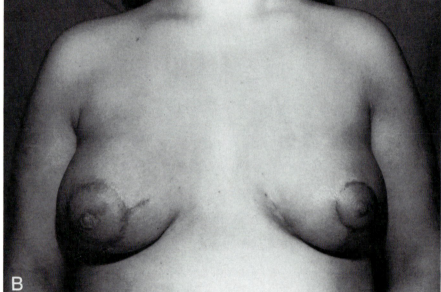

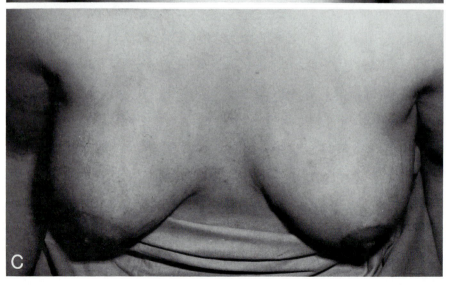

FIGURE 48–12
A, A 22-year-old patient is shown with multiple breast deformities associated with the tubulotuberous breast. *B,* The same patient 6 months after use of the technique described in Figures 48–10 and 48–11. A 250-gm Meme prosthesis was used. *C,* A bird's-eye view of the corrected breast 6 months later showing the normal lateral extension of the base from the medial to lateral aspect, compared with the normal breast.

Conclusion. The tubulotuberous breast deformity comprises several varied anatomic deformities. Each component of the deformity should be addressed individually. The common denominator in all cases appears to be the missing skin element, which is believed to be best managed by the transfer of a medially based full-thickness flap from the submammary fold.

CASE 4 (Contributed by Walter R. Mullin, M.D., and D. Ralph Millard, Jr., M.D.)

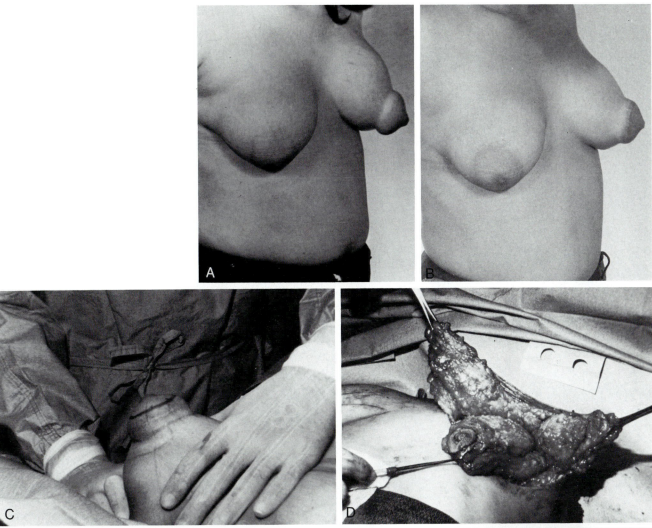

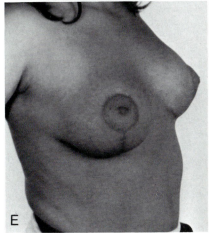

FIGURE 48–13

A, A 13-year-old girl is shown with abnormal development of the breasts over a 2-year period. She was particularly concerned with the abnormal shape of the left breast. *B,* The patient is shown 1 year after the "doughnut" of epithelium was decreased by excision of the epithelium surrounding the areola, which decreased the size of the areola. The nipple side of the areolar rim was de-epithelialized and fitted under the peripheral circumference in an effort to readjust the nipple areola and provide a better shape and balance. It was noted that there was only a slight improvement over a 6-month period. *C,* Herniated nipple-areola complex is shown prior to a secondary surgical intervention. *D,* This intraoperative photograph demonstrates the column of glandular tissue carrying the nipple and the areola complex along with the medial and lateral flap of breast tissue forming a cone. This technique allowed a precise telescoping and adjustment of the desired nipple projection. At the same time, the neurovascular component was kept intact. The medial and lateral breast flaps designed by keyhole patterns preoperatively allow the medial and lateral breast flaps to be firmly approximated at the three-point closure area. Utilizing a central column technique can create greater nipple viability problems. However, such problems did not occur in this patient. *E,* The patient is shown 5 months after reconstruction of the left breast. A reduction mammaplasty had been carried out on the right breast.

CASE 5   (Contributed by John Q. Owsley, M.D.)

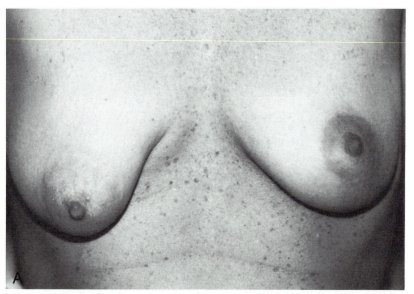

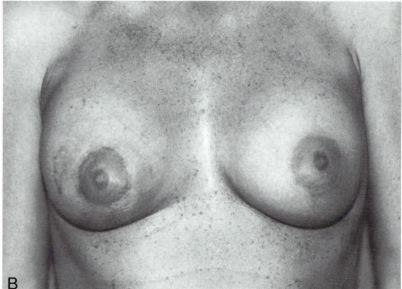

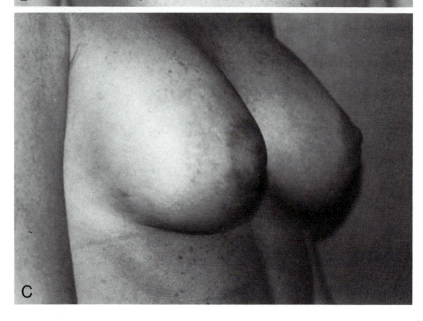

FIGURE 48–14

A, A 33-year-old patient is shown with asymmetry of the breasts. She appeared to have a mild form of a tuberous breast on the right. She desired larger, symmetric breasts. Preoperatively, with the patient in an upright position, the anticipated superior margin of the right areola was marked. *B* and *C,* The same patient is shown 5 weeks after reconstruction with an aesthetically pleasing result.

Procedure. The left breast was augmented through an inframammary incision. A 235-cc polyurethane-covered silicone gel–filled prosthesis was inserted in the retromammary pocket. The right areola was marked to match the left areola. At the 6 o'clock position along the areola a vertical incision was extended to the inframammary fold. The skin was undermined circumferentially after excision of the excess amount of areola. Undermining was extended in all directions 6 to 8 cm. An incision was made on the opposite breast just above the inframammary fold and a retromammary pocket developed. A similar-sized 230-cc prosthesis was inserted on the left side. The skin at the 12 o'clock position of the areola was excised superiorly to the preoperative marking. To match the superior edge of the left areola, a new keyhole matching was then developed to accommodate the newly sized areola matching the opposite areola. After satisfactory matching of the contour with the opposite breast, the medial and lateral inferior flaps were adjusted and sutured. Excess skin was trimmed, and the dog-ears created in the inframammary fold were corrected.

CASE 6 (Contributed by Ronald Riefkohl, M.D.)

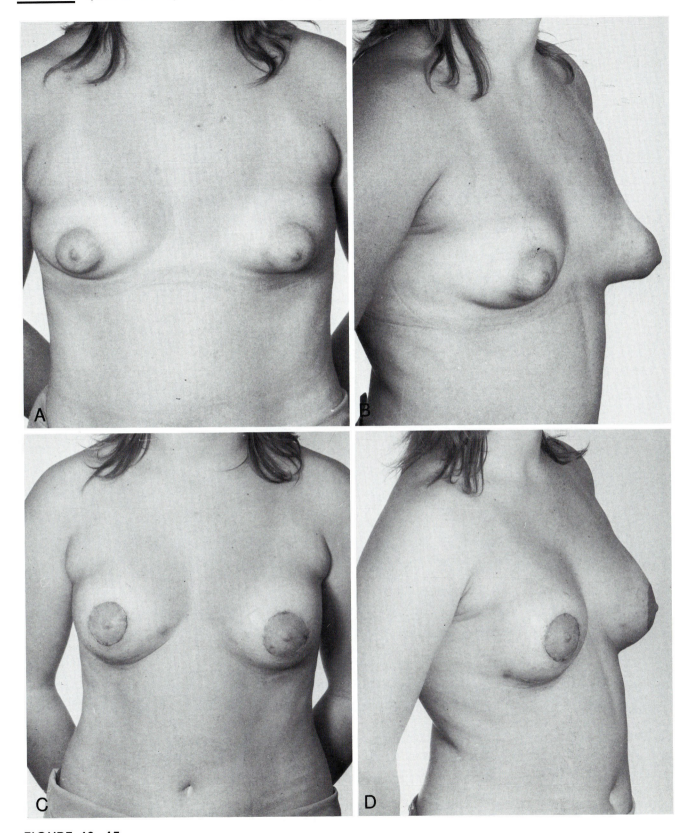

FIGURE 48–15

A and *B,* A 17-year-old patient is shown with hypomastia and tuberous breasts. An augmentation mammaplasty with 165-cc gel prostheses was carried out, and a 1.5-cm width of areola was excised in a doughnut fashion, decreasing the diameter of the areola. *C* and *D,* The same patient is shown 6 weeks after surgery.

CASE 7   (Contributed by Stephan Ariyan, M.D.)

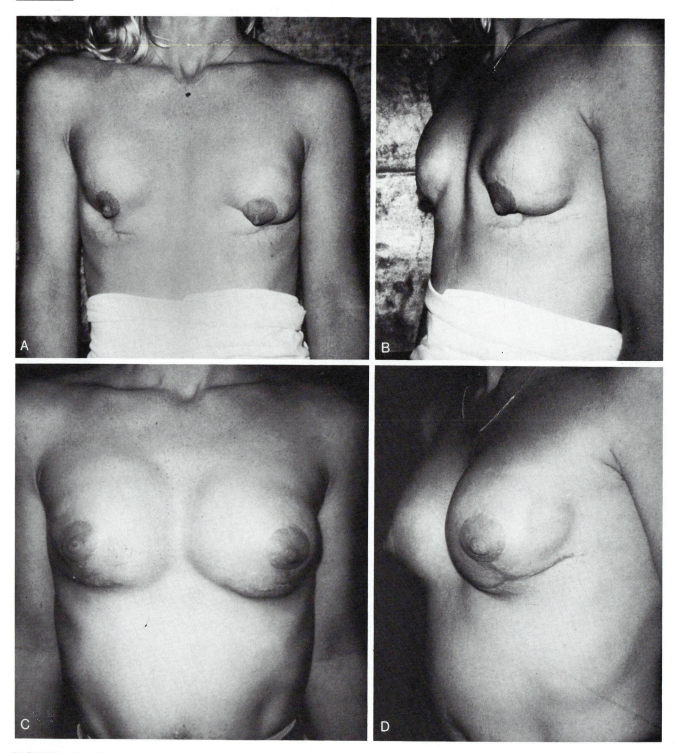

FIGURE 48–16

A and *B,* A patient is shown 18 months after a subcutaneous mastectomy with immediate subpectoral gel implants. The prostheses were noted to be superiorly displaced, with associated capsular contracture and ptosis. *C* and *D,* The same patient is shown 6 months after reconstruction, which was carried out by removal of the prostheses, undermining the skin over the pectoral muscle, releasing the inferior portion of the pectoralis major muscle, and deepening the pockets inferiorly beneath the subserratus anterior and anterior rectus sheath; 275-cc silicone gel prostheses were inserted in these pockets, and the previously undermined skin was redraped. Excess skin was excised in the inferolateral positions.

CASE 8   (Contributed by Dale P. Armstrong, M.D.)

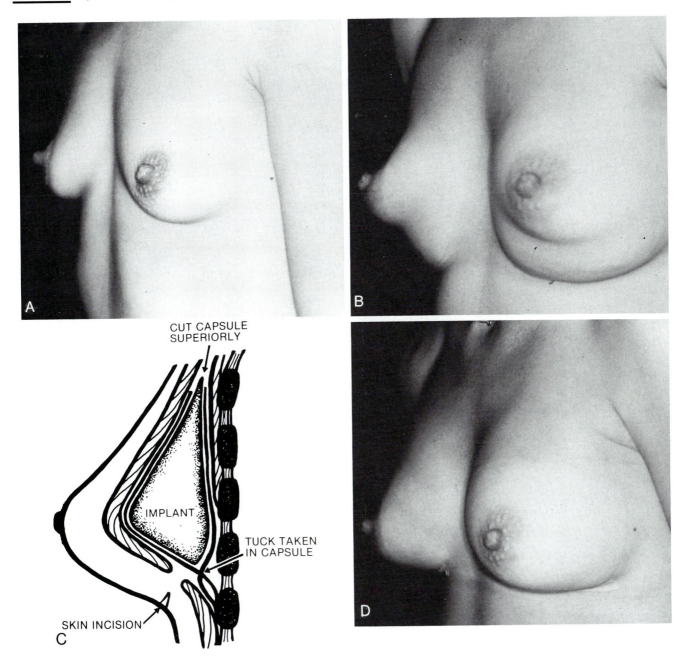

FIGURE 48–17

A, A patient is shown in an oblique view prior to augmentation mammaplasty. *B,* The same patient is shown 6 months after augmentation mammaplasty. The implants have been placed too low, thus obliterating the inframammary crease. *C,* The problem was corrected by excising a measured strip of the inferior capsule and reapproximating the capsule edges with 3-0 Mersilene running sutures. This procedure is shown in *C. D,* The postoperative result 1 year later.

CASE 9   (Contributed by Carson M. Lewis, M.D.)

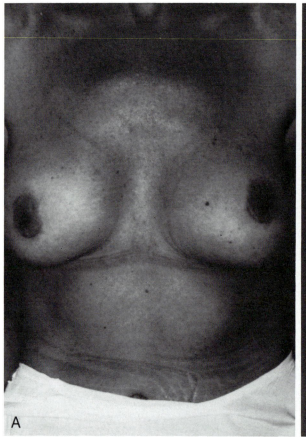

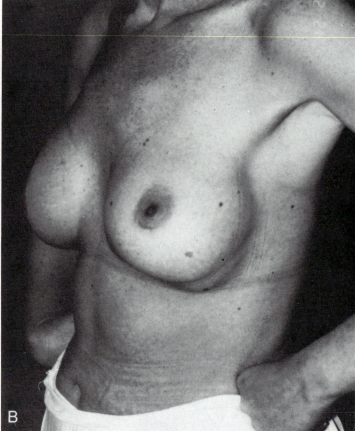

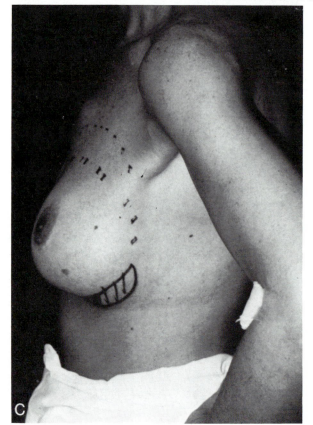

FIGURE 48–18

A to *C*, A 42-year-old female is shown after augmentation mammaplasty at age 25. She subsequently had four additional operative procedures for capsular contractures and asymmetry.

Treatment. Treatment consists of exploration of the capsule and excision of inferior lateral distorted portions of the capsule and repair with multilayered closure to prevent recurrent ptosis. The patient is placed in an upright position on the operating table for visualizing the result and comparison with the opposite breast. Postoperatively, supportive tape was applied for a 2-month period, together with the constant use of a brassiere.

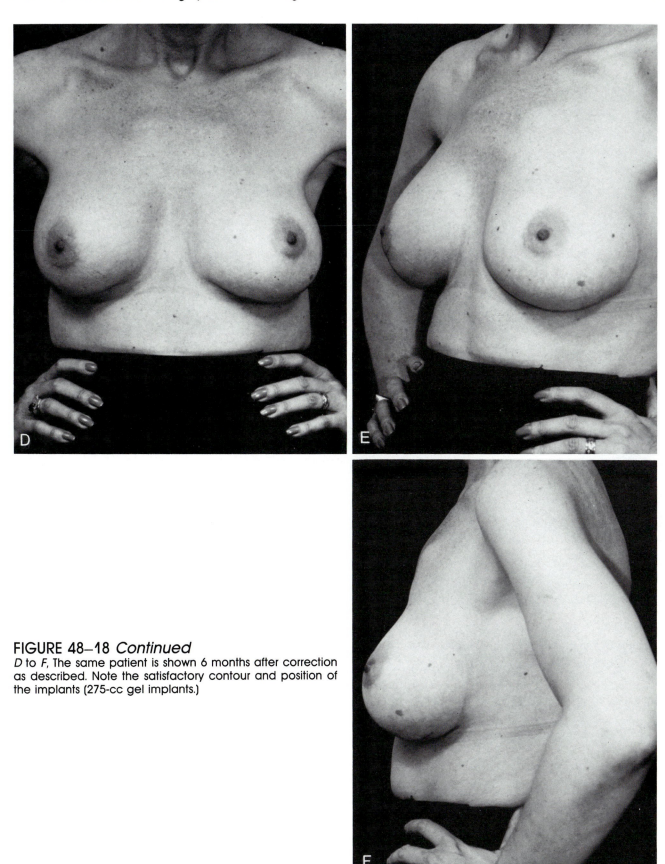

FIGURE 48–18 *Continued*
D to *F*, The same patient is shown 6 months after correction as described. Note the satisfactory contour and position of the implants (275-cc gel implants.)

CASE 10 (Contributed by Kenna S. Given, M.D.)

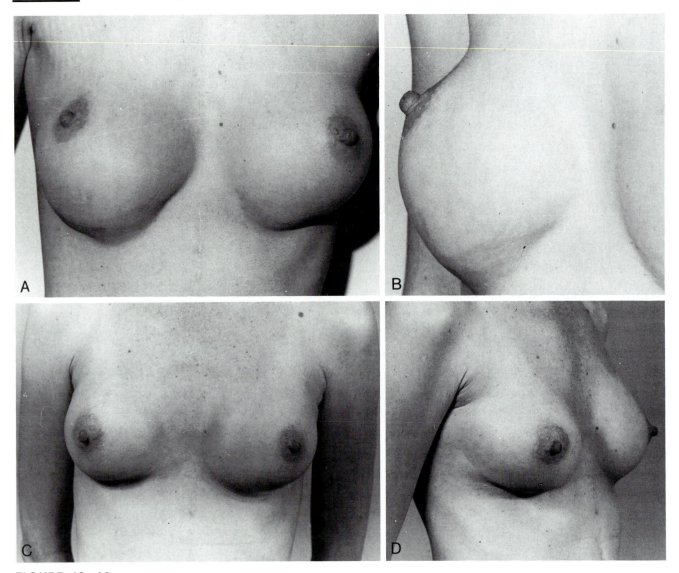

FIGURE 48–19
A and *B,* This patient is shown with marked displacement of the nipple-areola complex superiorly and descent of the implants below the inframammary crease after three previous procedures, including capsulotomies and reimplantation of double-lumen prostheses containing 10 mg of methylprednisolone sodium succinate (Solu-Medrol). *C* and *D,* Correction of the deformities included revision of both breasts by obliterating the excess of capsules and pockets inferiorly with 3-0 Prolene sutures. A new inframammary fold was created at a higher level, and the pockets were extended superiorly. This patient is shown 18 months later; no further problem has occurred.

CASE 11 (Contributed by Dale P. Armstrong, M.D.)

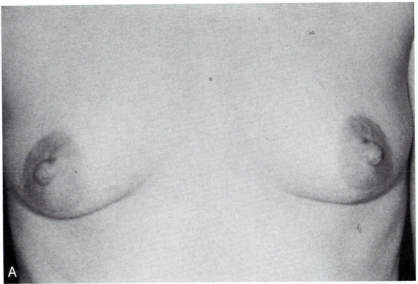

FIGURE 48–20

A, This young patient is shown prior to subpectoral augmentation mammaplasty. *B,* The same patient is shown postoperatively with superior displacement of the prostheses, resulting from an incomplete release of the pectoral muscle inferiorly and an early inappropriate wearing of brassiere postoperatively. *C,* The same patient is shown after extension of the subpectoral pockets inferiorly and abstinence from brassiere support for 4 to 6 weeks postoperatively.

Editor's Note. Occasionally, additional pressure may be helpful, utilizing a 4-inch elastic bandage wrapped around the chest superior to the prostheses to maintain a more normal inferior position.

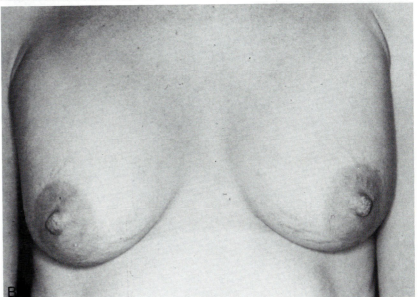

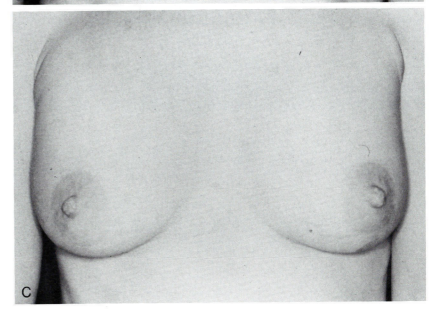

CASE 12   (Contributed by Richard A. Mladick, M.D.)

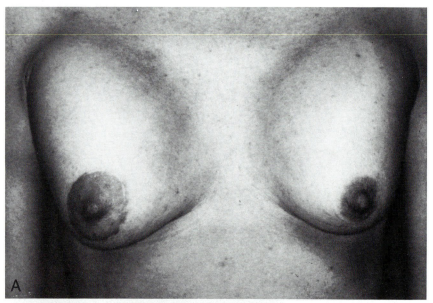

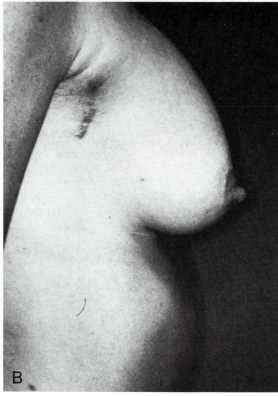

FIGURE 48–21

A and *B,* This woman underwent a submuscular augmentation mammaplasty through axillary incisions, with resulting capsular contractures and marked superior displacement of the prostheses. There are also prominent axillary scars as a result of the operative procedure.

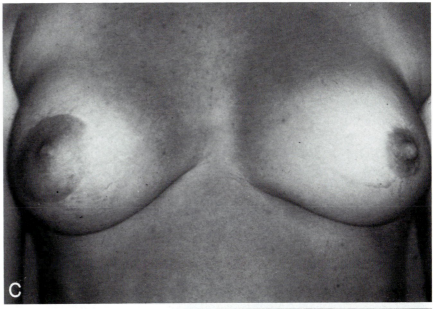

FIGURE 48–21 *Continued*

C and *D,* Correction of the problem was carried out with the use of inframammary incisions bilaterally, with capsulotomies, deepening of the muscle pockets, and replacement of the prostheses in a more inferior position.

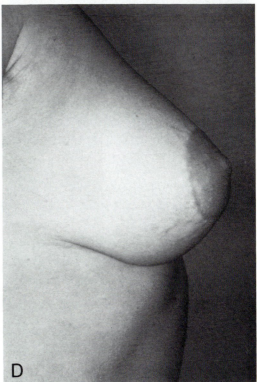

CASE 13 (Contributed by Saul Hoffman, M.D.)

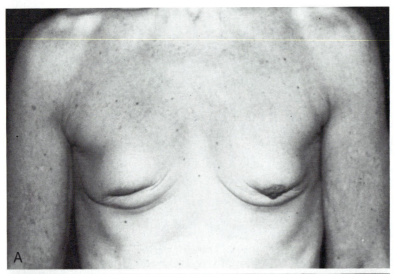

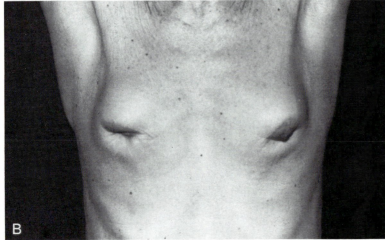

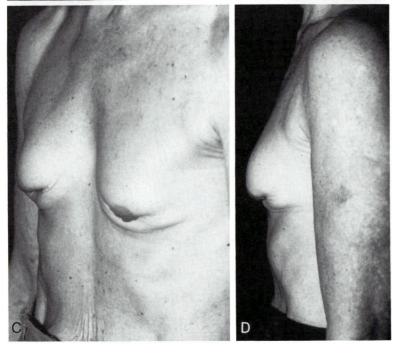

FIGURE 48–22

A to *D*, A 60-year-old woman is shown 8 years after augmentation mammaplasty. She had a capsulotomy and replacement of silicone gel implants 3 years previously. The prostheses were subsequently removed because of further encapsulation and rupture of the implant. Notice the circumareolar scars with severe depression of the nipples inferiorly.

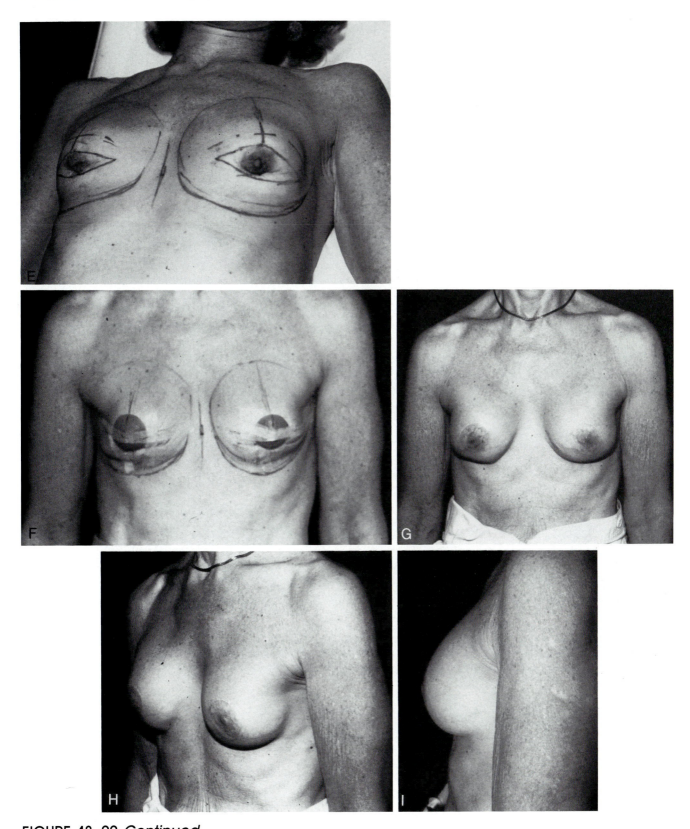

FIGURE 48–22 *Continued*

E and *F,* Excision of the depressed scars, including the nipple-areola complex, and simultaneous submuscular augmentation with the replacement of the nipple-areola complex bilaterally as full-thickness skin grafts. *G* to *I,* The patient is shown 2½ years following reconstruction and insertion of double-lumen teardrop implants containing 140 cc gel on the right and 125 cc gel on the left. A slight capsular contracture was noted on breast compression.

CASE 14   (Contributed by O. Gordon Robinson, Jr., M.D.)

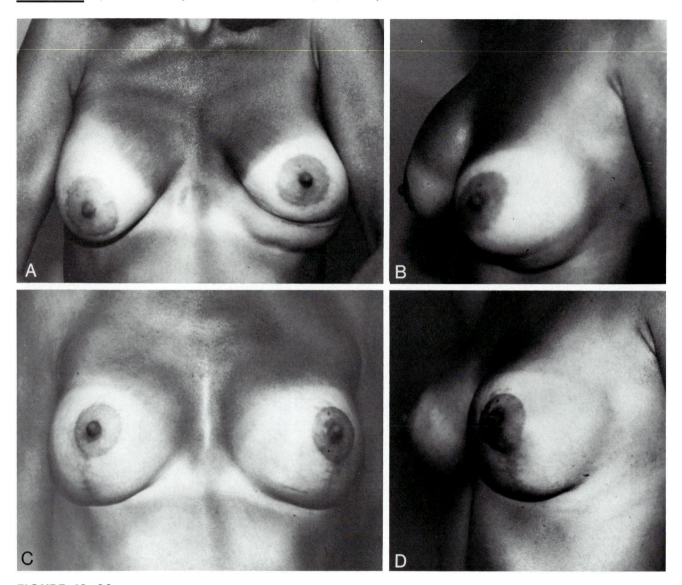

FIGURE 48–23
A and *B*, A 39-year-old patient underwent two prior submuscular augmentation mammaplasties. Examination revealed bilateral ptosis and prostheses that were too high. She had bilateral capsular contractures with a significant contracture band across the midinferior mammary area of the left breast. *C* and *D*, The patient is shown 6 months postoperatively. Her breasts have an excellent contour and softness.

Treatment. Both prostheses were removed. Four months later, the submuscular pockets were enlarged, and extensive capsulotomies were carried out. Prostheses were inserted, and a mastopexy was carried out bilaterally.

CASE 15 (Contributed by Walter R. Mullin, M.D., and D. Ralph Millard, Jr., M.D.)

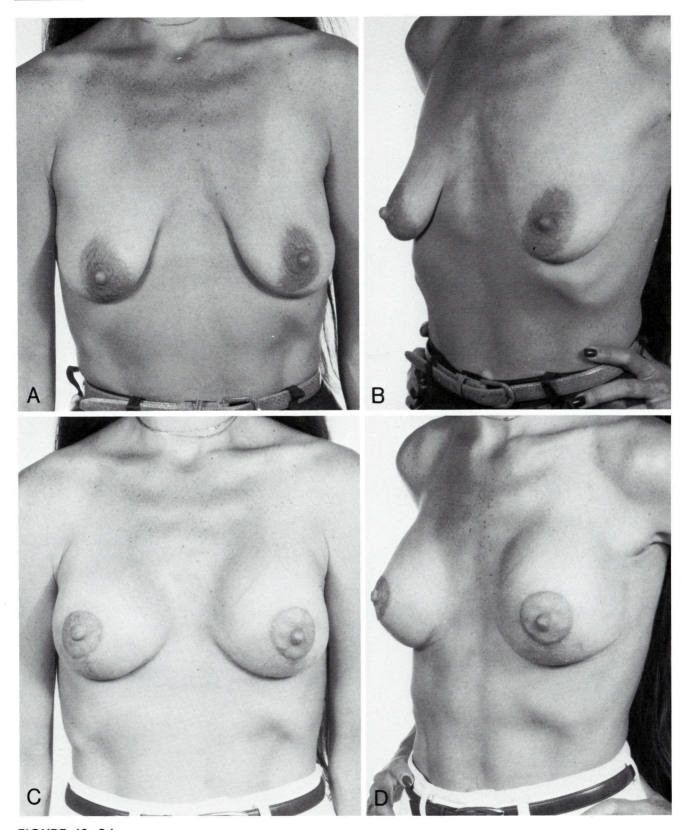

FIGURE 48–24

A and *B*, A 30-year-old patient is shown after two full-term pregnancies with loss of breast substance and associated development of ptosis. *C* and *D*, The same patient is shown 6 weeks after a superiorly based nipple-areola flap mastopexy and insertion of 100-cc gel implants above the pectoral muscle. An adjustment of the excess skin envelope was carried out in the inframammary area.

CASE 16 (Contributed by Walter R. Mullin, M.D., and D. Ralph Millard, Jr., M.D.)

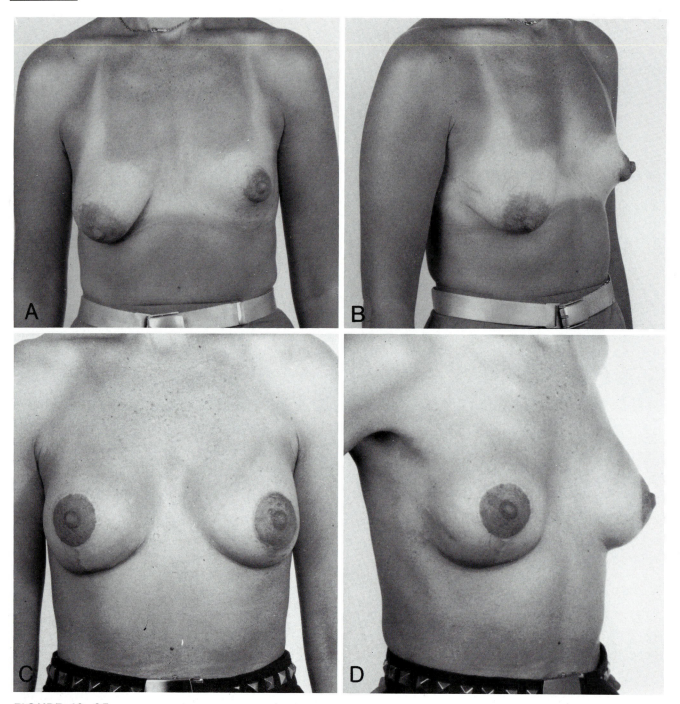

FIGURE 48–25
A and *B,* A 42-year-old patient is shown with marked breast asymmetry. She subsequently had a mastopexy procedure on the right, and a right submammary 160-cc gel implant was inserted. A second procedure was carried out, adjusting the size of the right areola to conform to the left nipple areola. A final procedure involved replacement augmentation mammaplasty utilizing a slightly smaller 120-cc gel prosthesis above the muscle, replacing the previously inserted 160-cc gel implant. *C* and *D,* The same patient is shown 14 months after the above-mentioned procedures.

Contributors' Note. It is important always to prepare the patient for a possibility of multiple stages over several months. This enables the tissues to settle and stretch to what will approach the final position and contour, allowing a more precise control of the final result.

CASE 17   (Contributed by John H. Hartley, Jr., M.D.)

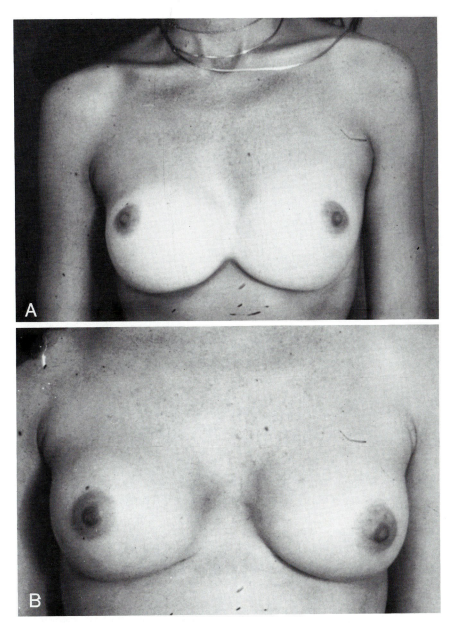

FIGURE 48–26
A, This patient is shown following an augmentation mammaplasty with extensive undermining of the submammary pockets in close proximity to each other. Shortly after augmentation, these pockets became connected, with contact of the prostheses. Note the high position of the nipple relative to the inferiorly placed prostheses. *B,* The same patient is shown approximately 5 months later. Notice the cleavage and new position of the prostheses, with a satisfactory appearance.

Treatment. The pockets were approached through previous incisions in the inframammary areas. The capsule was divided anteriorly and posteriorly in the midsternal line. This allowed enough capsule on each side to be reflected laterally in each direction. The capsule was then repaired with a "vest over pants" type of procedure separating the two pockets. At the same time, the implants were elevated slightly, recreating a normal medial fold, or cleavage.

CASE 18 (Contributed by William R. N. Lindsay, M.D.)

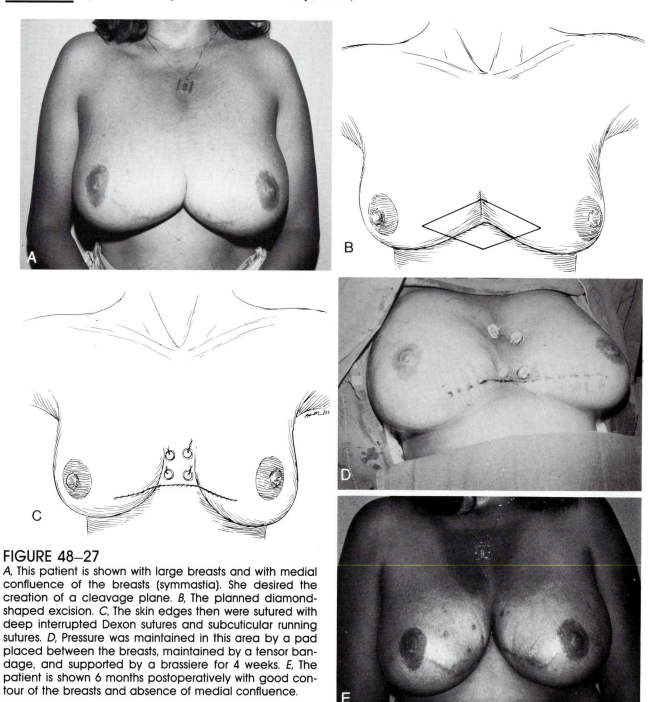

FIGURE 48–27

A, This patient is shown with large breasts and with medial confluence of the breasts (symmastia). She desired the creation of a cleavage plane. *B*, The planned diamond-shaped excision. *C*, The skin edges then were sutured with deep interrupted Dexon sutures and subcuticular running sutures. *D*, Pressure was maintained in this area by a pad placed between the breasts, maintained by a tensor bandage, and supported by a brassiere for 4 weeks. *E*, The patient is shown 6 months postoperatively with good contour of the breasts and absence of medial confluence.

Treatment. A diamond-shaped excision of skin and breast tissue was planned. Note that the long axis of the diamond is in a horizontal direction and centered at the midpoint of the intermammary skin bridge and fatty tissue. The length of the diamond is usually 5 to 7 cm and varied, depending on the amount of skin and breast tissue requiring excision. This triangular portion of skin was excised with a medial wedge of breast tissue from each side. This excision tends to reshape the medial and inferior portions of the breast into a more attractive shape and corrects the sagging in the medial part of the inferior breast. The superior skin flap was undermined in the midline for 5 cm and partially defatted. The flap was then sutured to the underlying periosteum and muscle utilizing 3-0 Dexon mattress sutures, which were all inserted and then tied individually. Also, several No. 30 stainless steel wire sutures were placed laterally and brought through the skin, then later twisted tightly over buttons with protective underlying plastic foam.

CASE 19 (Contributed by Robert A. Fischl, M.D.)

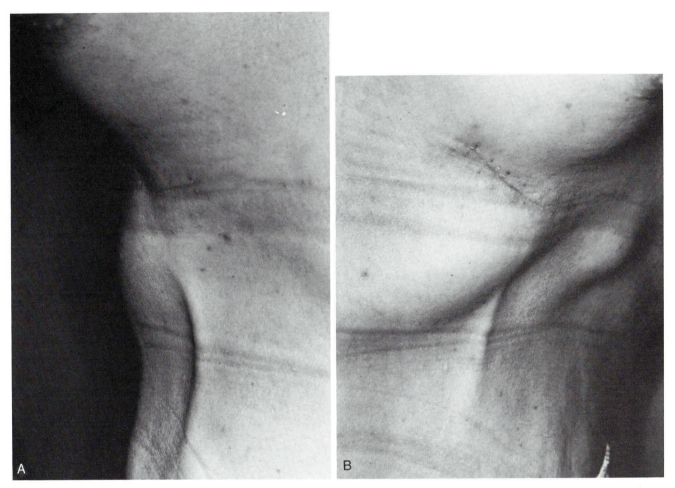

FIGURE 48–28

A and *B*, This patient had had an augmentation mammaplasty 3 months previously. Raised, tender, cordlike bands had developed; the condition was diagnosed as superficial phlebitis. Mondor's disease, a self-limiting, benign problem that gradually disappears without residual deformity over a period of weeks, may be associated with transient hyperemia and sensory changes in the skin.

Editor's Note. Mondor's disease is superficial thrombophlebitis of the chest wall and breast. This phenomenon was described over 100 years ago; however, it was better recognized after Henri Mondor's publication in the French literature in 1939. There is thrombosis usually of the thoracoepigastric vein or occasionally the lateral thoracic vein or the superior epigastric vein; however, the medial aspect of the breast is not involved. The condition is characterized by the appearance of a cordlike thrombosed vein as shown in these photographs. Initially this band may be tender and erythematous, but the discomfort gradually subsides, leaving a cordlike band for a period of months that gradually disappears. The pathologic process is that of a nonspecific thrombophlebitis. The occurrence appears to be related to trauma, e.g., surgery. The usual treatment for Mondor's disease is expectant.

References

Mondor, N.: Tronculite sous-cutaneé subaigué de la paroi thoracique antero-laterale. Mem. Acad. Chir. (Paris) 65:1271, 1939.

Johnson W. C., Wallrich, R., Helwig, E.: Superficial thrombophlebitis of chest wall. J.A.M.A. 180:103, 1962.

CASE 20 (Contributed by Michael E. Jabaley, M.D.)

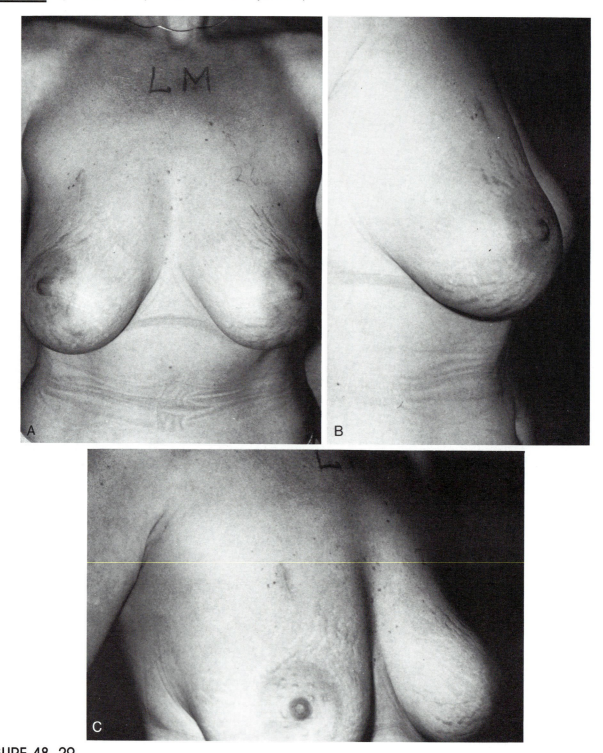

FIGURE 48–29
A to C, This patient is shown 2 years after an augmentation mammaplasty when her breasts were enlarged from a C+ brassiere cup to a D cup.

There was a 2-year history of intermittent to constant mastodynia after the augmentation. Upon examination, the patient had bilateral breast tenderness on palpation, particularly along the anterior axillary line and over the intercostal spaces. She had associated ptosis.

Procedure. The implants, with an approximate volume of 230 cc, were removed, and bilateral mastopexies were performed without removal of breast tissue.

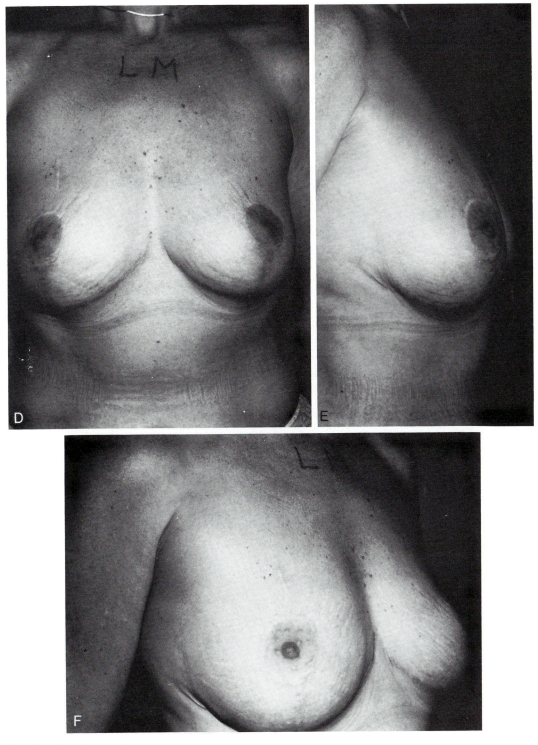

FIGURE 48–29 *Continued*
D to *F*, The patient is shown 1 year after the removal of the prostheses and mastopexy.

Contributor's Note. A common feature, in patients with the above-mentioned complaints and findings without any response to medication and other forms of treatment, is that they appear to be overaugmented initially, with progressive ptosis and increasing size over the postaugmentation years. Removal of the prostheses, decreasing the mechanical forces on the breasts, and associated mastopexy appear of benefit in this type of patient.

CASE 21 (Contributed by David W. Furnas, M.D.)

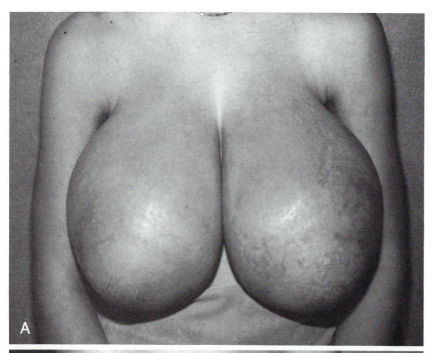

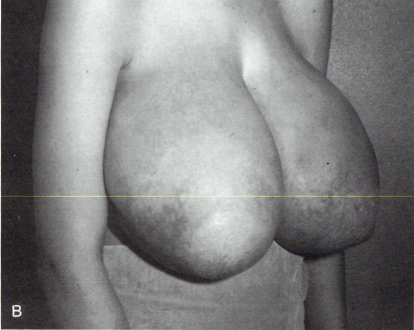

FIGURE 48–30
A and *B*, A 12-year-old patient is shown with severe juvenile hypertrophy.

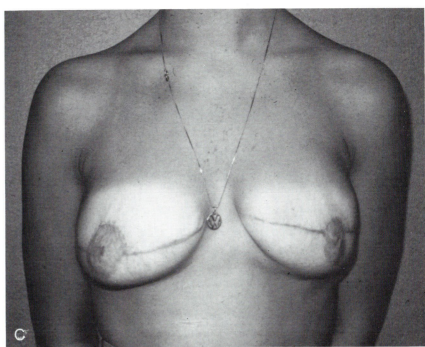

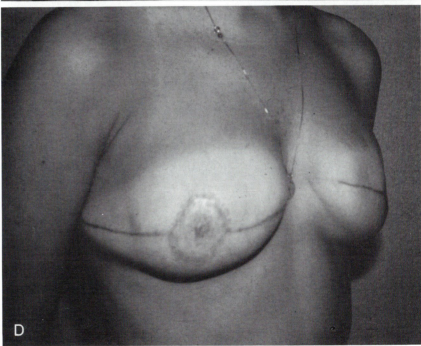

FIGURE 48–30 *Continued*
C and *D*, The patient is shown 6 years postoperatively after a bilateral subcutaneous mastectomy and insertion of 200-cc gel-filled implants.

CASE 22   (Contributed by Richard C. Schultz, M.D.)

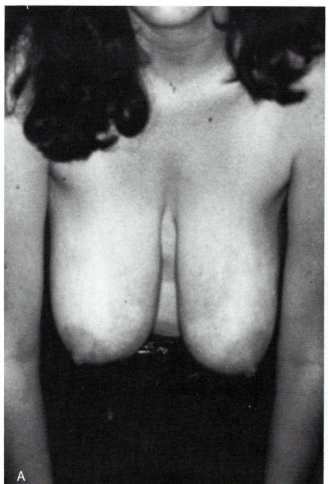

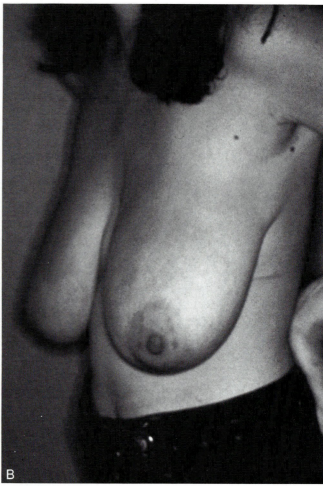

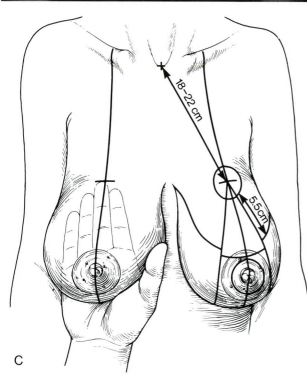

FIGURE 48–31

A and *B,* A 19-year-old patient is shown with symptomatic breast hypertrophy, compounded by an unusual degree of ptosis for her age. *C,* The markings for correction of the breast hypertrophy and ptosis are outlined. The proposed nipple placement is shown on the right breast and determined by the height of the inframammary fold. The proposed location of the nipples was established by a measurement from the suprasternal notch to the inframammary crease. A 4.5-cm diameter is established for the new areola size. The vertical heights of the lateral breast flaps are 5.5 cm from the inferior border of the new areola position. A de-epithelialized inferior pedicle technique was utilized for parenchymal resection. To obtain maximum nipple projection, a de-epithelialized dermal platform was created at the location of the new nipple. Six hundred forty-three grams were removed from the right breast and 645 gm were removed from the left breast.

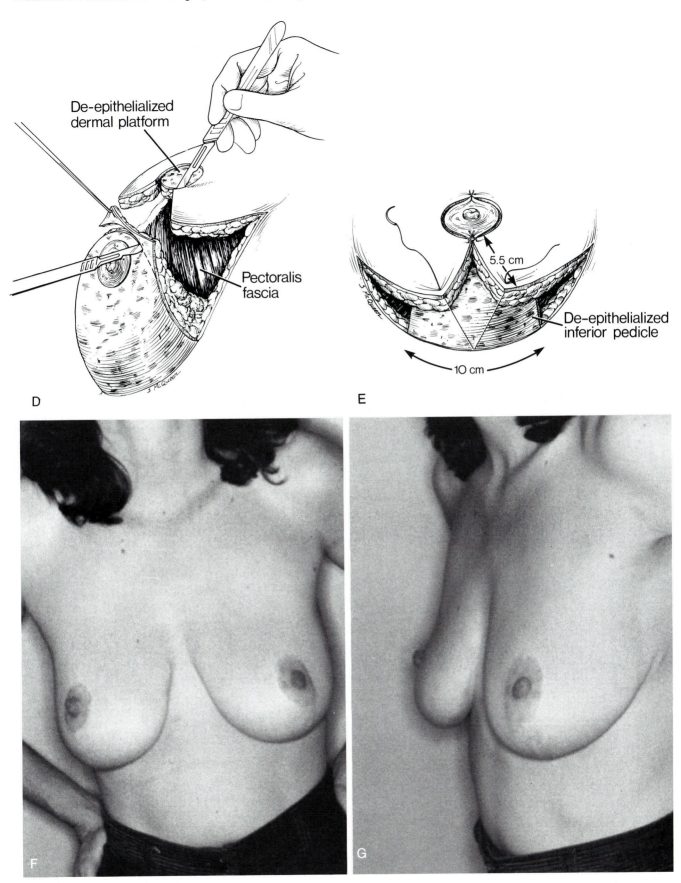

D

De-epithelialized dermal platform

Pectoralis fascia

E

5.5 cm

De-epithelialized inferior pedicle

10 cm

F

G

FIGURE 48–31 *Continued*

D and *E*, The positioning of the inferior dermal flap over the platform is shown prior to approximation of the medial and lateral flaps to the inframammary position. *F* and *G*, The same patient 2 years after reduction mammaplasty and mastopexy as described. Although she had some inframammary protrusion, she was quite satisfied with her result.

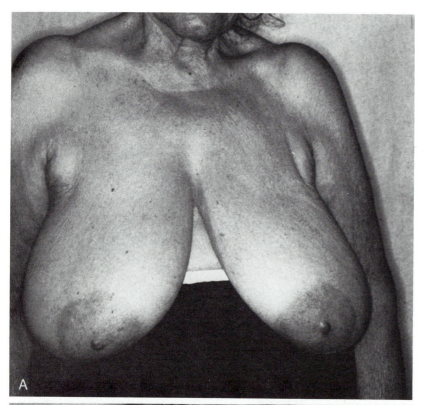

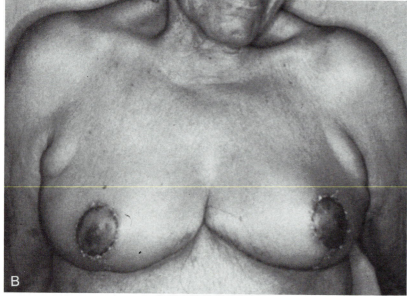

FIGURE 48–32

A and *B*, A 74-year-old patient is shown with symptomatic breast hypertrophy and ptosis. A procedure similar to that described above with a 950-gm reduction of the right breast and a 1000-gm reduction of the left breast was done to preserve maximum sensation and superior breast configuration. She is shown 1 month after surgery with a satisfactory aesthetic result and sensitivity of the nipples intact.

CASE 23   (Contributed by Jean-Paul Bossé, M.D., F.R.C.S.)

Contributor's Comments. Regarding correction of the misplaced nipple after reduction mammaplasty, a nipple too high or too medial is probably the most difficult problem. Patients are bitterly disappointed with their appearance, disenchanted with the surgeon because they realize he has made a mistake, and appalled by the prospect of the added scarring of a secondary procedure.

They will often seek a second opinion or even get legal expertise. The second surgeon may not be comfortable with the problem because he knows that the prospect for a good aesthetic result is slim.

Very little has been said or written about the correction of the misplaced nipple except for brief anecdotes regarding the difficulty, the poor aesthetic result, and the inevitable visible scar.

Most techniques remain closely limited to the nipple area in order to minimize scarring. We have tried to establish a standardized correction that would involve most of the original surgical area, or more or less start over and try to place the additional scar where it will be well concealed by clothing. This pattern would adapt ideally to any kind of problem, whether the nipple is too high, too medial, or both.

The technique is easy, even for an inexperienced surgeon. We believe that we have found a pattern that can be extended to any width or length; it does involve wide undermining and eventual reposition of the nipple.

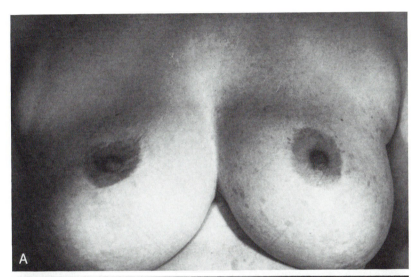

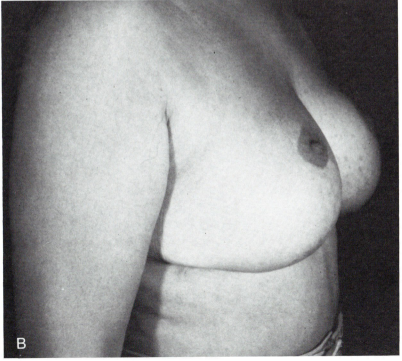

FIGURE 48–33
A and *B*, This patient is shown after reduction mammaplasty with markedly superiorly displaced nipple-areola complexes.

The markings are made with the patient in a sitting position. The position of the normal nipple is used as a point of reference and measured from the sternal notch. If the deformation is bilateral, we use a point 19 to 22 cm from the sternal notch. A horizontal line is drawn for further reference to the ultimate upper position of the nipple (Fig. 48–34). The patient is then anesthetized and prepared in the usual way. A curved downward incision, 4 to 6 cm long, is made at the inner portion of the breast. This incision will contact the nipple on the outside and will be brought downward in a lazy-S fashion and include the original scar (Fig. 48–35). A drawing of the proposed lower portion of the S is then traced according to the amount of excess skin to be removed (Fig. 48–36A and B). This can be quite variable but easy enough to assess by pinching the skin. The nipple is then incised and the excess marked skin dissected. A moderate to extensive undermining of the whole peri-areolar area is then undertaken, mostly at the upper and external areas, being more conservative at the inner and lower portion. Depending on the amount of tension on the skin edges, the wound can be loosely closed, completely burying the nipple under it. If there is too much skin tension, the wound is left open at the approximate site of relocation of the nipple. The inner upper portion of the incision is closed completely, preferably with intradermal sutures, with an attempt to avoid any dog-ear at the end (Fig. 48–37). The next step is to decide and measure the exact reposition of each nipple by using the contralateral nipple, if normal.

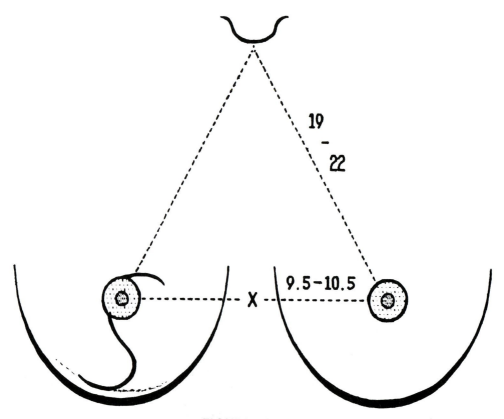

FIGURE 48–34

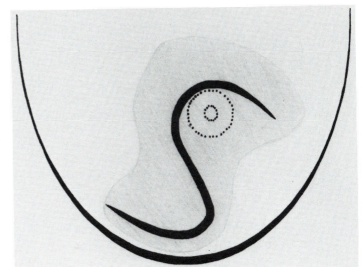

FIGURE 48–35

If both nipples have to be corrected, we follow the classic concept for nipple position; use our point of reference of 19 to 22 cm as the highest point of the nipple, then mark the inner point of the nipple between 9.5 and 10.5 cm from the midline with the patient in the reclining position. While using these two points of reference, we outline a full circle 4 to 4.5 cm in diameter. This can be modified according to the actual preoperative diameter of the nipple. This skin circle is then excised. The nipple is exteriorized and sutured. We use intradermal 5.0 Dexon and Steri-Strips. There are no specific postoperative recommendations.

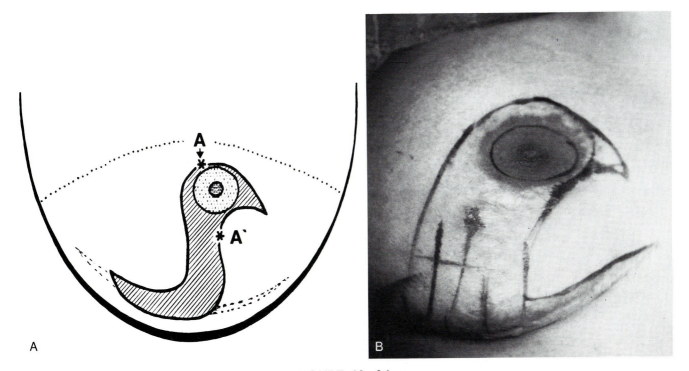

A

B

FIGURE 48–36

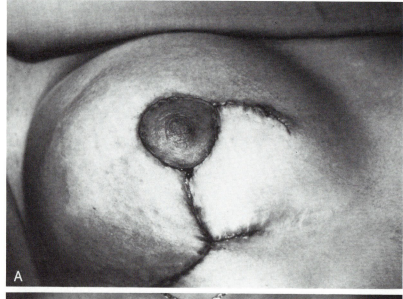

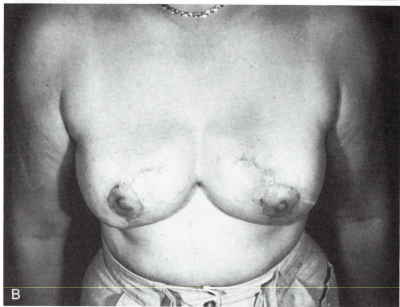

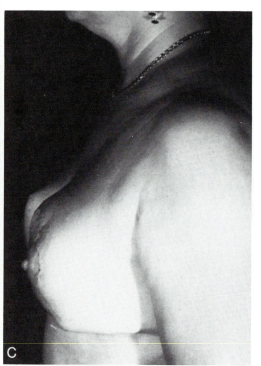

FIGURE 48–37

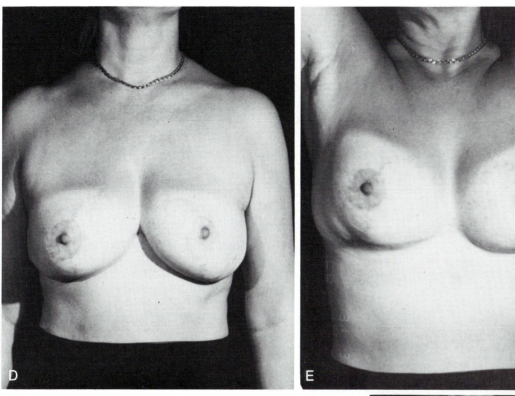

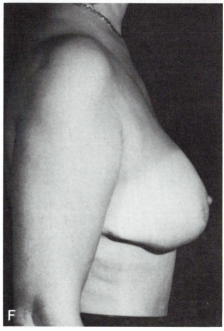

FIGURE 48–37 *Continued*

At the beginning, the nipple-areola complex can tend to look somewhat flattened (Fig. 48–37A to C), but it will eventually round itself and blend into a normal protruding curve (Fig. 48–37D to F). If there is a dog-ear at the inner portion of the incision, it can be corrected after 3 to 4 months. Only one such correction was needed in our limited experience of four cases. This inner scar has otherwise healed well, without hypertrophy, and has remained well hidden in the brassiere. The patients were pleased to recover some symmetry and accepted the additional scar.

Discussion. Because a new technique is rarely invented in surgery, other experienced surgeons probably have used more or less the same design for correction of this difficult problem. The technique could be a standardized procedure quite adaptable and modifiable to many situations and with predictable results.

CASE 24   (Contributed by Namik K. Baran, M.D., and Cemalettin Celebi, M.D.)

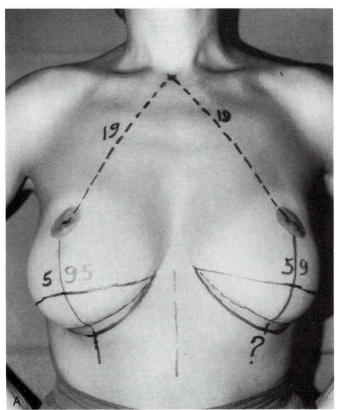

FIGURE 48–38

A and *B,* This 42-year-old patient had undergone reduction mammaplasty 6 years previously. There are markedly superiorly displaced nipple-areola complexes with extensive inframammary scarring. The distance from the midsternal notch to the nipple was 19 cm. In contrast, the distance from the areola to the inframammary fold was 9 cm on the left breast and 9.5 cm on the right breast. Inversion and upward projection of both nipples are also obvious *(B).*

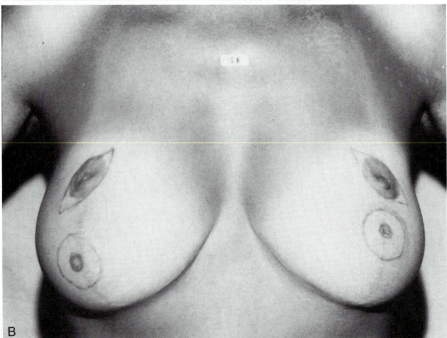

Discussion. The first and easier procedure to consider is to transfer the nipple-areola complexes to a more acceptable lower position as free grafts. The closure of the "doughnut" area could then be managed by excising the skin in a fusiform shape along an oblique line. However, this procedure would probably result in two additional unacceptable scars.

The second procedure for consideration is an excision of 4 to 4.5 cm of excess skin and breast tissue from the inframammary area, if one realizes that a secondary procedure might be necessary in approximately a year to further decrease the areola inframammary distance and bring the nipple-areola complexes into an even more favorable position (Fig. 48–38C).

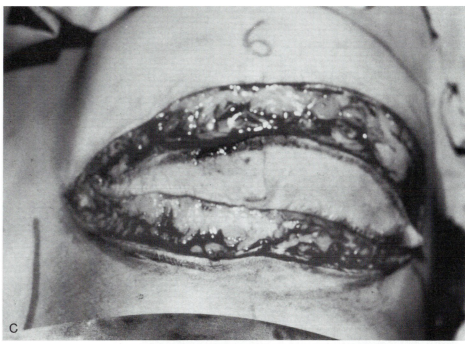

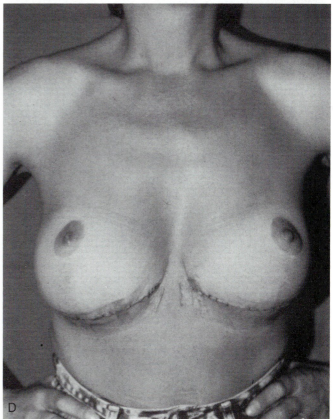

FIGURE 48–38 *Continued*

C, See Discussion. *D,* The patient is shown 10 days after excision of the excess inframammary tissue. The patient has a satisfactory result but may need further tailoring, particularly on the right breast. Note that the nipples now protrude satisfactorily.

CASE 25   (Contributed by Robert M. Goldwyn, M.D.)

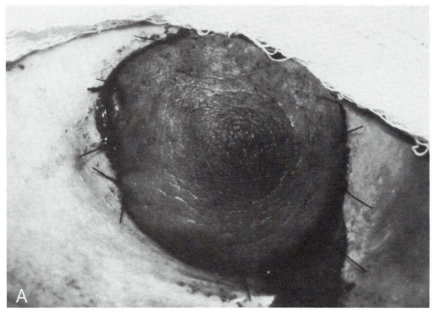

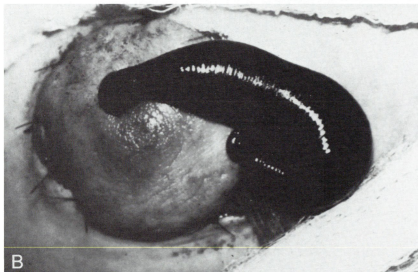

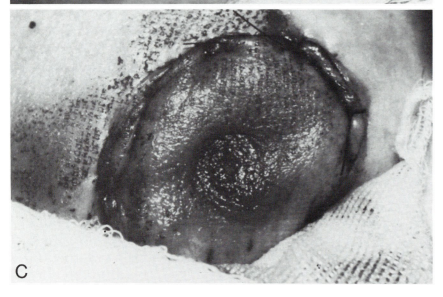

FIGURE 48–39

A, The nipple-areola complex of a 50-year-old woman is shown. She had a preoperative history of heavy smoking and underwent a bilateral breast reduction by the inferior pedicle technique with removal of 460 gm of tissue on the right side and 360 gm on the left side. Intraoperatively, on the left nipple, progressive duskiness and decreased capillary filling developed. The areola became blotchy. The appearance of the nipple-areola complex 4 hours after the operation is shown. *B,* Medicinal leeches were applied, with rapid restoration of excellent vascularity to the nipple and areola. The leeches were maintained for 72 hours. The patient was given tetracycline to prevent infection by *Aeromonas hydrophilia,* present in the leech's gut. *C,* Appearance of the nipple-areola complex 1 week postoperatively. The patient healed uneventfully without necrosis; her nipple-areola complex has normal sensation.

Reference

Whitlock, M. R., O'Hare, P. M., Sanders, R., Morrow, N. C.: The medicinal leech and its use in plastic surgery: A possible cause for infection. Br. J. Plast. Surg. 36:240, 1983.

CASE 26 (Contributed by Liacyr Ribeiro, M.D.)

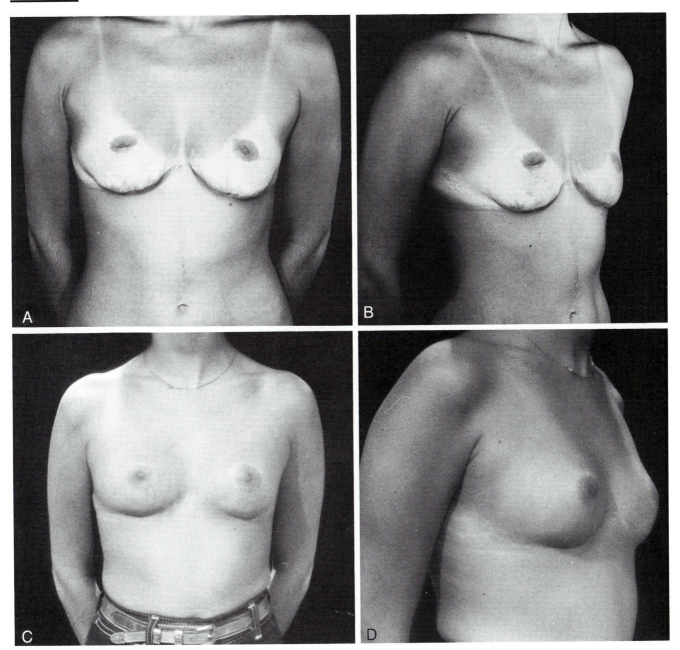

FIGURE 48–40

A and *B,* This patient is shown having undergone reduction mammaplasty with resulting asymmetrical invagination of the nipples, hypertrophied scars, disparity in volume of the residual breast tissue, redundant skin envelopes, and malpositioned nipple-areola complexes. Management included excision of the hypertrophic scars and the excess tissue at the inframammary crease area and shifting the nipple-areola complex inferiorly into a more normal position. At the same time, reconing of the breast was carried out. *C* and *D,* The postoperative results in the same patient are shown approximately 1 year later.

CASE 27   (Contributed by Richard A. Mladick, M.D.)

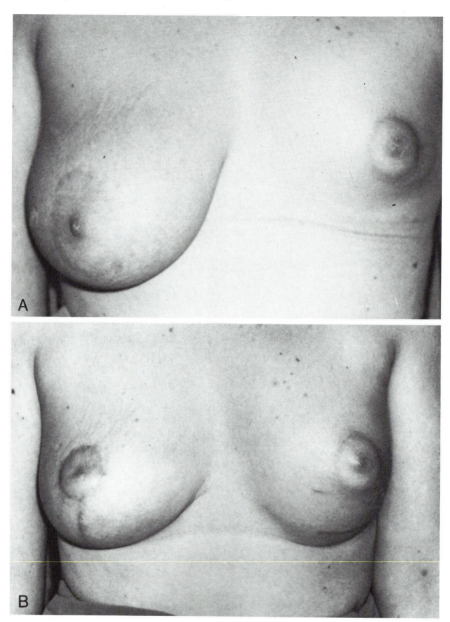

FIGURE 48–41

A, This young patient is shown with left hypomastia and right hypermastia with associated ptosis. Management consisted of a right breast reduction utilizing the superior pedicle technique and a left augmentation mammaplasty via an inframammary incision with insertion of a 225 cc saline prostheses inflated to 240 cc. *B,* Postoperative appearance approximately 6 months after reconstructive surgery.

CASE 28   (Contributed by Edgar A. Altchek, M.D.)

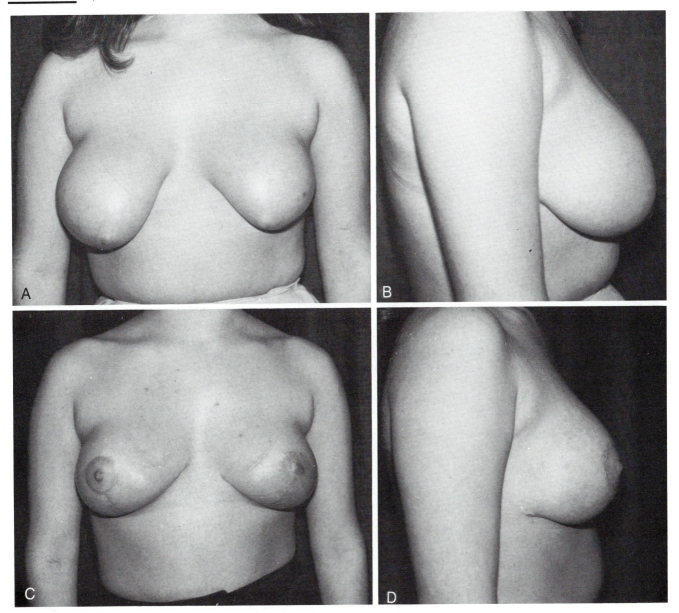

FIGURE 48–42

A and *B*, A young female patient is shown with marked breast asymmetry, consisting of a moderately hypertrophied and pendulous right breast with an unusual inframedial location of the nipple-areola complex. The left breast was unusually shaped and ptotic and varied considerably in size and contour from the right breast. Note the unusual inframedial location of the nipple-areola complex. *C* and *D*, The patient is shown approximately 1 year after correction involving a left mastopexy with repositioning of the nipple-areola complex as a free graft and a right reduction mammaplasty utilizing an inferior pedicle technique.

CASE 29   (Contributed by T. Ray Broadbent, M.D.)

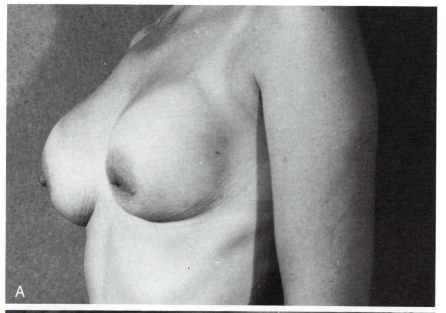

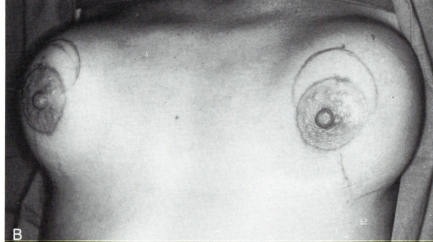

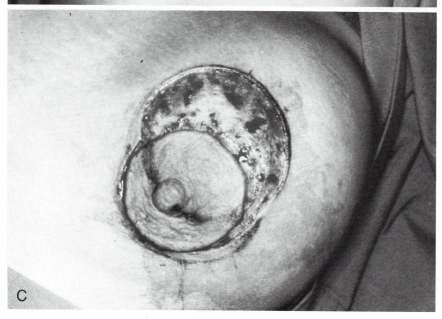

FIGURE 48–43
A, This patient is shown following a subcutaneous mastectomy and immediate reconstruction. Note the residual ptosis. *B*, The areas marked represent the new positions of the areolae after de-epithelialization. *C*, The area of de-epithelialization in the superior lateral position is shown.

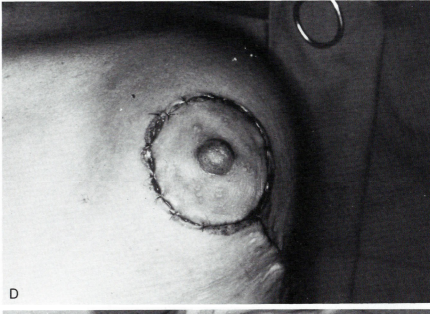

FIGURE 48–43 *Continued*
D, The postoperative appearance of
the nipple-areola is shown. Excision of
the residual skin is carried out in the
inferior lateral position. *E,* The patient is
now shown postoperatively with a satisfactory aesthetic result.

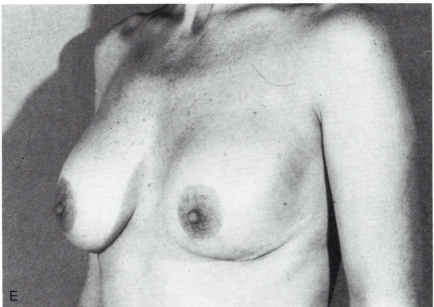

CASE 30 (Contributed by Henry W. Neale, M.D.)

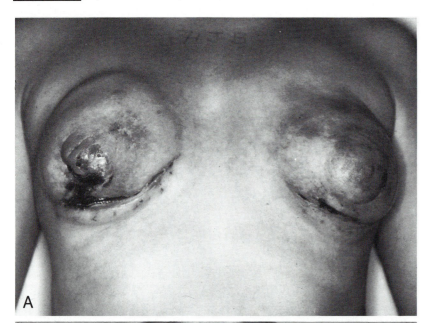

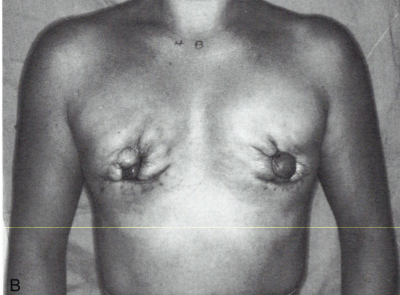

FIGURE 48–44

A to *B*, This patient is shown during early and late stages of bilateral skin necrosis of the breast and areola area after an attempt at a subcutaneous mastectomy and immediate prosthesis replacement.

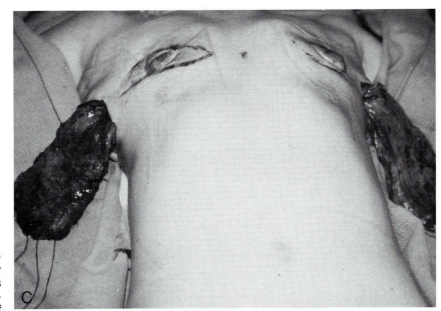

FIGURE 48—44 *Continued*
C, It was necessary to remove the prostheses (suprapectoral); after a few months of healing, bilateral latissimus dorsi musculocutaneous flaps were elevated and transferred into the area of defect after release of the scar contracture bilaterally. *D,* Postoperative appearance of the patient after submuscular insertion of implants and a nipple-areola reconstruction.

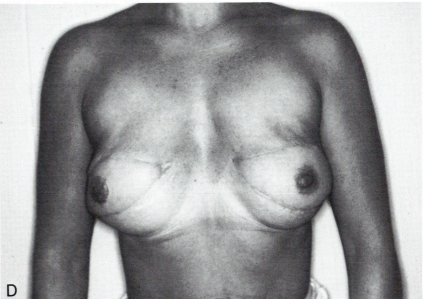

CASE 31   (Contributed by Louis C. Argenta, M.D., and Malcolm W. Marks, M.D.)

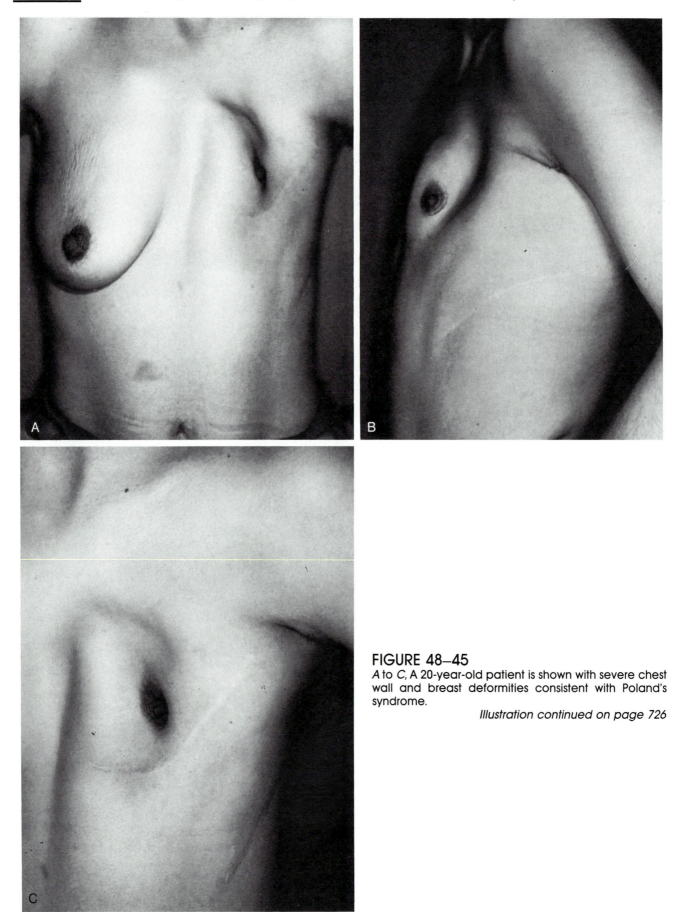

FIGURE 48–45

A to *C*, A 20-year-old patient is shown with severe chest wall and breast deformities consistent with Poland's syndrome.

Illustration continued on page 726

Editor's Note. Poland's syndrome is characterized by variable congenital deformities of the chest wall, ipsilateral upper extremity, and vertebral bodies. Although Poland's original description of a patient with this complex deformity included hand and chest wall maldevelopment (Poland, 1841), the current literature usually includes cases with absence of or deficiency of the pectoralis major muscle as Poland's syndrome, regardless of the presence or absence of other anomalies. Other chest wall abnormalities, in addition to pectoralis major muscle deficiency, include deficiencies of the subcutaneous tissue and nipple-areola complex, aplasia or hypoplasia with cephalad malposition, abnormalities of the costal cartilages and anterior portion of the ribs—particularly the second through fourth ribs—and a variable deficiency of the latissimus dorsi, deltoid, supraspinatus, and infraspinatus muscles (Ravitch, 1977; Haller et al., 1984; Hester and Bostwick, 1982; Anderl and Kerschbaumer, 1986).

The associated chest wall deformities result in a serious aesthetic deformity of the female breast (Argenta et al., 1985). Correction of the physical deformity should be appropriately timed to minimize psychosocial problems in the adolescent patient.

Preoperative Considerations. Determination of the operative approach is based on a careful evaluation of the deformities, the degree of chest wall depression, the associated abnormal projection of costochondral junctions, whether there is absence of the anterior axillary folds, the degree of breast development and associated breast asymmetry, and the nipple-areola complex position. The amount of skin and subcutaneous tissue is also carefully evaluated. At the time of puberty and in the ensuing years, young women deposit a considerable amount of subcutaneous tissue in the chest wall area. In patients who present prior to or during puberty, it is beneficial to postpone the definitive reconstruction until the amount of subcutaneous tissue has stabilized and the exact extent of deformity can be evaluated. Once a breast starts developing on the contralateral side, a tissue expander is placed beneath whatever muscle exists on the thorax or in the subcutaneous pocket and inflated at a rate to maintain symmetry with the opposite side. This helps alleviate psychosocial problems that may result from breast asymmetry during the period of development. Once the patient achieves physiologic maturity, definitive reconstruction can be carried out.

Definitive reconstruction depends on the severity of the chest wall deformity. A mild deformity, characterized primarily by absence of the muscle and a hypoplasia or aplasia of the breast, can, in most cases, be managed by expansion, followed by placement of a permanent implant. We have noted that pre-expansion in these patients provides enough stretching of skin and subcutaneous tissue to facilitate placement of an adequately sized breast implant. When the areolar complex is present, it tends to be in a superiorly displaced position, and pre-expansion also helps to bring the nipple-areola complex down to a more normal position.

With a moderate deformity with greater deficiency of subcutaneous tissue, it is advantageous to cover the permanent implant with latissimus dorsi muscle. Even though the muscle subsequently undergoes considerable atrophy, the muscle aids in restoring a fullness to the upper part of the chest above the level of the implant and provides a better general contour to the breast. Transfer of the latissimus dorsi muscle is carried out as described by Hester and Bostwick, with an approach through an incision at the upper anterior border of the latissimus (Hester and Bostwick, 1982). If there is deficiency of the anterior axillary fold, the insertion of the latissimus dorsi muscle may be detached and then reinserted through an axillary incision to the periosteum of the humerus just below the insertion of the clavicular head of the pectoralis major muscle.

With a severe deformity characterized by an actual contour depression of the chest wall due either to posterior displacement of ribs or actual absence of rib segments, the latissimus dorsi muscle is not adequate to provide bulk once it atrophies. A custom-made Silastic implant must be used to correct the contour deformity. These implants are fabricated in the same fashion as those used for correction of pectus excavatum deformities (Marks et al., 1980).

If there is also a significant subcutaneous tissue deficiency, latissimus dorsi muscle is used to cover the chest wall implant to prevent visible and palpable edges of the prosthesis. Serous fluid collects around chest wall implants for several weeks postoperatively and will require serial percutaneous aspiration. The fluid may allow displacement, with subsequent malposition of breast implants, and aspiration will risk puncture of the breast implant. Therefore, a breast prosthesis is better placed at a secondary procedure after all fluid formation has ceased. The breast prosthesis is placed either in a subcutaneous pocket or in the plane between the latissimus muscle and the capsule that forms with the chest wall implant.

Many of these patients have an abnormal projection of the costochondral junction associated with the chest wall deformity. Although this projection is generally on the involved side, occasionally there is also an associated malposition of the costochondral junction on the normal side. The costochondral projections are primarily cartilage in nature and can be shaved down during any of the stages of chest wall reconstruction. Bony projections can be taken down with a rongeur. During these maneuvers care must be taken not to enter the pleural cavity.

The following patient represents a severe deformity requiring a multi-staged procedure for reconstruction.

Case Report. The patient shown in Figure 48–45A to C did not have any abnormalities of the extremity or vertebral column. There was a severe contour deformity of the anterior chest wall with absence of segments of the anterior second through fourth ribs. The breast was hypoplastic, with a well-formed nipple-areola complex that was displaced cephalad. The subcutaneous tissue of the chest wall was significantly atrophied. There was also a scar from the failed previous rib graft to the defect when the patient was a young child (Fig. 48–45D).

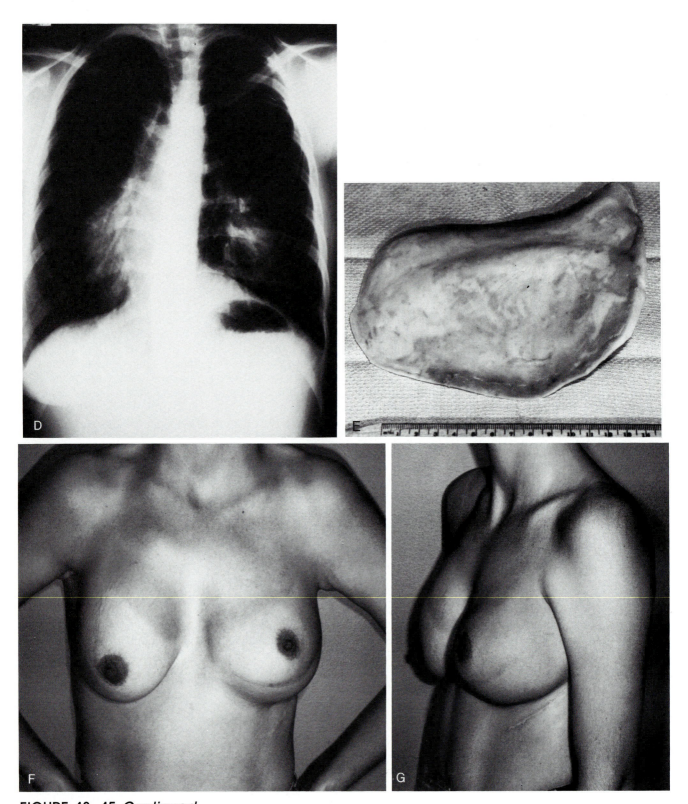

FIGURE 48–45 *Continued*
D, A chest roentgenogram revealed dextrocardia with absence of the second through fourth ribs anteriorly. An electrocardiogram revealed no abnormality. *E,* Appearance of the tissue expander is shown at the time of removal and replacement by a custom Silastic implant. *F* and *G,* The same patient is shown 3 years after a three-stage procedure.

Procedure. A moulage was taken of the chest wall deformity from which a custom Silastic implant was fabricated to correct the contour. A tissue expander placed beneath the subcutaneous tissues was later inflated to a volume of 500 cc slowly over a 12-week period. The implant was left in position for another 2 months to aid in developing breast ptosis. At a second procedure it was removed, and the custom Silastic implant was inserted in the capsule that had formed around the expander. A capsulotomy was performed to allow accurate positioning of the implant. No fixation of the implant was employed. Postoperatively, after the swelling had resolved, the outline of the implant was quite noticeable because of the paucity of the overlying soft tissue. Four months later, a latissimus dorsi muscle was transferred to completely cover the implant, and a silicone breast implant was also placed beneath the latissimus dorsi muscle. The patient had ptosis of the opposite breast; however, she was reluctant to have additional scars on that breast and elected to improve the ptosis with a subpectoral breast implant. The patient is shown 3 years after reconstruction following the three-stage approach, including (1) skin expansion, (2) placement of a custom Silastic implant, and (3) coverage of the custom implant with a latissimus dorsi muscle and placement of a breast implant between the capsule overlying the custom Silastic implant and the latissimus dorsi muscle. A contralateral augmentation mammaplasty was carried out at this time to improve symmetry (Fig. 48–45E to G).

Conclusion. As in all cases where multiple deformities exist, careful preoperative definition of specific problems allows prioritization and appropriate correction. The multiple deficiencies and abnormalities that exist in Poland's syndrome are remediable with proper planning and execution of well-described techniques.

References

Anderl, H., Kerschbaumer, S.: Early correction of the thoracic deformity of Poland's syndrome in children with the latissimus dorsi muscle flap: Long term follow-up of two cases. Br. J. Plast. Surg. 39:167, 1986.

Argenta, L. C., Vanderkolk, C., Friedman, R. T., Marks, M. W.: Refinements in reconstruction of congenital breast deformities. Plast. Reconstr. Surg. 76:73, 1985.

Haller J. A., Jr., Colombarri, P. M., Miller, D., Manson, P.: Early reconstruction of Poland's syndrome using autologous rib grafts combined with a latissimus muscle flap. J Pediatr. Surg. 19:423, 1984.

Hester T. R., Jr., Bostwick, J.: Poland's syndrome: Correction with latissimus muscle transposition. Plast. Reconstr. Surg. 69:226, 1982.

Marks, M. W., Argenta, L. C., Lee, D. C.: Silicone implant correction of pectus excavation: Indications and refinement in technique. Plast. Reconstr. Surg. 74:52, 1980.

Poland, A.: Deficiency of the pectoralis muscle. Guy's Hospital Reports 6:191, 1841.

Ravitch, M.: Poland's syndrome: A study of an eponym. Plast. Reconstr. Surg 59:508, 1977.

CASE 32 (Contributed by Saul Hoffman, M.D.)

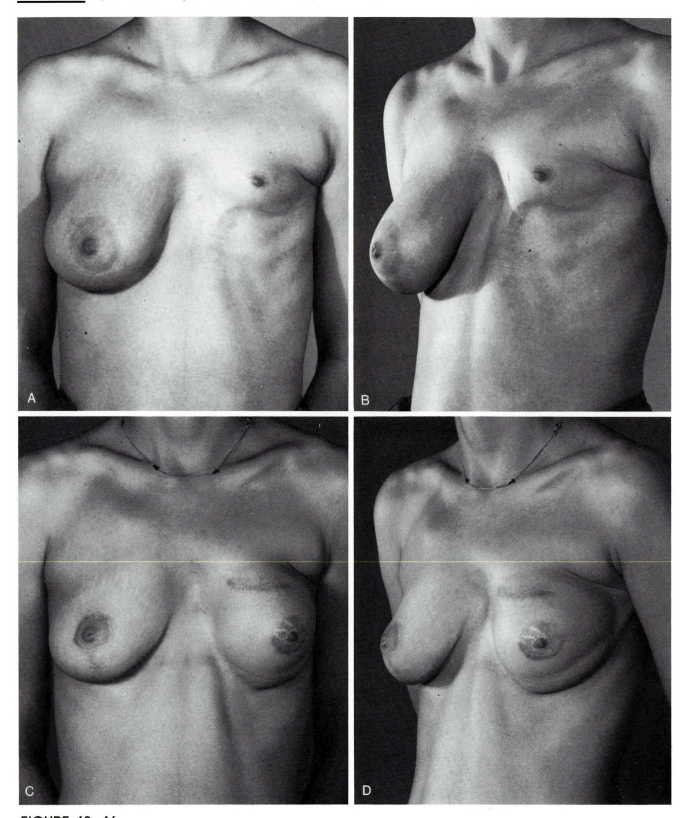

FIGURE 48–46

A and *B*, This patient with Poland's syndrome has a markedly underdeveloped left breast and a rudimentary nipple with an abnormally high position. *C* and *D*, An augmentation mammaplasty was performed and the nipple repositioned simultaneously. Reconstruction of the nipple-areola complex was done with a full-thickness skin graft. A mastopexy was carried out on the opposite breast.

CASE 33 (Contributed by Nicholas G. Georgiade, M.D.)

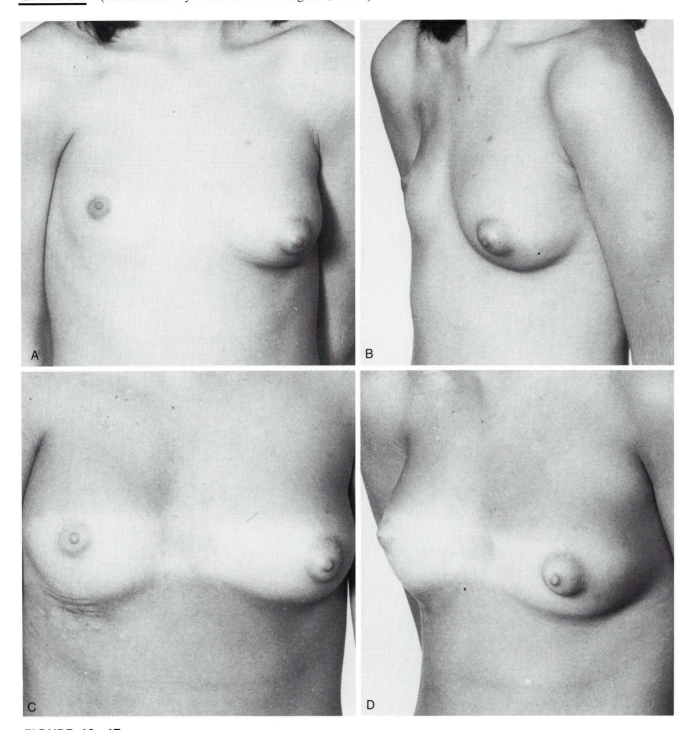

FIGURE 48–47

A and *B*, A 16-year-old patient is shown with right Poland's syndrome. She had a one-stage transfer of the entire latissimus dorsi muscle on its vascular pedicle to the right chest area with transfer of the head of the latissimus muscle to the subclavicular area. Medial sternal sutures were used to secure the latissimus dorsi muscle in place. A 185-cc gel prosthesis was inserted beneath the latissimus muscle during the initial operative procedure. *C* and *D*, Six-month postoperative views are shown.

CASE 34 (Contributed by Gilbert B. Snyder, M.D.)

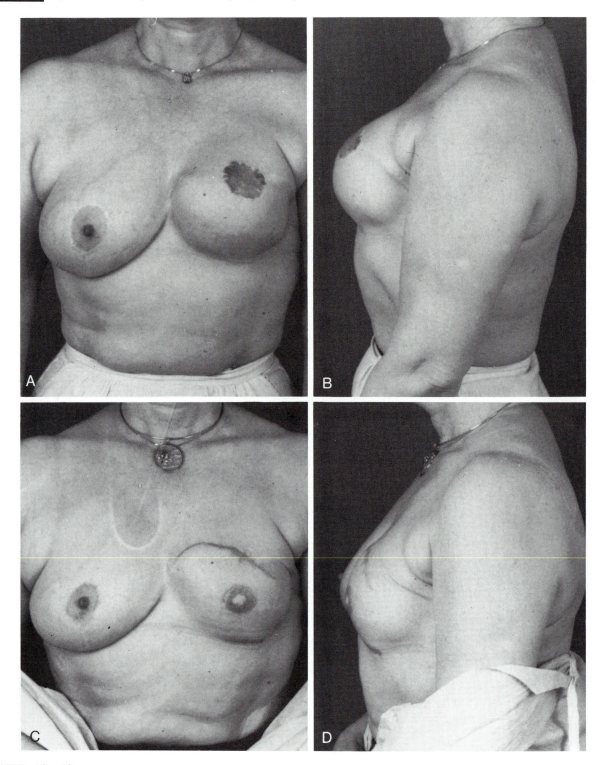

FIGURE 48–48
A and *B*, A 50-year-old patient is shown after an unsatisfactory attempt at left breast reconstruction. Note the markedly elevated and malpositioned labial graft for areola reconstruction accompanied by a superiorly displaced prosthesis. *C* and *D*, After treatment.

Treatment. Instead of an attempt to use the labial graft, which had a poor color match with the opposite nipple-areola area, it was excised, and the wound was closed primarily. The implant was replaced and matched with the opposite breast mound. A new nipple-areola com-plex was constructed in an appropriate position, utilizing the nipple-areola from the contralateral breast. Nipple tattooing is a consideration for future increased pigmen-tation of the nipple area if the patient so desires.

CASE 35 (Contributed by Saul Hoffman, M.D.)

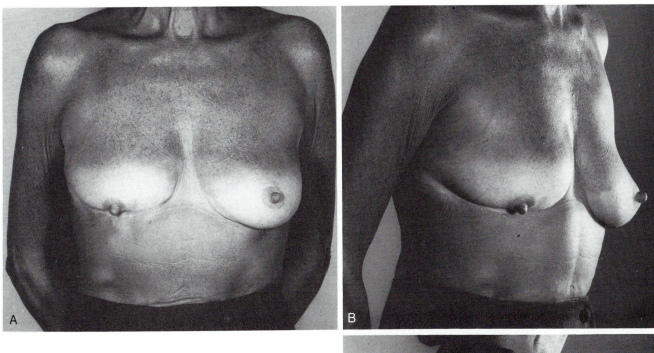

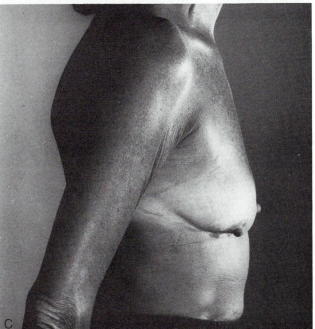

FIGURE 48–49

A to *C,* This 51-year-old patient had a right partial mastectomy. She had refused a modified radical mastectomy for a well encapsulated, low grade malignancy. The resultant deformity is shown.

Illustration continued on following page

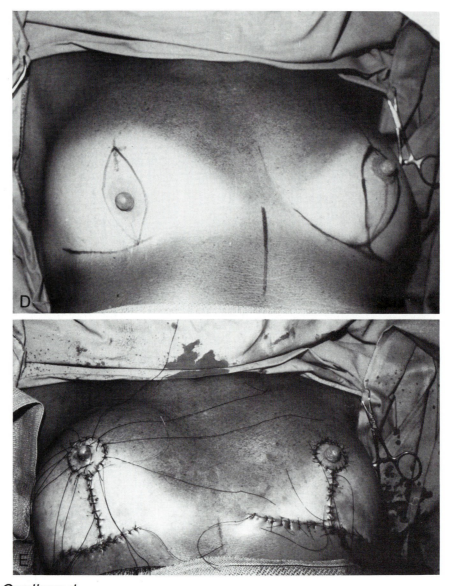

FIGURE 48–49 *Continued*

D and *E*, Augmentation and relocation of the nipple-areola complex via a vertical excision mastopexy and augmentation of the right breast were performed. The left breast required both vertical and transverse skin excision to approximately match the opposite breast.

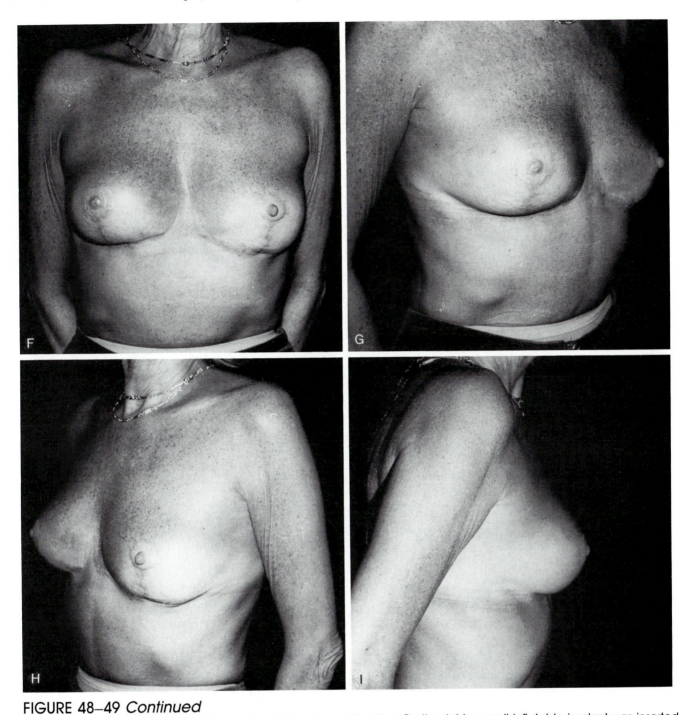

FIGURE 48–49 *Continued*

F to *I,* The same patient is shown 1 year after bilateral reconstruction. On the right a small inflatable implant was inserted with 85 cc of saline providing volumetric symmetry. Because of the extensive scarring in the periareolar area, repositioning of the right nipple was impossible, and a free full-thickness nipple-areola graft was used to place the new nipple-areola complex in a satisfactory position. The final result shows good symmetry and contour with a class 2 capsular contracture.

CASE 36   (Contributed by O. Gordon Robinson, Jr., M.D.)

This 35-year-old patient had a subcutaneous mastectomy in 1975 for fibrocystic disease. Two years later she subsequently had the prostheses replaced but developed bilateral capsular contractures (Fig. 48–50). Because of increasing capsular distortion, the prostheses were removed, capsulotomies were done, and bilateral submuscular tissue expanders were inserted. An expansion to 1000 cc was done over a period of 4 weeks. Four months later these expanders were replaced with 800-cc permanent prostheses (Fig. 48–51). The breasts were larger than desired, and 18 months later, mastopexy was performed, and 550-cc prostheses were inserted. The patient is shown 9 months postoperatively in Figure 48–52.

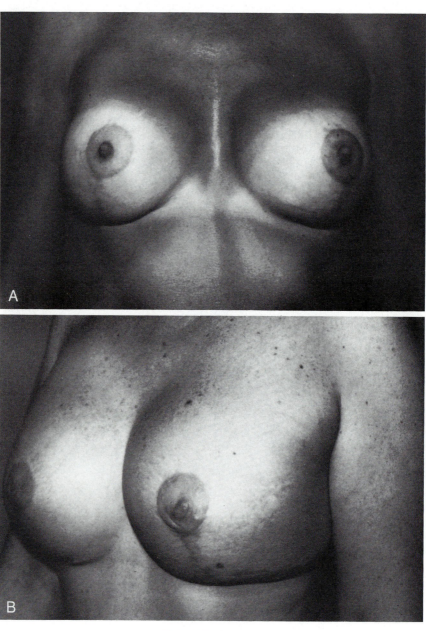

FIGURE 48–50

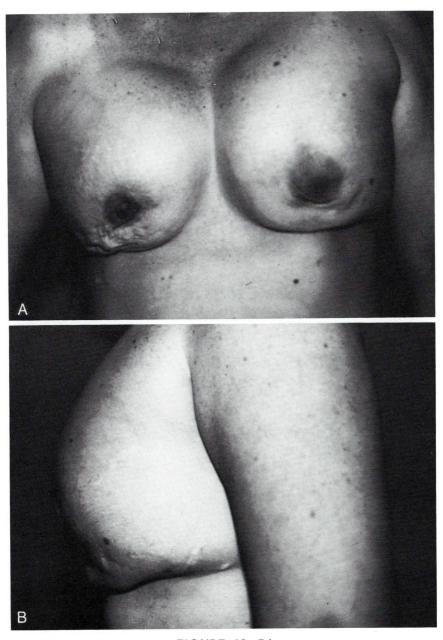

FIGURE 48–51

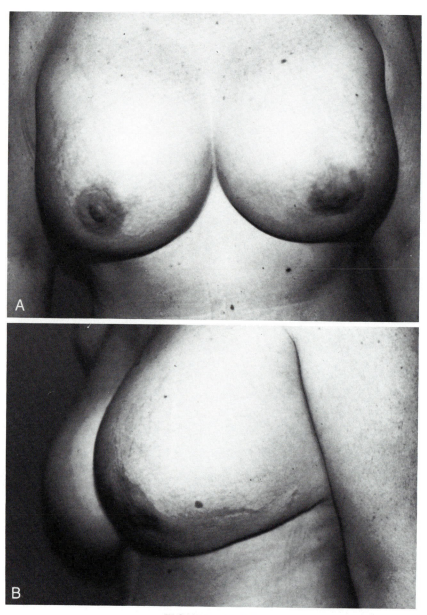

FIGURE 48–52

CASE 37 (Contributed by O. Gordon Robinson, Jr., M.D.)

A 43-year-old patient is shown with fibrocystic disease, having had multiple previous breast biopsies (Fig. 48–53). A subcutaneous mastectomy and skin reduction was done, and postoperatively the nipples became necrotic. Subsequently both nipples and areolae were lost (Fig. 48–54). Complete healing with resultant scarring oc-

curred by 4 months (Fig. 48–55). At 6 months, the scars were revised, and the nipple-areola complexes were reconstructed with skin grafts from the groin for the areolae and labia majora grafts for the nipples. Subpectoral 285-cc implants were inserted. The patient is shown 5 months following reconstruction in Figure 48–56.

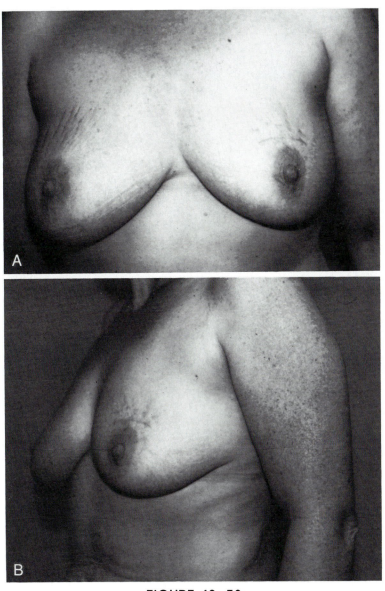

FIGURE 48–53

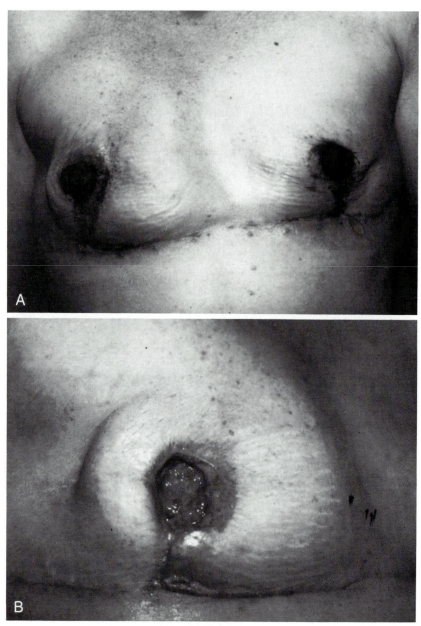

FIGURE 48–54

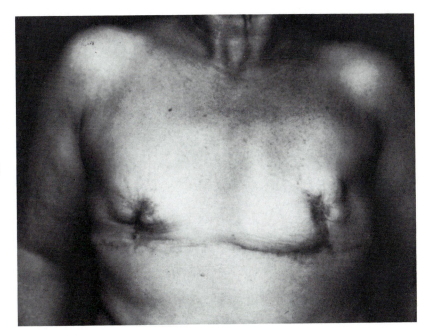

FIGURE 48–55

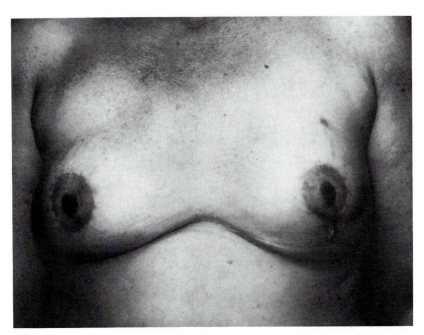

FIGURE 48–56

CASE 38   (Contributed by Nabil I. Elsahy, M.D.)

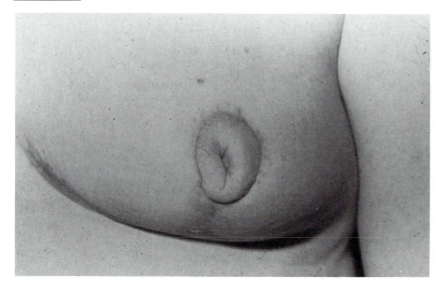

FIGURE 48–57
A 35-year-old patient who had undergone a Strömbeck type reduction mamma-plasty that resulted in a deformed areola and an invaginated nipple.

FIGURE 48–58
A to C, The Elsahy technique for correction of inverted nipples was done. Note the use of two "turned down" dermal flaps sutured beneath the nipple to maintain the nipple in an upright position. (From Elsahy, N. I.: Alternative operation for inverted nipple. Plast. Reconstr. Surg. 57: 438, 1976.)

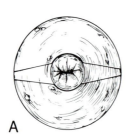 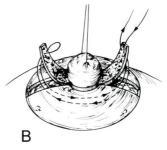 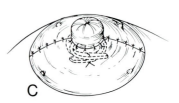

A   B   C

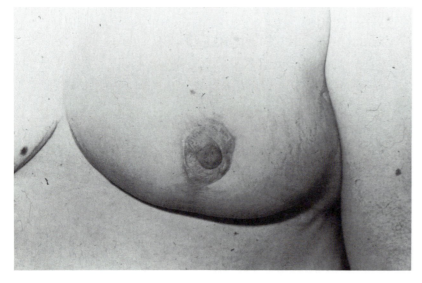

FIGURE 48–59
This patient 1 year after correction of the invaginated nipple with the two dermal flaps and revision of the irregularity of the areola by excising the periphery of the areola.

Reference

Elsahy, N. I.: Alternative operation for inverted nipple. Plast. Reconstr. Surg. 57:438, 1976.

CASE 39 (Contributed by Henry W. Neale, M.D.)

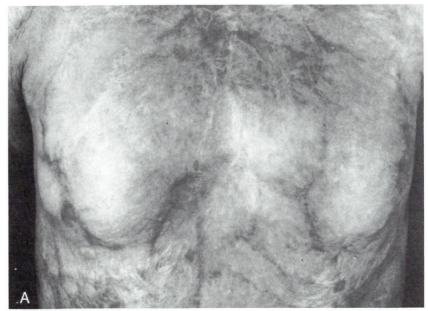

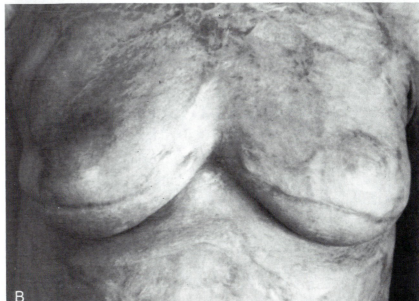

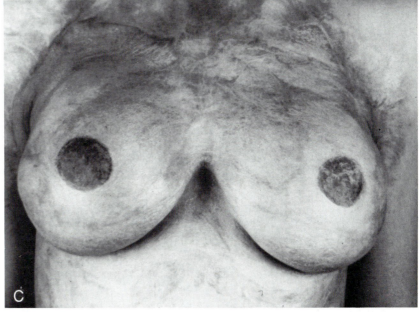

FIGURE 48–60

A, This 14-year-old girl sustained a 40% full-thickness thermal burn when her nightgown caught fire at age 6. Split-thickness skin grafts had been applied to the chest and breast. Breast development is restricted by the scar contractions. *B,* Appearance of this patient at age 16 after inframammary release of the scar contractures and thick skin grafts. The nipple and areola were reconstructed with toe pulp composite grafts and full-thickness skin grafts from the inner thigh. The patient was still dissatisfied with the size of her breasts. *C,* At age 18, Becker prostheses were placed subglandularly through inframammary incisions. Over a 4-month period 300 cc of saline were added to 100 cc of gel every other week. This same patient is shown after 200 cc of saline were withdrawn, ports were removed, and tattooing was done of the nipple-areola complex. Note the natural degree of ptosis produced even in the previously burned chest wall.

741

CASE 40 (Contributed by O. Gordon Robinson, Jr., M.D.)

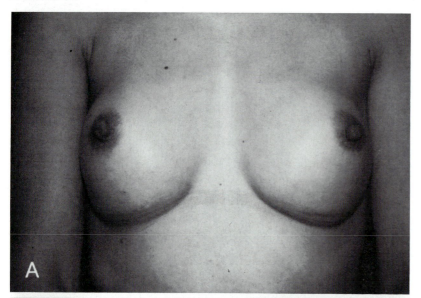

A

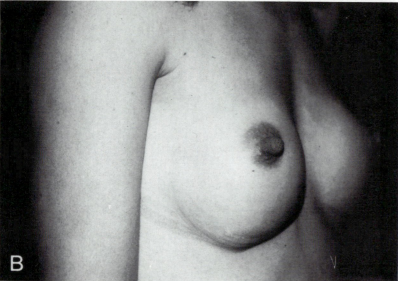

B

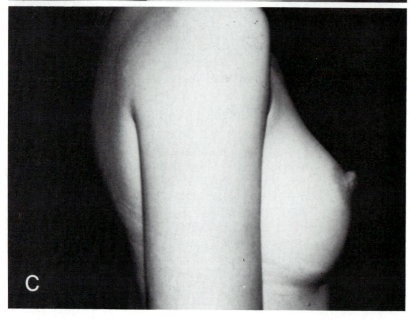

C

FIGURE 48–61

This woman had undergone augmentation mammaplasty 3 years previously, and she subsequently developed bilateral capsular contractures. The capsules were released by closed capsulotomy, and afterward there was upward rotation of the nipple and descent of the breast mass (Fig. 48–61A to C). Approximately 1 year later the inflatable prostheses were replaced with 285-cc Surgitek low-profile gel-filled prostheses, and the "droopy" appearance was simultaneously corrected by suturing Scarpa's fascia with a row of 3-0 Mersilene to the underlying muscle fascia.

Photographs taken approximately 2 months postoperatively show a satisfactory result (Fig. 48–61D to F). This problem appears to occur commonly with saline-filled prostheses and probably is preventable by carefully suturing Scarpa's fascia during augmentation mammaplasty.

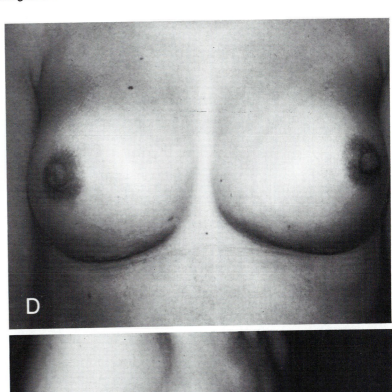

FIGURE 48–61 Continued

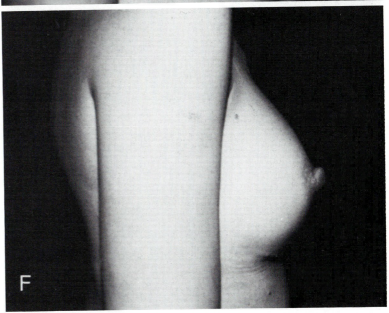

NEWER TECHNIQUES

*The Benelli Periareolar Mammaplasty: The Round Block Technique**

In all types of mammaplasty, a main concern is to limit the scar. The scar in the submammary fold is visible particularly in the supine position. The ideal scarring is confined to the periareolar area.

Periareolar dermopexy and retromammary mastopexy appear to have been first described by Hinderer in 1972 (Hinderer, 1972). Others also report this type of peri-areolar mastopexy (Bartels, 1976; Erol, 1980; Gruber, 1980; Gasperoni, 1988). The indications and use to the present appear to have been limited to moderate ptosis of small breasts (Hinderer, 1972), because of the risk of enlarging or distorting the areola by the excessive tension on the areolar skin. The round block technique eliminates tension on the areola, thus avoiding any enlargement of it (Benelli, 1984, 1988, 1989, 1990; Faber, 1988, 1989; Faivre, 1984; Felicio, 1989).

Indications for Use of the Round Block Technique

The round block technique is indicated for the following:

1. All mammary ptosis and mild to moderate associated hypertrophy.
2. Mammary ptosis corrected by augmentation mammaplasty and mastopexy. Insertion of the prosthesis is easily managed by a crosswise incision on the lower part of the de-epithelialization area. In augmentation mastopexy, it is generally unnecessary to perform plication of the gland. The former projection of the breast is obained by the positioning of the prosthesis.
3. Areolar hypertrophy. A too-large areola (whether due to constitutional or postoperative causes) and unsightly periareolar scars are good indications for the round block technique, which corrects the deformity.
4. The tuberous breast. The round block technique permits a definitive correction of the tuberous breast deformity.
5. Correction of moderate gynecomastia.

APPLICATION OF THE ROUND BLOCK TECHNIQUE TO MAMMARY HYPOPLASIA AND ASSOCIATED PTOSIS

In cases of mammary hypoplasia, the round block technique provides simultaneous correction of the ptosis and easy access for insertion of the prosthesis, regardless of size, by an incision in the horizontal diameter of the de-epithelialized periareolar area, leaving only a periareolar scar.

Principle

The aim of this operation is to obtain a pleasing breast shape with the areola in its proper location and, above all, free from any tension that would cause postoperative enlargement of the incision. The round block technique produces a very solid, circular dermis-to-dermis scar around the areola, fixed by a nonresorbable suture. This suture, which encircles the areola and fixes definitively its diameter, should preferably be of woven nylon fiber to allow the "anchoring" at the breast of the periareolar scar block. The remodeling of the breast curve is completed by a crisscrossed periosteal mastopexy. This mastopexy is used to increase the breast projection, to refine the lower quadrants, and to add to the upper quadrants. The glandular unions and anchorings should be performed with a nonresorbable suture of monofilament nylon 2-0. The round block technique has as its keystone the supradermal and subdermal periareolar blocked suture, which is nonresorbable and fixed. It ensures the permanence of the result.

Technique

The preoperative markings (Fig. 49–1) are adapted to the specific deformity to be corrected and consist of the following:

1. Outline of the breast meridian.
2. Identification of the tip of the new areola—point A.
3. Identification of the base of the new areola—point B.

---

*This chapter was previously published (Benelli, L.: A new peri-areolar mammaplasty: Round block technique. Aesthetic Plast. Surg. 14:93, 1990) and is used here, revised, by permission of the publisher and editor.

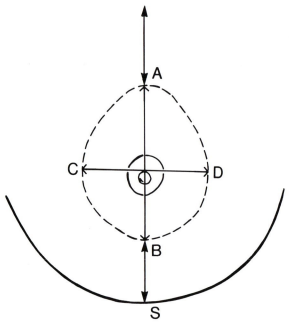

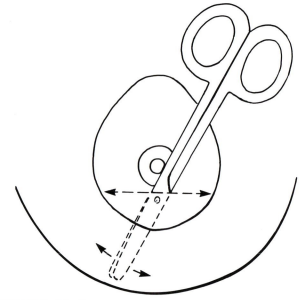

FIGURE 49–1

Outline of the measurements for elevating the nipple-areola complex to point A is shown. The base of the new areola is point B. The amount of de-epithelialization (points C-D) for removal of the excess skin is estimated. S, Submammary fold. (From Benelli, L.: A new periareolar mammaplasty: Round block technique. Aesthetic Plast. Surg. 14:93, 1990.)

FIGURE 49–2

Subcutaneous dissection of the inferior and medial areas of the mammary gland is carried out but is not extended inferior to the submammary fold. (From Benelli, L.: A new periareolar mammaplasty: Round block technique. Aesthetic Plast. Surg. 14:93, 1990.)

4. Outline of the limit of the de-epithelialized zone according to the amount of cutaneous excess. There is no need to be wary of outlining very large areas of de-epithelialization. The fixed nature of the "round block" avoids all postoperative areolar deformity. A large amount of excess skin, linked to accentuated ptosis, of 14 cm vertically (A-B) by 12 cm laterally (C-D) (or more, if necessary), can be excised.

5. Outline of the circumference of the new areola, the diameter of which is about 4 cm (to be adapted according to breast size).

The operative technique begins with careful de-epithelialization of the area between the areola and the peripheral outline, necessary in order to keep the underlying dermis intact; horizontal incision of the skin at the lower side of the de-epithelialized area (B); deep subcutaneous dissection of the lower and median parts of the mammary gland extending to, but not beyond, the submammary fold (Fig. 49–2); and careful hemostasis (a hematoma could easily form where dissection has taken place).

Mastopexy is then carried out at the aponeurotic prepectoral level and sutured into the periosteal structure for the purpose of maintaining the new position of the breast.

A periosteal crisscrossed mastopexy is here described (Fig. 49–3). Retroglandular detachment is in the prepectoral area above the submammary fold. This maneuver creates a large glandular flap with a superior base. The nipple-areola complex is then freed from its lower

attachments and supported only by a vertical dermoglandular flap with a superior base.

The large glandular flap beneath the areola is separated into two parts, external and internal, by a vertical incision in the center of the flap. A crisscrossed periosteal mastopexy is then performed by attaching the medial part of the external flap to the presternal periosteum over the submammary fold. The periosteum is secured

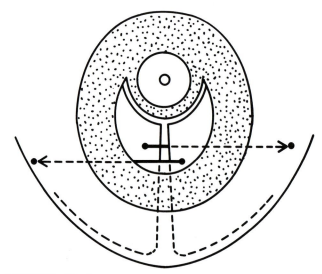

FIGURE 49–3

After dissection of two glandular flaps, the external flap is crossed under the internal flap and anchored to the presternal periosteum. The internal flap is crossed over the external flap and anchored to the costal periosteum.

with a large curved needle, which is pushed to the bone through the sternal insertion of the large pectoral muscle. In this way, the external glandular flap is firmly fixed in the paramedian position under the internal glandular flap. The internal glandular flap is then fixed at the costal periosteum laterally over the submammary fold. This crisscrossing of the flaps fixed at the periosteum constitutes a crisscrossed periosteal mastopexy. Several inverted sutures are placed along the line where the glandular flaps cross. The suture used for all of these points is monofilament 2-0 nylon.

This crisscrossed periosteal mastopexy provides very strong support of the mammary cone. The anterior projection of the breast is maintained by this maneuver. In the case of mammary hypertrophy, either minimal or moderate, an excision of glandular volume can easily be performed by resection of glandular tissue on the external and/or internal glandular flaps before performance of the mastopexy.

In the case of moderate hypertrophy, the excision can be extended to the upper pole of the gland in the pectoral area with an easy elevation of the flap supporting the areola.

The subcutaneous dissection can be extended laterally and medially if desired, with careful lysis of any adhesions that might appear after mastopexy.

Alternate supradermal and subdermal positioning of the periareolar suture is used at the edge of the de-epithelialized area. This closure is made with a nonresorbable woven thread of strong quality (0 or 1 according to the amount of traction to be performed). It is initiated in the subdermal location of the incision made for performing the mastopexy and terminates at the starting point (Fig. 49–4).

Even distribution of the redundant skin is achieved by sliding the excess skin along the suture, thus evenly dispersing it (see Fig. 49–4B).

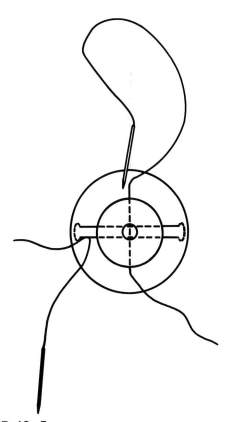

FIGURE 49–5
Vertical and transversal U sutures, which protect against postoperative protrusion of the areola.

The suture is circumferentially positioned (blocked) to achieve the desired areolar diameter, usually about 4 to 5 cm.

A drain is then placed. In order to avoid a protrusion of the areola due to the inframammary pressure, two crossed sutures are placed—one in the horizontal diameter of the areola and the other in the vertical diameter. These points of the braided nylon 2-0 are threaded onto a straight needle and crossed under the nipple in the center of the areola. These stitches are simply put into place and should not be tied tightly. A tuberous appearance of the areola is prevented by these sutures (Fig. 49–5).

A cutaneous suture is utilized after positioning the four cardinal points of the areola. No dermis-to-dermis uniting suture is necessary, because the round block technique ensures the fixed state of the structure. The cutaneous suture can be applied easily and without tension. Continuous horizontal mattress resorbable sutures allow eversion of the edges, producing a skin closure without tension and resulting in minimal scarring.

The dressing is held in place by a supportive brassiere.

Postoperative Care

The breast is supported by a brassiere worn day and night for a month. The suture line is cleaned every day with an antiseptic, and covered with a dressing.

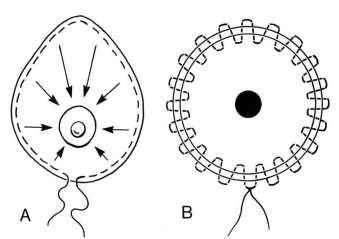

FIGURE 49–4
A, The position of the periareolar nonabsorbable suture is shown alternating in the supradermal and subdermal levels along the de-epithelialized margin. The skin is evenly distributed along this suture. (From Benelli, L.: A new periareolar mammaplasty: Round block technique. Aesthetic Plast. Surg. 14:93, 1990.) *B,* Cutaneous suture by continuous horizontal mattress suture with Vicryl 4-0.

FIGURE 49–6

A cross-section view shows the relationship of the closure to the underlying excess de-epithelialized tissue. (Redrawn from Benelli, L.: A new periareolar mammaplasty: Round block technique. Aesthetic Plast. Surg. 14:93, 1990.)

The periareolar skin "pleats" will disappear in some weeks. Bruising is common on the lower part of the breast, and exposure to the sun is not advisable until its complete disappearance. The periareolar diameter is well fixed. The suture encircling the areola at a depth supports any subsequent skin tension, thus giving a circular form to the areola (see Fig. 49–4; Fig. 49–6). Healing is generally good because of the absence of any cutaneous tension (Figs. 49–7 and 49–8).

Complications

Hematoma can be avoided by meticulous hemostasis and an aspiration drain or "gluing" with human biologic fibrin glue.

If the residual periareolar skin pleats fail to disappear after 6 months, these can be easily eliminated by a reopening of the periareolar scar, with the use of local anesthesia. This should not happen if the excess skin

has been distributed evenly by sliding it along the suture uniformly.

Separation of the suture surrounding the areola is unknown in our experience. The solidity of the fibrous scar "block" penetrated by the woven nylon suture renders such an occurrence unlikely. In the case of suture separation after a healing period of 1 year, the round block unit has become so fixed that the presence of the deep periareolar suture is no longer of importance.

APPLICATION OF ROUND BLOCK TECHNIQUE TO HYPERTROPHY

The excess breast volume is corrected by excision of the cutaneous glandular triangle, located inferior to the areola. This excision of tissue can easily be extended to all the glandular area extending to the posterior surface in the retroglandular prepectoral space for the purpose of achieving the desired volume (Fig. 49–9).

Technique

The preoperative markings (see Fig. 49–9) consist of the following:

1. Classical points of reference: submammary fold, meridian, median axis, areolar perimeter (dotted line).
2. The summit of the new areola—point A.

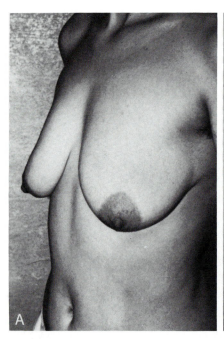
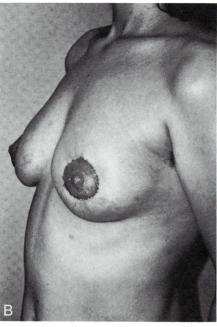
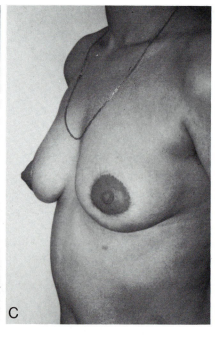

FIGURE 49–7

A, Preoperative view of a patient with mammary ptosis. B, Postoperative view 15 days after use of the round block technique without modification of volume. C, Postoperative view 1 year later, showing minimal periareolar scarring, good maintenance of the breast contour, and no distortion of the areola. (From Benelli, L.: A new periareolar mammaplasty: Round block technique. Aesthetic Plast. Surg. 14:93, 1990.)

FIGURE 49–8

A, Preoperative view of a patient with hypomastia with associated ptosis. *B*, Postoperative view 3 years later of the same patient after mastopexy by the round block technique and insertion of a 160-cc prosthesis. *C*, Postoperative view of the same patient 3 years after surgery, showing the scar. (From Benelli, L.: A new periareolar mammaplasty: Round block technique. Aesthetic Plast. Surg. 14:93, 1990.)

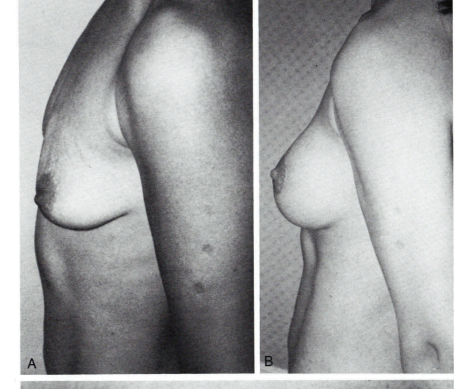

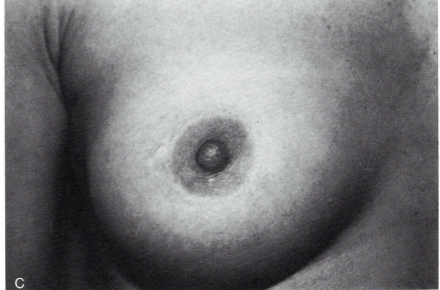

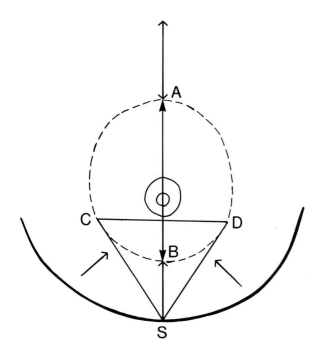

FIGURE 49–9
The previously described critical points of reference. The submammary fold (S) marks the farthest point of the cutaneous glandular triangle. Points C and D denote the most medial and lateral of the periareolar de-epithelialization. These points will vary, depending on the amount of cutaneous glandular excess to be excised. (From Benelli, L.: A new periareolar mammaplasty: Round block technique. Aesthetic Plast. Surg. 14:93, 1990.)

3. The inferior location of the cutaneous glandular triangle—point S in the submammary fold.
4. Points C and D, the lateral and medial limits of the ellipse of periareolar de-epithelialization, depending on the amount of cutaneous-glandular excess.
5. The limits of the incision uniting points C and D. The location of the superior ellipse of periareolar de-epithelialization depends on the amount of cutaneous-glandular excess to be excised.

De-epithelialization of the entire periareolar ellipse and a band of 1 cm of dermis along the border of the inferior triangle permits a satisfactory location of the inferior portion of the suture for a strong dermis-to-dermis approximation.

Excision of the cutaneous-glandular block is made following the premarked triangle. The cutaneous triangle can be de-epithelialized to preserve the subdermal vascularization of the inferior skin flap.

Dissection of the retroglandular prepectoral space and excision of the excessive breast tissue at the posterior surface of the gland are carried out until the desired volume is obtained.

The dermoglandular flap to support the areola will be vertical, allowing a better mobilization of the areola.

Crisscrossed periosteal mastopexy is performed as described previously. Additional de-epithelialization of periareolar surface can be carried out to obtain a perfectly round breast form.

Placement of the supradermal and subdermal suture follows the same principles as those described for breast ptosis. The suture is drawn up until the desired areolar diameter is achieved. The suture is then tied at this point, and aspirative drains are placed. Cutaneous intradermal suturing of the vertical incision is done as previously described for ptosis.

The dressings are maintained by a brassiere providing good breast support.

SUMMARY

Editorial Comment

A new, simplified technique has been described that is useful in the management of patients with mammary ptosis with or without associated slight to moderate breast hyperplasia and gynecomastia (Figs. 49–10 and 49–11). Postoperative results up to 3 years have shown that correction of the mammary problems described by the author have yielded satisfactory aesthetic results with minimal scarring. This procedure appears to yield satisfactory long-term results.

Guest-Editorial Comments (Carson Lewis, M.D., F.A.C.S.)

What obstacle plagues the aesthetic breast surgeon? The presence of unsightly scars.

When repositioning the nipple is required, present techniques place incisions on the skin of the breast. In many instances, resultant scars are conspicuous and evidence of our ineptitude.

Surgeons have attempted to solve this problem in several ways, including reduction of the length of the inframammary crease incision, elimination of the inframammary crease incision, making the vertical incision shorter, and changing the position of the vertical incision to run obliquely. However, in all instances, scars are present on the skin of the breast. Another approach was the doughnut mastopexy, which enlarged the areola. Again, the scars widened. The enlarged areola was aesthetically unacceptable to surgeons and patients.

Dr. Benelli devised a method of performing most procedures through a periareolar incision with his round block technique. A segment of skin around the present

FIGURE 49–10

A, Preoperative view of a patient with hypertrophic ptosis. *B*, Preoperative marking—an ellipse 15 cm in vertical diameter and 11.5 cm in horizontal diameter. *C*, Postoperative view of the same patient 3 days after surgery. Note the regular distribution of the small pleats around the areola. *D*, Postoperative view of the same patient 3 months after surgery. *E*, Preoperative view of a patient with hypertrophy with associated ptosis. *F*, Postoperative view 3 months after surgery of a 400-gm reduction in each breast. *G*, Preoperative lateral view of same patient. *H*, The same patient 3 months after surgery, shown in profile. (From Benelli, L.: A new periareolar mammaplasty: Round block technique. Aesthetic Plast. Surg. 14:93, 1990.)

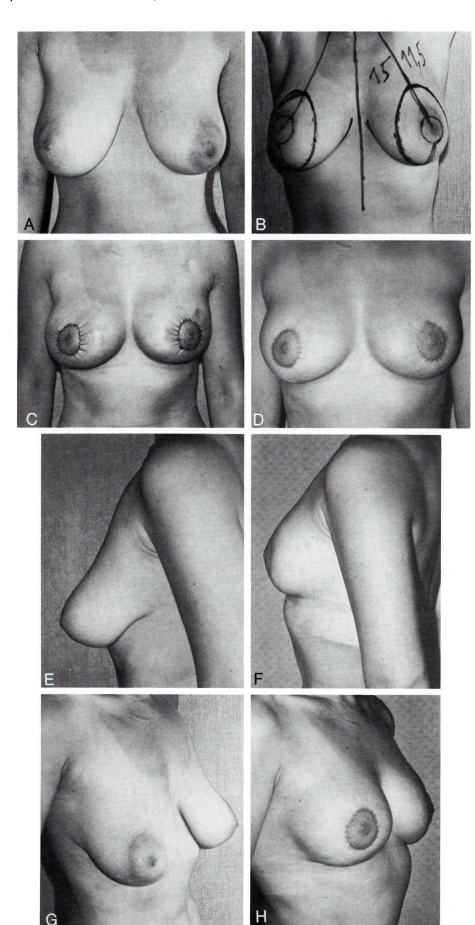

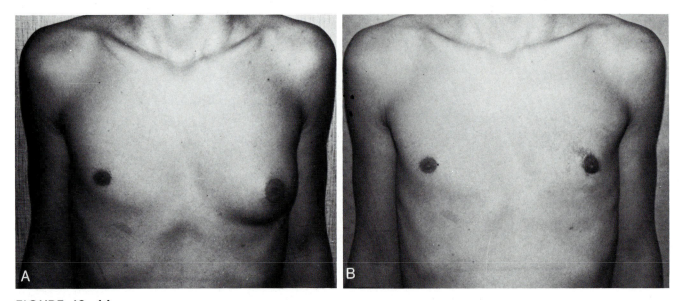

FIGURE 49–11

A, Preoperative view of a patient with unilateral gynecomastia with areolar hypertrophy. *B,* Postoperative view of same patient after correction of the asymmetry and reduction of the left areola utilizing the "round block" technique to correct the gynecomastia and areolar hypertrophy. (From Benelli, L.: A new periareolar mammaplasty: Round block technique. Aesthetic Plast. Surg. 14:93, 1990.)

areola is de-epithelialized, and surgery is performed through the skin in this de-epithelialized segment. A permanent purse-string suture is then utilized to reposition and to close the skin around the nipple-areola complex. Initially there is a pleating of the skin, which smooths out after several months. These incisions leave a scar in the periareolar area only; and, in most instances, the scars remain narrow and inconspicuous.

I met Dr. Benelli in January 1989; subsequently, I have been to Paris and watched him operate. I have seen several of his patients postoperatively as well as numerous photographs of many of his patients having various procedures performed. Some of the results I saw were 4 years after surgery. Subsquently, Dr. Benelli came to La Jolla, California, and helped me do a mastopexy procedure with his technique. I have used the technique on several occasions throughout the year and have been pleased with the results.

In my opinion, it is a major breakthough in breast surgery. It is applicable to mastopexy, mastopexy with augmentation and reduction mammoplasty, and treatment of gynecomastia, as well as some tumor removal procedures. It is a technique that allows the surgeon to eliminate the presence of incisions on the skin of the breast.

References

Bartels, R. J., Strickland, O. M., Douglas, W. M.: A new mastopexy operation for mild or moderate breast ptosis. Plast. Reconstr. Surg. 57:687, 1976.

Benelli, I., Faivre, J.: Traitement chirurgical des lésions inesthétiques de l'aréole et du mamelon. Chirurgie Esthétique, Paris, Maloine, 1984.

Benelli, L.: Technique de plastie mammaire le round block. Revue Française de Chirurgie Esthétique 50:7, 1988.

Benelli, L.: Technique du round block. Revue Française de Chirurgie Esthétique 52:9, 1988.

Benelli, L.: Periareolar mammoplasty técnica round block. International Symposium Recent Advances in Plastic Surgery. Sao Paulo, Brazil, March 3, 1989.

Benelli, L.: Une technique personnelle de plastie mammaire périaréolaire: "round block." Eléments techniques permettant d'élargir les indications. Revue Française de Chirurgie Esthétique 57:27, 1989.

Benelli, L.: A new periareolar mammaplasty: Round block technique. Aesthetic Plast. Surg. 14:99, 1990.

Erol, O., Spira, M.: Mastopexy technique for mild to moderate ptosis. Plast. Reconstr. Surg. 65:603, 1980.

Faber, C.: Plastie mammaire: La technique round block réduit au minimum la cicatrice. Le Quotidien du Médecin, No. 4082, May 18, 1988.

Faber, C.: Plastie mammaire: Le "round block" evite l'élargissement de l'aréole. Le Quotidien du Médecin, No. 4202, January 17, 1989.

Faivre, J., Carissimo, A., Faivre, J. M.: La voie péri-aréolaire dans le traitement des petites ptoses mammaires. Chirurgie Esthétique, Paris, Maloine, 1984.

Felicio, Y.: Periareolar reduction mammaplasty: A single incision technique. International Symposium Recent Advances in Plastic Surgery. Sao Paulo, Brazil, March 3, 1989.

Gasperoni, C., Salgarello, M., Gargani, G.: Experience and technical refinements in the "donut" mastopexy with augmentation mammaplasty. Aesthetic Plast. Surg. 12:111, 1988.

Gruber, R. P., Jones, H. W., Jr.: The "donut" mastopexy: Indications and complications. Plast. Reconstr. Surg. 65:34, 1980.

Hinderer, U.: Plastia mamaria modelante de dermopexia superficial y retromamaria. Rev. Esp. Cir. Plast. 5:521, 1972.

INDEX

Note: Page numbers in *italics* refer to illustrations; page numbers followed by *t* refer to tables.